Clinical Nursing Handbook

A David T. Miller Book

Clinical Nursing Handbook

Ellen Baily Raffensperger, R.N., C.C.R.N., B.A. in Nursing
Staff Nurse, Progressive Care Unit
Sibley Memorial Hospital
Washington, D.C.

Mary Lloyd Zusy, R.N., B.A. and M.A. in Nursing
Formerly Clinical Instructor
Montgomery Community College
Takoma Park, Maryland

Lynn Claire Marchesseault, R.N., B.S.N., M.S.N.
Senior Staff Nurse
Visiting Nurse Association of Northern Virginia
Arlington, Virginia

1792

J. B. Lippincott Company *Philadelphia*
London, Mexico City, New York, St. Louis, São Paulo, Sydney

Sponsoring Editor: David T. Miller
Manuscript Editor: Marianne Zajdel
Indexer: Bernice Eisen
Art Director: Tracy Baldwin
Design Coordinator: Charles Field
Designer: Adrianne Onderdonk Dudden
Production Supervisor: J. Corey Gray
Production Coordinator: Charlene Catlett Squibb
Compositor: University Graphics, Inc.
Printer/Binder: R. R. Donnelley and Sons

6 5 4 3 2

Library of Congress Cataloging-in-Publication Data

Raffensperger, Ellen Baily.
Clinical nursing handbook.

"A David T. Miller book."
Includes bibliographies and index.
1. Nursing—Handbooks, manuals, etc. 2. Medicine, Clinical—Handbooks, manuals, etc. I. Zusy, Mary Lloyd. II. Marchesseault, Lynn. III. Title. [DNLM: 1. Nursing—handbooks. WY 39 R137C]
RT51.R25 1986 610.73 85-18234
ISBN 0-397-54461-8

The authors and publisher have exerted every effort to ensure that drug selection and dosage set forth in this text are in accord with current recommendations and practice at the time of publication. However, in view of ongoing research, changes in government regulations, and the constant flow of information relating to drug therapy and drug reactions, the reader is urged to check the package insert for each drug for any change in indications and dosage and for added warnings and precautions. This is particularly important when the recommended agent is a new or infrequently employed drug.

To my husband, Maurey,
and our daughters, Maura and Karen EBR

To Fred with deep affection.
His encouragement and support were vital elements
in the production of the book MLZ

To my children, William and Daniel LM

Reviewers

We wish to express our appreciation to our reviewers, whose comments and insights have strengthened the book.

Nurse Reviewers

Annette Aicheson, RN, BSN, MA
Susan Dempsey, RN, BSN, MSN
Hetty L. deVroom, RN, BSN
Gita Dhillon, BSN, MEd
Janet Lobatz Epstein, RN, MSN, CNM
Mary Ellen Galloway, BA, RN
Anne Garrett, RN, MA
Margaret Geiger, RN
Dorothy Goodman, RN, ET
Catherine Rice Gorrell, RN, MSN
Nancy Hart, RN, MSN
Pat Hewitt, RN
Sharon Johnson, RN, ET
Catharine Kopac, RN, C, Ph.D
Susan Ludington, PhD, CNM
Jayne Melrose-Smith, RN, MSN, PNP
Jean Muir, RN, BSN
Betty Orner, RN
Claire R. Pettrone, CPNP, NNP, MSN
Sylvia Hasmelek Reid, RN
Daniel A. Sands, RN, BSN
Carole Stone, MSN, PNP

Pharmacist Reviewers

Freddy Grimm, Pharm D
Joel Kahn, RPh

Physician Reviewers

George J. Cohen, MD
Jack Dalton, MD
Thomas Havell, MD
Fred R. T. Nelson, MD, FAOS
Norman Odyneic, MD, FACS
Arnold Oshinsky, MD
Richard Pollen, MD, FACP
Neel J. Price, MD
Joy Samuels-Reid, MD
Yolanda S. Reid, MD
Giulio I. Scarzella, MD, FACS, FICS
Timothy J. Tehan, MD, FACP
Eliot Wilner, MD
Anthony Yenson, MD

Librarian

Annie B. Footman

Contributor

Joan Andrews Kramer, BSN, ET

Preface

Clinical Nursing Handbook is a book for use in the clinical area. Our goal has been to present information that fills the immediate needs of nurses working in general hospitals, nursing homes, or the community. Common problems that come up in day-to-day nursing practice are addressed.

In order to keep the book compact and portable, we have made difficult decisions as to what information to include and what to exclude. Because of this limitation on size, we have concentrated on the information we believe to be most needed in solving immediate clinical problems.

We assume that nurses, as professionals, will go to references of greater depth when time allows. Textbooks, journals, and the wealth of nursing literature now available provide the depth required for professional nursing. Many of these are listed in the bibliographies that accompany each section.

The book is divided into several sections with cross referencing. The first section, Clinical Laboratory Tests, Their Implications and Related Nursing Responsibilities (LAB), is a practical adjunct to the hospital lab manual.

Management in Special Nursing Situations (MNS) includes information on how to handle common problems that have mental health aspects but are more often seen on the general, rather than the psychiatric, units of hospitals. This section also includes a useful section on evening and night duty for the beginner.

Although the hospital procedure book is the first source, Nursing Responsibilities for Diagnosis and Treatment (NR) presents material on how to make procedures work and how to prepare patients for common diagnostic tests.

The Medical-Surgical Nursing (MSN) section highlights nursing care of patients and is organized according to organ systems. The care of the elderly and children is integrated throughout. However, there is a separate pediatrics section (PED), that presents information that applies solely or primarily to children.

Obstetrics (OB) stands alone, although where medical disorders coexist with pregnancy the reader is referred to other appropriate sections.

In the Pharmacology (PH) section, whenever possible, drugs are presented in families or prototypes to emphasize their common characteristics. Therefore, it is essential to read the presentation for the family of drugs before going to specifics of dosages, common side effects, and nursing implications of individual ones.

The Appendix contains useful information that does not seem to fit elsewhere. We call special attention to the list of Poison Control Centers. In the event of poisoning, these centers can be called upon to provide accurate information immediately.

Topics in each section are arranged alphabetically, with the exception of obstetrics. In that section, because of its nature, they are arranged sequentially. Some topics may appear under one of several names (*e.g.,* urinary calculi, renal calculi, kidney stones). Therefore, the general index is the ultimate source for quick referral.

We wish to express our appreciation to our reviewers, whose comments and insights have strengthened the book.

We wish to express our appreciation also to the Harper/Lippincott team. Our special thanks go to David T. Miller, Vice President, Diana Intenzo, Editor-in-Chief, and Patrick O'Kane, Manuscript Editor, whose editorial assistance was invaluable.

To our families, who have tolerated our absorption in the project and have given us support in many ways during the production of the book, we give heartfelt thanks.

Clinical Nursing Handbook is written for nurses engaged in direct patient care. It is our conviction that hands-on care is the heart of nursing practice.

Ellen Baily Raffensperger, RN, BA, CCRN
Mary Lloyd Zusy, RN, BA, MA
Lynn Marchesseault, RN, BSN, MSN

Contents

Clinical Nursing Handbook

1
Clinical Laboratory Tests, Their Implications and Related Nursing Responsibilities (LAB)

LABORATORY EXAMINATIONS OF BLOOD AND URINE

Laboratory examinations of blood and urine are done to obtain a biomedical evaluation of the patient.Tables 1-1 to 1-5 include frequently performed tests, values, and pertinent comments. The values may vary depending on the equipment and techniques used; therefore, know what is normal for the specific laboratory.

ARTERIAL BLOOD GASES (ABGs)

Description

Arterial blood gas (ABG) measurements are done to determine the ability of the lungs to perform oxygen and CO_2 transfer. ABGs also establish the kidneys' levels of function in the secretion or absorption of bicarbonate ions, which aid in maintaining the acid-base balance of the body. The following table lists ABGs and normal values.

Gas	Normal Values at Sea Level	Comments
pO_2	80–100 mm Hg partial pressure (room air)	Higher altitude = lower pO_2 Older ages = lower pO_2
pCO_2	38–42 mm Hg partial pressure	The average is 40.
HCO_3	24–28 mEq/liter	The bicarbonate is regulated by kidneys.
pH	7.35–7.45	Above 7.45 = alkalosis Below 7.35 = acidosis
O_2 Sat	95%	Higher altitude = lower O_2 Sat.

TABLE 1-1 RELATION BETWEEN COMMON BLOOD CHEMISTRY EXAMINATIONS AND BODILY FUNCTIONS AND DISEASE

Blood Tests		
LDH SGOT	Necrosis and infarction	Hepatic function
Bilirubin, total		
Bilirubin, direct (if total is elevated)		
SGPT		
Total protein		
Albumin		
Globulin		
A/G ratio		
Alkaline phosphatase		
Calcium Phosphorus	Parathyroid disease	Bone and joint conditions
Uric acid	Gout	
Urea nitrogen (BUN) Creatinine	Kidney	
Glucose	Diabetes	
CO_2 Chloride Sodium Potassium	Electrolytes	
Triglyceride Cholesterol	Lipid metabolism	

(Courtesy of Central Diagnostic Laboratory, Tarzana, California)

Alkalosis

Patients can tolerate a mild alkalosis, which may result from either respiratory or metabolic imbalance. Respiratory alkalosis results from blowing off too much CO_2. It is treated by building up CO_2 by breathing into a bag or decreasing the respiratory rate. The primary indicator of respiratory alkalosis is a significant decrease in CO_2, with lesser decrease in HCO_3, and a slight increase in pH. Typical symptoms include the inability to concentrate and dizziness. Patients with central nervous system (CNS) disease or injury who may have uncontrolled rapid breathing must be watched. Metabolic alkalosis results from too much base that may be caused by excessive ingestion of antacids, the loss of too much acid by way of the gas-

(Text continues on page 12)

TABLE 1-2 BLOOD CHEMISTRY

Test	Normal Value*	Comments
Albumin	3.5 g–5.0 g/dl	Necessary to keep fluid in vascular space. It is produced by the liver and kept in the vascular space by the kidney. It is decreased in chronic liver and kidney diseases, and increased in dehydration, shock, and so forth.
Alkaline phosphatase	30 IU–90 IU/L	Produced in the bone and hepatobiliary system. It is increased in bone and liver diseases. Children have much higher levels because it increases with new bone formation. Levels also are increased during pregnancy.
Bilirubin, total	0.5 mg–1.2 mg/dl	Increased in liver damage, biliary obstruction, and eclampsia. It is increased in the first month of life.
BUN (blood urea nitrogen)	7 mg–21 mg/dl	Increased in renal disease, gastrointestinal hemorrhage, or high protein diet. It may be slightly decreased in children, and slightly increased in the aged.
Calcium	8.6 mg–10.7 mg/dl	Slightly higher in newborns and children. Hypercalcemia from cancer affecting the bones. It is increased in hyperparathyroidism and decreased in hypoparathyroidism.

(continued)

TABLE 1-2 BLOOD CHEMISTRY

Test	Normal Value*	Comments
Cholesterol	150 mg–300 mg/dl	Levels may increase during pregnancy. It is very low in the newborn, and gradually increases with age. Currently, it is felt that the level should be maintained at less than 200 mg/dl for those over 30; 180 mg/dl or less for those under 30
Creatinine	0.7 mg–1.3 mg/dl	End-product of muscle activity, slightly higher in males because of larger muscle mass. Excellent test of filtration ability of the kidneys. Only reliable test of creatinine level in the elderly in a 24-hour creatinine clearance urine.
Glucose (fasting, FBS)	70 mg–110 mg/dl	Levels in newborns are usually as low as 20 mg to 80 mg/100 ml; levels in children are about the same as in adults.
Glucose (2 hours postprandial [after meal])		Results should be the same as the pre-meal FBS. Older people tend to have slightly higher postprandial levels.
Phosphorus	2.5 mg–4.5 mg/dl	Slightly higher in children and slightly lower in the aged. It is increased in hypoparathyroidism and slightly lower in hyperparathyroidism.
Protein, total	5.9 g–8.0 g/dl	Total of serum albumin and globulin. It is increased in dehydration and diabetic acidosis, and decreased in patients with severe burns and hemorrhage.

Uric acid	F, 2.0 mg–7.0 mg/dl M, 2.5 mg–8.0 mg/dl	Levels are increased in gout, leukemia, and toxemia of pregnancy. Drugs may cause an increase. See PH, diuretics.
Electrolytes (See NR, Electrolyte imbalance)		Measurements to determine fluid and electrolyte balance
CL (chloride)	95 mEq–109 mEq/liter	
CO_2 (carbon dioxide, indicates bicarbonate level)	20 mEq–33 mEq/liter	
Na (sodium)	135 mEq–145 mEq/liter	
K (potassium)	3.4 mEq–5.0 mEq/liter	
Enzymes		
Amylase	30 IU–130 IU/liter	Synthesized and secreted from parotid and pancreatic glands. Damage in these areas cause elevations, *e.g.,* pancreatitis and mumps.
CPK (creatine phosphokinase)	F, 10 IU–100 IU/liter M 20 IU–140 IU/liter	An intramuscular injection will cause an elevated CPK. Blood specimens should be drawn before, or at least one hour after an injection.

(continued)

TABLE 1-2 BLOOD CHEMISTRY

Test	Normal Value*	Comments
CPK has the following three isoenzymes:		
CPKBB (CPK-1) is elevated in brain tissue damage		
CPKMB (CPK-2) is elevated in cardiac injury		*CPKMB (CPK-2) is the first enzyme to rise after myocardial infarction (MI).* It rises in 2–6 hours, peaks at about 6 hours, and then returns to normal in 24–48 hours.
CPKMM (CPK-3) is elevated in muscle damage		
LDH (lactic dehydrogenase)	90 IU–200 IU/liter	After an MI the elevation of the *total* level of LDH rises slowly in 24–72 hours, and stays elevated for 10–14 days. However, LDH_1 rises within 4 hours of the event. Normally, it is lower than LDH_2. Increased levels are found in newborns.

Isoenzymes		
LDH_1 elevated in	20%–30% of total	
LDH_2 cardiac necrosis	27%–37% of total	
LDH_3 may be elevated in pulmonary infarct	16%–24% of total	
LDH_4 increases in liver damage	7%–15% of total	
LDH_5 increases in muscle damage	9%–17% of total	
SGOT (serum glutamic oxaloacetic transaminase) or APT (aspartate amino transferase)	8 IU–36 IU/liter	Found in heart muscle, liver, kidney, and cerebral tissues. It rises in 6–12 hours after an MI, peaks in 24–48 hours, and returns to normal in 4–6 days. It may also rise with liver disease. Newborns have increased levels.
SGPT (serum glutamic pyruvic transaminase) or ALT (alanine amino transferase)	2 IU–32 IU/liter	Primarily present in liver tissue. Newborns have increased levels.

*Values vary with laboratory
*M = men; F = women.

TABLE 1-3 HEMATOLOGY EXAMINATIONS THAT RELATE TO THE STRUCTURE AND FUNCTION OF BLOOD CELLS

Test Description	Normal Value*	Comments
RBC (red blood cells, or erythrocytes)	M, 4.6–6.2 million F, 4.2–5.4 million	Increased in newborn, varies with the age of child.
Reticulocytes (immature erythrocytes)	0.5%–1.5% of erythrocytes	Increased with bleeding because the body attempts to replace RBCs as quickly as possible.
HCT (hematocrit): volume percentage of erythrocytes in 100 ml blood	M, 42%–52% F, 37%–47%	Increased in newborn; gradually lowers during early childhood.
Hgb (hemoglobin): oxygen-carrying pigment of erythrocytes reported in grams per 100 ml blood.	M, 14 g–18 g F, 12 g–16 g	Increased in newborn; gradually lowers during childhood.
MCV (mean cell volume): refers to the size of an RBC. Reported in cubic microns (μm^3)	M and F, 87 $\pm$ 5 μm^3	Decreased in some anemias, *e.g.*, pernicious, iron deficiency. It increases in liver disease.
MCH (mean cell hemoglobin): the hemoglobin content of the individual RBCs. It is reported in micromicrograms ($\mu\mu g$)	M and F, 29 $\pm$ 2 $\mu\mu g$	Increased in macrocytic anemias; decreased in microcytic anemia.
MCHC (mean corpuscular hemoglobin concentration): the concentration of hemoglobin in 100 ml of erythryocytes reported as a percentage	M and F, 34% $\pm$ 2%	Decreased in some anemias.

WBC (white blood cells):	4,800–10,800 cu mm	May be greatly increased in newborn. Differential varies in children.
Differential (the percentage of major types of WBCs comprising the total count)		
Granulocytes		
Neutrophils (also called polys, segs)	40%–60%	First responder to bacterial infection and necrotic tissue.
Bands (immature neutrophils, also called "stabs")	2%–6%	Elevated in acute infection. The expression "shift to the left" refers to an increase in the percentage of immature cells, and is indicative of infection.
Eosinophils	1%–3%	Elevated in allergic conditions.
Basophils	0%–1%	Uncertain function. They contain histamine and heparin.
Lymphocytes	20%–40%	Two types are found, T cells and B cells. Eighty percent of circulating lymphocytes are T cells. T cells are the initial responders to viral infections. B cells are antibody-producing cells.

(continued)

TABLE 1-3 HEMATOLOGY EXAMINATIONS THAT RELATE TO THE STRUCTURE AND FUNCTION OF BLOOD CELLS

Test Description	Normal Value*	Comments
Monocytes	2%–8%	Responders to infection.
Platelets: necessary for coagulation of the blood	150,000–350,000/cu mm	
ESR (erythrocyte sedimentation rate): rate at which erythrocytes settle in uncoagulated blood (Wintrobe test)	M, 0 mm–8 mm in 1 hour F, 0 mm–15 mm in 1 hour	Usually marked increase during pregnancy.

*M = men; F = women.

TABLE 1-4 URINALYSIS EXAMINATIONS

Urinalysis (UA) examinations describe the color of the urine and consist of pH, specific gravity (SG), presence or absence of glucose, ketones, protein, and blood, along with a microscopic evaluation of sediment.

Characteristic Examined	Normal Values	Comment
Color	Yellow	Dark urine suggests bile or blood. Many drugs result in colored urine.
pH	4.6–8.0	Alkaline urine with an elevated pH is present with urinary tract infections or when the urine is left standing at room temperature. pH measurement is inaccurate with hematuria, diuresis, and contrast media. Urine pH is normally acid.
Specific gravity (SG)	1.025–1.035	SG is obtained by comparing the weight of urine to an equal amount of water. Lowered SG reflects the kidneys' inability to concentrate urine. If kidneys lose their ability to function, the excreted urine will become fixed at 1.010.
Glucose	None	Blood glucose levels are usually greatly increased before glucose appears in the urine.
Ketones	None	These occur in diabetes and starvation
Protein	0–trace	When more than a trace of protein is present, a 24-hour urine is usually done.
Blood	0	May occur in cystitis or renal calculi.

Microscopic UA

- RBC casts: seen in cases of active glomerulonephritis.
- WBC casts: seen in infectious process.
- Hyaline casts: a few are normal; the number is increased in proteinuria.
- Renal tubular casts: seen in cases of acute renal failure.

Crystals: seen in diseases of stone formation.

TABLE 1-5 MISCELLANEOUS TESTS
These miscellaneous tests are examinations of blood to determine the toxicity or effect of certain drugs on the blood.

Test	Normal Value	Therapeutic Boundaries
Barbiturates	0	
Digoxin level	0	0.6 ng–2.0 ng/ml
Dilantin (Phenytoin)	0	10 μg–20 μg/ml
Gentamicin level	0	4 μg–12 μg/ml
Lithium	0	0.5 mEq–1.5 mEq/liter
PT (prothrombin time)	12–14 seconds	1.5–2 times the normal level
PTT (partial thromboplastin time)	35–45 seconds; prolonged in infants until 4–6 months of age	1.5–2 times the normal level
Quinidine level	0	3 μg–6 μg/ml
Theophylline (aminophyllin) level	0	10 μg–20 μg/ml

(continued from page 2)

trointestinal (GI) tract or kidneys, nasogastric (NG) suction, vomiting, or excessive diuretics with resulting low potassium. The treatment consists of correcting the cause. Be certain that IVs run on time in patients with NG suction. An adequate potassium level is necessary to correct alkalosis resulting from a loss of HCl. The primary indicator of metabolic alkalosis is a significant increase in HCO_3, with lesser increases in CO_2 and pH. Typical symptoms are muscle weakness, confusion, or paralytic ileus caused by abnormal losses of potassium.

Acidosis

Patients cannot tolerate acidosis, which may result from either respiratory or metabolic imbalance. The condition requires immediate correction. Respiratory acidosis results from CO_2 retention, which may be caused by chronic obstructive lung disease or chest trauma. The treatment is improved air exchange. Intubation or tracheostomy may be necessary. The primary indicator of respiratory acidosis is a significant increase in CO_2, with a lesser increase in HCO_3, and some decrease in pH. Typical symptoms are restlessness, confusion, and tachycardia. If untreated, acidosis leads to coma and death. Metabolic acidosis results from diabetic ketoacidosis, uncontrolled diarrhea, shock, or renal failure. The treatment is to correct the specific cause. The primary indicator is a significant decrease in HCO_3, with some decrease in CO_2 and pH. The HCO_3 bicarbonate may fall so low in its effort to correct acidosis that IV replacement usually is given. Typical symptoms are stupor, deep rapid breathing, and fruity odor of the patient's breath.

Nursing Considerations

- If the patient is on oxygen, check with the physician as to whether ABGs are to be drawn when the patient is breathing oxygen or room air. If they are to be taken when the patient is on oxygen, the correct liter flow must be maintained for 30 minutes before the blood is drawn. Mark on the lab slip the number of liters. If the patient is on room air, write "room air."
- A special kit is usually provided for this procedure. The blood is drawn by designated personnel in each hospital, *e.g.*, nurses and respiratory therapists.
- Alert the laboratory when the ABGs are about to be drawn.
- The specimen must be immediately placed in a container of ice, and the specimen should arrive in the laboratory within 5 minutes.
- Pressure should be maintained on the withdrawal site for at least 5 minutes.
- When anticoagulants are in use, prolonged bleeding at the withdrawal site may occur.

CULTURES AND SPECIMEN COLLECTION

Description

Cultures of body fluids or secretions are done in order to identify bacteria. Sensitivity determinations are usually done concurrently to identify the antimicrobial drugs effective in destroying the bacteria.

Nursing Considerations

- Use sterile technique in obtaining all cultures, except those for stool examination. Specimens contaminated with normal skin flora are misleading and another culture may be required.
- Do not contaminate the outside of the container.
- Send cultures immediately to the laboratory for accurate examination results. Specimens that have been allowed to dry out or stay at an incorrect temperature are useless.
- Label the container as well as the laboratory slip. Include the time when the specimen was obtained.
- If an infectious disease is suspected, write this on the label.
- No antibiotic should be started until after a culture specimen is obtained. If this is not possible, the antibiotic should be noted on the laboratory slip.

TABLE 1-6 SPECIMEN COLLECTION

Site	Amount Required	Container	Pathogens	Procedure
Throat	Thorough swabbing	Swab replaced in sterile container	Group A *Streptococcus*, β-hemolytic	Inspect throat with a flashlite before swabbing to identify both tonsils and posterior pharynx.
Wound (decubitus ulcer)	The applicator should go as deeply as possible into the wound, and then be swabbed on tissue surfaces.	Swab replaced in sterile container	*Staphylococcus aureus;* Group A *Streptococcus* β-hemolytic	Avoid swabbing pus on the skin surface. Wash off the skin with saline to lessen contamination with normal skin flora. If a large area is involved, take specimens from different sites.
Stool	Size of a pea	Clean container	*Salmonella, Shigella, Campylobacter* species, ova and parasites	A rectal swab may be sufficient; check with laboratory. Stool must be free of barium for parasite studies. Stool should not be more than 1 hour old.
Urine	5 ml	Syringe or sterile container. See clean catch urine.	Any organism greater than 50 to 100,000 ml, excluding flora generally found in perineal area	When the tip of an indwelling catheter is sent to culture, cleanse the meatus before withdrawing the catheter. Cut off the catheter top with a sterile

				scissors. Never collect a specimen from a urinary drainage bag. Specimens may be taken from an indwelling catheter by first cleansing the specimen port in the catheter with alcohol. Specimens should not be more than 1 hour old. There is an extremely high incidence of urinary tract infections (UTI) after 3 days of use of an indwelling catheter.
Sputum	3ml–5ml	Sterile container	Any predominant organism	Preferably, early AM bronchial secretion (not saliva) obtained after a deep cough. May be obtained by suctioning or a Lukens tube. Tuberculosis bacilli may not grow out for several weeks.
Cerebrospinal fluid (CSF)	10 ml or more	Three sterile containers marked 1, 2, 3	Any organism	Must be sent to lab *immediately*.

(continued)

TABLE 1-6 SPECIMEN COLLECTION

Site	Amount Required	Container	Pathogens	Procedure
Blood	Usually done by lab personnel	Check with lab if to be done by other than lab personnel	Any organism	Blood usually taken three or four times at 30-minute intervals to avoid missing an organism and confirm the diagnosis. Should be taken between chill and fever spikes.
Body fluids (*e.g.*, pleural fluid)	Check with the lab.	Sterile container. Check with the lab. May require special container	Any organism	Should be processed immediately.

- A tentative identification of organisms takes 24 hours, and final results 48 hours or more, with the exception of tuberculosis bacilli, which may take several weeks.
- Physicians should be notified immediately of pathogens appearing in cultures. Call the laboratory for assistance in interpreting culture reports.

TESTING FOR OCCULT BLOOD

Description

Blood need not be visible in body secretions or stool; it may be present as occult blood. Testing for occult blood may be done on the unit using a variety of testing material. Read the manufacturer's directions carefully. If there is any question, send the specimen to the laboratory.

Nursing Considerations

- In preparing a patient for a routine laboratory examination of the stool for occult blood, the diet should be restricted for two days. During this time no meat, turnips, horseradish, or aspirin, and no more than 250 mg of vitamin C per day should be consumed.

URINE SPECIMEN COLLECTION AND TESTING

CLEAN CATCH METHOD

When possible, all urine specimens should be collected in this manner to ensure an uncontaminated specimen. If patient cooperation is not possible, an in-and-out catheterization may be necessary. In the case of infants, a needle aspiration of the bladder may be performed.

Nursing Considerations

- This should be the first morning specimen after the bladder has been emptied initially on awakening.
- Instruct the patient to wash his or her hands, and then to cleanse the periurethral meatus thoroughly with two antiseptic towelettes. The patient starts the urine stream, stops, and then voids directly into a sterile container.
- This specimen should go directly to the laboratory.

FRACTIONAL URINE METHOD

A fractional collection of a urine specimen before meals (ac) and at bedtime (hs) is done with diabetic patients to test for glucose and acetone.

Nursing Considerations

- Specimen should be from the *second voiding* at the hour specified. The patient empties his or her bladder approximately 30 minutes before the time of specimen collection.
- At the time of collection, the patient voids again, and this specimen is tested for glucose or acetone. The test indicates whether glucose or acetone is being excreted at that time, not what accumulated in the bladder over several hours.
- If the specimen is being collected from an indwelling catheter, one collection is sufficient since the bladder is essentially empty at all times.
- A specimen from an indwelling catheter is aspirated through the collection port, *never* from the drainage bag.
- A report from a patient or nursing assistant that a urine test indicates more than a trace of glucose is present requires another test by the nurse before insulin is given or the physician notified.

TIMED URINE METHOD

These urine collections are done to determine metabolic and kidney functions.

Nursing Considerations

- Obtain a container that will accommodate the entire specimen.
- Add the preservative in the laboratory if it is necessary for the test.
- Refer to Table 1-7 for the tests requiring a preservative.
- Instruct the patient to start the collection by voiding and discarding this specimen. Mark the time on the container.
- Instruct the patient to save all urine voided during the time period required.
- Complete the collection by having the patient urinate the last specimen at the closing time.
- Caution the patient not to void directly into the container.
- All timed specimens must be kept on ice or refrigerated during their collection.
- Notify the laboratory if any urine is lost during the collection period.

TESTING FOR GLUCOSE AND KETONES

Description

Urine obtained from diabetic patients as stat specimens or fractionals is tested for acetone and glucose. The results help determine daily insulin doses and additional insulin coverage as necessary.

Testing Methods

Acetest

Tablet test for acetone

- Place one tablet on paper towel.
- Place one drop of urine on tablet.
- Wait 30 seconds.
- Read by Acetest color chart. Values are in shades of purple. Results indicate negative, small, moderate, or large amounts of acetone in the urine.

Ketostix

For ketones

- This estimates the amount of ketones in urine as small, moderate, or large. Test for ketones, when urine glocuse measures 1% or more. L-Dopa, phenylketones (PKU), or brom-sulphalein (BSP) may cause false-positive results.

Dip and Read Reagent Strips

For glucose and ketones

- Throwaway strips of reagent paper are passed through urine stream or dipped into urine, then compared with accompanying color chart to estimate amounts of glucose and ketones in urine.

Diastix

For glucose

- Large quantities of ketone bodies, ascorbic acid, or L-dopa may depress color development.

Clinistix

For glucose

- This 10-second test only shows whether glucose is present or absent, so it is most useful for well-controlled diabetic patients who need only periodic checks for glucose in urine. High doses of aspirin or vitamin C may affect test results.

Keto-Diastix

For ketones and glucose

- This test is designed for diabetic patients whose control is uneven enough to warrant regular ketone (acetone) testing at the same time as glucose testing. (For occasional ketone testing, use Ketostix or Acetest.)

Tes-Tape

For glucose

- A dip and read test for glucose that comes in a tape dispenser. The tape is sometimes difficult to read.

Clinitest

Tablet test for glucose (five- and two-drop methods)

- Except for the use of either five drops or two drops of urine, the procedure is the same, although one must compare the specimen with the appropriate (*i.e.,* five-drop or two-drop) color chart. The two-drop method is more accurate and is used especially for the patient whose diabetes is difficult to control. It estimates glucose concentration from 0%–5%. The five-drop method estimates glucose concentrations from 0%–2%, and is usually reported in terms of negative, trace, and pluses.

PROCEDURE

- Collect urine in clean receptacle. Place five (or two) drops of urine in a clean test tube. Rinse dropper and add 10 drops of water to test tube.
- Drop one tablet into the test tube. Watch the reaction as it takes place. If color should rapidly "pass through" from bright orange to dark brown or greenish brown, it indicates that the glucose level is over 2%. Record as such or try the two-drop method for more accurate results.
- Do not shake the test tube during or for 15 seconds following the reaction.
- After a 15-second waiting period, shake test tube gently and compare with color chart.
- Record and report results. Check the physician's orders for appropriate insulin coverage.

Nursing Considerations

- Clinitest tablets are *poisonous* and may cause chemical burns. Don't touch them with wet fingers. They should be kept in a dry, dark, safe place.
- Clinitest tablets will react with any sugar in the urine (not only glucose). Clinistix or Diastix are specific for testing presence of glucose, so they could be used as a second test as necessary.
- Large quantities of ascorbic acid, nalidixic acid (Neg Gram), cephalosporins (Keflin, Keflex, Loridine), and probenecid (Benemid) may cause false-positive results with Clinitest. Use another method when patients are receiving these drugs.
- Be consistent in the method used to test urine on each individual patient.
- A report from a patient or nursing assistant that a urine test indicates more than a trace of glucose requires another test by the nurse before insulin is given or the physician notified.

TABLE 1-7 PRESERVATIVES FOR 24-HOUR URINES

Use No Preservative	No Preservative Necessary, However, 10-ml Concentrated HCl Will Not Interfere	Miscellaneous Preservatives	
Amylase	Estrogen	VMA	10 ml concentrated HCl
BUN	Follicle-stimulating hormone	Aldosterone	15 ml 30% acetic acid, or 4.5 ml glacial acetic acid plus 10.5 ml water
Calcium	17-Hydroxycorticosteroids		
Creatinine	17- Ketogenic steroids		
Glucose	17-Hydroxysteroids	5 HIAA	25 ml glacial acetic acid
Heavy metals	17- Ketosteroids	Metanephrine	5 ml concentrated HCl
Hydroxy-proline	Pregnanediol	Porphyrins	5 g sodium carbonate
LDH		Uroporphyrins	5 g sodium carbonate
Oxalates		Coproporphyrins	5 g sodium carbonate
Phosphorus		Cortisol	2 boric acid tablets
Porphobilinogen		Catecholamines	10 ml concentrated HCl
Potassium			
Pregnanetroil			
Quantitative HCG			
Sodium			
Uric acid			
Urine total protein			

TESTING FOR SPECIFIC GRAVITY

Description

The specific gravity (SG) of urine is its weight compared with the weight of an equal volume of water. It indicates the kidney's ability to concentrate and dilute urine. A low SG occurs with overhydration or renal failure. A high SG indicates a low fluid intake or excessive fluid loss. The normal range of urine SG is 1.001 to 1.035.

Nursing Considerations

- The equipment to test SG includes a cylinder to contain the urine (about 10 ml) and a urinometer.
- Use a freshly voided specimen and fill the cylinder about three-fourths full of urine.
- Place the urinometer into the cylinder; gently spin it; when it comes to rest, read at eye level where the meniscus crosses the scale on the urinometer. This is the SG reading.
- Record and report results.

BIBLIOGRAPHY • Clinical Laboratory Tests

JOURNALS

Cohen J, Pantaleo N, Shell W: What isoenzymes can tell you about your cardiac patient. Nursing 82 12(4)46, April 1982

Hargiss C, Larson E: Infection control. How to collect specimens and evaluate results. Am J Nurs 81(12):2166, Dec 1981

CONFERENCES

Bancroft B: Clinical Interpretation of Lab Tests. Bethesda, Maryland Oct 26, Nov. 3, Nov. 14, 1983

BOOKS

Corbett J: Laboratory Tests in Nursing Practice. Norwalk, Conn, Appleton–Century—Crofts, 1982

Fischbach F: A Manual of Laboratory Diagnostic Tests, 2nd ed. Philadelphia, JB Lippincott, 1984

McFarland M, Grant M: Nursing Implications of Laboratory Tests. New York, John Wiley & Sons, 1982

Strand M, Elmer L: Clinical Laboratory Tests, 2nd ed. St. Louis, CV Mosby, 1980

Tietz N: Clinical Guide to Laboratory Tests. Philadelphia, WB Saunders, 1983

Tilkian S, Conover M, Tilkian A: Clinical Implications of Laboratory Tests, 2nd ed. St Louis, CV Mosby, 1979

2
Management in Special Nursing Situations (MNS)

MENTAL HEALTH

ALCOHOLIC PATIENT IN WITHDRAWAL

Description

Recognizing the symptoms of alcohol withdrawal may be a matter of life or death. More than 15% of patients who experience delirium tremens (DTs) die despite treatment. Patients admitted to the hospital with alcohol on their breath and showing symptoms of intoxication are easy to identify. Suspect those admitted with diagnoses of diseases that are alcohol-related; those with burns, evidence of falls, and bruises; or those who do not respond in the usual way to normal doses of medications, particularly sedatives. Often, alcoholics are also heavy smokers, and addictions to controlled substances ranging from diazepam (Valium) to street drugs (e.g., cocaine, and heroin), are not uncommon.

The goal of treatment is to avoid the toxic crisis of DTs by staying ahead of symptoms with medication. Accurate, continuous assessment is vital.

Observations

- Evidence of accidental injuries—bruises, burns,—or symptoms of disorders that may be alcohol-related (*e.g.*, cirrhosis; see MSN, Gastrointestinal, Liver)
- Evidence of poly drug abuse
  1. Check arms for "track marks" (veins darkened by frequent injections).
  2. Check patient's belongings for concealed drugs.
- A history of the patient's alcohol-use habits should be included in all nursing histories. Question the patient in a matter-of-fact way. Be nonjudgmental.
  1. Avoid the use of the word "alcoholic," which may put patient on the defensive.
  2. Ask the question, "When did you have your last drink?" The answer is important because if it was 4 hours ago, you have a little time. If it was 8 hours ago, he or she may already be in withdrawal and will need to be medicated immediately.

3. Ask, "What happens when you stop drinking?" "How much alcohol do you drink each day?" Follow by saying that it makes a difference in determining the dosage of drugs he or she will be receiving. Assume that an alcoholic does not want to reveal the amount of alcohol he or she actually consumes.

- Early symptoms of alcohol withdrawal include
  1. Headache, slurred speech, poor coordination, staggering gait, nausea and vomiting, diarrhea, insomnia, failure to respond to average dose of tranquilizers or sedatives
- Later symptoms include
  1. A fluttery feeling, minor anxiety, tremulousness (difficulty lighting a cigarette or holding a cup of coffee), tachycardia, disorientation, agitation, nausea and vomiting, diaphoresis, hallucinations (may be visual, auditory, or tactile), seizure
- Symptoms of delirium tremens (DTs) include the following, in addition to all of the above:
  1. Fever over 100°F or 38°C, pulse rate over 120, diaphoresis, thrashing, and extreme psychotic behavior
  2. One of the keys to the differential diagnosis between a withdrawal reaction to alcohol and to drug overdose is that in alcohol withdrawal all vital signs are elevated; in drug overdose they are depressed.
  3. DTs may occur anytime from the third to the seventh day after withdrawal, or sooner if trauma or injury is present. DTs may occur as a result of reduction of alcohol use from heavy to moderate, rather than total cessation of drinking, thereby modifying the time of onset of the delirium.

Treatment

- Sedatives in sufficient doses to control the symptoms. The patient should be sedated to the point where he exhibits no symptoms but can still be aroused. Drugs must be given around the clock (if necessary, patient must be wakened to take medication). Diazepam (Valium), chlordiazepoxide hydrochloride (Librium), or thioridazine hydrochloride (Mellaril) may be given PO or parenterally.
- Anticonvulsant medications (Valium is one of the best anticonvulsants. Phenytoin [Dilantin] is also frequently prescribed.)
- Antiemetics
- Maintenance of fluid and electrolyte balance
- Reestablishment of adequate nutrition—regular diet, high in vitamins
- Early involvement in an alcohol rehabilitation program

Nursing Considerations

- Provide a calm, safe, nonstressful environment. Delirious patients may be very frightened by their hallucinations; they can become very agitated, sometimes even suicidal.
- Give quiet reassurance. Help the patient stay in touch with reality. Keep the room well lit 24 hours a day.
- Stay with the patient, if possible, or have a member of the family come in to stay with him. Keep directions simple.
- Restrain with a Posey vest, if needed. Use leather wrist cuffs only if absolutely necessary.
- Have a padded tongue blade available. Try to protect patient from head injuries.
- Monitor vital signs and for alertness and responsiveness every two hours (q 2 hr). Assess for response to drug therapy q 4 hr. Remember, medications are given around the clock. Communication and follow-up between nursing shifts are essential.

Sources of Information

Alcoholics Anonymous, Grand Central Station, P.O. Box 459, New York, NY 10163, or local chapters

Al-Anon Family Groups, Inc., Madison Square Station, P.O. Box 182, New York, NY 10159-0182, or local chapters

National Council on Alcoholism, 733 3rd Ave., Suite 1405, New York, NY 10017

ATTEMPTED SUICIDE

Description

A person attempting suicide is one who voluntarily and intentionally tries to take his or her own life. The individual may not really want to die, but may be desperately seeking help for an intolerable situation. All verbal indications of suicide must be taken seriously, because for every 10 persons who kill themselves, eight had given definite warnings of their intentions.

More men than women commit suicide, but women attempt suicide more frequently than men. Men tend to use more violent methods such as firearms, hanging, jumping, and drowning. Women frequently use drugs and poisons. The actual suicide rate is high for individuals 55 to 64 years of age, but the highest *attempt* rate is among those 24 to 44 years old. Other high-risk groups include adolescents, the elderly, the sick, and the mentally ill. Suicide rates fluctuate seasonally, with the highest number occurring in the spring.

Observations

- Factors that increase suicidal potential are concrete plans or pervasive thoughts about suicide, male sex, older age, social isolation, lack of plans for the future, contemplation of a violent method, history of previous attempts, no apparent secondary gain, severe depression, active psychosis, command hallucinations, history of alcohol or drug abuse, and a family history of suicide.
- Factors that are associated with a suicidal crisis are
  - Suicidal ideas and behavior
  - Depression with feelings of helplessness and hopelessness
  - Anxiety
  - Isolated life-style
  - Agitated or panic state
  - Previous suicidal behavior (25% of individuals who have made a previous attempt ultimately succeed)
  - Recent, significant loss
  - Psychic pain, intolerable stress
  - High-risk life-style
  - Severe, chronic physical illness

Treatment and Prevention

It is extremely important to assess the lethality and suicidal risk of the threat.

- The major predictor of a lethal suicide attempt is a previous attempt.
- A concrete plan also indicates lethality:

  Has the individual decided on a method?

  Are the means available to the individual?

  Has he or she decided when and where to accomplish the act?
- Be alert for verbal clues as well as direct or indirect feelings and behaviors:

  Making or changing a will

  Putting affairs in order

  Giving away cherished personal items

  Unexpected changes in behavior (unusual calmness in adverse situations, sudden withdrawal from emotional ties, sudden appearance of tranquility after an agitated depression)
- Ask pointed questions:

  How is your life going?

  How do you feel in general?

  Do you wish you could be out of it, away from it all?

  Would you sometimes like to give up?

Have you ever wished you were dead?

Have you thought of ending your life?

How close to suicide are you now?

How would you do it?

What is your plan?

- If you suspect your patient is suicidal, do not leave him or her alone until appropriate mental-health support and protection have been provided.

Depression is present in about 95% of all suicidal cases and must be alleviated to help prevent future suicide attempts. (See MNS, Depression.)

Nursing Considerations

- Depressed individuals have their strongest suicidal tendencies when they are just entering into or recovering from an attack of depression because they have the energy to carry out the suicidal act.
- Persons who abuse drugs or alcohol may increase their consumption to get the courage to act.
- Talk of suicide or actual attempts may be a cry for help. Prevention and treatment frequently involve families as well as mental-health personnel.
- Most communities have mental-health and suicide prevention hotlines. Be aware of the resources in your area.
- Support groups are also available for family members and friends of suicide victims. Normal feelings of grief, guilt, anger, and shame are common and frequently overwhelming.
- Suicide prevention resources are seldom directed to the elderly population, yet each year the elderly quietly and methodically kill themselves in larger numbers than any other age group. Most elderly people who attempt suicide complete the act. Those who do not complete the suicide are frequently found to have some degree of dementia that appeared to interfere with coordination, planning, determination, and awareness of reality.
- Many suicidal risk factors can be present in the life of an individual elderly person:

  Social isolation

  Financial difficulties

  Multiple chronic illnesses

  Depression

  Loss of role and status resulting from retirement

  Threats of dependency or institutionalization

  Multiple losses of family and friends

- The number of suicides among adolescents and children is increasing. The high accident rate in this group may reflect suicides masked by accidental death or homicide.
- Approximately 90% of adolescents who attempt suicide are girls. The method of choice is frequently an overdose of drugs, usually medications prescribed for parents. Firearms and hangings account for the largest number of deaths in the 10- to 14-year age group for both boys and girls. Suicide is rare under age 9, but incidence rises sharply after age 14.
- Disrupted family life is involved in the majority of adolescent suicides. Divorce, separation, alcoholism, and death of a significant other are frequently found in the youth's history. Intact families tend to be marked by marital discord, disturbed communication, physical aggression, abnormal patterns of interaction, and a lack of unity.
- Suicidal gestures in adolescents frequently are impulsive acts designed to force parents or other significant persons to pay attention to the adolescent's need for help.
- Children and younger adolescents may desire to punish others who will be grieved by their death.
- Social isolation appears to be a significant factor in distinguishing those adolescents who will kill themselves from those who will not. Teachers may be aware of behavioral problems, and older children may begin using drugs and alcohol.

DEPRESSION

Description

Depression is a severe, persistent episode of depressed mood. There is a change in the way the person feels about himself or herself, and he or she loses interest or pleasure in the usual activities of life.

Depression can be described as endogenous or reactive. Endogenous depression is thought to have biochemical and genetic causes. It is usually deeper and longer lasting, and may be a lifelong characteristic. The individual's history demonstrates the lack of a recent precipitating event, and the depression runs its course without apparent relation to the environment.

A reactive depression is a reaction to a stress or loss. The onset can usually be traced. The onset of a serious physical illness can precipitate depression.

Observations

- Feelings of hopelessness, despair, and that nothing in life makes sense or matters
- Low self-esteem

- Irritability or anger
- Apathy and fatigue
- Painful sadness and crying
- Confusion
- Regression
- Pessimism, especially about the future
- Inability to concentrate
- Memory loss and complaints of memory impairment
- Loss of appetite, weight loss, or weight gain
- Sleep disturbances (*e.g.,* inability to fall asleep, early morning awakening)
- Constipation
- Psychomotor retardation or agitation
- Diminished interest in sex
- Recurrent thoughts of death or suicide

Treatment

Three modes of therapy are commonly used, either separately or in combination.

Psychotherapy

Both individual and group psychotherapy are available in hospital settings and in the community. Marital and family therapy should also be considered. Therapy involves unqualified acceptance and protection of the individual. He or she must be assisted to hope, to try new ways, and to plan to have a future.

Pharmacotherapy

Drugs of choice are frequently the tricyclic antidepressants. Monoamine oxidase inhibitors (MAOI), tetracyclics (*e.g.,* Trazadone), and antipsychotic drugs are also used. It is very important that the health-care provider prescribing these medications be familiar with their actions, uses, and adverse effects. Because it may take from 2 to 6 weeks for the individual to experience improvement, the patient needs a great deal of support to ensure compliance with the regimen. These medications can be lethal in relatively small amounts. Patients should be discharged on the lowest effective dosages, and with only a small supply of the drug.

Electroconvulsive Therapy (ECT)

ECT may be considered when the patient is depressed with psychotic symptoms or behaviors, has severe insomnia and weight loss that threaten physical health, or has medical problems that are more safely treated with ECT than with medication. ECT is also the treatment of choice when the patient has not responded to medication and other treatments.

Nursing Considerations

- The use of prescription drugs can precipitate depression, and the individual's drug history should be reviewed when symptoms of depression are evident. Examples of such drugs are tranquilizers, antihypertensives (*e.g.,* hydralazine, methyldopa, reserpine), beta-blockers (*e.g.,* propranolol), and the antiarrhythmic drug procainamide.
- Depression is the most common emotional illness found in older people. It can occur at any time in the elderly person's life and is characterized by insomnia, despair, lethargy, anorexia, loss of interest, and somatic complaints.
- The older depressed person is more likely to report somatic complaints than a younger individual (*e.g.,* physical illness, difficulty in family and social relationships, dissatisfaction with economic circumstances). However, he or she is less likely to indicate feelings of depression.
- Depression may not be as cyclic in the older individual, and while he or she is waiting for the depression to go away, dangerous factors can intervene (*e.g.,* social isolation, immobility, decreased nutrition).
- Depression in older adolescents is similar to that seen in adults. However, in early adolescence and childhood the depression may be masked by a variety of behaviors. It may manifest itself as delinquency, aggression, truancy, bullying younger children, promiscuity, running away from home, school failure, and accident proneness. Children may express boredom, restlessness, fatigue, and difficulty in concentrating.

DISORIENTATION

Description

A mild degree of disorientation can be expected in any patient since the hospital environment is quite different from the one normally encountered. This type of mental confusion is very common in older patients who become perturbed when their established daily routine is disrupted. Also, patients with brain damage are very vulnerable to psychoses and inability to perceive reality. Serious disorientation can occur as a result of metabolic changes or imbalances caused by an illness. Imbalance of electrolytes, BUN, blood glucose, ABGs, elevated temperature or blood pressure, or withdrawal from alcohol and other drugs, are common causes of disorientation. Almost any drug can produce an adverse psychologic effect in a sensitive elderly patient. Mental confusion may be evident shortly after admission; or, as in the case of alcohol withdrawal, may not occur until two or three days after admission.

Nursing Considerations

- It is important to obtain a nursing history that gives details of medications presently being taken and the amount of alcohol normally consumed daily. The probability of mental confusion occurring increases with the number of medications being taken.
- Explain the hospital routine and attempt to learn the patient's daily routine, especially at night (*e.g.,* frequency of use of the bathroom, and usual pattern of sleep). Emphasize that nurses and other hospital personnel will be entering the patient's room at night.
- Schedule medications, treatments, and procedures as much as possible so that they don't interrupt sleep.
- Early symptoms of confusion may appear gradually. These include increasing restlessness, emotional irritability, apprehension, difficulty in identifying familiar people or objects, and picking at air or bedding. Sometimes these result from anoxia, and oxygen administration is helpful.
- A bed near a window, a calendar on the wall, and a clock that the patient can see promote contact with reality. A day-night reversal pattern can develop.
- Confusion is most severe in twilight or darkness. Feelings of loneliness, despair, and longing for home increase. The addition of flashing lights on an IV pump, suction machines, and unfamiliar noises in a dark room heighten anxiety.
- Keep normal lights on, since partial darkness causes shadows. Keep hearing aids, eyeglasses, and dentures in place on the patient. Patients with eye patches have an increased tendency to disorientation. The head of the bed should be kept elevated; hallucinations increase when a patient is flat in bed. A radio left on day and night is helpful in providing a feeling of companionship.
- The hospital intercom may be left on to monitor activity, but don't use it to talk to the patient. A disembodied voice increases confusion.
- A gentle, caring touch may help because it communicates a feeling of "I care."
- In cases of extreme agitation, a family member or friend should be asked to sit with the patient, especially at night. Restraints should be a last resort.
- The common drug of choice in controlling severe agitation and hallucinations is haloperidol (Haldol). It should be regularly scheduled around the clock, *never* just prn. It should be discontinued gradually over a period of several days.

EVENING AND NIGHT SHIFT

Description

In hospital nursing, the management of patient care during the evening and night shifts must rely more completely on the individual nurse, as contrasted to receiving support from the hospital staff that is generally available during regular daytime hours.

Nursing Considerations

- After day or evening report, the oncoming nurse should make rounds and do patient assessments. Dressings need to be checked and drainage stains outlined with pencil for future reference. Levels of fluid in IV or drainage containers and the IV flow rate should be noted. Be sure that oxygen settings are correct and humidifiers have sufficient water. Call lights should be in place, side rails up, and restraints applied to those needing them.
- A roll of one-inch tape, scissors, an alcohol sponge, a Band-Aid, and a small flashlight carried in a pocket can be invaluable.
- Be familiar with the duties of nurse's aides. Make out a work sheet and discuss it with each aide. Point out the patients who need assistance with eating, including any special orders for increased or limited fluid intake, as well as those patients who need intake and output recorded. Clearly identify to the aide those patients who require specimen collection, fractional urines, or timed collections, elevated temperature procedure, and ambulation or turning or positioning.
- Bedside tables and the areas around patients' beds should be cleared because dim lighting and unfamiliar surroundings increase the possibility of accidents.
- Tell patients early in the evening if they are going to be NPO after midnight.
- At around 8:00 P.M., check the temperatures of patients who have had elevations (99.4°F or 37.5°C orally or 100.4°F or 38°C rectally). After this time, schedule assessments of vital signs to coincide with the administration of medications to minimize interruptions of patients' sleep.
- The day's postoperative patients, or any patients who have had an indwelling catheter removed, should have orders covering the possibility of their not voiding spontaneously within 8 hours.
- An adequate supply of individual patient's medicines should be on hand for the entire night. To avoid late night calls to the physicians, orders for sedation or sleep should be obtained as early as possible in the evening.
- Sleep medications should be withheld until midnight if there are other medications or treatments scheduled for that hour. Repeat sleep medication should generally not be given after 3 A.M.

- Ideally, noisy or disoriented patients should be in private rooms. It often helps if bright lights and radios or TVs are left on to alleviate darkness and loneliness. When this is not possible, move the patient for the night into any available room (*e.g.*, treatment room) or to a wheelchair at the nurse's station.
- When there is any doubt about calling a physician at night, first call the nursing supervisor. When a physician is called, know the patient's current and previous vital signs.

BIBLIOGRAPHY • Management in Special Nursing Situations

Alcohol Withdrawal

Bluhm J: When you face the alcoholic patient. Nursing '81 11(2):71, Feb 1981
Crovella A: When your patient's an alcoholic. RN 47(2):50, Feb 1984
Kurose K, Anderson T, Bull W: A standard care plan for alcoholism. Am J Nurs 81(5):1001, May 1981
The hospitalized alcoholic. Continuing Education. Am J Nurs 32(12):1861, Dec 1982
Brodsley L: Avoiding a crisis: the assessment, p 1865
Cohn L: The hidden diagnosis, p 1862
Scherwerts P: An alcohol treatment team, p 1878

Attempted Suicide

Cohen M: The suicidal patient on the surgical ward: A multidisciplinary case conference. Gen Hosp Psychiatry 5:65, 1983
Cohen-Sandler R, Berman A: Life stress and symptomatology: Determinants of suicidal behavior in children. J Am Acad Child Psych 21:178, 1982
Farberow N: Suicide prevention in the hospital. Hosp Community Psychiatry 32:99, 1981
Garfinkel B, Froese A, Hood J: Suicide attempts in children and adolescents. Am J Psychiatry 139:1257, 1982
Grollman E: Suicide, Prevention, Intervention, Postvention. Boston, Beacon Press, 1971
Hendin H: Suicide in America. New York, Norton, 1982
Keidel G: Adolescent suicide. Nurs Clin North Am 18:323, 1983
Miller M: Suicide after Sixty: The Final Alternative. New York, Springer, 1979
Valente S: Suicide in school-aged children: Theory and assessment. Pediatr Nurs 9:25, 1983

Depression

Blazer D: Depression in Late Life. St Louis, CV Mosby, 1982
Bowden C: Unipolar depression: Common sense treatment that really helps patients. Consultant 22:113, 1982

Butler R, Lewis M: Aging and Mental Health. St Louis, CV Mosby, 1982
Goodstein R: The diagnosis and treatment of elderly patients: Some practical guidelines. Hosp Community Psychiatry 31:19, 1980
Hazle N: Postpartum blues: Assessment and intervention. J Nurse Midwife 27:21, 1982
Petti T: The assessment of depression in young children . . . infant, preschool and early school age. J Child Contemp Soc 15:19, 1982
Salzman C: Basic principles of psychotropic drug prescription for the elderly. Hosp Community Psychiatry 33:133, 1982
Talley J: Depression: Differentiate the endogenous variety from the look-alikes. Consultant 23:105, 1983
Vogel C: Anxiety and depression among the elderly. J Gerontol Nurs 8:213, 1982

Disorientation

JOURNALS

Castledine G: A confusing age-old problem. Nursing Mirror 154(18): 38, May 5, 1982
Chisholm S, Deniston O, Igrisan R, Barkes A: Prevalence of confusion in elderly hospitalized patients. J Gerontol Nurs 8(2): 87, Feb 1982
Kroner K: Dealing with the confused patient. Nursing '79(11):71, Nov 1979
Langland R, Panicucci C: Effects of touch on communication with elderly confused clients. J Gerontol Nurs 8(3): 152, March 1982
Lippman S: The treatment of dementia. Med Times 110(5):95, May 1982
Massey E, Riley T: Managing the patient with dementia. Postgrad Med 71(5):207, May 1982
Taylor R: Psychological masquerades. The Stanford Magazine, Winter 1983

CONFERENCE

Drug Therapy for the Elderly: Nursing Implications. Peter P. Lamy, Ph.D. FCP. George Mason University, May 4, 1981

3
Nursing Responsibilities for Diagnosis and Treatment (NR)

BONE MARROW ASPIRATION AND BIOPSY

Description

The bone marrow has, as its principal function, the manufacture of normal erythrocytes, leukocytes, and platelets. Bone marrow aspiration and bone biopsy are done to determine the effectiveness of this function.

Nursing Considerations

- A physician does these at the bedside and usually the patient's signed consent is required.
- Contact the laboratory for a proper container and preservative.
- A bone marrow aspiration may be done on the sternum or iliac crest; the sternum is avoided in infants and small children. When a bone biopsy is done, the iliac crest is used.
- The site is anesthetized with a local anesthetic.
- This procedure causes momentary but sharp pain when the marrow or bone is withdrawn.
- Apply pressure to the site for 3 to 5 minutes to prevent bleeding.
- Check again in 15 minutes for any bleeding.
- A pneumothorax is a possible complication of a sternal puncture, the result of inadvertantly entering the pleural cavity.

CARDIOPULMONARY RESUSCITATION (CPR)

Procedure

Adults

1. Place the unconscious person flat on his back on a *firm* surface. If no respirations are observed, open airway by either head-tilt or chin-lift methods (see Fig. 3-1*A* and *B*). The head tilt cannot be used for patients who have had spinal injury or surgery, or for those who are in traction. The necessary modifications of CPR technique must be included in their nursing-care plan.

2. If the person is not breathing, begin artificial respirations with four quick breaths, mouth to mouth and with the person's nose pinched closed (see Fig. 3-1*C*). If readily available, a manual resuscitation bag may be used. If the patient has a tracheostomy, artificial breathing is applied directly to the stoma; in this case, a head tilt is unnecessary. Watch for the chest to rise and fall signifying an open airway. CPR cannot continue until the victim's airway is open.
3. If the airway *is* obstructed, turn the patient toward you and, with the heel of your hand, give four back blows to the midscapular area. If obstruction persists, turn the patient on his or her back and deliver four abdominal or chest thrusts. The rescuer's hands should be between the waist and rib cage for

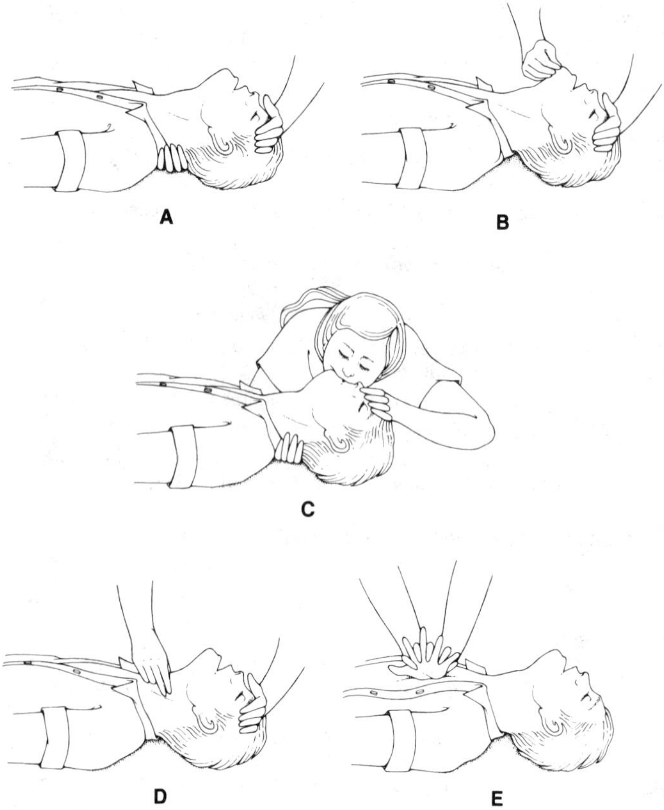

Fig. 3-1. *Cardiopulmonary resuscitation.*

inward and upward abdominal thrusts. The hand position for chest thrusts is the same as that for chest compression. A finger sweep of the mouth, using the index finger, may be done on an adult. Be careful not to push an object into the throat.

4. After the airway is open, reposition the head and give four quick breaths.
5. Check for carotid pulse (see Fig. 3-1*D*).
6. If a pulse is absent, begin chest compressions about 2 inches up from the xiphoid process. Depress sternum 1.5 to 2 inches (see Fig. 3-1*E*). With one rescuer 15 compressions (counting 1 and 2 and 3 and 4 and . . up to 15), two quick breaths, making the compression rate 80/minute. With two rescuers: five compressions (counting "one one thousand, two one thousand, three one thousand, four one thousand, five one thousand"), one quick breath. The rate of compression is 60/minute. Continue until advanced life support arrives or the patient is pronounced dead by a physician.

NR

Children (Considered Those 1 to 8 Years of Age)

1. Proceed through step 2 of adult CPR. Sealing the nose and mouth of a small child may be more appropriate than ventilating through the mouth.
2. If the airway is obstructed, the rescuer should kneel and position the small child over the rescuer's thighs, face down with the head lower than the trunk. Deliver four back blows with the heel of the hand in the midscapular area. If obstruction persists, return to back and with the head lower than the trunk deliver four chest thrusts with the heel of one hand in the midsternal area. Attempt to ventilate. If unsuccessful, repeat above sequence until an open airway is obtained. Abdominal thrusts are not recommended for children, because of a greater possibility of internal injuries.
3. Check for a carotid pulse.
4. If no pulse is present, begin chest compressions in the *midsternal* area. Children require 1 to 1.5 inches of compression done with the heel of *one* hand. One breath with every fifth compression is the correct ratio; counting 1 and 2 and 3 and 4 and 5, breathing on the upstroke of 5. The rate of compression is 80/minute.

Infants (Under 1 Year of Age)

1. The back must be supported on a *firm* surface, *e.g.*, place the infant on a table.
2. Do not hyperextend the neck of an infant because of possible injury; support it in an extended position with one hand.
3. If the infant is not breathing, both the nose and mouth are covered with the rescuer's mouth. Give four quick puffs. Watch for the chest to rise and fall indicating an open airway.

4. If the airway *is* obstructed, straddle the infant over the rescuer's arm, supporting the head and neck. The head should be lower than the trunk. Deliver four back blows between the scapula with the heel of the hand. If the obstruction persists, return to back position with the head lower than the body. Deliver four chest thrusts with the tips of the index and middle fingers to the midsternum. Again attempt to ventilate. If unsuccessful, repeat above sequence until the airway is open. Abdominal thrusts are not recommended in infants.
5. Check for *brachial* pulse.
6. If the pulse is absent, begin chest compressions in the *midsternal* area, 0.5 to 1.0 inch with the tips of the index and middle finger. One breath every fifth compression is the correct ratio; counting l, 2, 3, 4, 5, breathing on the upstroke of 5. The rate of compressions is 100/minute.

CAST BRACE

Description

Usually following a period of traction providing acceptable alignment, a cast brace may be used to reduce rehabilitation time for fractures of the femoral shaft or tibia. The cast brace makes early ambulation and weight bearing possible. A thigh cuff is made of plastic or plaster, and is joined with metal hinges to a short-leg walking cast at the knee. This provides not only fracture stability, but also joint movement and muscle function. It promotes more rapid healing (see Fig. 3-2).

The cast brace is applied usually after the fracture site is stable and initial pain and edema have subsided. Skeletal fraction may be applied until time for cast brace application (see NR, Traction).

Nursing Considerations

- Once the brace is applied, watch for swelling of the knee. If swelling is apparent, elevate the extremity. Apply ice packs, if ordered.
- Watch for signs of circulatory or neurological impairment caused by the cast. They are pallor, pulselessness, pain, paralysis, or paresthesia (tingling or numbness).
- Protect the cast from soiling with urine or feces, since the cast may extend to the groin.
- Vigorous quadriceps and hamstring exercises started during the period of traction are continued throughout treatment.
- Provide assistance to the patient with exercises and ambulation.
- Inspect knee hinges for firm attachment.
- If ordered, teach the patient how to inspect and tighten screws with the special instruments provided by the manufacturer. Some physicians prefer to make all such adjustments themselves.

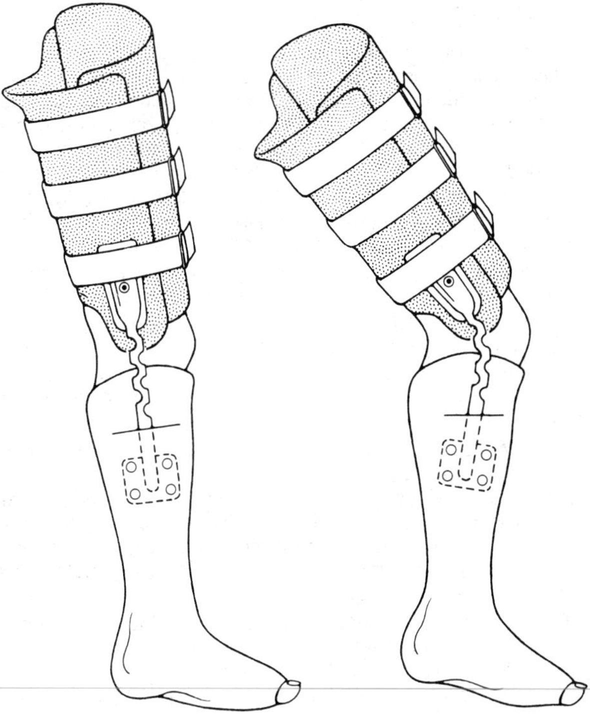

Fig. 3-2. Example of a cast brace with adjustable quad socket. (Pope brace, orthopedic division of Parke, Davis).

- Unless specifically ordered, neither nurse nor patient should attempt to adjust the brace. Its function is that of a cast.

CAST CARE

Description

Casts are used to immobilize a bone or joint in alignment, to hold reduction in fractures, and to correct and prevent deformities. They may be made of layers of plaster-of-paris bandages or synthetic materials including polyester/cotton knit, fiberglass, and thermoplastic.

Compared to casts made of plaster of paris, synthetic casts are quick setting, lightweight, less bulky, and immersible in water. They are more expensive, and have more potential for skin irritation and maceration.

Observations

- Unrelieved pain, pallor, pulselessness, paralysis, or paresthesia (tingling or numbness) are all signs of possible neurovascular impairment caused by edema under the unyielding cast. After application of a fresh cast, observe the patient frequently during the first 48 hours, at the beginning of each shift, and prn thereafter. Report the presence of any of the above symptoms immediately. The cast may need to be altered, bivalved (split in half), or removed. Pain must always be investigated. Do not mask it with medication until the cause is determined.
- All toes and fingers should be warm and pink, should have feeling, and should be capable of flexion and extension.
- Check for decreased capillary filling in nail beds: test by applying pressure to finger nail or toe nail. Normally, when pressure is released, the nail almost immediately becomes pink. A delay in return of normal color indicates impaired circulation. Report immediately.
- *Caution:* Compartment syndrome leading to Volkmann's contracture is a dreaded complication of compromised blood supply (ischemia) to a muscle group (usually in the arm or hand). If unrelieved, it can cause permanent disability within 6 hours. The cast must be released. The cast can be changed, the contracture cannot (See MSN, Fractures, and Postoperative nursing tips for more about compartment syndrome).
- Check for bleeding. Circle the outer border of the area of apparent bleeding and mark the time. Check underside of cast; blood tends to pool at the bottom of a cast.
- "Hot spots" felt on a dry cast or a musty odor coming from the cast could be signs of skin breakdown underneath it.
- Watch for signs of pressure on the heel or Achilles' tendon (burning sensation over heel area) in patients in leg casts.
- Watch for signs and symptoms of complications of immobility (*e.g.,* pneumonia, constipation, renal calculi, or neurovascular problems).

Nursing Considerations

- Skin under the cast should be clean, dry, and in good condition.
- Patient should be told that as a plaster-of-paris cast sets, it will give off heat for about 20 minutes. It will then cool, dry, and grow lighter.
- Casting may be postponed to allow for reduction of swelling. Provide pain medication and gentle handling in the interim.
- Elevate the affected part a little above the level of the heart in an effort to reduce edema.

Care of New Casts

- Plaster of paris may require 24 to 48 hours to dry, depending upon variables such as humidity and the thickness of the cast.
- To promote drying of the plaster-of-paris cast:
  1. Expose all sides of the cast to the air. Cast dryers are dangerous; if ordered, use on cool setting only. Lamps and lights are discouraged; if used they should be placed 15 to 18 inches away from the cast.
  2. Keep cast uncovered. Provide extra covering for the rest of the body if patient feels chilly.
  3. For a large body cast (*e.g.*, a hip spica), turn the patient every three hours.

     Turn carefully as a unit with three or four people supporting the areas of greatest strain.

     In most cases, turn with the affected limb up (*i.e.*, turn toward the unaffected side).

     Handle only with the palms of your hands.

     Never place wet cast on flat, hard surface or where there are sharp edges that will alter the shape of the cast.

     Ice bags, if ordered to reduce edema, should be filled only one-third full and placed with care against the sides of the cast so as not to dent it.

     Do not use the abduction bar on a hip-spica cast for turning. When patient is prone, toes should hang over end of bed.
- Pillows not covered with plastic (plastic retards drying) should support the curves of the cast, so that it will not become flattened over bony prominences (*e.g.*, sacrum or heel).
- A firm mattress with a bed board, overbed frame, and trapeze is useful when the patient has a hip spica or a large body cast.
- If surgeon cuts a window in a cast to expose a wound, save the cut-out piece; the surgeon may replace it later.

Protection of the Cast

- "Petal" the edges of the cast with short strips of adhesive with rounded corners on one end. Tuck rounded end under; secure it; pull other end over the edge of the cast and secure it. The next petal will overlap slightly.
  1. The cast edges of a fiberglass cast, if sharp, can be smoothed with nail file or emery board.
- To clean the cast
  1. Plaster-of-paris casts may be dry cleaned by using a damp cloth and scouring powder on small areas of the cast. Care must be taken not to dampen it.

To decrease odor, a 1:750 solution of benzalkonium chloride (Zephiran) may be sponged lightly on soiled areas.

2. Synthetic casts can be cleaned with soap and water. Thorough rinsing and drying of the cast is essential to prevent build up of soap film.

- Synthetic casts vary in how they dry, how they mold, and how they should be dried if they become wet. Ask the physician about the specifics of their care.
- The large body or hip spica cast
  1. Protect it from soiling by feces or urine by lining the area of the cast around the buttocks and perineum with plastic.
  2. A fracture bed pan should be used. Place a small pillow under the patient's back to prevent cracking of the cast. Raise the head of the bed slightly.
  3. Try to prevent the patient becoming constipated by providing high roughage diet and stool softeners, if ordered.

Itching Under the Cast

- A gauze strip placed next to the skin and under the cast may be moved back and forth, up and down.
- Air may be blown under the cast with a large syringe or a hair dryer with a "cool" setting.

Patient Teaching for Patients with Synthetic Casts

- Do not engage in excessive physical activities.
- If cast becomes wet, it must be thoroughly dried to prevent skin irritation and maceration.
  1. Blot the cast with towels.
  2. Use hand blower on cool or warm setting to dry cast and stockinette under it thoroughly. It may take an hour.
  3. Patients should avoid the beach, where sand can get under the cast and cause irritation. If sand or dirt particles should get under the cast, they must be rinsed out thoroughly.
- Casts are sometimes rough, snagging clothing or scratching furniture, so rest cast on towel or pillow.

Cast Removal

- Equipment required
  1. Cast cutter (a saw that oscillates rather than one that uses a continuous circular motion), cast knives, spreaders
  2. Solution of one part vinegar and four parts water may be used to soften cutting line on plaster-of-paris casts.
- Advise patient that procedure is noisy and produces feelings of warmth, but will not hurt.

- Elevate and support the affected body part after cast removal. There is always some swelling.
- Gently clean the skin with lanolin or lotion, followed with mild soap and water.
- Never force movement in a joint.
- Physiotherapy or hydrotherapy, or both, usually is ordered to help the patient regain motion and to learn crutch walking, if required.

CATHETERIZATION, URINARY

Description

Recognition of the high incidence of bladder infection associated with catheterization has made this a procedure that is ordered only if it is absolutely necessary. Nursing measures that promote normal emptying of the bladder should be used (*e.g.,* a warm bed pan, a comfortable position for the patient, privacy, and the sound of running water). When all else fails, catheterization is still ordered in some cases to relieve urinary retention, to measure for retention, occasionally to collect a sterile urine specimen, and to insert an indwelling or retention catheter for continuous urinary drainage or irrigation, especially following genitourinary (GU) surgery. It is essential to maintain sterile technique during the procedure. Avoidance of contamination of the closed urinary drainage system and hand washing before handling catheter or drainage equipment are also necessary.

Equipment

- Prepackaged catheterization kits with sterile contents that are available in most hospitals contain the catheter, cotton balls, lubricant, disposable forceps, cleansing solution, specimen cup, gloves, and drapes. Kits with urinary drainage bags and tubing may be requested. Instructions on how to do the catheterization procedure are usually included in the kit.
- Take a second catheter and pair of sterile gloves with you to the patient's bedside for use if needed. They can be returned, if they are not contaminated.
- When catheterizing for residual urine, be sure patient has voided first.
- Have tape available if a retention catheter is being inserted.
- Commonly used types of catheters
  1. French or Robinson: usually used in "in-and-out" catheterization.
  2. Foley: a two-lumen (one lumen is for a balloon), or three-lumen (the third lumen is for irrigant)—the most commonly used retention catheter.

3. Coude: a stiffer catheter with a curved tip. It is especially useful for relieving retention caused by an enlarged prostate because the tip rides over the prostate.

- Size in the French, Robinson, or Foley catheters
  1. The larger the number, the larger is the catheter.
  2. For women, usually sizes 14 to 16 are used.
  3. For men, usually sizes 16 to 18 are used, although some urologists recommend sizes 18 to 20 because the larger, blunter tip causes less damage to an enlarged prostate.
- Material: rubber, latex, 100% silicone, and silicone-coated latex
  1. The 100% silicone or silicone-coated latex catheter is preferred if it is to be retained for more than a week.

Nursing Considerations

Catheterization Procedure

- See hospital procedure book and/or directions included in the kit.
- Sterile technique is essential.
- Cut the tape, if it will be needed, before starting the procedure.
- For the female patient
  1. Side lying or lateral position makes the procedure technically simpler for the nurse and more comfortable for the patient.
  2. Before opening the sterile kit, put on unsterile gloves and find the landmarks: the urinary meatus, the clitoris, and the vagina (see Fig. 3-3). Be sure you can see the urinary meatus clearly.
  3. If the first catheter goes into the vagina, leave it there as a landmark. Insert the second catheter into the meatus.
- For the male patient
  1. Grasp the penis firmly (grasping it too lightly may stimulate an erection). With the patient's legs drawn up slightly, hold the penis at a 60° to 90° angle slightly toward the legs.
  2. Insert the well-lubricated catheter into the urinary meatus using scrupulous sterile technique. Slight resistance may be felt as the catheter passes the internal urethral sphincter. Use gentle constant pressure. *Never* force the catheter.
- Decompression of the bladder should be done slowly. The maximum amount of urine to be withdrawn at one time is 300 ml, unless the physician has stated otherwise. Allow another 300 ml to escape 15 minutes later. Continue in this fashion until the bladder is empty.

Indwelling or Retention Catheter

- Try to reduce the incidence of infection.
  1. Wash hands before touching catheter or any part of the urinary drainage system.

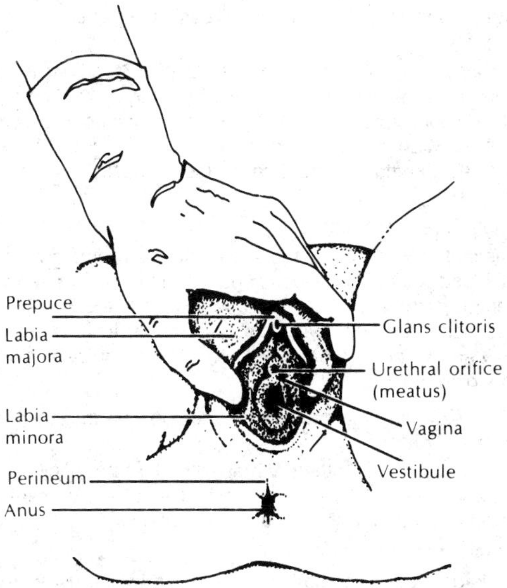

Fig. 3-3. *Female structures in the perineal area.*

2. Force fluids, unless otherwise contraindicated. Carefully monitor intake and output.
3. Never place a patient with a closed urinary drainage system in a room with another patient with any kind of infection. Try to avoid placing two patients with closed urinary drainage systems in the same room.
4. Catheter care varies from institution to institution. Check your agency's procedures.

   The meatus-catheter junction should be cleansed as part of daily hygiene.

   Do not pull on the catheter and expose a part of the catheter that will slip back into the urethra, thereby contaminating it.
5. When long-term indwelling catheter use is anticipated, ascorbic acid 1 g qd may be ordered to acidify the urine. Cranberry juice will acidify urine, but the amount needed to be effective (six to eight glasses per day) makes it impractical.
6. Some recent studies indicate that periodic instillation of hydrogen peroxide into the urinary drainage bag significantly decreases incidence of catheter-related urinary tract infections. If ordered, 3% hydrogen peroxide, 30 ml, is introduced into the bag, either through the outlet tube or through closed additive

sites found in some new bags, each time after it has been emptied.

7. Signs of urinary tract infections (UTI) in a patient include a burning sensation around the catheter, fever, chills, and cloudy, foul-smelling urine. If a UTI is suspected, the physician usually will order a specimen sent for culture and sensitivity before beginning treatment (see MSN, Urinary tract infections).

- Taping the retention catheter

1. The catheter should be taped so that it has some give, will not pull, and will not be directly against the skin. This can be accomplished by running the tape around the catheter before applying it to skin. Physicians' preferences vary somewhat on how and whether to tape. Inquire. General guidelines include the following:

   Female patient: the catheter is taped against the inner aspect on the thigh.

   Male patient: the catheter is taped so that the penis rests on the abdomen or laterally, preventing fistula development or abscess formation at the penal scrotal angle (Fig. 3-4).

- Leaking around the catheter

1. Leakage around the catheter is caused by the use of a catheter that is too small, by inadequate inflation of the balloon, or by bladder spasms, usually following surgery of the prostate (See MSN, Prostate enlargement).
2. Balloon sizes vary: They usually hold between 5 ml and 30 ml water. Most standard Foley kits contain catheters with 10-ml

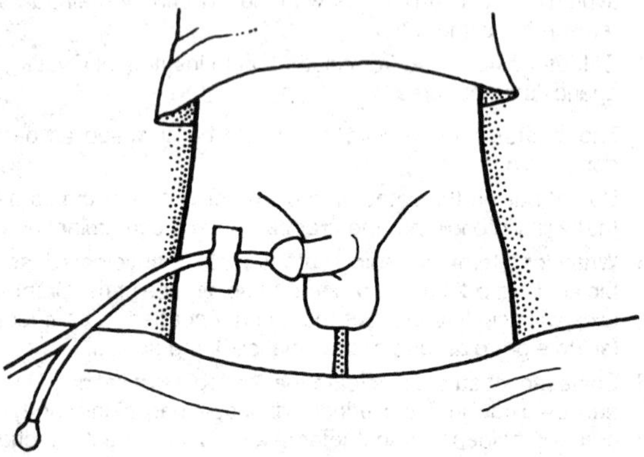

Fig. 3-4. *Method of taping catheter in a male patient.*

balloons. Larger balloon sizes may be ordered by the physician.

3. Check the balloon by withdrawing water from it through its port with a syringe. Refill with sterile water to its ordered capacity. If leakage continues, the physician may order a balloon with increased capacity.

- Any problem with a retention catheter inserted during genitourinary surgery should be reported to the physician.
  1. The catheter should never be removed or manipulated without a physician's order.
- Urinary drainage bags: receive urine in a closed system; usually attach to bedside or chair. Smaller "leg" bags may attach to an ambulating patient's leg.
  1. Wash hands before touching catheter or urinary drainage system.
  2. Never lift the bag above the level of the bladder. Avoid reflux (the backward flow of urine from the system into the bladder). Teach the patient to carry the bag below the level of the bladder when walking, and instruct him or her not to lay it on the floor while sitting.
  3. Keep the bag on the side to which the patient is turned. Avoid occluding the tubing by preventing kinks in it and by positioning the patient so he or she is not lying on the tubing.
  4. A urine meter, as part of the drainage system, makes accurate hourly measurement of urinary output possible.
  5. Empty the bag at least every eight hours, and record output. Wash your hands. Keep the emptying tube clean and away from the side of the graduate into which urine is being emptied. Use a separate, labeled disposable graduate for each patient. Wipe the tip with alcohol before reinserting it into its holder.
  6. Check and follow agency procedure as to when bags are to be changed. If there is white sediment in a bag, or if the tubing feels sandy when rubbed between fingers, it is time to ask. Always use a new bag and tubing when a catheter is changed.
- Collection of specimens from closed urinary drainage systems
  1. Never violate the integrity of a closed system by disconnecting the catheter from the tubing to collect a specimen.
  2. Avoid clamping tubing for specimen collection. Let urine collect in the tube as it lies on the bed.
  3. Sponge the trap of the area between balloon arm and connecting tube on a rubber catheter with an alcohol wipe. (Silicone and plastic catheters are not self-sealing, so the trap is the only place where urine can be withdrawn.)
  4. Withdraw the amount of urine needed with a sterile needle and syringe. In many hospitals, if the specimen is for culture, it is

sent to the laboratory in the syringe in which it was collected, with the needle covered. Chances of contaminating it by putting it into another container are thus avoided.

a. If a urine specimen is to be put into a container, remove the needle, thus avoiding damage to cells and casts that may breakdown if forced through the needle.

- Removal of the indwelling catheter
  1. Remove water from the balloon through its port with a syringe (do not cut the end), and gently withdraw catheter.
  2. Encourage fluid intake, if not otherwise contraindicated.
  3. Accurately measure and record intake and output.
  4. Encourage ambulation (if allowed) to reinstate normal voiding patterns.
  5. Record the amount of urine in a patient's first voiding after catheter removal. Note position of the bladder. Some patients void but incompletely empty the bladder (retention). If a patient has not voided or shows evidence of a distended bladder six hours (or at a time specified by the physician) after the catheter's removal, notify the physician.

CONTINUOUS BLADDER IRRIGATION

Description

Continuous bladder irrigation may be ordered following surgery of the prostate or bladder to reduce clot formation and to prevent obstruction. Its use to prevent multiplication of bacteria in a closed urinary drainage system is now under question. A three-way catheter (one lumen for drainage, one for inflation of the balloon, and one for the irrigating solution) is used. Antimicrobial solution (usually 1 ml Neosporin GU irrigant added to 1000 ml sterile, normal saline, intravenous solution) is delivered by intravenous tubing or special GU irrigant tubing at approximately 125 ml/hr, or at a rate specified by the physician.

Nursing Considerations

- Irrigating solution should be at room temperature, unless otherwise ordered. ("Iced" GU irrigant is sometimes ordered during heavy bleeding or clot formation.)
- Care of the catheter and the system is like that of any retention catheter and closed urinary drainage system (see Catheterization).
- Calculate the urinary output by subtracting the amount of irrigating solution that has gone in from the total amount in the drainage bag. Bags should be emptied, and output should be recorded at least every eight hours.

INTERMITTENT BLADDER IRRIGATION

Description

Intermittent bladder irrigation may be ordered to flush clots and to keep the catheter patent following GU surgery.

Nursing Considerations

- Aseptic technique is essential.
  1. Wash your hands and put on sterile gloves.
  2. Cleanse junction of catheter and tubing with povidone-iodine or 70% alcohol before disconnecting.
  3. Cover the end of the tubing with a sterile cap.
  4. Use a new sterile syringe for each irrigation.
  5. Use small bottles (200 ml to 500 ml) of irrigant so that it can be used in 24 hours. Refrigerate leftover solution between uses to reduce bacterial growth. Warm before using by placing bottle in warm water in a basin or sink.
- Insert 30 ml to 50 ml of irrigant into catheter at one time. Allow this to drain, or use gentle suction to aspirate. This procedure is usually done two or three times. If there is no return from the catheter, notify the physician immediately. Never use force to aspirate a catheter unless specifically ordered.
- Note character and color of aspirated bladder contents. Chart.

INTERMITTENT SELF-CATHETERIZATION

Description

Intermittent self-catheterization may be ordered for the patient who has had a spinal cord injury and has lost bladder control. This technique reduces the risk of urinary tract infection, and makes the patient more independent.

While in the hospital, sterile technique is required because of the danger of nosocomial infection. At home, clean technique can be used.

Nursing Considerations

- In the hospital, a sterile catheterization kit should be provided.
- Teach catheterization with sterile technique.
  1. Help the female patient locate her labia majora, labia minora, vagina, and meatus with a hand mirror. (After she becomes used to catheterizing herself, she will be able to do it without one.)

2. After catheterization, when the urine stops draining, have the patient press on the abdomen to be sure the bladder is empty. Then, the catheter should be pinched near the tip, to prevent urine leaking into the urethra as it is being slowly withdrawn.

- The patient *must* follow a regular schedule for self-catheterization.
- Modifications for clean technique (to be done at home) follow:
  1. Hand washing is essential. Area around the meatus may be washed with a clean washcloth, soap, and water. (Downward strokes are important in the female patient.)
  2. Following catheterization, wash the catheter in warm, soapy water. Rinse it well, inside and out, dry it with a clean towel, and put in a plastic storage bag for used catheters. Use each catheter only once.
  3. When the patient has used all but the last one or two clean catheters, the washed used catheters should be boiled for 20 minutes in a pan of water, drained, and stored in a covered pan or a freshly laundered towel.
  4. New catheters should be purchased when old ones become brittle.
- Patients should leave the hospital with instructions regarding catheterization schedule, required fluid intake, and prescribed medications.
  1. Some physicians want patients to keep accurate records of fluid intake and output.
  2. Urine should be checked for changes in amount, color, odor, clearness, particles, and blood.
  3. Dietary restrictions designed to prevent urinary calculi formation may be prescribed. These may include limits on calcium- and phosphorus-rich foods (*e.g.,* dairy products, organ meats, shellfish, cereals, beans, dried fruits, eggs, and dark green vegetables). (See MSN, Urinary calculi.)

SUPRAPUBIC CATHETERS

Description

Suprapubic catheters are inserted directly into the bladder through the abdomen about two inches above the symphysis, under strict aseptic technique. Several types of catheters may be used (*e.g.,* the dePezzer (mushroom), the Bonanno, and the Cystocath). Sutured into place, these catheters are started by siphonage, and they drain directly into closed systems. They are being used in a variety of gynecologic, bladder, and prostate surgeries because they are relatively infection free and pain free, and seem to promote earlier spontaneous voiding.

Nursing Considerations

- Distinguish between obstruction and bladder spasms the first postoperative day by checking hourly.
  1. Obstruction, indicated by decreased urinary output, distention, and tenderness, is dangerous and must be corrected immediately. The catheter must remain patent.
  2. Bladder spasms usually subside in 48 hours. They are painful, but do not affect urinary output, and may be relieved with Sitz bath or an antispasmodic agent (see PH).
- Continue to monitor the amount of urine flow and its character.
- Prevent undue tension on the catheter or tubing. Avoid kinks or other occlusion of the tubing.
- Protect skin around the catheter, apply antimicrobial ointment, and maintain a sterile, dry dressing.
- The physician may order intermittent clamping of the tubing to restore bladder tone and function while preparing patient for the removal of the catheter.

CENTRAL VENOUS PRESSURE MONITORING

Description

Central venous pressure (CVP) describes the pressure in the right atrium of the heart, which receives the venous blood returning from all parts of the body. This pressure is determined by the volume of blood, the condition of the heart muscle, and vascular tone. CVP is useful for monitoring the administration of fluid into the vascular system.

Starting and Maintaining the CVP Measurement

- The physician inserts an IV catheter through the basilic, subclavian, or internal jugular vein into the superior vena cava or right atrium. A chest X-ray is done to verify catheter placement. The catheter then is connected to IV tubing that has a manometer connected to it by way of a three-way stopcock. This IV tubing must be filled (primed) with fluid, usually D_5W, prior to connecting it to the catheter.
- The manometer must be taped on a pole in an upright position with the zero point on the manometer at the level of the right atrium. Mark this atrium location on the patient with a permanent ink mark at the midaxillary line. Check for proper alignment at every reading.
- A three-way stopcock, at the base of the manometer, allows IV fluid to flow to the patient, usually at a slow keep vein open (KVO)

rate (20 ml to 30 ml per hour), when readings are not being taken. This keeps the tubing patent (open).

- To obtain a reading, place the patient flat in bed. When this cannot be done, be certain that all readings are taken at the same head-of-bed elevation. These readings will not be as accurate as when the patient is flat in bed.
- Adjust the stopcock so that the IV fluid fills the manometer to about the 20-cm level; then the stopcock is opened to the patient. The fluid level will fluctuate with respirations. A lack of fluctuation indicates a kink or a clot in the tubing. Read the fluid level in the manometer where the meniscus stabilizes. This is the CVP reading.
- Return the stopcock to resume KVO IV to the patient.
- A CVP reading ranges between 5 cm to 12 cm H_2O in adults, 3 cm to 10 cm H_2O in children. Changes in the reading are more important than a one-time value. To establish values for a patient, begin taking CVP readings every 15 minutes for one hour, and then as often as ordered.
- A significant decrease in pressure may indicate hypovolemia; an increased pressure may indicate hypervolemia or right ventricular failure. The changes indicate blood volume, fluid replacement needed, and the effect on the heart muscle of cardiac drugs.

Nursing Considerations

- False CVP readings may be caused by a misplaced venous catheter, use of intermittent positive pressure breathing (IPPB) or respirators (these must be momentarily disconnected while the CVP is read), or a kink in the tubing.
- Hourly urine outputs are recorded when a CVP is being monitored.
- Sepsis is always a risk with IV catheters. IV tubing and dressing must be changed with strict aseptic technique every 48 hours. Check each individual institution's policy.
- Establish with the physician the CVP reading changes that will necessitate his attention.

CHEST TUBE DRAINAGE (THORACIC DRAINAGE)

Description

Drainage of air and fluid from the pleural cavity is accomplished by gravity flow or aided by suction. A water-seal bottle system or disposable plastic unit (*e.g.*, Pleur-evac) is used to collect air and fluid. Either system must be kept 2 to 3 feet below the patient's chest. The mattress may be kept at the elevated position to ensure that the 2- to 3-feet difference between the patient and the collection unit is maintained. Bottles should be in a rack or taped to the floor. The plastic unit, Pleur-evac, hangs from the bedframe at the patient's feet. All connections within any system should be taped to avoid air leakage. These drainage systems rely on a seal that acts as a one-way valve to prevent the evacuated air and fluid from flowing back into the pleural space. Commonly used systems have a water seal, and the fluid in the water seal tube will normally fluctuate approximately 6 cm between inspiration and expiration, but excessive bubbling in the water seal indicates a leak in the system. An obstructed chest tube may stop the fluctuation. These water-seal systems have an opening to the atmosphere to either vent evacuated air or to allow automatic control of the amount of suction. *Do not obstruct this opening.*

ONE-BOTTLE WATER-SEAL GRAVITY DRAINAGE

Drainage is collected and air expelled using just the one container. See Figure 3-5(*A*). Evacuated air is released into the atmosphere through an air vent. The end of the glass tube connected with the patient must always be submerged 1 inch to 2 inches into sterile water or saline to produce a water seal. This allows air and fluid to leave the pleural space, but makes it impossible for outside air and fluid to reenter. Mark the level of sterile fluid before drainage enters for accurate I–O monitoring. As the fluid level rises from the accumulating drainage, the glass tube needs to be raised so that it continues to be submerged 1 inch to 2 inches, thereby maintaining a low pressure that the drainage must overcome. This is the principal disadvantage of a one-bottle system. Remember, the end of the glass tube must always be 1 inch to 2 inches below the fluid level.

TWO-BOTTLE WATER-SEAL GRAVITY DRAINAGE

In a two-bottle water-seal system, drainage collection and water seal are in two separate bottles. They are connected as shown in Figure 3-5(*B*). The water seal is independent from the drainage collection, which provides an advantage over a one-bottle system.

SUCTION WITH WATER-SEAL DRAINAGE

Suction creates negative pressure within the closed system. See Figure 3-5(*C*). This negative pressure sucks air and fluid from the pleural space faster than the gravity drainage system. In addition to a 1- or 2- bottle drainage and water-seal system as described earlier, this suction method includes another bottle for suction control. The former air vent opening on the gravity system water-seal bottle is attached as shown in the figure to the suction bottle. The long glass tube in the suction bottle is the suction control tube. The upper end must always be kept open to atmospheric air. The depth that the tube is submerged beneath the fluid level establishes the suction

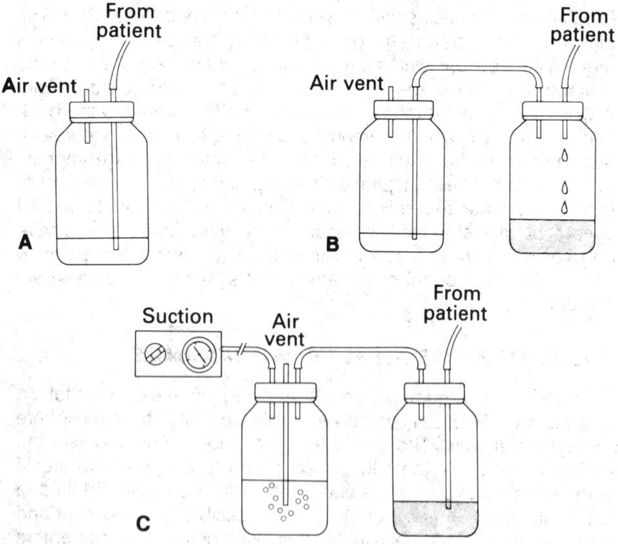

Fig. 3-5. *Types of water seal drainage: (A) 1-bottle water seal gravity drainage; (B) 2-bottle water seal gravity drainage without suction; (C) suction with water seal drainage, 2 bottles.*

pressure, which is always ordered by the physician as "10, 15, or 20 cm H_2O." It is prudent to mark the fluid level at the beginning of suction and then check hourly that the tube remains submerged the proper number of centimeters. There will be continuous bubbling in a suction control bottle since this is what maintains the desired amount of suction. The other bottles function the same as described earlier for the gravity system.

Nursing Considerations

- Frequent coughing and deep breathing are painful but necessary to prevent respiratory complications.
- Remember, continuous, as contrasted to intermittent, bubbling in the water-seal bottle in either gravity or suction sets probably indicates an air leak. Check all connections starting at the chest catheter site. This air leak must be stopped because air is entering the system and the pleural cavity. Notify the physician if an air leak cannot be stopped.
- When you receive a report on a patient with a chest tube, find out how much and where bubbling is occurring.

- Two large clamps should be kept taped to the head of the bed of any patient with chest tubes. They are to be used only in an emergency situation to prevent outside air from entering the pleural space. They are clamped as close to the chest as possible, *never* covered up, and clamped for as short a period of time as possible. The danger of clamped chest tubes is that trapped air in the pleural space will cause a tension pneumothorax. Sudden chest pain, dyspnea tachycardia, cyanosis, and chest pain are indicative of a pneumothorax.
- Vertical loops of chest tubing hanging from the mattress or kinks in chest tubing defeat gravity drainage. Coil any loops of tubing horizontally on the mattress, but *never pin* directly on the tubing. A kink or pressure on suction tubing lessens the suction.
- Chest tubes with draining fluid may develop clots. These tubes must be "milked" every hour for the first 24 hours and then every four hours. This may be uncomfortable for the patient. Stabilize the tube at the chest insertion site with one hand and gently squeeze down the tube with the other hand. Move hands, as necessary, all the way to the drainage collection unit.
- The drainage from chest tubes will be bloody at first, gradually changing to serosanguineous. Mark the level of drainage each hour for the first 24 hours and then every four hours. If there is more than 200 ml per hour the surgeon must be notified.
- Following a pneumonectomy there may be a chest tube, but it is never on suction.
- A plastic disposable unit (*e.g.*, Pleur-evac), duplicates in one unit a three-bottle system. The same principles apply regarding keeping the Pleur-evac 2 feet to 3 feet below the patient's chest. Read the manufacturer's directions carefully.
- When starting suction, increase it until steady bubbling appears in the suction bottle or chamber. Do not increase suction beyond this point since proper operation is established when steady bubbling occurs.
- Always keep a spare bottle set or Pleur-evac ready for replacement usage when either is in use.
- The removal of chest tubes is very painful; medicate the patient for pain at least 30 minutes before this is done. During the removal, the patient must perform the Valsalva maneuver of holding her breath and bearing down.

CRUTCH MEASUREMENT

Nursing Considerations

- When measuring for crutches, make sure the rubber tips are on the crutches.

- With the patient standing, measure 2 inches from the axillary fold to a position on the floor 4 inches in front of the patient and 6 inches to the side of his toes. (There should be two finger widths between the axillary fold and the arm piece.)
- With the patient lying down, measure from the anterior fold of the axilla to the sole of the foot, and add 2 inches.
- The location of the handgrip should allow 20° to 30° flexion of the elbow.

CT SCAN (COMPUTED TOMOGRAPHY)

Description

The x-ray CT scanner was initially developed in 1973 for noninvasive examination of the brain. It was so successful that present-day scanners are designed to examine any portion of the body. CT scans (also referred to as CAT scans) require that the patient remain completely immobile while x-ray pictures are taken sequentially by the x-ray mechanism from different angles around the body. As many as 180 x-ray pictures, each at a different angle, may be used. A mathematical technique, using a computer program, compares and combines the density of small parts (called pixels) of each x-ray film. The resulting composite pictures, produced by mathematically analyzing some 30,000 pixels, reveal the internal organs and structures in cross sections, or tomographs. These tomographs have sufficient detail to show abnormalities that would not be apparent from the individual x-rays. In some cases, a contrast material is injected that selectively increases the x-ray density of body structures or organs so as to obtain even more detail in the tomograph. Because of the x-ray technique used in CT scans, the body effectively receives no more radiation than when it is exposed to the more classical x-ray studies. CT scans are replacing many of the invasive studies (*e.g.*, pneumoencephalograms, cerebral angiograms, and myelograms). Also, CT scan is now the preferred procedure in traumatic head injuries, because of the speed and definitiveness of the resulting tomography. It is also the only diagnostic test that demonstrates cerebral edema. Tomographs of other parts of the body are becoming more common, and are now capable of supplanting some exploratory surgery using needle biopsy technique to obtain tissue samples.

Nursing Considerations

- Always schedule CT scans before barium studies of organs.
- A contrast substance may be given to enhance visualization; therefore check for allergy to seafood or iodine. Biopsies are also sometimes done. Therefore, patients are asked to sign an informed consent when the procedure is explained to them.

- CT scans may be done with or without a contrast substance given orally, rectally, or intravenously (IV). Contrast usually is given for scans involving the abdominal organs to improve visualization of highly vascular organs.
- Patients should know that with the IV injection they may experience, momentarily, a flushed face and have a strange taste in their mouth. Also, the hypertonic contrast agent can act as a diuretic, with the amount of urine increased for several hours.
- Children may require sedation because it is necessary to remain motionless for as long as 30 minutes.

DEEP BREATHING TECHNIQUES

Abdominal breathing may be taught by having the patient place one hand on the chest and one on the abdomen to determine proper abdominal movement. When breathing is done correctly, the abdomen moves, while the chest remains immobile. The most complete lung expansion occurs when arms are placed above the head. This technique is especially useful for the patient with chronic obstructive pulmonary disease (COPD). (See MSN, Chronic obstructive pulmonary disease.)

Incentive spirometers are especially useful in promoting deep breathing because they enable the patient to actually see and measure the effectiveness of deep-breathing efforts. Directions for the use of incentive spirometers usually come with the product and vary slightly according to manufacturer.

Intermittent positive pressure breathing (IPPB) is administered by the respiratory therapy department. (The usefulness of IPPB is currently being questioned; some evidence links the treatment to spread of infection through the equipment.)

Sustained maximal inspiration (SMI) is essentially a yawn technique. The patient is instructed to draw in one or more slow, deep breaths in succession before exhaling.

Forced expiration (coughing) should only be done when the incision is splinted either with a pillow or with both hands. Increasingly it is being encouraged only if secretions are auscultated in the chest.

Cooperation in deep-breathing efforts postoperatively is improved if nursing care can be planned so that the patient will have been medicated for pain a few minutes before deep breathing is attempted.

DIALYSIS

Description

Renal dialysis is used to perform the functions of normal kidneys in cases of acute or chronic kidney failure. This includes correction of electrolyte and acid-base abnormalities, removal of toxic substances, and the removal of excessive body fluid when diuretics are not effective. The process of dialysis involves osmosis, filtration, and diffusion of solutions across a semipermeable membrane. In peritoneal dialysis the prescribed dialysate solution is infused into the peritoneal cavity through a catheter. The peritoneal membrane serves as the semipermeable membrane between blood vessels and the dialysate. When the dialysate is drained, it contains waste products normally excreted by the kidneys. Hemodialysis circulates the patient's blood through a machine in which the blood and dialysate are separated by a synthetic semipermeable membrane, which allows transfer between blood and dialysate. In both peritoneal and hemodialysis the objective is the same; however, hemodialysis is faster in achieving fluid or chemical correction. Both types of dialysis may be performed in the home by carefully selected patients.

HEMODIALYSIS

- Hemodialysis is a procedure carried out in special units or, in some cases, at home. It usually takes from four hours to six hours, repeated as indicated by the patient's condition. Patients receiving this treatment may enter the hospital for other reasons. Their artificial access to the circulatory system requires special attention.
- Direct access to the circulatory system is usually obtained by an internal fistula or by an arteriovenous shunt with a cannula connection brought out to the skin surface. (See Fig. 3-6.) In either case, do not take a blood pressure reading, start an IV, or draw

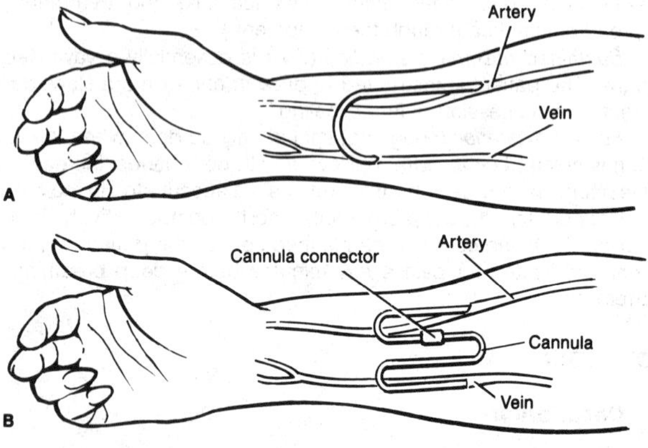

Fig. 3-6. *(A) An internal fistula is formed by joining an artery to an adjacent vein. The "arterialized" vein will gradually enlarge and thicken allowing repeated veinpunctures. (B) A shunt (cannula) between an artery and an adjacent vein provides permanent external access to a dialysis machine by means of a connector that may be opened and attached to the machine.*

blood from an involved extremity.

- An internal fistula can be created by anastomosing a vein to an artery in either a leg or, preferably, an arm. It takes several weeks before the vein enlarges. Vein puncture is necessary for each dialysis treatment. A fistula lasts longer and is less susceptible to infection and clotting than the external shunt. Report any redness or tenderness over the fistula site, absence of a bruit, or ischemia distal to the fistula. A bruit is the turbulence of arterial blood heard with a stethoscope over the fistula.
- The cannulas of an arteriovenous shunt are connected by a plastic bridge when not attached to the kidney machine. Vein puncture is not necessary for each dialysis. There is, however, the possibility of infection on the skin site and the danger of hemorrhage if the cannulas are accidentally disconnected, and clotting may occur in the cannulas. The shunt site usually has to be changed every few months.
- Observe for clotting in the cannula immediately following its insertion. Report the absence of a bruit, a sudden change from bright red blood to dark-colored blood in the cannula, or a cannula that becomes cold to the touch.
- Daily site care around the cannula is necessary using strict aseptic technique. Any sign of a wound infection requires immediate treatment.
- Two clamps should *always* be kept wrapped in the exterior covering over the shunt site in case of the separation of the cannula. A blood pressure cuff positioned above the site and inflated to greater than systolic pressure can be used as an emergency tourniquet.
- Patients on hemodialysis have an increased incidence of hepatitis B because of blood contamination; those caring for these patients are at a high risk of acquiring the disease.
- Coordinate nursing care plans with the dialysis nurse, dietitian, and other personnel involved in the patient's care.

Nursing Considerations

- Accurate daily weights taken before and after dialysis, or at the same time each day when not receiving dialysis, are necessary in planning and evaluating the treatment.
- Intake and output records must include *all* oral and parenteral fluids, as well as any form of output, including stools and emesis.
- Patients on dialysis have a lowered resistance to infection.
- There is an increased bleeding tendency because of the heparinization of blood during hemodialysis.
- Urine should be checked regularly for glucose levels during peritoneal dialysis. Hyperglycemia can result from absorption of glucose in the dialysate.

- Blood tests are done routinely for serum electrolytes, creatinine, BUN, phosphorous, calcium, and glucose, as well as for partial thromboplastin time (PTT), hemoglobin, and hematocrit (HCT). It is very important that the blood be taken when ordered and that blood samples be labeled "before" or "after" dialysis.
- The diets of these patients are individualized depending on serum chemistry and whether peritoneal dialysis or hemodialysis is used. Close cooperation with the dietitian is essential. Serum potassium and sodium are retained in renal failure, so their intake needs to be restricted; serum phosphorous levels usually are high, while serum calcium levels are low. The fluid intake allowed is determined daily according to urine output.
- In renal failure the patient's kidneys are not a route for excretion of drugs. Know the reason for administration as well as the action and side effects of each medication given. Be certain that any medication ordered is approved by the nephrologist. Also, understand when each medication is to be given, pre- or postdialysis.

PERITONEAL DIALYSIS

- Explain the procedure to the patient and have the appropriate permit signed. The patient must void or be catheterized to prevent accidental perforation of the bladder. Also, a baseline weight, vital signs, and central venous pressure (if ordered) are taken.
- Using aseptic technique, the physician inserts a catheter into the peritoneal cavity, which is then sutured in place. A sterile dressing is applied, which must be kept dry and is changed as necessary.
- The prescribed container of dialysate is warmed to body temperature and is connected to administration tubing. This tubing is flushed to prevent air from entering the peritoneal cavity, and is then connected to the peritoneal catheter. Heparin is added to the dialysate to keep any fibrin from clotting in the tubing.
- The physician will order the type and amount of dialysate to be infused and the schedule to be followed. The irrigation schedule, also called the exchange cycle, is divided into inflow, dwell, and outflow time. These times are periods allowed for the dialysate to run into the peritoneum, dwell there, and then drain into a collection container. Usually, two liters are used for each exchange cycle in an adult; this procedure takes about one hour. In children, the amount of dialysate is determined by body weight. The exchange cycle is repeated continuously until the necessary clinical response is achieved. Peritoneal dialysis can be continuous, lasting from 6 hours to 48 hours. It may also be done at home by

chronic renal patients with an extended dwell time allowing for sleep.

- Meticulous aseptic technique is absolutely necessary throughout the entire peritoneal dialysis procedure. Peritonitis is the most common complication. Culturing drainage is done frequently or when there is any indication of infection. Also, the patient's temperature should be taken every four hours.
- Frequent assessments of the abdominal catheter site are necessary to check for signs of redness or leakage. When cared for with proper aseptic technique, a catheter can remain in place indefinitely.
- The initial exchange drainage fluid may be blood tinged as a result of the catheter insertion. It should then clear and be straw colored. Any variation must be reported immediately to the physician.
- Stop dialysis and notify the physician if dyspnea occurs during dialysis. A sudden severe diarrhea or sudden increase in urine volume in the first cycle may indicate a bowel or bladder perforation.
- Keep a continuing record of each exchange at the bedside. Repositioning the patient may help if all of the fluid does not drain at the end of an exchange cycle. If fluid continues to be retained after two or three exchanges, report this to the physician.
- Vital signs and lung assessment are important in assessing the patient for symptoms of overhydration or for shock resulting from fluid loss. Take the blood pressure and pulse every 15 minutes during the first exchange cycle and then between each cycle. Hypotension may follow a rapid loss of a large amount of fluid. Do not place the patient in the Trendelenburg position when fluid is still in the abdomen. Respiratory distress can result because of compression of the thoracic cavity; the fluid also will press on the inferior vena cava and decrease the blood supply to the heart.
- Be aware of the possibility of changes in neurological status resulting from metabolic imbalances.
- The possibility of skin breakdown is increased with long periods of immobility and altered tissue nutrition.

ELECTROCARDIOGRAM (ECG) LEADS AND HOW TO PLACE THEM

Description

A standard 12-lead ECG (also called EKG) includes six limb leads and six chest leads. The six limb leads are obtained from only four limb electrode placements. The electrodes are applied to the right and left arms and right and left legs. (See Fig. 3-7.)

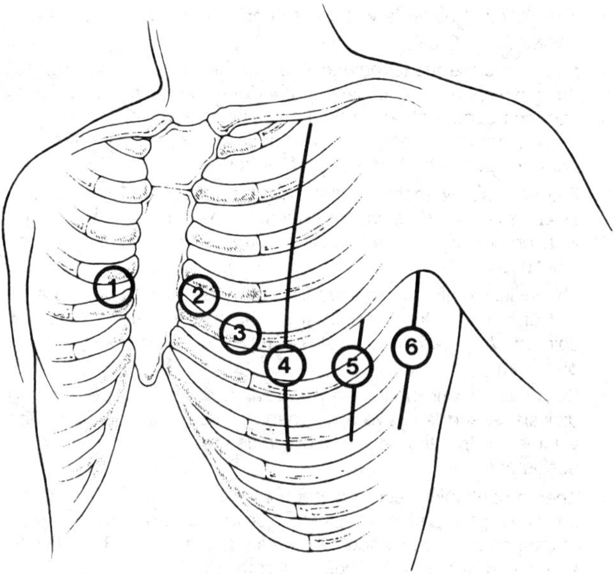

Fig. 3-7. *Standard positions for "C" (also called "V") chest leads: (1) 4th intercostal space to right of sternum; (2) 4th intercostal space to left of sternum; (3) midway between V_2 and V_4; (4) 5th intercostal space midclavicular line; (5) 5th intercostal space between V_4 and V_6; (6) 5th intercostal space midaxillary line.*

Procedure

- Tell the patient you are preparing for an ECG. Also, state that the attached wires do not conduct electricity to the body. If possible, keep the bed flat.
- Emphasize the importance of not moving during this procedure, since movement interferes with the electrical signals being measured.
- The limb electrodes are metal and are attached with wide rubber bands to the patient's extremities. A saline pad or electrode gel should be placed between the patient's skin and the electrode.
- Place the electrodes on the insides of the forearms and ankles. If these areas are unavailable, any area on an extremity may be used. The cables that connect the electrodes to the machine are color-coded on the plug ends that insert into the electrodes. They are marked as follows:

  RA (right arm) with white letters

  LA (left arm) with black letters

RL (right leg) with green letters
LL (left leg) with red letters

- The cable–electrode connection should be tight. Twisting or bending of the cable should be avoided.

ELECTROENCEPHALOGRAM (EEG)

Description

An electroencephalogram (EEG) is a recording on paper of electrical activity within the brain. It is diagnostic for seizure disorders and brain death, and also may indicate changes related to other brain abnormalities.

NR

Nursing Considerations

- The diet should contain no caffeine for the 24 hours preceding the test. The physician may decide to withhold medications during this period. If not, the technician should be informed of the medications that have been taken by the patient.
- Patients being evaluated for seizure disorders should be sleep deprived, and the EEG obtained during sleep. Sedation may be given to achieve sleep. Some abnormal brain waves are only present during sleep.
- It is important that the patient know that there will be no electric shock. The electrodes attached to the head are for recording electrical activity within the brain. It is possible to insert the electrodes through the nose to the nasopharynx to better record activity in the temporal lobe of the brain. Find out if this is to be done, so that the patient can be informed.
- The procedure takes one hour or longer if a sleep study is done.
- The conduction paste used on the head should be either shampooed out or removed with nail polish remover as soon as possible after the EEG is done.

ENDOSCOPIC PROCEDURES

Description

Endoscopic procedures refer to the viewing of hollow organs or body cavities with a tubular metal instrument having a light source. Flexible fiberoptic endoscopy (FFE) describes a technique using special plastic-coated scopes that are very maneuverable and have excellent optics. They contain bundles of light fibers that conduct light to an area, and other bundles that send magnified images back to the viewer, a camera, or a TV screen. There are channels in the scope for insertion of a variety of instruments. Some of these instruments are grasping devices, biopsy forceps, and electrocautery tools. There are also air, water, and suction channels. Malfunction and disease may be seen clearly and special procedures performed with these scopes.

Diagnostic Tests

- Bronchoscopy provides a visual examination of the lungs and permits a biopsy. FFE allows a more complete viewing of the respiratory tree, compared to the inflexible metal bronchoscope.
- Proctoscopy or sigmoidoscopy provides a visual examination of the sigmoid or lower colon and also permits a biopsy.
- Colonoscopy, using FFE, may be used to view as far as the sigmoid or all the way to the cecum. Polyps frequently are removed this way.
- Cystoscopy provides a visual examination of the bladder and permits a biopsy.
- Mediastinoscopy provides a visual examination of organs and lymph nodes in the mediastinum, and permits a biopsy. The instrument is inserted through a small suprasternal incision. A mediastinotomy is a similar procedure; the incision is done on either side of the sternum.
- Peritonoscopy/laparoscopy is essentially useful in viewing the anterior surface of the liver and gallbladder and for obtaining a biopsy. The instrument is inserted through a small incision in the abdomen.
- Panendoscopy (or EGD), using FFE, permits the viewing of the esophagus, stomach, and duodenum where ulcers, tumors, hiatal hernia, esophageal varices, and origins of bleeding may be seen. Biopsies often are done.
- Endoscopic retrograde cannulation of the papilla of Vater (ERCP) is done with a special side-viewing FFE instrument. It is passed down into the duodenum. A small catheter is then passed in the scope, through the papilla of Vater and into the opening of the pancreatic duct, and positioned in the common bile duct. A contrast material is ejected to enable fluoroscopic viewing of the pancreatic duct or biliary tree. If stones are seen, an electrocauterizing wire may be introduced to open the sphincter of Vater, and the stones withdrawn using a basket adaptor.
- Arthroscopy is used to view the interior surface of a joint, but most commonly to look at the knee. This procedure permits diagnostic and surgical procedures (*e.g.,* biopsy and removal of loose bodies).
- The nasopharyngolaryngoscope has greatly improved viewing of the ear, nose, nasopharynx, and larynx.

Nursing Considerations

- Endoscopic procedures must be fully discussed with the patient by the physician and a signed permit obtained. Informed consent forms include the explanation of the possibility of complications. These are rare, but include perforation, bleeding after biopsies, or mucosal irritation. If there is a possibility of a polypectomy, or stone removal, this should be included on the consent form.
- Always find out if the patient is taking aspirin products or an anticoagulant.
- Frequently a PT, PTT, and type and cross-match are done beforehand (see Lab).
- In lieu of special orders the evening before, keep the patient NPO after midnight of the day of the examination.
- An IV often is started beforehand to allow immediate vein access in case medication is needed after the procedure is started.
- Laxatives and enemas are given in preparation for bowel examination. It is usually a two-day preparation.
- When a scope is introduced through the mouth, the throat is anesthetized. Nothing by mouth is allowed afterward until the gag reflex has returned, usually in about 2 hours. A sore throat lasts a day or two.
- In order to permit better viewing, carbon dioxide or air is insufflated into the bowel during a colonoscopy, causing spasm-like pains. This is also done in the abdomen when peritonoscopy/laparoscopy is performed, and abdominal distention and cramping may result.
- The incisions for a mediastinoscopy or peritonoscopy/laparoscopy are often covered with only a Band-Aid. However, the complications following these procedures may be extremely serious. These patients should be monitored closely following these procedures. Subcutaneous emphysema, pneumothorax, or recurrent laryngeal nerve injury may follow a mediastinoscopy; peritonitis and abdominal bleeding are complications of peritonoscopy/laparoscopy.
- It is imperative that the nurse know when the patient returns to the floor whether or not an operative procedure such as a liver biopsy or polypectomy was done in order to be alert to possible complications. The patient needs to know of any limitations to activity following any procedure.

EXTERNAL FIXATION DEVICES

Description

An external fixation device provides for reduction and immobilization of complex fractures, especially open fractures with extensive soft tissue trauma. Transfixing pins inserted percutaneously through bone are attached to an external metal frame (Fig. 3-8). It may be used for upper or lower extremities or for the pelvis in fractures that will not hold position with conservative treatment (*e.g.*, casts, cast bracing, or traction). (See NR sections on Casts, Cast Brace, Traction.)

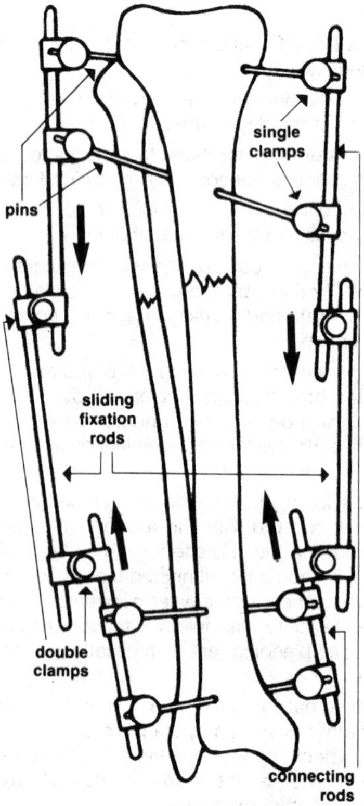

Fig. 3-8. *External fixation site. Pins inserted through the bone proximal and distal to the fracture site are connected in pairs with metal rods and clamps. Adjustable sliding fixation rods join the pins and, as they tighten, pull the pins toward each other (see arrows). The resulting pressure holds the pieces of bone in proper alignment.* (Meredith S: Formidable—that's the only word for the external fixation device—and the care it demands. RN December 1979. Courtesy Lou Bory Assoc.)

Nursing Considerations

- Elevate affected body part postoperatively. Support foot to prevent foot drop.
- Watch for signs of neurovascular impairment, pallor, pulselessness, pain, paralysis, or paresthesia (tingling or numbness).
- Until the patient is able to move the extremity by himself, move it by grasping the frame of the fixator, not by grasping the limb itself.
- Wound and pin-site care require meticulous aseptic technique—great care is required to avoid cross contamination between them.
- Protocols for pin care vary, so check your physician's orders or hospital's policy. A commonly accepted one includes the following:
  1. Inspect pin sites for tension or motion at the site (believed to increase possibility of infection), and for signs of infection (*e.g.*, redness, swelling, tenderness, or drainage).
  2. Cleanse each pin site, removing crusts (if in the protocol), two or three times a day at first. (Later, cleansing once a day may be sufficient.)

     Using a separate sterile applicator for each pin site, cleanse with hydrogen peroxide solution.

     Rinse with sterile normal saline.

     If ordered, apply nonocclusive antibacterial agent (*e.g.*, Neosporin ointment) with sterile applicator. (Use of povidone-iodine is discouraged because it tends to corrode the metal.)
- If pin loosening occurs, notify the physician.
- Cleanse fixator daily with alcohol wipes.
- Encourage self-care of pin sites and fixator.
- Active motion of adjacent joints usually is begun after the initial swelling has gone down, through an exercise program developed by a physiotherapist. Early weight bearing usually is not allowed.
- Care for soft-tissue wounds, if present. (See MSN, Open fracture)

GASTROINTESTINAL INTUBATION

Description

Intubation of the stomach or intestine is done for the following reasons:

- To empty or decompress, by removing gas and stomach or intestinal contents by suction (done especially in cases of bowel obstruction)

- To diagnose certain conditions by analysis of aspirated material
- To wash out the stomach (lavage) following ingestion of poisonous substances, or to constrict blood vessels in the stomach lining in cases of gastrointestinal bleeding (iced lavage)
- To provide nutrition by gavage (enteral feeding) for the patient who is unable to take food by mouth

The tube is usually passed through the nose in an adult, but it may be introduced by mouth—and is usually done in this way in infants.

Nasogastric, or *NG* (from nose to stomach), and *nasointestinal* or *nasoenteric* (from nose to intestine) are terms commonly used to describe these tubes. A *gastrostomy* tube is inserted directly into the stomach from an opening made in the abdominal wall; an *enterostomy* tube is inserted into the intestine; and an *esophagostomy* tube is inserted into the esophagus.

Equipment

- Short tubes are for placement in the stomach, and are usually about 127 cm (approximately 4 ft) long.

1. *Levin tube:* this is a single-lumen tube that comes in several sizes; 16 French (Fr) is used most commonly for adults, 6 Fr to 12 Fr for children, and 5 Fr for neonates. Low, intermittent suction is used when suction is required.

   Rubber Levin tubes should be chilled to stiffen them before insertion by putting the tubes in the refrigerator or a pan of chipped ice.

   Plastic Levin tubes do not require chilling.

2. *Gastric sump tube* (*e.g.,* Salem, Ventrol): this is a double-lumen tube (tube within a tube) with two ports, one for suction and the other a "pigtail" port to allow for the flow of air.

   Continuous low suction (30 mm Hg) is preferred. If unavailable, intermittent suction should be set at "high."

   The vent tube (pigtail) should give off a hissing sound. If it does not, or if fluid comes out of the vent, reposition the patient to reposition the port of the tube. Then—only with a physician's order—gently irrigate the vent tube with 10 ml normal saline followed by 10 cc to 20 cc of air.

   The vent lumen must be kept above the patient's midline (*i.e.,* pinned to gown on upper chest). The collection trap must be kept below the midline.

3. Newer, smaller, softer, more pliable tubes for NG feedings are available. The placement of these tubes usually is confirmed by x-ray before feedings are started.

Keofeed: this is a silicone tube weighted at the end. Sizes 7.3 Fr to 9.6 Fr are used most commonly. Most formulas will drip by gravity. Patient cooperation is required for insertion. Keofeed Tube Guide (made of gelatin) may aid in passing tube. In an average adult, the Keofeed tube is in the stomach at the 50-cm mark, in the small bowel, at the 75-cm mark.

Dobbhoff tube: this is made of polyurethane and weighted at the end.

Med Pro: this is a silicone tube enclosed in a stiff, outer polyvinyl chloride tube, which is withdrawn after the tube is passed. This tube is easier to pass in patients who are unable to cooperate. It usually requires a pump for continuous infusion.

Small Levin tube: this is a 6 Fr to 8 Fr tube.

NR

- Long tubes: these are used to decompress the bowel (usually 6-ft to 10-ft long).
  1. *Miller-Abbott:* a double-lumen tube is passed; then, the balloon is inflated with air, or partially filled with mercury, to facilitate passage of the tube through the pylorus into the small intestine. The suction lumen should be marked so that it can be differentiated.
  2. *Cantor:* this is a single-lumen tube with a small rubber bag at the distal end that is filled with mercury before insertion.
- *Gastrostomy tube:* a large rubber catheter (20 Fr to 22 Fr or Malecot) may be sewn into place in the stomach at first (enterostomy tube goes directly into intestine). After the wound has healed, the tube may be withdrawn and reinserted prn.
- *Sengstaken-Blakemore tube:* this tube is used for compression of bleeding esophageal varices.
- *Suction:* suction is used for decompression. It should also be available for the unconscious patient or one in danger of aspirating regurgitated enteral feeding.
  1. Wall suction: this is a suction device built into the wall at the patient's bedside.
  2. Portable suction machines (*e.g.,* Gomco) in most cases provide intermittent suction at "high" and "low" settings.
- A pump for volumetric or drop administration is required for some enteral formulas.
- For enteral feedings
  1. An administration set (manufactured or improvised), with an IV pole for continuous feeding
  2. A 50-ml syringe and a cup of water for intermittent feeding
  3. Formula containing balanced nutritional elements and electrolytes appropriate to patient's needs (*e.g.,* Isocal, Ensure Plus, Vivonex)

Nursing Considerations

- Check your agency's procedure book for step-by-step instructions regarding these procedures. The following are suggestions for how to make them work.
- Mark the level of fluid drainage in the container at the beginning of each shift.
- Serious electrolyte imbalances may occur with gastric suctioning if IV fluid replacement is not administered correctly. Be certain to maintain IV at ordered rate.

Inserting the Tube

- Place the patient in high Fowler's position, unless contraindicated, and maintain for at least one hour after feeding to prevent regurgitation and aspiration of stomach contents.
- In adults, measure distance between bridge of nose and earlobe plus distance from earlobe to top of xiphoid process, and mark tube with tape. This represents the approximate distance the tube should be inserted for placement in the stomach. In children, measure to a point between the xyphoid and the umbilicus.
- Choose the nostril with greatest air flow, unless you are changing the tubing (when you will use the other naris). When the tube is passed through the mouth (the last choice), the patient's dentures must be removed.
- Curve the end of the tube by curling it around your finger. Lubricate the tube with sterile water or lubricating gel. With the patient's head back against the pillow, insert the tube, trying to point the end downward toward the ear. Once the tube is past the back of the nasopharynx (where there may be slight resistance), pause; have the patient bring his head forward; rotate the tube 180° and advance it down the esophagus as the patient swallows sips of water or sucks in air through a straw.
- Using a flashlight, check the back of the throat to be sure that the tube is advancing correctly. Unusual discomfort or resistance during insertion may indicate that the tube is curled up in the back of the throat.
- Excessive coughing, cyanosis, and the patient's inability to talk during the insertion of the tube are signs that the tube has gone through the vocal cords and is in the trachea. Withdraw the tube.

Checking the Placement of the Tube in the Stomach

- Check the placement of the tube immediately upon insertion, before each intermittent gavage feeding, and at least every 4 hours when the patient is on continuous enteral feeding.
  1. Inject 10 cc of air while auscultating over the stomach. If tube placement is correct, you will hear a "swoosh" sound.

2. Aspirate stomach contents. If nothing is aspirated and there are no other signs that suggest that the tube is in the respiratory tree, advance the tube a little and attempt to aspirate again. Some fluid should be returned.

Taping the Tube

- Never tape the tube to the forehead. Pressure on the naris can cause tissue necrosis. Use hypoallergenic tape to secure the tube as shown in Figure 3–9. Attach the end of the tube (if it is free) to the patient's gown with a rubber band and a safety pin.
- Long tubes used for intestinal decompression are never taped while they are being advanced.
- Tubes are seldom left in place in infants. They are reinserted through the mouth for each feeding.

Gastric Analysis

- Specimens are taken of stomach contents. This procedure is prescribed by the physician, depending upon diagnostic needs.

Lavage

- To wash out the stomach, fluid (usually water or normal saline) is repeatedly introduced and aspirated.
- Iced lavages are used to remove clots and to reduce and stop gastric bleeding by constricting blood vessels of the stomach by chilling.

1. The physician will order the specifics.
2. A gastric tube will be passed into the stomach.

   Large tubes (36 Fr to 40 Fr) will be passed orally. (A smaller tube would become occluded with clots.)

   A double-lumen gastric tube provides for more rapid continuous lavage. Iced solution is fed through a smaller tube; suction is attached to the larger port. A bag within a bag (one for ice and one for solution) may be used for delivery of iced solution.
3. If a single-lumen gastric tube is used, instill at least 200 ml of cold solution (iced saline or water), and allow it to remain in the stomach for one to two minutes; then aspirate.
4. Manual irrigation will remove clots more effectively than intermittent suction. Note and record the amount, color, and consistency of aspirated fluid.
5. Monitor patient's vital signs.
6. Keep patient warm during the procedure.

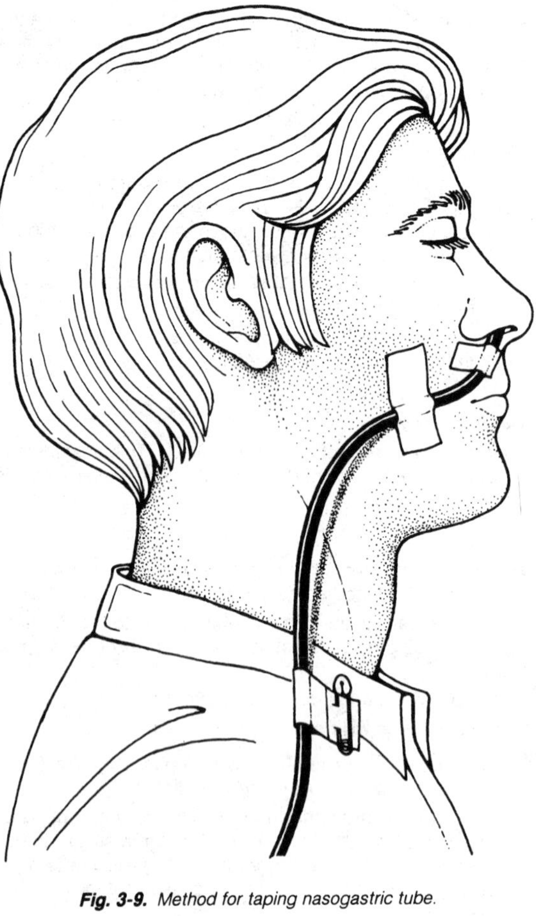

Fig. 3-9. *Method for taping nasogastric tube.*

The long tube intestinal intubation for decompression of the intestines (See MSN, Obstruction of the GI tract) involves the following:

- Position patient on his right side to facilitate the tube's passage through the pylorus, with specific changes of position ordered after an x-ray confirms that the tube has passed into the small intestine. Ambulation may then be encouraged.
- Advance the tube 2 inches to 4 inches at a time according to physician's order. Slow advance decreases the possibility of kinks.

- Never tape tubing until it has reached its destination.
- Attachment of tubing to suction as it advances or after it reaches the obstruction may be ordered.
- If irrigation of the tube is ordered, irrigating fluid may be difficult to aspirate. Irrigating fluid that goes in is counted as intake. All drainage, including what is aspirated, is counted as output. Observe and record character and color of drainage, as well as amount.
- Mouth care is essential. An antibiotic mouthwash may be ordered.

Removal of Gastrointestinal Tubes

- Clamp tube to prevent aspiration of drainage.
- A nasogastric tube is pulled out in one continuous, moderately rapid motion with the patient exhaling slowly and deep breathing.
- An intestinal tube is withdrawn slowly. Patient may feel nauseated. Deep breathing may be helpful.
  1. A weighted tip may be brought out through the patient's mouth for removal. The rest will be pulled out through the nose.
  2. The tube may have a fecal odor. If so, give mouth care immediately.
  3. If the tube has passed through the ileocecal valve, the tube may be allowed to pass out through the rectum.

Keeping the Tube Open

- Vomiting around the NG tube, unrelieved gastric distention, and no drainage are signs that suction is not functioning properly.
  1. Repositioning the patient may help by moving the tube's sucking port away from the stomach or intestinal wall.
  2. Check suction mechanism by disconnecting the tube and testing to see whether or not water can be sucked up. If it cannot, replace suction machine.
  3. Milk NG tube toward the machine, then check its patency by gentle aspiration. Irrigation with 30 ml normal saline may open the tube, but a doctor's order is required. What goes in is counted as intake; what is aspirated, as output.

Relieving Discomforts of Intubation

- Dry lips and mouth, sore throat, hoarseness, earache, and dry nose are common complaints. Relieve them with lip pomade, Vaseline applied to lips and nose, gargles, throat sprays, lozenges, and antibiotic mouthwashes prn and as ordered. Try to prevent parotitis (surgical mumps) by giving excellent regular mouth care.

Gavage (Enteral Feeding)

- Elevate the head of the bed at least 30° during and for one hour following gavage feeding if not contraindicated for other reasons. Hold an infant and "burp" him frequently.
- Check placement of the tube before each intermittent feeding and every 4 hours with continuous feeding.
- Check for residual during continuous feeding in adults by aspirating every 2 to 4 hours. Residual over 150 ml is indicative of delayed gastric emptying; the rate should be decreased, and the physician should be notified. In infants and children, check for amount of residual allowed before refeeding. Aspirated residual should be refed slowly.
- Restrain the hands of restless or disoriented patients to prevent their removing the nasogastric tube.
- Intermittent enteral feeding
  1. Administer slowly by gravity (never with pressure), taking 15 to 20 minutes for 250 ml of formula, followed by 50 ml of water. The formula should be at room temperature.
  2. Too-rapid administration may cause nausea and vomiting and other gastrointestinal symptoms.
- Continuous enteral feeding (the safety and correctness of this are now being questioned)
  1. Infusion rate should be consistent. Check q 30 minutes if it is being administered by gravity. Check every hour if administered by pump.
  2. Delivery sets vary in the number of drops per milliliter (gtt/ml) they deliver. Check tubing package. Label tubing with gtt/ml delivered by this set.
  3. Calculate gtt/min as with intravenous sets.

     $$\frac{\text{gtt/ml}}{\text{60 min/hr}} \times \text{ml/hr} = \text{gtt/min}$$

     Example problem:
     Physician's order: Continuous gavage feeding at 75 ml/hr. Delivery set delivers approximately 20 gtt/ml.

     $$\frac{20}{60} \times 75 = 25 \text{ gtt/min}$$

  4. Do not hang more than a 4-hour supply of formula at one time. Don't add new formula to old.
  5. Mark the bag with tape showing the expected level of the formula at each hour if administration is on schedule. Never attempt to catch up on volume. Retape bag with new times when necessary.

Recognizing and Preventing Complications

- Gastrointestinal intolerance to a formula may cause diarrhea, vomiting, and cramps.
  1. Slower infusion rates or smaller, more dilute feedings may help, but antidiarrheal agents (*e.g.* diphenoxylate hydrochloride with atropine sulfate, [Lomotil], Paregoric) may be ordered.
- Metabolic disturbances because of the high glucose content of many formulas may cause
  1. Diarrhea, nausea, dehydration
  2. Glucosuria with diuresis
  3. Hyperosmolar hyperglycemic nonketotic coma (see MSN, diabetes mellitus, HHNC), preceded by symptoms of lethargy, thirst, glucosuria, and polyuria
- Glucose intolerance may be seen, particularly in diabetic patients or those on steroid therapy.
  1. Urine should be checked for sugar q 4 6 hr (see LAB).
  2. Those with glucosuria should have periodic blood glucose tests (see LAB). They may be done by finger stick.
  3. Insulin may be ordered.
- Aspiration pneumonia
  1. Have suction equipment at the bedside of unconscious or semiconscious patients. Suction prn to prevent aspiration of regurgitated formula.
  2. Interrupt continuous feedings while patient is receiving other treatments (*e.g.*, respiratory therapy). Resume feeding 30 minutes later.
  3. Gastrostomy and enterostomy feeding are being used in some cases both for patient comfort and in the attempt to avoid this common complication of gavage feeding.
- Monitor for electrolyte imbalances (see LAB).
- Watch for gastric distention; prevent it by periodically aspirating for residual (see above).

Administration of Medications Through the Nasogastric Tube

- Liquid medications or crushed nonenteric-coated tablets mixed with a small amount of water may be given by NG tube, using the same precautions as with enteral feedings. Always follow by injecting 30 ml water.
- Discontinue suction, if it is being used, for 30 minutes after the administration of medication, so that the medication can be absorbed.

HYPOTHERMIA BLANKET

Description

A hypothermia blanket is made from rubber or plastic. A cooled solution of alcohol and water circulates in coils within the blanket. The blanket is attached to a refrigeration machine which is set, by physician's order, at the body temperature to be maintained. A rectal probe connects to the machine and indicates on a control panel a continuous body temperature reading. Hypothermia blankets are used to reduce highly elevated and prolonged body temperatures; the temperature is lowed by about 1°F per hour. The blanket usually is placed under the patient; however, two blankets may be used, with one covering the patient.

Starting and Maintaining the Hypothermia Blanket Procedure

- Bathe and oil the patient's skin before using the blanket. Baths are not given during hypothermia blanket use; however, the skin should be kept well oiled during the procedure.
- Prior to using the blanket, an intravenous or nasogastric tube should be in place. These patients will be NPO. Also, an indwelling urinary catheter should be inserted, and a cleansing enema given prior to the hypothermia procedure.
- Wrap or pad areas of pressure (*e.g.*, heels, elbows, and sacrum) to prevent tissue breakdown.
- Secure rectal probe with paper tape.
- Take baseline vital signs prior to starting the procedure.
- Read the manufacturer's directions for proper use of the machine.
- Set the machine at the temperature to be maintained. Check for correct placement of the rectal probe every hour. Take a rectal temperature reading with another thermometer every 2 hours to verify the rectal probe's accuracy.
- Shivering must be avoided because it increases metabolism and prolongs the time necessary to decrease temperature. Chlorpromazine hydrochloride (Thorazine) is often given to prevent shivering.
- Turn the patient every hour and check the skin for areas of irritation.
- Blood pressure, pulse, and respirations must be taken every 30 minutes for the first two hours and then at least every 2 hours. Heart rate, respirations, and urinary output decrease during hypothermia. Cardiac irregularities and respiratory depression may develop at low body temperatures.

- Hypothermia blankets may be used for several days. When they are removed, continue to check the patient's temperature every 2 hours until it stabilizes.

INFECTION CONTROL (ISOLATION PRECAUTIONS)

CONTACT ISOLATION

Contact isolation is designed to prevent transmission of highly transmissible or epidemiologically important infections (or colonization) that do not warrant strict isolation. All diseases or conditions included in this category are spread primarily by close or direct contact. Thus, masks, gowns, and gloves are recommended for anyone in close or direct contact with any patient who has an infection (or colonization) that is included in this category. For individual diseases or conditions, however, one or more of these three barriers may not be indicated. For example, masks and gloves generally are not indicated for care of infants and young children with acute viral respiratory infections; gowns generally are not indicated for gonococcal conjunctivitis in newborns; and masks generally are not indicated for the care of patients infected with multiply-resistant microorganisms, except those with pneumonia. Therefore, some degree of "over-isolation" may occur in this category.

Specifications for Contact Isolation

1. A private room is indicated. In general, patients infected with the same organism may share a room. During outbreaks, infants and young children with the same respiratory clinical syndrome may share a room.
2. Masks are indicated for those persons who come close to the patient.
3. Gowns are indicated if soiling is likely.
4. Gloves are indicated for touching infective material.
5. Hands must be washed after touching the patient or potentially contaminated articles, and before taking care of another patient.
6. Articles contaminated with infective material should be discarded or bagged and labeled before being sent for decontamination and reprocessing.

Diseases or Conditions Requiring Contact Isolation

Acute respiratory infections in infants and young children, including croup, colds, bronchitis, and bronchiolitis caused by respiratory syncytial virus, adenovirus, coronavirus, influenza viruses, parainfluenza viruses, and rhinovirus, require contact isolation.

Conjunctivitis, gonococcal, in newborns

Diphtheria, cutaneous

Endometritis, group A *Streptococcus*

Furunculosis, staphylococcal, in newborns

Herpes simplex, disseminated, severe primary or neonatal

Impetigo

Influenza, in infants and young children

Multiply resistant bacteria, infection, or colonization (any site) with any of the following require contact isolation:

1. Gram-negative bacilli resistant to all aminoglycosides that are tested (In general, such organisms should be resistant to gentamicin, tobramycin, and amikacin for these special precautions to be indicated.)
2. *Staphylococcus aureus* resistant to methicillin (or nafcillin or oxacillin if they are used instead of methicillin for testing)
3. *Pneumococcus* resistant to penicillin
4. *Haemophilus influenzae* resistant to ampicillin (beta-lactamase positive) and chloramphenicol
5. Other resistant bacteria may be included if they are judged by the infection control team to be of special clinical and epidemiologic significance.

Pediculosis

Pharyngitis, infections, in infants and young children

Pneumonia, viral, in infants and young children

Pneumonia, *S. aureus* or group A *Streptococcus*

Rabies

Rubella, congenital and other

Scabies

Scalded skin syndrome, staphylococcal (Ritter's disease)

Skin, wound, or burn infection, major (draining and not covered by dressing or dressing does not adequately contain the purulent material) including those infected with *S. aureus* or group A *Streptococcus*

Vaccinia (generalized and progressive eczema vaccinatum)

RESPIRATORY ISOLATION

Respiratory isolation is designed to prevent transmissions of infectious diseases primarily over short distances through the air (droplet transmission). Direct and indirect contact transmission occurs with some infections in this isolation category, but it is infrequent.

Specifications for Respiratory Isolation

1. A private room is indicated. In general, patients infected with the same organism may share a room.
2. Masks are indicated for those who come close to the patient.
3. Gowns are not indicated.
4. Gloves are not indicated.
5. Hands must be washed after touching the patient or potentially contaminated articles, and before taking care of another patient.
6. Articles contaminated with infective material should be discarded or bagged and labeled before being sent for decontamination and reprocessing.

Diseases Requiring Respiratory Isolation

Epiglottitis, *H. influenzae*
Erythema infectiosum
Measles
Meningitis
    H. influenzae, known or suspected
    Meningococcal, known or suspected
Meningococcal pneumonia
Meningococcemia
Mumps
Pertussis (whooping cough)
Pneumonia, *H. influenzae,* in children (any age)

STRICT ISOLATION

Strict isolation is an isolation category designed to prevent transmission of highly contagious or virulent infections that may be spread by both air and contact.

Specifications for Strict Isolation

1. A private room is indicated; the door should be kept closed. In general, patients infected with the same organism may share a room.
2. Masks are indicated for all persons entering the room.
3. Gowns are indicated for all persons entering the room.
4. Gloves are indicated for all persons entering the room.
5. Hands must be washed after touching the patient or poten-

tially contaminated articles, and before taking care of another patient.

6. Articles contaminated with infective material should be discarded or bagged and labeled before being sent for decontamination and reprocessing.

Diseases Requiring Strict Isolation

Diphtheria, pharyngeal

Lassa fever and other viral hemorrhagic fevers, such as Marburg virus disease*

Plague, pneumonic

Smallpox*

Varicella (chickenpox)

Zoster, localized in immunocompromised patient or disseminated

TUBERCULOSIS ISOLATION (AFB ISOLATION)

Tuberculosis isolation (AFB isolation) is an isolation category for patients with pulmonary tuberculosis (TB) who have a positive sputum smear or a chest x-ray that strongly suggests current (active) TB. Laryngeal TB is also included in this isolation category. In general, infants and young children with pulmonary TB do not require isolation precautions because they rarely cough, and their bronchial secretions contain few AFB (acid-fast bacilli) compared to adults with pulmonary TB. On the instruction card, this category is called AFB. Isolation is to protect the patient's privacy.

Specifications for Tuberculosis Isolation (AFB Isolation)

1. A private room with special ventilation is indicated; the door should be kept closed. In general, patients infected with the same organism may share a room.
2. Masks are indicated only if the patient is coughing and does not reliably cover mouth.
3. Gowns are indicated only if they are needed to prevent gross contamination of clothing.
4. Gloves are not indicated.
5. Hands must be washed after touching the patient or potentially contaminated articles, and before taking care of another patient.
6. Articles rarely transmit TB. However, articles should be thoroughly cleaned and disinfected, or discarded.

*A private room with special ventilation is indicated.

BLOOD/BODY FLUID PRECAUTIONS

Blood/body fluid precautions are designed to prevent infections that are transmitted by direct or indirect contact with infective blood or body fluids. Infectious diseases included in this category are those that result in the production of infective blood or body fluids, unless the disease is included in another isolation category that requires more rigorous precautions, for example, Strict Isolation. For some diseases included in this category, such as malaria, only blood is infective; for other diseases, such as hepatitis B (including antigen carriers), blood and body fluids (saliva, semen, and so forth) are infective.

Specifications for Blood/Body Fluid Precautions

1. A private room is indicated if the patient's hygiene is poor. A patient with poor hygiene does not wash hands after touching infective material, contaminates the environment with infective material, or shares contaminated articles with other patients. In general, patients infected with the same organism may share a room.
2. Masks are not indicated.
3. Gowns are indicated if soiling of clothing with blood or body fluids is likely.
4. Gloves are indicated for touching blood or body fluids.
5. Hands must be washed immediately if they are potentially contaminated with blood or body fluids, and before taking care of another patient.
6. Articles contaminated with blood or body fluids should be discarded or bagged and labeled before being sent for decontamination and reprocessing.
7. Care should be taken to avoid needle-stick injuries. Used needles should not be recapped or bent; they should be placed in a prominently labeled, puncture-resistant container designated specifically for such disposal.
8. Blood spills should be cleaned up promptly with a solution of 5.25% sodium hypochlorite diluted 1:10 with water.

Diseases Requiring Blood/Body Fluid Precautions

Acquired immunodeficiency syndrome (AIDS)

Arthropod-borne viral fevers (for example, dengue, yellow fever, and Colorado tick fever)

Babesiosis

Creutzfeldt-Jakob disease

Hepatitis B (including HBsAg antigen carrier)

Hepatitis, non-A, non-B
Leptospirosis
Malaria
Rat-bite fever
Relapsing fever
Syphilis, primary and secondary with skin and mucous membrane lesions

DRAINAGE/SECRETION PRECAUTIONS

Drainage/secretion precautions are designed to prevent infections that are transmitted by direct or indirect contact with purulent material or drainage from an infected body site. This newly created isolation category includes many infections formerly included in wound and skin precautions, discharge (lesion), and secretion (oral) precautions, categories, which have been discontinued. Infectious diseases included in this category are those that result in the production of infective purulent material, drainage, or secretions, unless the disease is included in another isolation category that requires more rigorous precautions. For example, minor or limited skin, wound, or burn infections are included in this category, but major skin, wound, or burn infections are included in contact isolation. (If you have questions about a specific disease, refer to the infection control book kept on each patient care unit.)

Specifications for Drainage/Secretion Precautions

1. A private room is not indicated.
2. Masks are not indicated.
3. Gowns are indicated if soiling is likely.
4. Gloves are indicated for touching infective material.
5. Hands must be washed after touching the patient or potentially contaminated articles, and before taking care of another patient.
6. Articles contaminated with infective material should be discarded or bagged, and labeled before being sent for decontamination and reprocessing.

Diseases Requiring Drainage/Secretion Precautions

The following infections are examples of those included in this category provided they are not (1) caused by multiply resistant microorganisms; (2) major (draining and not covered by a dressing or dressing does not adequately contain the drainage) skin, wound, or burn infections, including those caused by *S. aureus* or group A *Streptococcus;* or (3) gonococcal eye infections in newborns. See Contact Isolation if the infection is one of these three.

Abscess, minor or limited
Burn infection, minor or limited
Conjunctivitis
Decubitus ulcer, infected, minor or limited
Skin infection, minor or limited
Wound infection, minor or limited

ENTERIC PRECAUTIONS

Enteric precautions are designed to prevent infections that are transmitted by direct or indirect contact with feces. Hepatitis A is included in this category because it is spread through feces, although the disease is much less likely to be transmitted after the onset of jaundice. Most infections in this category primarily cause gastrointestinal symptoms, but some do not. For example, feces from patients infected with "poliovirus" and coxsackieviruses are infective, but these infections usually do not cause prominent gastrointestinal symptoms.

Specifications for Enteric Precautions

1. A private room is indicated if the patient's hygiene is poor. A patient with poor hygiene does not wash hands after touching infective material, contaminates the environment with infective material, or shares contaminated articles with other patients. In general, patients infected with the same organism may share a room.
2. Masks are not indicated.
3. Gowns are indicated if soiling is likely.
4. Gloves are indicated if touching infective material.
5. Hands must be washed after touching the patient or potentially contaminated articles, and before taking care of another patient.
6. Articles contaminated with infective material should be discarded or bagged, and labeled before being sent for decontamination and reprocessing.

Diseases Requiring Enteric Precautions

Amebic dysentery
Cholera
Coxsackievirus disease
Diarrhea, acute illness with suspected infectious etiology
Echovirus disease
Encephalitis (unless known not to be caused by enteroviruses)

Enterocolitis caused by *Clostridium difficile* or *Staphylococcus aureus*

Enteroviral infection

Gastroenteritis caused by the following:

Campylobacter species

Cryptosporidium species

Dientamoeba fragilis

Escherichia coli (enterotoxic, enteropathogenic, or enteroinvasive)

Giardia lamblia

Salmonella species

Shigella species

Vibrio parahaemolyticus

Viruses—including Norwalk agent and rotavirus

Yersinia enterocolitica

Unknown etiology, but presumed to be an infectious agent

Hand, foot, and mouth disease

Hepatitis, viral, Type A

Herpangina

Meningitis, viral (unless known not to be caused by enteroviruses)

Necrotizing enterocolitis

Pleurodynia

Typhoid fever (*Salmonella* typhi)

Viral pericarditis, myocarditis, or meningitis (unless known not to be caused by enteroviruses)

INFECTION CONTROL (ISOLATION TECHNIQUE)

Description

Isolation technique prevents the spread of communicable diseases among patients, hospital personnel, and visitors. The Joint Commission on Accreditation of Hospitals requires all accredited acute-care institutions to have an infection control program, implemented by an infection control committee. An isolation manual with information on establishing and maintaining isolation technique must be available on each patient care unit. Category-specific isolation includes seven categories: strict, contact, respiratory and tuberculosis (AFB) isolation, and drainage/secretion, enteric, and blood/body fluid precautions. Each category is described on a card. The front of the card lists the type and essential requirements pertaining to a private room, gown, mask, hand care, gloves, and care of articles. The back of the card lists diseases or conditions requiring the particular type of isolation. The card specific to the isolation needed is placed on the patient's bed or door. It also may be put on the front of the patient's chart. A disease-specific category of isolation is also approved, although not as frequently used. With this, the isolation manual describes the required isolation/precaution for each specific disease.

Nursing Considerations

- Remember, isolation is for the disease. These patients are often very sensitive about being considered contaminated.
- When conditions appear to warrant isolation, the physician should be contacted. In the event this is not possible, notify the infection control nurse. It is better to "over isolate" than "under isolate," but always consider the mode of transmission.
- Handwashing is the most important method of preventing nosocomial (hospital-acquired) infections. Handwashing should be done before significant contact with any patient, and after contact with any excretions or secretions. Vigorous scrubbing with soap and water for at least 15 seconds, followed by thorough rinsing, constitutes proper handwashing. The faucet should be turned off with a clean paper towel. The use of an antiseptic hand cleaner is recommended before performing an IV or urinary catheterization.
- Common sources of nosocomial infections are urinary and IV catheters. Urinary tract infections are the most common nosocomial infection.
- Gowns, masks, and gloves must be used only once. Gloves must be changed after contact with secretions and excretions, even if patient care is not completed.
- All wounds should be dressed using one pair of gloves to remove soiled dressings and another pair to apply the new dressing. The use of gloves does not excuse handwashing.
- Patients who are immunosuppressed because of therapy or disease are at great risk of infection from others, and especially from organisms present on their own bodies. For this reason, patient care should include a bath twice a day, including a complete linen change, and mouth care after meals and before sleeping. Obviously, anyone with an infection should avoid contact with these patients.
- Specimens sent to the laboratory must be clearly labeled "isolation."
- When culture reports are used as a criterion for discontinuing isolation, the negative cultures must be specimens obtained after antibiotic therapy has been terminated.

INTRAVENOUS THERAPY

Description

Intravenous (IV) administration is necessary when taking fluids by mouth is impractical or contraindicated for a patient, or when direct access to the bloodstream is required. The type, amount, and flow rate of IV fluid and electrolyte replacement are determined in accordance with the physical needs of the patient. It is very important to maintain the prescribed flow rates to prevent fluid and electrolyte imbalances. An IV also may be used to provide vein access for routine or emergency medication administration. The solution commonly used for the keep vein open (KVO) IV is D_5W (5% dextrose in water). The KVO delivery rate in an adult is 50 ml or less per hour, depending on the cardiac or renal status of the patient. Infant and children KVO delivery rates are always ordered by the physician.

Starting and Maintaining the IV

- Handwashing with an antiseptic agent is absolutely necessary before this procedure to prevent infection.
- Preoperative IVs in adults should always be started with an #18 or #19 needle or catheter in case a blood transfusion is necessary. A #22 or #23 scalp vein needle or a catheter often is used with children.
- An IV needle with a heparin lock is ideal for intermittent access to a vein.
- Use microdrop tubing for KVO IVs (60 gtt/ml).
- Solutions are ordered by the physician in milliliters per hour. When an infusion control device is not available the nurse manually regulates the flow rates in drops (gtt) per minute. The formula needed to convert from the ml/hr to the gtt/min is

$$\text{gtt/min (flow rate)} = \text{gtt/ml (from calibration of set)} \times \frac{\text{ml/hr}}{60}$$

- The size of the drop varies according to the calibration of the set. Standard or macrodrop sets are calibrated at 10 gtt = 1 ml; 15 gtt = 1 ml; or 20 gtt = 1 ml. Microdrop sets are calibrated at 60 gtt = 1 ml. This information is found on the package of the IV tubing.
- Fill the drip chamber half full before opening and priming the tubing. This will eliminate air bubbles.
- Always maintain a primary IV line into which an additive line (*e.g.*, piggyback tubing) may be connected.
- An infusion control device should always be used when the IV flow rates are extremely critical (*e.g.*, hyperalimentation, heparin, theophyllin). Check the equipment as well as the patient every 30

minutes. The control device should always be out of the patient's reach.

- In infants and individuals where fluid overload can be extremely hazardous, volume control chambers are often used. These are filled from above, and the tubing above is clamped allowing only the amount of fluid in the chamber to be infused.
- If the present container of IV solution contains less than 50 ml at the change of nursing shift, replace with a full container prior to the shift change.
- The IV site dressing and tubing must be changed according to hospital or unit policy. Both dressing and tubing must be marked with date and the nurse's initials.
- IV tubing often becomes permanently compressed by the mechanism in infusion pumps and the flow stops. To prevent this, change the tubing at least every 24 hours.
- The smallest possible container of IV fluid should be used to maintain a KVO IV. It must be discarded and a new container hung every 24 hours.
- Label IV tubing and container with the date it is hung.

The IV Site

- It is standard practice in adults to use arm veins; IVs in the lower extremities have a high risk of thrombophlebitis. When possible, start IVs in hand veins, which are satisfactory for KVO IVs. Use the larger veins above the hand for rapid infusions, blood, or when medications are going to be regularly added by piggyback. The antecubital vein should be saved for routine blood work.
- In infants scalp veins are preferred IV sites; the umbilical vein may be used in the first days of life.
- When stabilization of the limb is necessary to maintain the IV, a contour splint is more comfortable than an armboard.
- Be especially careful when taping down an IV needle so that blood flow is not obstructed.
- Wrapping the arm with warm towels for 15 minutes to 20 minutes is helpful in raising veins. Holding the arm below the heart level also helps identify veins.
- A blood pressure cuff is less traumatic to the skin than tourniquet tubing.
- The maximum time a needle may be in a vein without an increased incidence of infection and phlebitis is considered to be 72 hours. Metal needles should be changed every 48 hours, and plastic over-the-needle catheters every 72 hours, or as recommended by hospital or unit policy.
- After withdrawing an IV needle or catheter, apply pressure with a sterile pad to stop the bleeding. If the patient has been on anti-

coagulants, or if the platelet count is under 50,000, the bleeding may not stop immediately.

Factors Disturbing the Flow Rate

- The IV container should be at least three feet above insertion.
- When a clot occurs in a needle or catheter, *gently* irrigate with normal saline. If resistance is met, discontinue and start a new IV.
- If the needle or catheter position has changed, remove dressing and gently realign it into the vein and retape.
- Check for infiltration by applying a tourniquet above the insertion site. If the needle is in the vein, the IV will stop.
- Ambulatory patients should be instructed to keep the IV arm at waist level to prevent blood from backing up in the tubing. If blood does appear, increase the flow rate for a minute to flush it through.
- Blood appearing in the tubing, a wet IV dressing (infiltration or detached needle), pain at or above the insertion site, coldness, swelling, and redness in the arm are indicators of a disturbed flow rate. Instruct patients to alert a nurse if these symptoms occur.
- Patients may cause the IV to malfunction by handling the tubing. Keep it out of reach of children and confused patients.
- Infants and small children need special protection for IV sites, and this makes it difficult to see signs of infiltration.

Precautions when Medications Are Used in IVs

- Check the patient's allergies before giving or starting any IV medication. Watch carefully for any reactions during the first 15 minutes of any infusion.
- Always check with a pharmacist before adding anything to an IV solution for its compatibility with the solution. For instance, diazepam (Valium) and phenytoin sodium (Dilantin) are *never* given in an IV solution, but only as an IV bolus (see PH).
- Know the rate of infusion for medications by piggyback. In most adults, a delivery rate of 100 ml/hour is well tolerated for piggyback medications in a volume of 50 ml to 100 ml. The physician should specify rate for infants and small children. However, some antibiotics are particularly irritating (*e.g.,* penicillin, erythromycin, and the tetracyclines). They must be more dilute to be administered comfortably (see PH).
- When medications (*e.g.,* potassium or vitamins) are added, be sure to rotate the bottle to mix them in the solution. Attach a label with the name, date, and amount of additives. Avoid adding medication to hanging IV containers; use a new container.

Complications of IV Therapy

- Infections may result from skin bacteria entering at the insertion site because of poor aseptic technique. When a patient develops signs and symptoms of sudden systemic infection, such as chills, fever, and nausea, while receiving IV therapy, discontinue the IV and send tubing, needle, and container to the lab for examination. This also applies when an infection appears at the IV site (*e.g.*, purulent drainage).
- Speed shock may occur as a result of too rapid administration of drugs.
- Circulatory overload occurs with too rapid infusion. This may result in congestive heart failure or pulmonary edema. Be alert for shortness of breath, coughing, rales, dilation of neck veins, and decreased urine output in comparison to fluid intake.

Total Parenteral Nutrition IV Solutions

- Hyperalimentation therapy, also called total parenteral nutrition (TPN), provides necessary calories, amino acids, and electrolytes in small volumes. The solutions designed to meet an individual's need are prepared by pharmacists according to a physician's prescription.
- The solutions must be kept refrigerated until they are used. These solutions are highly concentrated, requiring the use of a large-size catheter or needle inserted into the large vein. The subclavian or internal jugular vein generally is used. A chest x-ray is necessary to ascertain proper catheter placement before TPN solution is administered.
- Sepsis and metabolic imbalance are potential risks. Check with the individual institution as to whether or not anything other than the TPN solution may be run into this IV line.
- An infusion control device must be used for delivery of TPN. Check the delivery system every 30 minutes. Microdrop tubing is often not suitable for these viscous solutions.
- The TPN dressing must be changed every 48 hours using strict sterile technique. Refer to the individual institution's procedure book concerning technique and frequency of filter and tubing change.
- TPN can provide about 1,000 calories per container. Metabolic and electrolyte abnormalities may occur. Hypoglycemia can result from the abrupt cessation of hyperalimentation. Hyperglycemia may be present as the body adjusts to the high glucose content of the TPN solution, even though insulin is included in the solution.
- Patients receiving TPN must have their temperature and fractional urines with specific gravity measured every six hours. In-

sulin coverage is usually ordered for 1% or 2% glucose. Daily weights done at the same time each day and intake and output (I–O) records are extremely important (see LAB).

- Check infusion site once a shift for signs of leaking, swelling of the neck, hand, face, or distention of neck or arm veins. Report any of the above to the physician.
- TPN solutions are prepared to be given in sequence. *Never* speed up or slow down the delivery rate, or change the sequence without an order from a physician.
- A complication of long-term TPN is a decrease in fatty acids. Thus, fat emulsions (*e.g.,* Intralipid) may be required one to two times weekly. There are 550 calories in 500 ml. This may be given in peripheral veins. Again, this line must not be used for any other solution. Use the tubing that comes with the solution. Do not use a filter.
- The initial flow rate for administering fat emulsions is 1 ml/min for 30 minutes, then proceed as ordered. Observe the patient closely during the first 30 minutes for allergic reactions.

BLOOD AND BLOOD-COMPONENT TRANSFUSION

Description

Blood transfusions are commonly used to replace blood losses or to correct an anemic condition. Blood is typed (A, B, AB, or O), and is classified further as Rh positive or Rh negative. Blood ordinarily is obtainable as whole stored blood, fresh whole blood, or as packed red blood cells (PBCs), which is whole blood that has 80% of the liquid plasma removed. Whole blood (stored or fresh) is given in cases of sudden and excessive blood loss because it restores volume. Whole blood may be stored in blood banks for up to 35 days, but stored blood has diminished clotting ability. Fresh whole blood is particularly useful in cases of massive hemorrhage, because fresh blood contains the necessary clotting factors. Fresh blood must be used immediately. PBCs have the advantage of the same amount of hemoglobin in a smaller volume. PBCs may be frozen and stored for up to three years but must be used within 24 hours of thawing.

Starting and Maintaining the Transfusion

- Blood transfusions require meticulous attention to detail. Death may result if the infused blood type does not match the patient's blood type. Therefore, two nurses together must verify the patient's name, by checking his wristband and asking his name. Also, they must double check the number on the lab slip, which must match the number on the container. The Rh type on the lab slip also must match that on the blood container. If there is any question, return the blood to the lab for investigation.

- Vital signs, including temperature, must be taken before, during, and after a transfusion.
- Start the IV with a #18 or #19 needle or catheter for adults; a #22 or #23 needle or catheter may be necessary for children or for patients with very small veins.
- Normal saline (never a dextrose solution) is started and infused through the blood administration tubing before the blood is obtained from the blood bank. When the blood arrives, it must be hung (transfusion started) immediately. Once the blood is released from the blood bank it cannot be returned.
- Blood and blood-product transfusions in adults should be started at 2 ml/minute for the first 15 minutes. This is the period when the most serious reactions are most likely to occur. If the patient's condition remains stable the flow rate may then be increased.
- While blood infusion rates may be adjusted to the patient's need for blood replacement, a unit of blood should be infused within 2 hours, and never longer than 4 hours. PBCs are commonly packaged in 250-ml containers. The blood bank can package smaller amounts when a slower infusion rate is required. The possibility of bacterial proliferation and hemolysis of red blood cells increases with time at room temperature.
- For patients who are susceptible to congestive heart failure, the infusion time of a unit should be lengthened, up to 4 hours. Check these patients frequently for signs of fluid overload, for example, coughing, SOB, rales, jugular vein distention (JVD) (see MSN, Congestive Heart Failure).
- Slow rates of infusion may cause the blood to stop running. To help prevent this, gently invert the bag two or three times while infusing. If it does stop, clamp the blood tubing and run saline through it for a minute before restarting the blood. Do not repeat this more than twice because it increases the patient's sodium intake.
- Never add any medications to the infusing blood or to the IV line.
- The IV tubing used to transfuse blood should be changed after two units are infused.
- A blood warmer is occasionally used for some patients who have antibodies that react to red blood cells at low temperatures. Blood should never be warmed to a temperature higher than 37°C.
- Blood pumping devices are used occasionally when blood needs to be transfused rapidly. Watch these patients extremely carefully for signs of congestive heart failure or infiltration from vein blowout at the needle site.
- Stop the blood immediately when *any* reaction is noticed. Reactions to blood transfusions produce a variety of systemic reactions: fever, chills, back pain, pruritis (itching), and urticaria. Notify the physician and change the tubing, keeping the vein open

with normal saline. Follow individual hospital procedures when there is any blood reaction. The blood product, saline solution, and tubing must be returned to the blood bank.

- Plasma, albumin, and dextran are volume expanders, and may be given in emergencies until blood is available.
- Plasma in 250-ml units is infused as rapidly as desired. A Y blood transfusion set is used, and normal saline may be run between units of plasma.
- Albumin comes with special tubing for its infusion, because of its high viscosity. The rate of infusion is 1 ml/minute, unless otherwise ordered, because of the possibility of fluid overload from rapid vascular volume increase.
- Dextran may cause a reaction, so the infusion rate should be 1 ml/minute for the first 15 minutes.
- Platelets are administered to adults at a rate of 10 minutes/unit by a special platelet transfusion set; their peak effect is in 2 hours. They must be given as soon as they become available because of their short life span of 1 day to 3 days. Six units of platelets raises the platelet count by about 50,000 cu mm.
- Multiple platelet transfusions become progressively less effective. Also, febrile reactions may begin to occur.

INDWELLING CENTRAL VENOUS CATHETER

Description

A minor surgical procedure using fluoroscopy allows the insertion of a subcutaneous, indwelling venous Silastic catheter (Fig. 3-10) into the patient. A Hickman or Broviac catheter is commonly used; the inside diameter of the Hickman catheter is slightly larger than that of a Broviac. A Dacron cuff anchors the catheter subcutaneously by stimulating adhesion formation. Direct access to a large vein permits the administration of IV fluid, medication, blood, and TPN formula through the cap of the catheter. Blood can be withdrawn and central venous pressure can also be monitored. The double-lumen Hickman catheter is a fusion of the Broviac and Hickman. With this system, TPN can be infused through the Broviac, and the larger-lumen Hickman is used to administer blood and medication, and to withdraw blood. When the catheter is not in use, it is flushed with heparin as ordered by the physician and kept closed with a smooth surface clamp. These catheters stay in place until they are no longer required. The need for repeated venipunctures is eliminated.

Nursing Considerations

- To prevent accidental cutting no scissors should be used near the catheter.

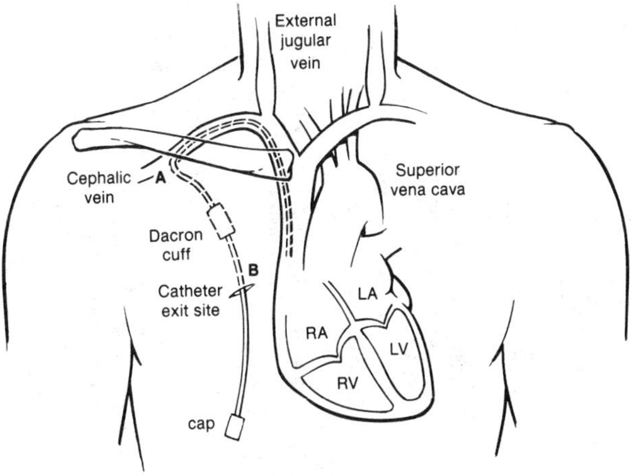

Fig. 3-10. *Indwelling central venous catheter.*

NR

- Institution guidelines vary as to the use and care of these catheters. Know what they are before instilling any solution or withdrawing blood. When drawing blood through the Hickman catheter, the first 6 ml usually are discarded.
- When the line is irrigated with a heparinized solution, the solution is injected as the clamp is released. Do not put a needle longer than one inch into the cap.
- Both entry and exit sites are dressed daily for about seven days, using sterile technique. The entry site should then be healed and only the exit site needs routine dressing changes unless the dressing becomes wet. Observe for redness, swelling, or leakage around the sites.
- Patients have great freedom of movement with these insertions; many are able to be cared for on an out-patient basis. However, arrangements must be made to teach the patient, caretaker, or visiting nurse how to flush the catheter, change the dressings, change and wrap the caps, and secure the catheter to prevent dislodgement.

INTRAVENOUS FLUIDS

The various kinds of IV fluids, their actions, and important considerations in their administration are listed in Table 3-1.

(Text continues on page 98)

TABLE 3-1 INTRAVENOUS FLUIDS

Fluid	Action	Comments
Dextrose in water		
5%	Replaces fluid Provides calories	Provides 170 calories per liter
10%	Replaces fluid Provides calories	Irritating to peripheral veins. Dextrose concentrations higher than 10% should not, in general, be given in peripheral veins.
50% as a 50-ml bolus	Corrects hypoglycemia. Osmotic diuretic	Given over a period of 5 minutes
Sodium chloride 0.9% (normal saline)	Isotonic fluid replacement. Corrects mild sodium depletion and precedes a blood transfusion	Use with caution in patients with congestive heart failure, or poor renal function
Sodium chloride 0.45% (½ normal saline)	Provides normal daily sodium and water needs	
Sodium chloride 3% or 5% (hypertonic)	Used to correct severe hyponatremia	May cause death if too much is administered. Always be sure of order before administering.
Dextrose/saline combination (*e.g.*, D_5½ NS, D_5NS, D_5¼ NS, D_5⅓ NS	Replaces fluid	May cause circulatory overload

Lactated Ringer's (Hartman's solution) (contains sodium, chloride, potassium, calcium, lactate, and water)	Balanced electrolyte solution, roughly equivalent to electrolyte concentration of potassium, calcium, sodium, and chloride in the plasma. Lactate is a bicarbonate precursor in persons with normal blood perfusion and normal liver function.	Can cause lactic acidosis in patients with poor perfusion (*i.e.*, shock) or liver disease
Ringer's solution	Higher concentrations of sodium and chloride than lactated Ringer's solution	Replaces electrolytes lost following surgery, burns, and other fluid losses
Balanced electrolyte solutions (*e.g.*, Ionosol, Isolyte-M)	Replaces fluids with approximately the normal serum electrolyte concentrations	These solutions have a fixed electrolyte concentration that does not allow for individual variations.
Amino acids (*e.g.*, Amigen, Aminosol)	Provides amino acids and calories for patients unable to eat or drink	May be given peripherally
Hyperalimentation solution	Depending upon the formulation, can provide approximately 1,000 calories per liter for patients who are unable to eat or drink, or who have an absorption deficiency	May cause severe metabolic and electrolyte imbalances. Solutions must be given in proper sequence as provided by pharmacy. Urine test for glucose, acetone, and specific gravity

NR

(continued)

TABLE 3-1 INTRAVENOUS FLUIDS

Fluid	Action	Comments
		every 6 hours because of high glucose content of fluid. *Do not add anything to bottle or piggyback into the same line without checking hospital policy.*
Fat emulsion	Concentrated amount of calories in small volume, 500 ml = 550 calories. Often given as an adjunct to hyperalimentation because this type of solution is deficient in fatty acids.	Don't use a filter. Run at 1 ml/min for the first 30 minutes to check for reaction (*e.g.,* nausea, dyspnea, allergic reaction). May deliver 500 ml in 4 hr to 6 hr. A peripheral vein may be used. Do not add anything to the solution.
Human serum albumin 5% iso-osmotic to plasma 25% hyperosmotic to plasma	Both solutions are used as plasma expanders. The osmotic pressure of the 25% solution will rapidly pull fluid into the bloodstream from surrounding interstitial spaces at a rate 3% times the amount infused in 15 minutes, causing hemodilution and diuresis in a	The 5% solution is administered at a rate of 2 ml to 4 ml, the 25% solution at 1 ml/min. However, they may be administered very rapidly in cases of hypovolemic shock. Monitor blood pressure. Watch for signs of circulatory overload (*e.g.,* SOB, chest pain). Note: Salt-poor albumin is a

	hydrated patient with normal renal function. The 25% solution is useful in patients whose fluid and sodium intake must be kept low.	misnomer used for 25% human serum albumin; the sodium content is approximately equivalent to that of blood.
Plasmanate 5%, iso-osmotic to plasma	Same actions as 5% albumin	Rapid infusion (greater than 10 ml/min) may cause hypotension and also vascular overload. Watch for chest pain and shortness of breath.
Dextran	Synthetic plasma expander (crossmatching of blood must be done prior to administration of dextran)	Watch for allergic reactions. Start at 1 ml/min.
Hetastarch (Volex, Hespan)	Synthetic volume expander	Does not interfere with blood typing. Causes fewer allergic reactions than dextran
Mannitol	Osmotic diuretic	Do not give if crystals are present in the solution. Use a filter.

NR

Nursing Considerations

- Isotonic IV solutions are given to expand plasma and interstitial fluid. A common isotonic solution is normal saline (0.9% sodium chloride).
- Hypotonic IV solutions cause blood cells to draw fluid inward and may cause them to burst (lyse). Hypotonic IV solutions also can cause fluid to move from the plasma to interstitial space. One-half normal saline (0.45% sodium chloride) is a common hypotonic solution.
- Hypertonic IV solutions draw fluid out of blood cells. They also can cause fluid to move into the plasma from interstitial space. Dextrose 10% in water ($D_{10}W$) is an example of a hypertonic solution.

KEGEL EXERCISES (PERINEAL MUSCLE STRENGTHENING EXERCISES)

Description

The patient consciously contracts and relaxes the perineal, gluteal, and abdominal muscles. Starting and stopping the urinary stream is one type of practice. Kegel exercises can be done frequently, at any time, and in any place. They are recommended for all women (especially postpartum) to prevent pelvic relaxation, and are prescribed in many situations postoperatively for both men and women.

LIVER BIOPSY

With local anesthesia, aspiration of liver tissue is usually done at the patient's bedside by closed-needle biopsy. Liver biopsy also is done frequently during peritonoscopy (see NR, Endoscopic procedures). With either method, the chief danger is hemorrhage.

Nursing Considerations

- Written permission (informed consent) usually is required.
- Typing and cross-matching is frequently done.
- "NPO after midnight" is frequently ordered preceding biopsy.
- For closed-needle biopsy, position patient on his left side with the right arm elevated, or in the supine position (lying on his back), according to the physician's preference. The needle is inserted into the liver through an intercostal space.
- To prevent movement of the chest wall, the patient is asked to take a deep breath, to exhale, and to hold the breath at the end

of the expiration while the needle is inserted, and until it is removed.

- Vital signs are taken preceding the procedure and q 15 min until stable, and q 4 hr for first 12 hours.
- Reposition patient on his right side with a pillow under the costal margin, a position to be maintained for several hours. Bed rest is necessary for 24 hours.
- Observe for signs of complications: hemorrhage, shock, peritonitis, and pneumothorax (see MSN, Postoperative care, hemorrhage, shock, peritonitis and MSN, Respiratory, pneumothorax).

NUCLEAR SCANS

Radioactive isotopes are used for diagnosis in nuclear medicine. They are given by mouth or injection, and emit a minute amount of radiation detected by a machine that measures or converts it into an image. It is preferable that scans be done before barium studies or x-rays that require dye injections, and that no other tests are scheduled for the same day. When a series of scans is requested, consult with the nuclear medicine department so that a proper sequence can be arranged.

Brain: to identify brain tumors, hemorrhage, hematomas, and abscesses. The patient should force fluids before and during the scan. An injection is given and a flow study is done. The patient returns to his room and at least an hour later returns for the second part of the scan, which takes about 30 minutes. If the patient has an indwelling catheter, the collection bag should be emptied every 2 hours to 4 hours. Pregnant nursing staff should not care for these patients on the day of their scan.

Blood volume: to determine fluid overload or dehydration. The patient's height and weight are necessary for this test.

Bone: to identify areas of increased bone metabolism associated with tumors and changes in bone metabolism. After an injection is given, the patient should drink at least three 8-oz glasses of liquid during the next 2 hours. Before going for the scan, 2 hours after the injection, the bladder should be empty. The scan takes one hour, and fluids should be forced for the remainder of the day. If the patient has an indwelling catheter, the collection bag should be emptied before the scan, and then every 2 hours to 4 hours for the rest of the day. Pregnant nursing staff should not care for these patients on the day of their scan.

Gallium: to detect tumors or inflammation in various organs or tissue. Check with the nuclear medicine department for specific instructions.

Gastrointestinal (GI) bleeding: demonstrates active bleeding sites in the GI tract.

Heart scan: uses thallium or technetium-99m isotopes to aid in diagnosing myocardial infaction or areas of ischemia.

Hepatobiliary scan: to analyze the function and diagnose acute and chronic gallbladder disease. The patient must be NPO for 6 hours to 8 hours. An IV injection is given, and the scan takes about 60 minutes.

Liver-spleen scan: to identify the size, shape, space-occupying lesions, or a ruptured spleen. This scan should be done before a barium enema x-ray or upper GI series, or after the patient is completely rid of the barium. There should be a one-day interval after a bone scan. The patient must be well hydrated. An IV injection is given, and the scan takes about 45 minutes. A liver/lung scan is done to identify a subdiaphragmatic abscess.

Lung: to determine pulmonary perfusion; an area of ischemia may be indicative of a pulmonary embolus. The patient should be well hydrated. An injection is given, and the scan takes about 20 minutes.

Pancreas: to identify size, shape, tumor, or pseudocyst. The patient is kept NPO. A special pancreatic meal ordered from the diet kitchen is given when the nuclear medicine department calls. If ordered by the physician, 1 ounce of whiskey is mixed with the meal to enhance pancreatic activity. The patient goes immediately to the nuclear medicine department. An injection is given, and the scan takes about 45 minutes.

Renal flow and scan: to demonstrate renal blood flow and identify size, location, and function of the kidneys and ureters. The patient should be well hydrated and sent for the scan with a full bladder. An injection is given, and the scan takes about 30 minutes. The patient should force fluids for the rest of the day. If the patient has an indwelling urinary catheter, the collection bag should be emptied before the scan, the day of the scan, and then every 2 hours to 4 hours for the rest of the day. Pregnant nursing staff should not care for these patients on the day of this scan.

Thyroid gland: for size, location, and shape of thyroid. The patient should be well hydrated. An injection is given, and a scan done after 20 minutes.

Thyroid uptake: to test the function of the thyroid. It must be established before this scan whether the patient is presently on thyroid or iodine medication or had an x-ray requiring IV contrast media in the past 5 years (*e.g.*, pyelogram). The patient must be able to take an ^{131}I capsule PO and go to the nuclear medicine department the next day for the 10-minute scan.

Xenon ventilation lung scan: to evaluate the air supply to pulmonary tissues. There is no injection. It is done by inhalation and takes about 20 minutes.

OSTOMIES, FISTULAS, AND DRAINING WOUNDS

Description

Ostomies, fistulas (abnormal passageways from a normal cavity to another or to the skin), and draining wounds present unnatural situations in which material from internal organs discharges directly onto the skin. Drainage from the upper gastrointestinal (GI) tract is especially irritating to the skin because of its high enzyme content.

Ostomies are created in an attempt to improve upon a pathologic condition. They may be temporary or permanent. The goal of treatment for fistulas and draining wounds is closure. These conditions are being considered together because of the commonalities of their nursing care: protection of the skin around the cutaneous opening; collection of drainage; prevention of odors; and emotional support for the patient.

Equipment

Select equipment from the many products available with individual patient's needs in mind. Read accompanying printed material for specifics about each product. The following will provide general guidelines (Fig. 3–11).

- Pouches or appliances
  1. One-piece disposable postoperative pouch with flexible adhesive-backed paper faceplate. This type of pouch is used in the hospital. It may be open-ended and drainable, or it may have a valve at the bottom to facilitate emptying (for the urinary stoma). Loop colostomies require an extra pouch at first, selected to fit over the support rod.
  2. Two-piece disposable pouch: This pouch has a skin-barrier wafer with an embedded flange that allows a pouch of the same size flange to be snapped into place.
  3. Disposable pouch with attached skin barrier gasket available with a pre-cut stomal opening. This is appropriate for the round or nearly round stoma. Select a stoma opening size 1/4 inch in diameter larger than the smallest opening on the measuring guide that will completely encompass, but not touch, the stoma. For example, a stoma measuring 1½ inch would require a 1¾-inch pre-cut pouch with attached skin-barrier gasket.
  4. Reusable pouch. This may be one unit (pouch and rigid faceplate) or a two-piece unit with separate rigid faceplate and pouch. It may be used at home after the stoma has shrunk to permanent size. The pouch may last several months with good care. If the patient brings one to the hospital, suggest that it be sent home. It is expensive and could be lost. Use of a dis-

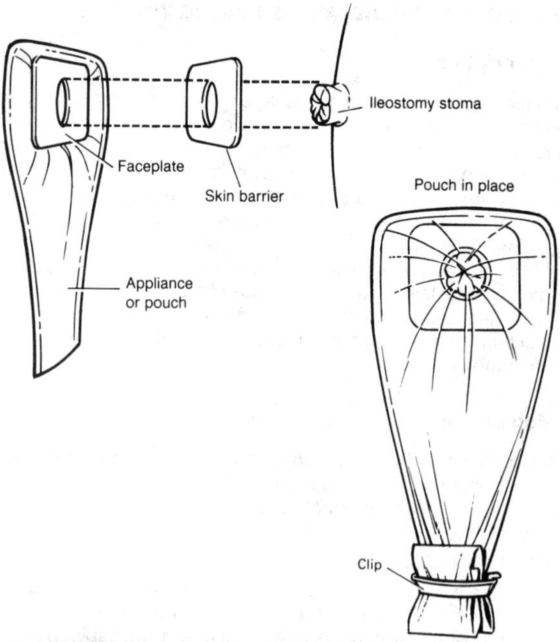

Fig. 3-11. *Components of ostomy appliance. The outlet of the pouch should be cuffed and doubled back twice. It either should be sealed with a clip or fanfolded and secured with a rubber band.*

posable pouch during hospitalization also saves the nurses 30 minutes to 40 minutes of clean-up time.

- Protective skin barriers
  1. Ostomy skin-barrier film. This coats and protects the skin. It is available as a spray, brush-on, or in wipes.
  2. Karaya

     Karaya powder

     Karaya paste comes in prepared form, but when large amounts are needed, karaya powder and glycerine can be mixed to the consistency of stiff peanut butter—almost to the point where the mixture can be worked with the hands.

     Karaya rings don't do well with urinary ostomies because urine melts them.
  3. Gelatin/pectin/cellulose preparations such as Stomahesive wafers (Squibb) are available as wafers, pastes, and powders. They can be used for urinary and fecal ostomies.

- Products for securing appliances
  1. Skin cement. The skin must be dry before application. Apply a light coat to the skin and to the adhesive surface of the pouch. Cement must be "dry" before applying pouch to body surface. Test dryness by touching lightly. The cement is "dry" when it does not come off on your fingertip.
  2. Solvents that are used to remove cement must be washed off.
  3. Belts may be used to support the weight of the pouch.
  4. Hypoallergenic tape is used to "picture frame" the faceplate to the skin for extra security.
  5. Double-faced adhesive discs may be used instead of cement. They usually are used with a reusable appliance, and should be applied over a skin barrier.

Nursing Considerations

- Patient teaching for the ostomate should begin preoperatively, and should resume after surgery as soon as possible. Mastery of the physical care of the ostomy comes first, and can be introduced in steps appropriate to the patient's condition, readiness, and capability. The goal is acceptance on the part of the patient of the body change, and independence in management of the ostomy.
- Sterile technique is used in dressing draining wounds.
- Montgomery straps facilitate ease of dressing changes in situations where a wound with copious drainage requires a large dressing (Fig. 3-12).

Basic Steps for Applying a Disposable Postoperative Pouch

1. Cleanse skin with water; pat and fan dry.
2. Lay the plastic wrapper from a skin-barrier wafer over the stoma and trace the stoma's shape with a pen. Cut out the pattern. The pattern should allow a ⅛-inch clearance around the stoma.
3. Place the pattern over the stoma. Lay the paper faceplate of the pouch on top of the pattern in the manner you want the pouch to be attached to the patient. Remove the pattern and pouch simultaneously. Invert and trace the pattern onto the faceplate. Cut out the pattern traced on the pouch.
4. Remove the protective paper from the faceplate of the pouch, and lay the pouch aside, sticky side up. Save the paper as a pattern.
5. After you carefully match the stomal openings, apply skin-barrier wafer down onto the pouch adhesive with the side of the wafer that is intended to go next to the skin facing up.

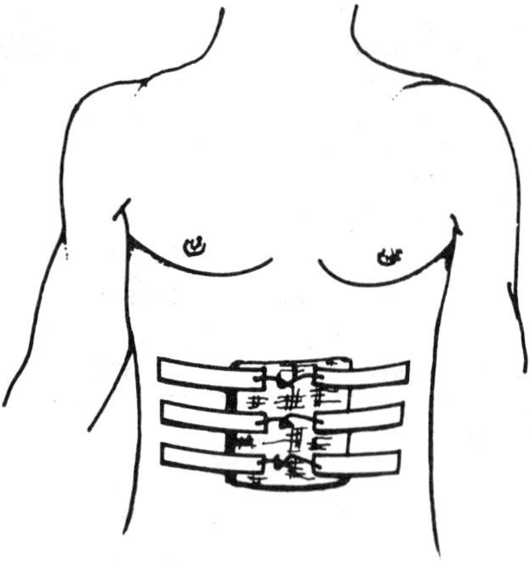

Fig. 3-12. *Montgomery straps are used for dressings that must be changed frequently.*

6. Apply the skin-barrier film to clean, dry, peristomal skin. Fan dry.
7. Remove the protective paper from the skin-barrier wafer and carefully apply the pouch.
8. Picture frame the pouch with hypoallergenic tape.
9. Add a capful of mouthwash to the pouch. Secure the end of the pouch with a clip or rubber band. Close the valve of the urinary pouch.

Prevention of Leaks Around Appliance

1. Proper fit of the appliance is essential.
2. A paper faceplate or skin barrier must be molded smoothly to the skin. The skin should be smooth and taut; this is best accomplished when the patient is either standing or reclining. (Concave defects in the skin around the stoma may be filled with skin-barrier paste to provide an even surface for application of the appliance.)
3. The skin around the stoma must be dry before application of faceplate or skin barrier. A tampon or a 4 × 4 gauze square may be held over the stoma to absorb drainage.
4. Have the patient lie quietly for 30 minutes after application of the pouch so that the seal can set.
5. Empty the pouch often enough to prevent unnecessary strain on the seal from the weight of drainage. (Rinse the pouch before closing it again.) Change the pouch often enough to prevent leaks—usually every 3 days to 5 days. Leaks cause skin

irritation. Patients can recognize leaks when they feel a burning or itching sensation under the appliance, and when they smell an odor coming from a clean pouch.

6. Always eliminate gas by emptying the pouch. The pouch is no longer odor or leak proof if a pin hole has been made in it.

For Skin Irritation

- Wash the skin with water, and dry thoroughly. Depending upon the degree of irritation, one or more of the following approaches may be helpful.

1. A shower, tub bath, and exposure to the air at the time the appliance is changed may be comforting to irritated skin.
2. Weeping skin may be washed with aluminum hydroxide antacid. This is soothing. Pour off the thin liquid at the top of the bottle and use the thick, pasty liquid at the bottom. Let dry. Dust with karaya powder. Spray lightly with skin-barrier film. Fan dry.
3. Karaya powder is an effective skin healer, but the patient should be warned that it will burn.
4. Large, excoriated areas may be covered by a thin application of skin-barrier paste applied with a tongue blade either at one time, or in several layers for quicker drying. Picture frame the faceplate of the pouch over the paste. Any exposed paste should be covered with paper tape, so that it does not stick to clothing or bedding.

NR

To Control Odors

1. The disposable fecal pouch should be rinsed well after emptying. Insert commercial pouch deodorant, a capful of mouthwash, or a drop of oil of peppermint or oil of cloves in the pouch.
2. Release gas by opening pouch in the bathroom.
3. Room deodorizers may be helpful. Plan time for colostomy irrigations and similar procedures with consideration for other patients in the room.

Colostomy Irrigation

- See hospital procedure book. Cones, the most popular irrigating tips, are easy to use and help avoid accidental perforation of the intestine.

Urinary Ostomies

- Any urinary diversion to the skin, for example, ileal conduit, cutaneous ureterostomy.

1. Karaya rings are dissolved by urine. Instead, use a gelatin pectic/cellulose skin barrier. If the skin becomes excoriated, use the technique described under skin irritation, above.

2. Disposable pouches are recommended. To prevent the buildup of odor and urine crystals, the pouch should be rinsed with a solution of ⅓ cup white vinegar and ⅔ cup tepid water every night, as follows:

   Snap night drainage adapter onto pouch tail closure.

   Using a catheter-tipped syringe, insert vinegar solution into pouch.

   Carefully remove the night drainage adapter, and close pouch. Have patient lie prone for 20 minutes. (For a child, this is a good time for a bedtime story.)

   Snap night drainage adapter onto pouch and connect it to night drainage.

   While patient is on measured intake and output, remember to subtract 8 ounces from urinary output.
3. Urostomy bags should be attached with tubing to a drainage bag at the bedside every night.
4. Threads of mucus in the urine of a patient with an ileal conduit are normal, but be alert for signs of urinary tract infection (*e.g.*, foul-smelling urine or pain in the back in the kidney region).

Sources of Information

- If your hospital has an enterostomal therapist, he or she is your nearest and most expert source of assistance in your care of patients with ostomies, fistulas, and draining wounds.
- United Ostomy Association, 2001 W. Beverly Blvd., Los Angeles, CA 90057. Telephone: 213-413-5510. Local branches of the association are in most cities.
- American Cancer Society, 777 Third Ave., New York, NY 10017. There are local branches of the society.
- Companies that are manufacturers of ostomy equipment will do inservice education programs on the use of their products. They offer good written material on their products and on ostomy care.

OXYGEN ADMINISTRATION

Description

Oxygen is a significant component of the air we breathe, and it is essential for sustaining life. When administered artificially, it must be handled and considered as a drug, and therefore considered capable of harm if misused. Oxygen must be administered at the prescribed flow rate, which should be governed by arterial blood-gas analysis. Oxygen should be humidified to prevent dryness of the respiratory tract. This humidification substitutes for the natural humidity in normal air. Oxygen is highly combustible, especially when concentrated. Specific precautions should be taken to avoid open flame or electrical sparks within any area where oxygen is being administered. Oxygen usually is administered to an adult by either a face mask that covers the nose and mouth, or by a nasal prong or catheter. An isolette, plastic hood, or tent may be used to deliver oxygen to an infant or small child. In the case of a tracheostomy, a "T" tube or special tracheostomy mask is used to introduce the oxygen into the trachea.

Starting and Maintaining Oxygen Therapy

Isolette Method

- The infant is placed inside the isolette, which has controlled temperature, humidity, and an oxygen flow.
- The level of oxygen may fluctuate, so a plastic hood is used inside the isolette to deliver precise oxygen concentrations.
- If a hood is not used, check the oxygen level frequently.

Oxygen Hood Method

- The infant's head is kept covered by the hood. If necessary, pad the edges to protect against contact with skin surfaces. Avoid having the oxygen flow directly onto the infant's face.
- A constant oxygen flow is delivered and a high concentration of oxygen can be delivered rapidly. Know the prescribed flow rate of oxygen and the method of monitoring it.
- High humidity within the hood will require keeping the linen dry, as well as frequent emptying of condensation buildup in the tubing.

Oxygen Tent Method

- Oxygen is delivered into a plastic tent. The patient is placed inside, and the tent must be snugly tucked into the bedding to prevent oxygen loss. Whenever the tent is opened, it will take 15 minutes to 20 minutes to restore the desired oxygen concentration.
- Know the prescribed oxygen flow rate, the method of monitoring it, and the temperature within the tent. The oxygen concentration must be analyzed frequently and the temperature and humidity controlled to keep the patient comfortable.

Nasal Prong Method

- The nasal prong has two small projections that hook onto the nose and direct oxygen into the nostrils.
- Turn the oxygen on at a low flow rate.
- Insert the prongs in the nose and the tubing over the ears.
- Turn the oxygen to the prescribed flow rate.
- Sinus pain, headache, and sore nostrils often occur as a result of the direct oxygen flow into the nostrils.

Nasal Catheter Method

- This consists of a tube that is inserted through one nostril and into the throat.
- Measure from the tip of the nose to the earlobe for the proper insertion length.
- Turn on the oxygen at a low flow rate.
- Insert the lubricated catheter into a nasal passage.
- The tip of the catheter should extend to slightly above the uvula.
- Turn the oxygen to the prescribed flow rate.
- Tape the catheter to the nose. Alternate nostril insertion every 8 hours.
- Check for possible abdominal distention resulting from oxygen flow to the stomach, which happens if the catheter is advanced too far.

Simple Face Mask

- This mask connects directly to the oxygen supply tubing.
- Turn on the oxygen at a low flow rate.
- Explain to the patient that to provide necessary oxygen, the mask must be fitted snugly. Exhaled air is expelled through vents in the sides of the mask.
- Turn the oxygen to the prescribed flow rate after the mask is in place.

Partial Rebreathing Mask

- This mask has a reservoir bag between it and the oxygen supply tubing.
- Turn on the oxygen at a low flow rate.
- Fill the reservoir bag with oxygen by momentarily closing the opening between the bag and the mask.
- Explain to the patient that the mask must be fitted snugly to provide the necessary oxygen. The reservoir bag should deflate slightly with inspiration.
- Turn the oxygen to the prescribed flow rate after the mask is in place.
- The patient rebreathes approximately 33% of expired air as a result of the reservoir bag. This air still contains a high percentage of oxygen.

Non-Rebreathing Mask

- This mask is similar to the partial rebreathing mask, except that two one-way valves ensure that only the source oxygen is delivered from the bag to the patient. This mask allows delivery of more concentrated oxygen than do other masks.

- Turn on the oxygen at a low flow rate.
- Fill the reservoir bag by momentarily closing the one-way valve between the mask and the bag.
- Explain to the patient that the mask must fit well.
- The one-way valves prevent rebreathing exhaled air. Be sure the oxygen delivery tubing is not obstructed. This is the only effective way the patient can receive any oxygen since outside air is shut off by the valve system.
- Set the oxygen at the prescribed flow rate.
- Empty any water that may accumulate in the bag.

Venturi Mask

- This mask functions by using the physics of the Bernoulli effect to maintain a constant mixture of air and source oxygen in the mask. No reservoir bag is required.
- Venturi masks are used to administer a carefully regulated flow of oxygen to patients who are extremely sensitive to oxygen concentrations.
- Turn on the oxygen at the prescribed flow rate, which is marked on the mask.
- Explain to the patient that room air is mixed wih source oxygen to deliver an accurate oxygen concentration.
- The mask must fit well.
- Be sure the air-entry openings on the mask are always clear and unobstructed.
- Separate humidification is not required because enough room air is mixed with the oxygen to provide humidification.

T Tube Method

- The base opening of a T tube is attached to an endotracheal or tracheostomy tube to conduct warm humidified oxygen. One arm is connected to the source oxygen nebulizer and the other arm is open to the atmosphere.
- A nebulizer is used to provide the high humidity necessary for patients with a tracheostomy. A continuous mist should exhaust from the T tube opening that goes to the atmospheric air. This shows that room air is not diluting the source oxygen.
- Water collects in the tubing and the tubing must be disconnected to empty the water.

Tracheostomy Mask

- This is similar to a simple face mask, except that it is shaped to cover the tracheostomy opening.
- See comments under "T" Tube Method, above.

Nursing Considerations

- Inspired oxygen should have minimal bacterial contamination. The oxygen delivery equipment must *never* be shared by other patients. Humidifiers and nebulizers must be kept scrupulously clean and filled with sterile water. Nebulizers are more apt to cause infection than are humidifiers.
- Continuous oxygen therapy, using a mask, should never be interrupted, except for short intervals, such as to wash and dry the patient's face in order to prevent necrosis of facial tissues.
- Nasal prongs can be substituted for masks when the patient is eating or drinking.
- Portable oxygen tanks should be used by patients on continuous oxygen therapy when they leave their beds.
- Never place oxygen delivery equipment on a patient before turning on the oxygen. This will avoid a sudden oxygen surge or aspiration of water in the tubing.
- Aspirations can be a problem with masks if the patient vomits.
- No electric razors should be used by patients receiving oxygen.
- Arterial blood gases should be done at least daily on patients receiving continuous oxygen.

POSTURAL DRAINAGE

Description

Postural drainage enables gravity flow of retained secretions from the lung segments into the bronchi and trachea, where they may be expectorated or suctioned. Each position is specific for draining of a bronchopulmonary segment (Fig. 3-13).

Nursing Considerations

- Make certain that the patient understands as much as possible about the procedure. Plan to stay with the patient during the first sequence of positions to determine the tolerance for the procedure which usually is done three to four times a day. *Never do the procedure immediately after meals.*
- Watch for symptoms of postural hypotension, and discontinue the procedure if dyspnea, tachycardia, or chest pain occurs.
- Inhalation therapy to help loosen secretions is beneficial when done before postural drainage.
- Auscultate the chest before and after the procedure to determine its effectiveness.
- Vital signs should be monitored before and, as indicated, during this treatment.
- Align the patient to be as comfortable and relaxed as possible in

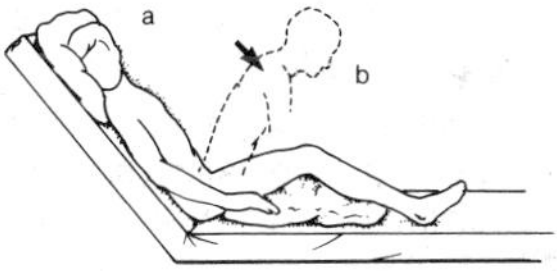

1 Upper lope: (a) apical segment (anterior)
(b) apical segment (posterior)

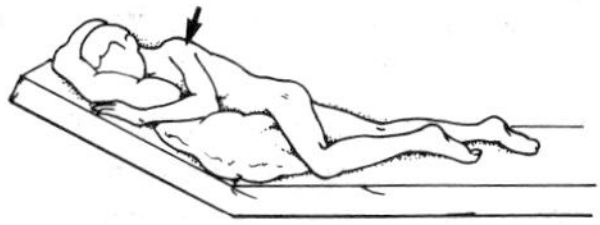

2 Left upper lobe: posterior segment

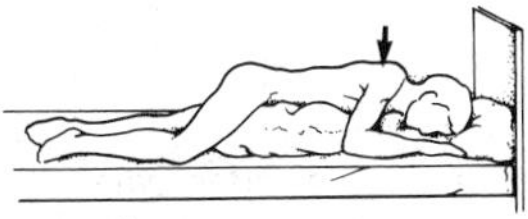

3 Right upper lobe: posterior segment

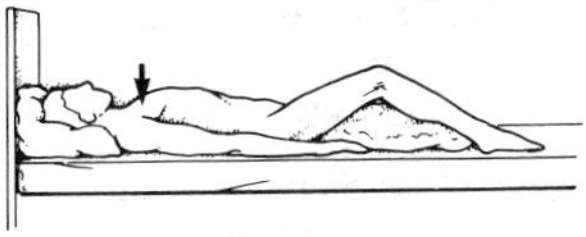

4 Upper lobes: anterior segments

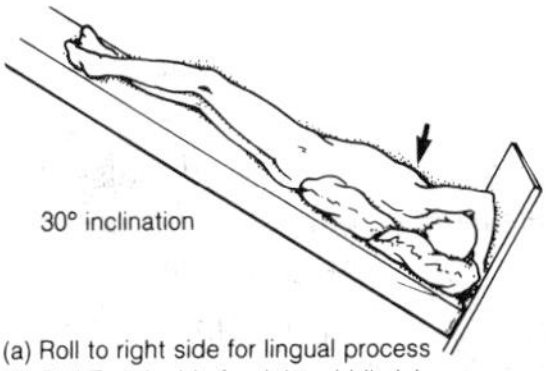

5 (a) Roll to right side for lingual process
(b) Roll To left side for right middle lobe

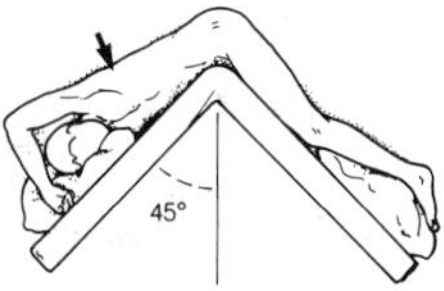

6 Lower lobe: lateral basal segment
(a) Roll to left for right lower lobe
(b) Roll to right for left lower lobe

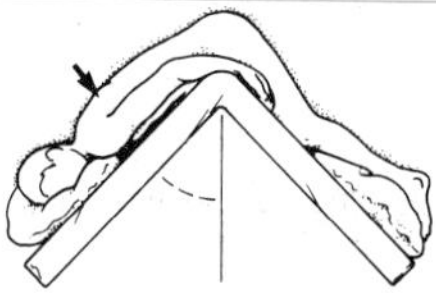

7 Lower lobes: posterior basal segments

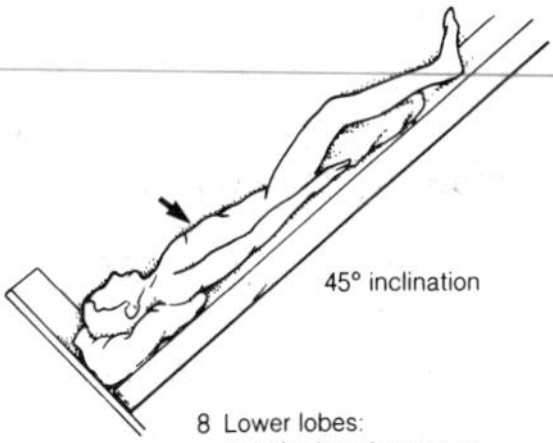

8 Lower lobes:
anterior basal segment

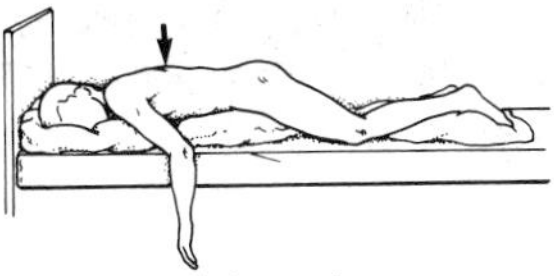

9 Lower lobes apical segments

Fig. 3-13. *Postural drainage positions.*

each position, using pillows or other supports. Infants usually are positioned while being held on the care-giver's lap.

- Coughing should be encouraged; be certain that paper tissues and a sputum collection container are available. Also, suction equipment may be necessary, especially for infants and small children.

POSTURAL HYPOTENSION (ORTHOSTATIC HYPOTENSION)

Description

Postural hypotension is an early sign of reduced blood volume, atherosclerotic vascular disease, or a possible effect of medication (*e.g.*, Aldomet) (see PH). It is indicated by a sharp drop in the patient's blood pressure when the patient assumes an upright position.

Observations

- Take the patient's blood pressure (BP) and apical pulse (AP) while the patient is lying down. Have the patient sit up and then stand beside the bed. Retake the BP and AP in these positions.
- An orthostatic drop of 10 mm Hg to 15 mm Hg in the systolic pressure may occur, but should not last longer than 3 minutes. However, a prolonged drop of 30 mm Hg is indicative of postural hypotension.
- Fainting may occur.

Nursing Considerations

- Advise the patient not to rise from the supine to the sitting or standing position too rapidly.
- Straining may cause changes in BP.
- Patients should consult with the pharmacist before using over-the-counter medications.
- Waist-high elastic stockings assist in blood return from the legs to the heart when the patient is standing. They should be removed while the patient is in bed, and replaced before the patient gets up.

RANGE OF MOTION EXERCISES

Description

Range of motion (ROM) exercises are done to maintain or restore full use of a joint or joints. Moving a joint through its normal ROM may be done actively or passively. In passive ROM, someone assists the patient. A physician's order is required if a pathological condition is present (*e.g.,* arthritis, fracture, or an acute cardiac condition).

Nursing Considerations

- Never move a patient's joint to the point of pain. Stop before pain or fatigue is felt.
- With the joint supported, move it slowly and rhythmically through its ROM about five times.
- When full ROM exercises are ordered, every joint should be moved: start with the head and neck, then the shoulder, elbow, wrist, and fingers; and then the hips to toes. Exercises usually are done three times a day.
- Progress from passive to active ROM as soon as possible by teaching the patient to do it himself. In case of paralysis, the affected extremity can be assisted by the good one.

RENAL BIOPSY

Description

A percutaneous needle biopsy of the kidney may make a definitive diagnosis possible by providing information about the glomeruli and tubules. Hemorrhage—causing hematuria, hematoma, or flank pain—is a serious risk with this procedure. Open renal biopsy (with specimen for electron microscopy) is also done.

Nursing Considerations

Percutaneous Needle Biopsy

- An informed consent is required.
- Pressure is applied to the area for 20 minutes following the procedure. A pressure dressing should remain on the site for 24 hours.
- Bed rest for 24 hours is usually ordered.
- Vital signs, color of urine, hemoglobin, and hematocrit must be checked frequently.
- Fluids should be forced.

Open Renal Biopsy

- The same nursing care as for kidney surgery is required.

ROTATING TOURNIQUETS

Description

Rotating tourniquets assist in the treatment of left ventricular heart failure by decreasing the work of the heart. These tourniquets are applied in a rotating sequence to the four extremities to decrease the amount of blood returning to the heart. This is an emergency treatment for pulmonary edema.

Establishing and Maintaining Rotating Tourniquets

- Place the patient in Fowler's position.
- Take the blood pressure before inflating the tourniquets, and then every 15 minutes.
- Apply the tourniquets as high as possible on all four extremities. Do not place a cuff on an arm with an IV line.
- Inflate three of the tourniquets to slightly less than the diastolic blood pressure. Distal pulses must always remain palpable. Arterial constriction from overly tight tourniquets must be avoided. Check skin color of extremities frequently.
- Rotate inflation of tourniquets so that each extremity has a 15-minute noninflated period out of every 60 minutes.
- Ensure that no extremity is compressed for more than 45 minutes. In elderly patients, tourniquets may be rotated every 5 minutes.
- Release the tourniquets in a clockwise pattern, and *never* all at the same time. Keep the 15-minute spacing between each release.
- Check and record urine output hourly.
- When a rotating tourniquet machine is used, the pressure adjustment of the cuffs should be in the 20-mm to 50-mm range to slow down venous return but not cut off arterial flow. The machine is not used for more than 3 hours to 4 hours.
- Assess the patient's heart and lungs frequently in the hour after removal of the tourniquets.

THORACENTESIS

Description

Needle aspiration of either pleural fluid or air from the pleural space may be done for either therapeutic or diagnostic purposes. In some cases, medications may be injected into the pleural space. The procedure is done with local anesthesia, using sterile technique. See your agency procedure book.

Nursing Considerations

- Informed consent must be signed.
- The patient's position will be designated by the physician. An upright position facilitates removal of fluid.

- Caution patient against sudden movements or coughing during the procedure.
- Monitor pulse and respirations. Observe for untoward symptoms during and after the procedure (*e.g.,* respiratory difficulties including dyspnea, uncontrolled coughing, and blood-tinged or frothy sputum; also, shock, pallor, cyanosis, weakness, diaphoresis, and pain).
- Possible complications include shock, pneumothorax (with possible mediastinal shift), infection, and electrolyte imbalances. (See MSN Postoperative complications; MSN, Respiratory system, pneumothorax)
- Fluid is removed slowly, the amount limited to 1,000 ml at one time.
- After the procedure:
  1. Apply small, sterile pressure dressing to the site.
  2. Position patient so that he or she is lying with the puncture site up to minimize leakage from it.
  3. Take vital signs every hour for 4 hours following the procedure, and longer if indicated.
  4. Record the amount and character of the withdrawn fluid. Care for specimens appropriately.

TRACHEO/ORO/NASOPHARYNGEAL SUCTIONING

Description

Suctioning of the trachea, along with the oropharynx or nasopharynx, is done to clear and maintain an open airway. The suction catheter may be inserted by way of the mouth or nose, or through an artificial airway (*e.g.,* tracheostomy).

Nursing Considerations

- Assess the need for suctioning by observing the patient's respirations and coughing, or by auscultating the chest.
- When possible, know the patient's arterial blood gases (see LAB), to best evaluate the respiratory status.
- Assess the patient's breath sounds and vital signs before and after suctioning.
- If the patient is able to comprehend the procedure, explain it before starting.
- Suction only when necessary and not as a routine procedure. There is a risk of excessive trauma with frequent suctioning. Also, hypoxemia and stimulation of the vagus nerve can lead to cardiac arrhythmias. Always have oxygen available.
- Suctioning should always be a sterile procedure in the hospital.

Always wear two gloves when suctioning although only the dominant hand needs to remain sterile; the other gloved hand is for the nurse's protection. Rinse the catheters with sterile saline during the procedure. Dispose of the catheter and remaining saline after completion of suctioning. If the mouth and nose need suctioning, use a separate catheter for suctioning the trachea.

- The setting of the suction apparatus should read between 80 mm Hg and 120 mm Hg when the suction port is occluded.
- *Never* apply suction (occlude the port) while inserting the catheter. Suction should not exceed 8 seconds to 10 seconds, and should be applied while withdrawing and gently rotating the catheter. After only 5 seconds of suctioning, there is a significant fall in oxygenation.
- Allow time for four or five breaths between each catheter insertion, or a self-inflating bag (*e.g.,* Ambu bag) may be used. Depending on the patient's condition, the bag may be connected to oxygen. Hyperinflation and oxygenation of the lungs prevents atelectasis and hypoxia, and should be done before and after the suctioning is completed.
- Note the color, amount, odor, and consistency of secretions, as well as the frequency of suctioning and vital signs. It is important to report any changes as well as any increase in the need for suctioning.

Oro/Nasopharyngeal Suctioning

- When there is suspected cerebrospinal fluid discharge from the nose, or when there is a bleeding disorder, do *not* pass the catheter through or do any nasopharyngeal suctioning.
- Oropharyngeal suctioning can stimulate the gag reflex. It may be difficult if the patient bites the tube; a padded tongue blade can be used to separate the teeth.
- For nasopharyngeal suctioning, lubricate the catheter (a size 14 or 16 French) and insert it 3 inches to 5 inches into the nares. If it is possible, ask the patient to take deep breaths and cough. This aids in allowing the catheter insertion past the nasopharynx and into the trachea. Alternate nares for repeated suctioning.
- With an unconscious patient, grasp the tongue and hold it out of the mouth for ease in passing the catheter from the nose to throat.

Tracheobronchial Suctioning Through a Tracheostomy

- When performing tracheostomy suctioning, a size 14 to 16 French catheter is used and it should not exceed one-third the diameter of the lumen of the tube.
- Insert the suction catheter toward the bronchus to be suctioned.
- When resistance is met, withdraw the catheter about 1 cm. The patient's head should be turned in the opposite direction from the

bronchus to be suctioned. Suction is not applied until the catheter is withdrawn, again using a pill rolling movement of the fingers to prevent it from adhering to the mucosal lining. Release the suction for a moment if it does adhere.

- When the secretions are very thick or cannot be aspirated and the patient is congested, it may mean that there is inadequate humidification. Be certain a mist collar is being used. A few drops of sterile saline solution may be instilled into the trachea to loosen the secretions; usually 0.5 ml is needed in infants, and 0.8 ml in adults.

Pediatric Nursing Considerations

- Suctioning should not exceed 5 seconds in an infant or small child. Again, allow time for three to four breaths before resuctioning, or use an Ambu bag connected to an oxygen source.
- A size 6 French suction catheter may be adequate for suctioning a neonate if the secretions are not too thick. A size 8 to 10 French may be used for children. *Never* occlude the total air passage with the catheter. *Never* exceed 100 mm Hg suction for infants.
- In tracheostomy suctioning, a catheter should not exceed one-third the diameter of the lumen of the tracheostomy. There must be room for adequate air passage around the catheter.
- Early signs of respiratory distress in an infant are tachycardia and restlessness.

TRACHEOSTOMY CARE

Description

A tracheostomy is a surgically provided, direct connection using a tube from a neck stoma to the trachea. When it is necessary to artificially maintain an open airway for longer than 72 hours, a tracheotomy is usually performed. An emergency, temporary open airway can be obtained without surgery by using an endotracheal intubation tube.

Maintenance and Care of a Tracheostomy

- The obturator to the tracheostomy tube in place must be kept in sight (*e.g.*, taped at the head of the bed).
- An extra tracheostomy set (same size) should be kept at the bedside. In case of accidental expulsion, keep the stoma open with a hemostat.
- A suction machine must always be at the bedside.
- Tracheostomy tubes are made of metal or plastic. Metal tubes have removable cannulas. Plastic tubes may or may not have removable inner cannulas.

- Tracheostomy care must be done with sterile technique in hospitals; however, clean technique is taught in home care. Pulmonary infection can be a serious complication of tracheostomies. Dust and lint enter directly into the lungs. Never use cotton-filled gauze for tracheostomy dressing.
- If there is a removable inner cannula, take it out and clean it as needed immediately following surgery, and then at least every 8 hours. Clean it with hydrogen peroxide, sterile water, and sterile pipe cleaners. Suction the outer cannula before replacing the inner cannula; replace and lock.
- Wash the skin around the stoma with hydrogen peroxide, rinsing with sterile water/saline at least every 8 hours. Replace a soiled dressing as needed, keeping the area as dry as possible. Observe for wound infections. Be gentle because the skin may be very tender.
- Mouth care should be provided at the same time as tracheostomy care. The mouth tends to be very dry.
- Since the upper airway is bypassed, air must be warmed and humidified. Often, a tube from a nebulizer is attached with a T tube or tracheostomy mask to the opening of the tracheostomy tube. Disconnect the tubing at the tracheostomy tube connection to empty the condensed water that accumulates in the tubing. Check the nebulizer at the beginning of every shift for an adequate water level. All water and medications to be nebulized must be sterile. Equipment and medication must *never* be shared with other patients.
- Some tracheostomy tubes have a built-in inflatable cuff that produces a tight seal in the trachea. These cuffs are deflated or inflated according to the physician's orders. It is common practice to inflate the cuff prior to an oral or tube feeding and for 30 minutes afterward to prevent aspiration.
- To prevent pressure necrosis on the tracheal wall, the cuff must never be overinflated; pressure usually is kept below 15 mm Hg. Know the exact pressures to be maintained in the cuff, and how to verify the pressure.
- Always suction the nose and mouth before deflating a tracheal cuff to prevent aspiration of mucus. Discard this suction catheter and use a new sterile catheter for removing tracheobronchial secretions.
- Leakage of food particles from a tracheostomy indicates a fistula between the esophagus and the trachea. Notify the physician immediately.
- It is important to teach the patient to cough in order to help prevent pulmonary infection. Often, taking a deep breath and momentarily covering the tracheostomy opening will produce a cough.

- Teach the patient to stabilize the tube with the fingers during a cough, and to cover the tracheostomy when coughing.
- When the tracheostomy ties are changed, one nurse should stabilize the tube to prevent accidental expulsion, while another nurse changes the ties.
- The ties should be tight enough to allow only two fingers beneath them.
- The ties must be knotted at the side of the neck. The gown should have snap closures or be tied in front to prevent accidental untying of the knot.
- Unless a laryngectomy has been done, speaking a few words can be accomplished by taking a breath and momentarily covering the tracheostomy opening.

Pediatric Nursing Considerations

- Restrain the hands of an infant or young child and never leave unattended.
- Provide support for an infant's head, so the chin does not cover the opening of the tracheostomy.
- Use half-strength hydrogen peroxide when cleaning the skin around the stoma, rinsing with sterile saline.
- The neck ties should be tight enough to only allow one finger tip between the ties and the neck, and should be changed daily or as often as necessary.
- Signs of respiratory distress in an infant or small child are cyanosis around the mouth and nose, tachypnea, tachycardia, and restlessness.

TRACTION

Description

Traction is a pulling force applied to a part of the body. It provides alignment and stability to a fracture site by reducing the fracture and maintaining correct position. It may prevent flexion contractures, reduce deformity (in scoliosis), and lessen muscle spasm (*e.g.*, back pain). If the part is elevated above the heart, it may reduce edema.

Countertraction is a pull in the opposite direction of the pull of the traction.

Most traction is continuously applied, although cervical and pelvic traction may be intermittent.

- In straight or running traction, the pull is in one plane, and the body supplies the countertraction (*e.g.*, Buck's traction; Fig. 3-15).
- In suspension or balanced suspension, there is a lifting force to the extremity as a whole (suspension), which allows the patient

movement while the line of traction is still being maintained (*e.g.*, skeletal traction with Thomas splint and Pearson attachment; Fig. 3-18).

- Manual traction is applied during cast application.
- Skin traction (Buck's or Russell's) is applied with tapes adhered to the skin and circumferential bandages, or a Buck's boot attached to a footplate or spreader with a hook on the bottom, which attaches to a rope, pulley, and weights.
- In skeletal traction, the traction is applied directly to the bone by inserting devices such as Steinmann pins, Kirschner wire, or Crutchfield tongs into the bones. It is used with balanced suspension.

Equipment

- A bed with a firm mattress, possibly a hinged headboard; and in most cases, an overbed frame with a trapeze
- Pulleys, ropes or cords, weights (with specific amount ordered by physician), and bars for attachment of the pulleys
- In addition to the above, special types of traction may require addition equipment

1. Traction for the lower extremity may include

   A footplate to maintain normal position of the foot

   A splint to support the part

      Thomas splint (supports the thigh), with Pearson attachment (supports the calf); it is used with skeletal traction

      Bohler-Braun is an inclined plane splint. The frame rests on the bed; it may be used with skin or skeletal traction of lower extremity

2. Pelvic traction

   A belt, measured to fit (See Nursing Considerations under Pelvic traction.)

   Straps that extend from belt to spreader, which is attached to traction rope

3. Cervical traction may be provided with one of the following:

   Head halter

   Crutchfield, Barton, Vinke, or Gardner Wells tongs for skull traction, with a bed frame that provides for turning. (*e.g.*, Foster or Stryker frame)

   Halo-skeletal traction

General Nursing Considerations

- The patient's body should be in good alignment; it should provide at least some countertraction. The patient's position in bed and the limitations of movement will be specified by the physician.
- The pull of the traction on extremities should be in alignment with the long axis of the bone.
- Keep the patient pulled up in bed. Footplate or knots should not touch pulley or foot of bed. Traction should be continuous (unless otherwise ordered).
- Teach the patient to use trapeze to lift back, buttocks, and shoulders off bed in a straight line.
- Eliminate possibilities of friction along the line from the patient to the weights.
  1. Weights must hang free. Never remove weights without a physician's order. Keep them off the floor and off the bed.
  2. Keep cords free of obstruction and free of linens.
- Be sure that ropes are not frayed, that knots are well tied (square knots) and taped, and that ropes are on center track of pulley.
- A sketch of the traction set-up in the nursing-care plan is extremely helpful.
- Bed making is usually easiest from top to bottom.
- Always investigate patient's complaints. Check for signs of neurovascular impairment: pain, pallor, pulselessness, paralysis, or paresthesia (tingling or numbness).
- Prevent complications of immobility.
  1. Pulmonary (See NR, Deep breathing techniques.)
  2. Circulatory (See MSN, Postoperative care, preventing vascular complication.)
  3. Constipation and fecal impaction
  4. Decubiti (See MSN.)
  5. Renal calculi (See MSN, Urinary tract and the prostate)
  6. Muscular atrophy/contracture
  7. Emotional problems: boredom, depression, and, sometimes, adjustment to changed body image

BRYANT'S TRACTION

Description

This is a skin traction applied to both legs that holds them in a vertical extension. (Fig. 3-14). It is used to reduce fractured femurs in small children.

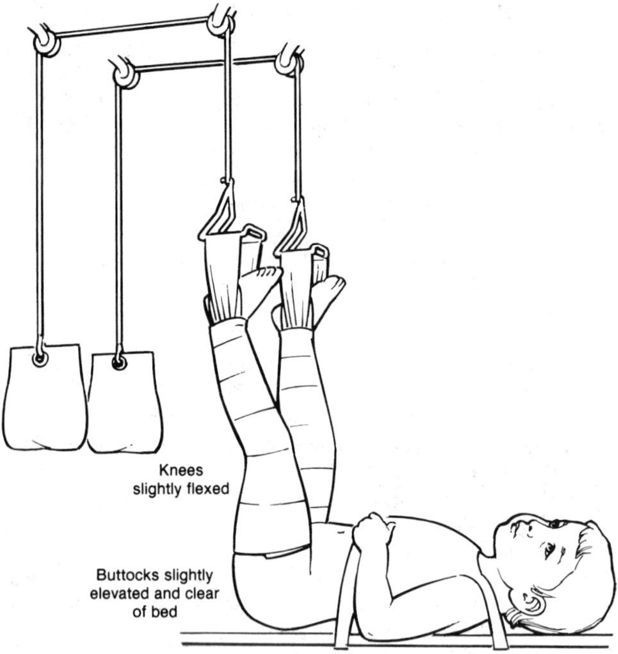

Fig. 3-14. *Bryant's traction.*

Nursing Considerations

- See general nursing considerations for traction.
- The hips and buttocks are kept elevated and clear of the bed. The child needs to be kept on the back and prevented from turning onto the side.
- The foot of the bed may be elevated on blocks to keep the child from being pulled down to the end of the bed; a jacket or harness may be used.
- Ace bandages are wrapped around the legs to keep the skin traction in place. Rewrap the legs twice a day. Observe the skin condition. Checks for circulation impairment should be done frequently. Pay particular attention to the inner aspects of the ankle and the heel. Be certain the heel is free of pressure.

BUCK'S EXTENSION

Description

As a running skin traction, Buck's extension may be applied with tapes that are adhered to the skin (secured by circumferential bandages, usually elastic) and attached to a footplate or spreader with a hook on the bottom (Fig. 3-15). But currently, it is most commonly applied with a prepadded "Buck's" boot. Either set-up attaches to a rope, pulley, and weights, with the specific amount of weight prescribed by the physician. Buck's traction can be applied for only short periods of time. Therefore, it usually is ordered for temporary immobilization of hip fractures (particularly subcapital fractures) before surgical fixation. It also may be used to immobilize the leg in abduction following total hip replacement.

Nursing Considerations

- See general nursing considerations for traction.
- Buck's boot must be the proper size. With the physician's order, Buck's traction is usually released every 8 hours for inspection of skin.
- Traction tapes can be applied only to skin in good condition. Circumferential bandages should be applied in spiral turns, be wrinkle free, and not too tight. Footplate or spreader must be wide enough to prevent tapes from rubbing ankle. Observe for, document, and report any of the following:
    1. Numbness, tingling, swelling, change in color, pain, decreased sensitivity to heat, cold, or touch, disturbance in the mobility of the foot—all are signs of neurovascular impairment. Avoid pressure on the peroneal nerve (3 inches below knee on outer aspect).
    2. Complaints of burning or irritation under the bandage, slipping of the tapes, a feeling of sponginess under the bandage (indicating possible skin breakdown)
    3. Tightness of elastic bandage caused by swelling

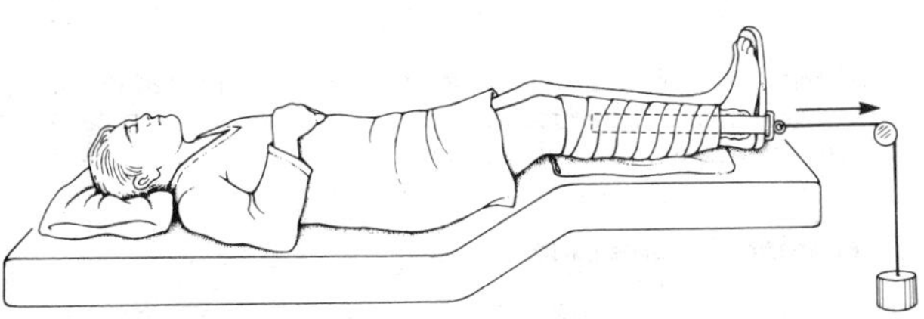

Fig. 3-15. *Buck's traction.*

- With either skin traction or Buck's boot, avoid pressure on the Achilles' tendon and the heel by placing a folded bath blanket under the calf or by using heel protectors. Cotton may be used to protect the malleolus.
- Keep patient pulled up in bed, with the body in alignment.
- The patient's position in bed and his limitations of movement will be specified by the physician.
- Usually, the patient may be turned to a 45° angle with a pillow between his legs for back care.
- Back care is very important. Massage with one hand while pushing mattress down with other. An egg-crate mattress is frequently ordered.

CERVICAL TRACTION: CERVICAL SKIN TRACTION

Description

Traction applied with a head halter is applied as tolerated. It usually is used for cervical myositis and minor fractures.

Nursing Considerations

See general nursing considerations for traction.

- The spreader must be wide enough to prevent pressure on the side of the head.
- Protect the patient's chin, ears, and back of head with padding. Give gentle massage, if permitted.
- Give frequent shampoos for cleanliness and stimulation of the scalp, if ordered by physician.
- Soft foods may be indicated to minimize chewing.

CERVICAL TRACTION: CRUTCHFIELD, BARTON, GARDNER WELLS, OR VINKE TONGS

Description

Crutchfield, Barton, Gardner Wells or Vinke tongs placed in the top of the skull make continuous skeletal traction possible in cases of severe cervical fractures or dislocation.

Nursing Considerations

See general nursing considerations for traction.

- A bed frame that provides for turning (*e.g.*, Roto Rest bed, Egerton Stoke Mandeville tilting and turning bed) is required.

- Motor sensory changes should be reported immediately (*e.g.*, loss of muscle strength, projectile vomiting, and respiratory distress).
- Check for bleeding around the tongs and for skin breakdown on the back of the head. (Protect the occipital area from pressure. Massage and shampoo prn if ordered.)
- Turn on frame every 2 hours. See hospital procedure for how to use Stryker frame or turning bed.
- Because of the difficulty the patient experiences in eating and drinking in the supine position and the consequent danger of aspiration, suction equipment should be at the bedside.
- Make the foundation of the bed with two drawsheets instead of one full-length sheet.
- Prism glasses for reading and for watching television will be helpful for the patient who must remain flat.

CERVICAL TRACTION: HALO-SKELETAL TRACTION

Description

The halo-skeletal traction device is another way to immobilize the cervical spine. A stainless steel ring fits around the head and is secured in place with four skull pins. The ring then is attached to a body vest of plaster or plastic to give it stability.

Nursing Considerations

- Assess neurovascular status at least q 8 hr
- Incentive spirometer
- Trained personnel should remove vest daily for skin care and inspection.
- Keep inner padding dry and clean.
- Range of motion exercises (See NR, Range of motion exercises.)
- Provide pin care as ordered to keep areas of pin insertion into the skull free from infection.
- Inspect the device to be sure that all screws are tight. Tools for adjustments should be at bedside or attached to the vest.

PELVIC TRACTION

Description

For possible herniated disc or back strain, traction is applied to the pelvis by means of a girdle or belt worn by the patient. The traction usually is applied on an "as tolerated" basis at 20 pounds to 30 pounds.

Nursing Considerations

- Proper fit of the girdle is essential. Measure pelvic circumference to ascertain size. The top edge of the belt should be at the iliac crest, and the lower part slightly below the greater trochanter.
- Watch for signs of skin irritation over iliac crests.
- Movement and position
  1. The back must be kept straight, level, and in proper alignment.
  2. A pillow may be allowed under the head, and the bed may be gatched at the knees with the angle of hips to knees from 45° to 60°, and with feet level with knees (Williams' position, Fig. 3-16) to provide countertraction.
  3. The patient should not bend or twist his back.
  4. A signal bell must be within easy reach.
- The spreader bar used to maintain equal pulling force on straps must be kept parallel to the foot of bed.
- Constipation can aggravate back discomfort. Plan an individualized bowel program to prevent it.
- Lack of sensation in legs should be reported to physician immediately.
- For reapplication of pelvic traction, apply belt carefully, and suspend weights slowly and smoothly.
- Keep the patient's feet, as well as belt straps, free of bed linens.
- Use fracture bedpan if bathroom privileges are not granted.

RUSSELL'S TRACTION

Description

This is a skin traction similar to Buck's, in which balanced suspension is provided by a sling under the knee (Fig. 3-17). Russell's traction is used in the treatment of some femoral fractures (preferred in intertrochanteric and subtrochanteric types), and for some knee injuries.

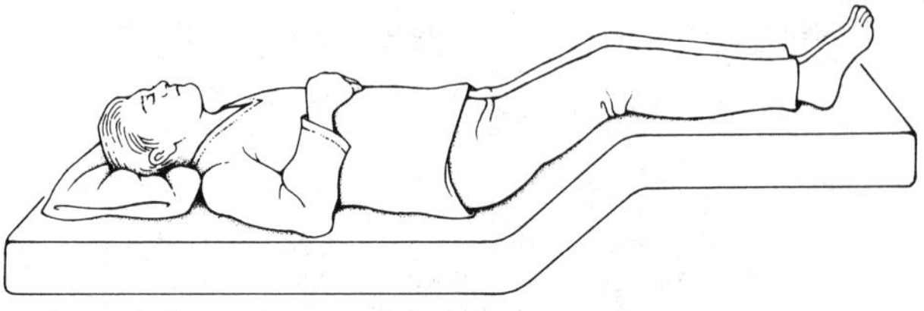

Fig. 3-16. *Williams' position. Degree of flexion at the hips may vary depending upon purpose of positioning.*

Nursing Considerations

See general nursing considerations for traction.

The physician will leave specific orders for the positioning of the patient and for the limits of movement. The following are general guidelines that usually will apply.

- The knee sling should elevate the calf enough to produce a 20° angle between the patient's hip and the bed, with the calf parallel to the bed. This relationship should be maintained in all positions. The heel should clear the bed.
- Movement
  1. The patient can lift with the trapeze, pushing downward with the unaffected leg while keeping the waist straight.
  2. External or internal rotation of the upper leg is prohibited.
  3. The lower body may be tilted, and movement of the whole body toward the foot or the head of the bed may be permitted for short periods of time only.
- Check popliteal space for evidence of pressure or skin irritation. The area may be padded with a piece of felt or sheepskin.
- Whether or not to have a pillow supporting the calf is part of the physician's traction plan. Find out what it is, and maintain as originally set up. Be sure it is noted on nursing-care plan.
- Check for color, warmth, sensation, and movement of the foot (ability to plantarflex and dorsiflex). Provide a footplate.
- Nursing considerations under Buck's extension traction apply here.

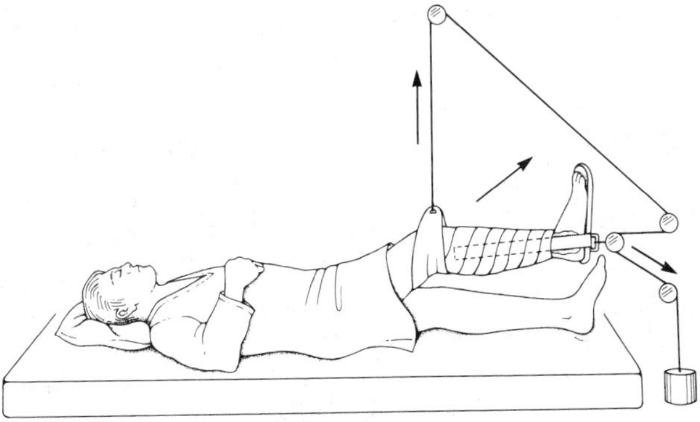

Fig. 3-17. *Russell's traction.*

THOMAS SPLINT WITH PEARSON ATTACHMENT AND SKELETAL TRACTION

Description

To reduce a fracture of the femur, hip, or lower leg, skeletal traction is applied by inserting a metal pin or wire (*e.g.*, Steinmann pin or Kirschner wire) into or through a bone distal to the fracture, and then applying traction directly to it. Balanced suspension is supplied by the Thomas splint, which supports the thigh, and the Pearson attachment, which supports the lower leg in a position parallel to the bed (Fig. 3-18). The knee is flexed about 45°. The advantage of this set-up is that the patient can lift his leg and move his body, furthering better circulation.

Nursing Considerations

See general nursing tips for traction.

The physician will leave specific orders for the patient's position in bed and limitations of movement. The following are general guidelines that will usually apply.

- Movement
  1. Most movements can be done within limits of patient's tolerance.
  2. External or internal rotation of the leg is prohibited.

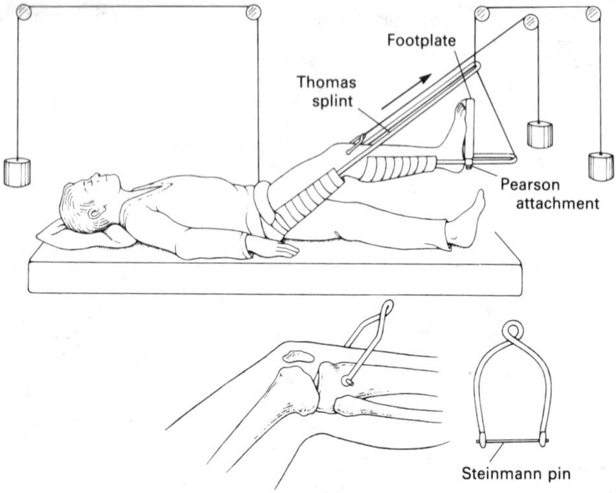

Fig. 3-18. *Skeletal traction with Thomas splint and Pearson attachment.*

3. When raising the body, the patient should push downward on the unaffected leg and keep the waist unbent.

- Check the color, pulse, temperature, and ability to plantarflex and dorsiflex both feet at least once each shift. Position footplate appropriately.
- Pressure points that require attention are the popliteal space, the Achilles' tendon, the heel, and the peroneal nerve (3 inches below knee on outer aspect), especially if the splint has tipped with movement. A tendency to invert the foot and difficulty in extending the toes are signs of peroneal nerve impairment.
- Material under the splint should be smooth; there should be no extra padding between the leather ring and the skin.
- Keep the ring of the Thomas splint dry and clean, with half-ring positioned over the anterior aspect of the thigh. Check groin and areas where ring might rub for signs of pressure or irritation.
- Inspect pin sites every shift for redness or other signs of infection. Give pin care, as ordered. Pin care varies, but one method consists of cleansing around the site with hydrogen peroxide solution, using a separate sterile applicator for each pin, at least every shift during the first postoperative days. After 4 or 5 days, use alcohol sponges to clean around the pin. The area may be allowed to remain exposed to the air. Some physicians prefer that the area be covered with a sterile dressing.
- Cleanse affected leg with either alcohol or lotion.
- Provide back care to prevent skin breakdown. An egg-crate mattress or alternating pressure mattress may be helpful.

TRANSCUTANEOUS ELECTRICAL NERVE STIMULATION (TENS)

Description

Transcutaneous electrical nerve stimulation (TENS) provides a noninvasive alternative to traditional pain management with narcotic analgesics. When it is used in combination with narcotic analgesia, the drug dosage usually can be reduced. One advantage of TENS is the reduction or elimination of narcotic side effects. Another is that the patient is in control.

TENS is being used more frequently for the relief of pain such as stump pain, phantom limb pain, sciatica, post-herpetic neuralgia, and postoperative pain.

It is not fully understood why TENS reduces pain perception, but it is believed that stimulation of large peripheral nerve fibers "closes the gate" to painful stimuli before they reach the central nervous system. Another theory is that nerve stimulation triggers the release of endorphins, the body's own opiates.

Equipment

- A battery–powered stimulator (generator) is connected by wires to electrodes on the skin. Control knobs on the stimulator adjust the electrical impulse. Adjustments can be made in the following:
  1. Amplitude: the intensity or amount of current delivered, described in milliamperes (mamps). Increasing amplitude is perceived by the patient as a flutter or tingling sensation. If the amplitude is too high, muscle contractions will occur.
  2. Pulse width: the duration of the impulse, measured in microseconds (μs). Increasing the width causes widening or deepening of the sensation. A burning or stinging sensation felt by the patient indicates that the pulse width is set too high.
  3. Frequency: the number of impulses delivered (also called the rate or repetition rate). With increased frequency, a smoother and less pulsating sensation is perceived.
- The stimulator may accommodate one set of two electrodes (single channel) or two sets of two electrodes (dual channel).
- At present, there are many TENS models on the market, and there is no standardization. Be sure to read package instructions carefully. If there are insolvable problems with one model, changing to another brand may be helpful.

Nursing Considerations

- Initial electrode placement usually is done by the physician or physiotherapist. When electrodes are temporarily removed, the site of their placement should be marked so that they can be replaced in the same position.
  1. Electrodes usually are not applied directly to the painful site, but are placed over areas where nerves supplying the affected area are nearest the surface, over the nerve trunk, or the painful derma. They usually are applied above and below, or on either side of the painful area.
  2. Electrodes should not be applied over hair, skin prep, or broken or irritated skin. They should not touch each other.
  3. They should be held firmly in place with adhesive supplied by the manufacturer or with a crepe bandage. Electroconductive jelly on the electrodes ensures good contact with the skin. (Be sure that wound drainage does not disrupt contact.)
  4. The stimulator should be removed when the patient is bathing.
  5. *Caution:* Electrodes should not be applied over the carotid sinus, laryngeal or pharyngeal muscles, or the abdomen of a pregnant woman. They also should not be used on a patient with a cardiac pacemaker.
- Adjustments to stimulator settings should be made by turning it up until it is mildly uncomfortable, and then turning it back slightly

to the place where stimulation is felt but is not uncomfortable. The area usually will feel numb after it accommodates to the tingling sensation.

1. Details of placement, regulation, and pain relief experienced should be charted carefully, so that needed adjustments can be made.

- Electrode sites should be checked twice daily for skin irritation. Should irritation occur, electrodes must be repositioned. See NR, Ostomy and draining wounds, for tips on care of irritated skin.
  1. To prevent skin irritation, be sure the skin is free of preoperative skin prep by rinsing the skin with sterile water, drying it thoroughly, and exposing it to air.
- If there is no stimulation, or if it cuts in and out, check batteries, electrodes, and connections to lead wires. Be sure that the amplitude is high enough, and that there is total contact between electrodes and skin.
- Unpleasant sensations such as itching, burning, prickling (without rash), nausea, or headache, indicate that adjustments need to be made in stimulator setting. The TENS specialist should be called if problems are unresolved.

ULTRASOUND (SONOGRAPHY)

Description

Ultrasound (sonography) uses sound waves with frequencies far above those that the human ear can detect to produce images of internal body organs and structure, and also to detect and measure internal movements, such as those produced by a beating heart.

- Ultrasound functions in the same way as radar and sonar. It produces no microwave or x-ray radiation and does not require injection of a contrast medium into the blood. It is safe and painless, and does not require invasive techniques.
- Ultrasound has a wide and growing range of application in medical diagnosis. It already has virtually replaced other imaging methods in obstetrics and the ultrasound noninvasive examinations of the heart (echocardiography) have been able to reduce the need for cardiac catheterization. Also, it is very useful in the detection of space occupying lesions in the abdomen, pancreas, and liver.
- Ultrasound scans can detect and locate deep venous thrombosis, stenosis (constriction in arteries), as well as plaque (fatty deposits) formations in the arteries.
- An ultrasound doppler stethoscope can detect blood flow and pulses that are undetectable by an ordinary stethoscope.

Nursing Considerations

- Barium studies, or any examination using air filling of an organ, should be done after ultrasonography.
- Patients scheduled for abdominal sonograms are NPO after midnight preceding the scan.
- A pelvic scan requires a full bladder; the patient should drink two to three glasses of water beforehand and not void until after the sonogram.
- Gallbladder scans necessitate a fat-free diet the day before and then NPO after midnight preceding the scan.

X-RAY PREPARATIONS

Nursing Considerations

Combined studies may be ordered without conflict of orders as outlined:

1. Gallbladder series, UGI
2. Gallbladder series, BE
3. Gallbladder series, IVP
4. IVP, BE, Gallbladder series

- Barium studies should be done, if possible, after other x-rays, scans, or sonograms, because barium tends to remain in the GI tract and obscures or distorts other studies.
- Notify the x-ray department and the physician before sending the patient for examination if the bowel preparation has not been effective.
- Never give castor oil to a weak, debilitated, or elderly patient without first discussing this with the physician. There are less severe bowel preparations.
- It is necessary to obtain a laxative or enema order following barium x-rays.
- X-ray series of the GI tract can take several hours. Be sure the patient is prepared for this with adequate covering and, if appropriate, reading or other diversional material.

BIBLIOGRAPHY • Nursing Responsibilities for Diagnosis and Treatment

Bone Marrow Aspiration and Biopsy

JOURNALS

Markus S: Taking the fear out of bone marrow examinations. Nursing '81 11(4):64, Apr 1981

Study	Preparation
Gallbladder series (oral cholecystogram)	1. 6.00 P.M., fat-free supper 2. 10:00 P.M., six (6) Oragrafin capsules 3. NPO after midnight 4. X-ray in A.M.
UGI (upper gastrointestinal tract, stomach, small bowel)	1. NPO after midnight 2. X-ray in A.M.
BE (barium enema, colon, lower GI)	1. Clear liquid diet on the day before examination 2. Laxative or enemas in the evening 3. NPO after midnight 4. X-ray in A.M.
Complete GI series	1. First day, barium enema as above 2. *Second day,* UGI as above
Intravenous Pyelogram (IVP)	1. Laxative @ 5 P.M. 2. May have liquids as desired 3. No solid food after midnight. 4. X-ray in A.M.
*IVC (bile ducts) (intravenous cholangiogram)	1. NPO after midnight 2. X-ray in A.M.
KUB (do before an IVP) (kidney, ureter, bladder)	1. No preparation necessary 2. On *call to x-ray*

*A contrast medium is used in this x-ray. Find out if the patient has ever had a reaction to any x-ray procedure, or is allergic to seafood or iodine.

NR

BOOKS

Waring W, Jeansonne L: Practical Manual of Pediatrics, 2nd ed. St Louis, CV Mosby, 1982

Cardiopulmonary Resuscitation (CPR)

A Manual for Instructors of Basic Cardiac Life Support. Texas, American Heart Association, 1981

Catheterization Urinary

BOOKS

Brunner L, Suddarth D: The Lippincott Manual of Nursing Practice, 3rd ed. Philadelphia, JB Lippincott, 1982

Nursing Photobook: Implementing urologic. procedures. Horsham, PA, Intermed Communications, 1981

JOURNALS

Bates P: A troubleshooter's guide to indwelling catheters. RN 44(3):62, Mar 1981

Bielski M: Preventing infection in the catheterized patient. Nurs Clin North Am 15(4):703, Dec 1980

Bradshaw T: Making male catheterization easier for both of you. RN 46(12):43, Dec 1983

Burke J, Garibaldi R, Britt M, et al: Prevention of catheter-associated urinary tract infections. Efficacy of daily meatal care regimens. Am J Med 70(3):655, 1980

Gordon R: Urinary catheter care may increase risk of infection. JAMA 246(1):30, July 3, 1981

Kennedy A, Brocklehurst J: The nursing management of patients with long-term indwelling catheters. J Adv Nurs 7(5):411, Sept 1982

Killon A: Reducing the risk of infection from indwelling urethral catheters. Nursing '82 12(2):84, May 1982

Kinney A, Blount M, Dowell M: Urethral catheterization. Geriatric Nurs 1(4):258, Nov/Dec 1980

Maizels M, Schaeffer A: Decreased incidence of bacteriuria associated with periodic instillations of hydrogen peroxide into the urethral catheter drainage bag. J Urol 123(6):841, June 1980

Steinert L: Urinary drainage need not lead to UTI: The use of hydrogen peroxide in urinary catheter drainage bags to prevent nosocomial infections. J Oper Room Res Inst 2(12):14, Dec 1982

West K: Foley catheter: Problems and management. Oper Room Res Inst 3(5):18, May 1983

Wong E: Guidelines for prevention of catheter-associated urinary tract infections. Am J Infec Control 11(1):28, Feb 1983

Central Venous Pressure

JOURNALS

Fisher R: Measuring central venous pressure. Nursing '79 9(10):74, Oct 1979

Ostrow L: Air embolism and central venous lines. Am J Nurs 81(11):2036, Nov 1981

Sedlock S: Interpretation of hemodynamic pressures and recognition of complications. Crit Care Nurse 1(1):39, Nov/Dec 1980

BOOKS

Abels L: Mosby's Manual of Critical Care. St Louis, CV Mosby, 1979

Guzzetta C., Dossey B: Cardiovascular Nursing Body Mind Tapestry. St Louis, CV Mosby, 1984

Sanderson R, Kurth C: The Cardiac Patient, 2nd ed. Philadelphia, WB Saunders, 1983

Chest Tube Drainage

JOURNALS

Bricker P: Chest tubes. The crucial points you mustn't forget. RN 43(11):21, Nov 1980

Erickson R: Chest tubes. Nursing '81 11(5):34, May 1981

Erickson R: Solving chest tube problems. Nursing '81 11(5):62, June 1981

Wooden L: Your patient with a pneumothorax. Nursing '82 12(11):50, Nov 1982

Dialysis

BOOKS

Abels L: Mosby's Manual of Critical Care. Unit 3. Fluid and Electrolytes. St Louis, CV Mosby, 1979

Hekelman F, Ostendarp C: Nephrology Nursing. New York, McGraw-Hill, 1979

Jackle M, Rasmussen C: Renal Problems. A Critical Care Nursing Focus. Bowie, Maryland, Robert J Brady Co, 1980

JOURNALS

Clarke B: Control and prevention of infection on hemodialysis units. Nurs Clin North Am 15(4):883, Dec 1980

Dennison D, Burns K: Home peritoneal dialysis. Am J Nurs 80(11):2022, Nov 1980

Gross S, Algrim C: Teaching young patients—and their families—about home peritoneal dialysis. Nursing '80 10(12):67, Dec 1980

Reed S: Giving more than dialysis. Nursing '82 12(4):58, Apr 1982

EEG—Electroencephalogram

BOOKS

Waring W, Jeansonne L: Practical Manual of Pediatrics, 2nd ed. St Louis, CV Mosby, 1982

JOURNALS

Bubb D: Neurodiagnostic care: Pre- and post-procedure care. RN 44(11):64, Nov 1981

EKG-ECG-Electrocardiogram Leads

BOOKS

Andreoli K, Fowkes V, Zipes D, Wallace A: Comprehensive Cardiac Care, 5th ed. St Louis, CV Mosby, 1983

Krovetz L, Gessner I, Schiebler G: Handbook of Pediatric Cardiology, 2nd ed. Baltimore, University Park Press, 1979

JOURNALS

Bubb D: Neurodiagnostic studies: Pre- and post-procedure care. RN 44(11):64, Nov 1981

Endoscopic Procedures

JOURNALS

Beck M: Preparing your patient physically for an esophagogastroduodenoscopy. Nursing '81 11(2):88, Feb 1981

Cameron T: Fiberoptic bronchoscopy. Am J Nurs 81(8):1462, Aug 1982

Fisher R, Kaplan W: The role of gastrointestinal endoscopy. Med Times 111(2):31, Feb 1983

Grossman M: Gastrointestinal endoscopy. Clin Symp 32(3):2, 1980

Hollen E, Toomey L: Mediastinoscopy. Nursing '83 13(2):140, Feb 1983

Overholt B: Colonoscopy and colon cancer: Current clinical practice. American Cancer Society, Professional Education Publication, 1981

Toben B, Kelly J: Flexible fiberoptic bronchoscopy. A guide for the respiratory therapist. Resp Ther 11(3):73, May/June 1981

Selkin S: Other Clinical Applications of FFE. The Cleft Palate Journal 21(1)29 Jan 1984

Stiklorius C: "Fair warnings" for patients facing esophagoscopy and gastroscopy. RN 45(6):64, June 1982

Gastrointestinal Intubation

BOOKS

Abels L: Mosby's Manual of Critical Care. St. Louis, CV Mosby, 1979

King E, Wieck L, Dyer M: Quick Reference to Pediatric Nursing Procedures. Philadelphia, JB Lippincott, 1983

Nursing Photobook: Performing GI Procedures. Horsham, PA, Intermed Communications, 1981

JOURNALS

Arnold C: Why that liquid formula diet may not work (and what to do about it). RN 44(11):34, Nov 1981

Grinde J, Voldeu C: Gastrointestinal intubation. Crit Care Update 9(3):5, Mar 1982

Hanson R: New approach to measuring adult nasogastric tubes for insertion. Am J Nurs 80(7):1334, July 1980

Jones S: Simpler and safer tube-feeding techniques. RN 47(10):40, 1984

Kostantinedes N, Shronts E: Tube feeding: Managing the basics. Am J Nurs 83(9) :1311, Sept 1983

Patterson R, Andrassy R: Needle-catheter jejunostomy. Am J Nurs 83(9):1325, Sept 1983

Persons C: Why risk TPN when tube feeding will do? RN 44(1):34, Jan 1981

Shea M, McCreary M: Early postop feeding. Am J Nurs 84(10):1230, 1984

Strange J: An expert's guide to tubes and drains. RN 46(4):34, Apr 1983

Volden C, Grinde J, Carl D: Taking trauma out of nasogastric intubation. Nursing '80 10(9):64, Sept 1980

Infection Control

JOURNALS

Arking L, McArthur B (eds): Symposium on infection control. Clin North Am 15(4), December 1980

Bass J: The spectrum of staphylococcal disease. Postgrad Med 72(5):58, November 1982

Bjark D, Tight R: Nursing home hazard of chronic indwelling urinary catheters. Arch Int Med 143(9):1675, 1983

Cunha B: Nosocomial urinary tract infections. Heart Lung 11(6):545, 1982

Garner J, Simmons B: Guidelines for Isolation Precautions in Hospitals. Centers for Disease Control. Infection Control 4(4) Special Supplement, July/August 1983

Hargiss C, Larson E: Infection Control: Guidelines for prevention of hospital acquired infections. Am J Nurs 81(12):2175, 1981

Larson, E: Infection Control issues in critical care: An update. Heart & Lung 14(2):149, March 1985

BOOKS

Benenson A (ed): Control of Communicable Diseases in Man, 13th ed. American Public Health Association, 1981

IV Therapy and Electrolytes

JOURNALS

Anderson M, Aker S, Hickman R: The double-lumen Hickman catheter. Am J Nurs 82(2):272, Feb 1982

Bjeletich J, Hickman R: The Hickman indwelling catheter. Am J Nurs 80(1):62, Jan 1980

Buickus B: Administering blood components. Am J Nurs 79(5):937, May 1979

Ellyatt T: The management of a patient with total parenteral nutrition. Nurs Times 78(41):1723, Oct 13–19, 1982
Freeman P, Boyer J: How to get the most out of OP-site. RN 45(1):37, Jan 1982
Friedman F (ed): KVOs: How fast is fast enough? RN 45(9):69, Sept 1982
Habel M: What you need to know about infusing plasma expanders. RN 43(8):30, Aug 1980
Hudson-Civella J, Banner T: Intravenous catheters: Current guidelines for care and maintenance. Heart Lung 12(5):466, Sept 1983
Hutchison M: Administration of fat emulsions. Am J Nurs 82(2):275, Feb 1982
Huxley V: Heparin lock: How, what, why. RN 42(10):36, Oct 1979
Johnston-Early A, Cohen M, White K: Venipuncture and problem veins. Am J Nurs 81(9):1636, Sept 1981
Koszuta L.; Choosing the right infusion control device for your patient. Nursing 14(3)55 Mar 1984
Piercy S: Children on longterm IV therapy. Nursing '81 11(9):66, Sept 1981
Querin J, Stahl L: Twelve simple steps for successful blood transfusions. Nursing '83 13(11)34, Nov 1983
Schmidt A, Williams D: The Hickman catheter. Sending your patient home safely. RN 45(2):57, Feb 1982

BOOKS

Hamilton H: Monitoring Fluid and Electrolytes Precisely. Horsham, PA, Intermed Communications, 1979
Kirkis E., Ettorre D.; Seven Sticky Problems (and their solutions) in Blood Transfusions RN 46(4)59 April 1983
West R: Managing I.V. Therapy. Nursing Photobook 80. Horsham, PA, Intermed Communications, 1980

Nuclear Scans

JOURNALS

Becher C, Maisey M: Nuclear medicine and nursing. Nursing Mirror 153(9):16, Aug 26, 1981; 153 (10):34, Sept 2, 1981; 153(11):22, Sept 9, 1981; 153(12):32, Sept 16, 1981
Gupta S: Nuclear scanning in the evaluation of hepatobiliary disease. Med Times 110(5):31, May 1982
Winzelberg G: Radionuclide detection of gastrointestinal bleeding. Am Fam Physician 25(2):191, Feb 1982

Ostomy

BOOK

Broadwell D, Jackson B: Principles of Ostomy Care. St. Louis, CV Mosby, 1982

JOURNALS

Brubacher L, Beard P: A helpful new handout for your ostomy patients. RN 46(8):34, Aug 1983

Brubacher L: To heal a draining wound. RN 45(3):30, Mar 1982

Mahoney JM: What you should know about ostomies: Guidelines for giving better post-op care. Nursing '78 8(5):74, May 1978

Taylor V: Meeting the challenge of fistulas and draining wounds. Nursing '80 10(6):45, June 1980

Oxygen Administration

BOOKS

Abelson L: Mosby's Manual of Critical Care. St Louis, CV Mosby, 1979

King E, Wieck L, Dyer M: Quick Reference to Pediatric Nursing Procedures. Philadelphia, JB Lippincott, 1983

Vincent M, Spence M: Commonsense Approach to Coronary Care, 4th ed. St Louis, CV Mosby 1985

JOURNALS

D'Agostino J: Set your mind at ease on oxygen toxicity. Nursing 13(7):54 July 1983

Fuchs P: Getting the best out of oxygen delivery systems. Nursing '80 10(12):34, Dec 1980

Moody A: Oxygen therapy. J Emergency Nurs 5(4):5, July/Aug 1979

Promisloff R: Administering oxygen safely. Nursing '80 10(10):55, Oct 1980

Rotating Tourniquets

BOOKS

Freitag J, Miller L: Manual of Medical Therapeutics, 23rd ed. Boston, Little, Brown & Co, 1980

Guzzetta C., Dossey B.; Cardiovascular Nursing Body Mind Tapestry. St. Louis, CV Mosby, 1984

Hincker E, Malasanos L: The Little Brown Manual of Medical Surgical Nursing. Boston, Little, Brown & Co, 1983

Tracheobronchial Suctioning and Tracheostomy Care

JOURNALS

Albanese A, Toplitz A: A hassle free guide to suctioning a tracheostomy. RN 45(4):24, Apr 1982

Brooks C: Suction, oxygen and ventilation: Getting it together. Crit Care Nurse 2(4):77, July/Aug 1982

Brown I: Trach Care? Take care—infections on the prowl. Nursing '82 12(5):45, May 1982

Fuchs P: Providing tracheostomy care. Nursing '83 13(4):139, Apr 1983

Grossbach-Landis I, McLane A: Tracheal suctioning: A tool for evaluation and learning needs assessment. Nurs Res 28(4):237, July–Aug 1979

Hennessy P (ed): Home care of your child with a tracheostomy. A handbook for parents. Children's Hospital National Medical Center, 1983

Kirilloff L, Maskiewicz R: Guide to respiratory care in critically ill adults. Am J Nurs 79(10):2005, Nov 1979

McFadden R: Decreasing respiratory compromise during infant suctioning. Am J Nurs 81(12):2158, Dec 1981

MacKenzie C: Compromises in the choice of orotracheal or nasotracheal intubation and tracheostomy. Heart Lung 15(5):485, Sept 1983

O'Donnell B: How to change tracheotomy ties—easily and safely. Nursing '78 8(3):66, Mar 1978

Pagana K: Teaching your tracheostomy patients to cope at home. RN 41(12):64, Dec 1978

Rindfleisch S, Tyler M: Duration of suctioning: An important variable. Resp Care 28(4):457, Apr 1983

Traction

JOURNALS

Agee B, Herman C: Cervical logrolling on a standard hospital bed. Am J Nurs 84(3):314, Mar 1984

Howard M, Corbo-Pelaia S: Psychological after-effects of halo traction. Am J Nurs 83(12):1839, Dec 1982

Howard M, Corbo-Pelaia S: A review of acute care (halo traction). Am J Nurs 82(12):1841, Dec 1982

Jabos R: Musculoskeletal assessment. Cranial nerve assessment with halo traction. Orthop Nurse 1(4):11, July/Aug 1982

Milazzo V: An exercise class for patients in traction. Am J Nurs 81(10):1842, Oct 1981

Rutechki B: Caring for a patient in a halo apparatus. Nursing '80 10(10):73, Oct 1980

Programmed instruction: Nursing care of a patient in traction. Am J Nurs 79(10):1771, Oct 1979

BOOKS

Farrell J: Illustrated Guide to Orthopedic Nursing, 2nd ed. Philadelphia, JB Lippincott, 1982

Transcutaneous Electric Nerve Stimulation (TENS)

Banyard S: New drug-free technique cuts postop pain. RN 45(4):31, Apr 1982

Frampton V: Pain control with the aid of transcutaneous nerve stimulation. Physiotherapy 68(3):77, Mar 1982

Meyer T: TENS: Relieving pain through electricity. Nursing '82 12(9):57, Sept 1982

Moore D, Blacker H: How effective is TENS for chronic pain? Am J Nurs 83(8):1175, Aug 1983

Taylor A, West B, Simon B, et al: How effective is TENS for acute pain. Am J Nurs 83(8):1171, Aug 1983

Tylor E, Caldwell C, Ghia J: Transcutaneous electric nerve stimulation: An alternative approach to the management of postoperative pain. Anesth Analg 61(5):449, May 1982

Ultrasound

JOURNALS

Donaldson R: Sounding out the heart. Nursing Mirror 152(8):40, Feb 19, 1981

Haughey C: Understanding ultrasonography. Nursing 11(4):100, Apr 1981

Hudson B: Sharpen your vascular assessment skills with a Doppler ultrasound stethoscope. Nursing '83 13(5):54, May 1983

Katerndahl D: General principles and applications of ultrasound. Postgrad Med 71(2):46, Feb 1982

Katerndahl D: Ultrasonic examination of the abdomen. Postgrad Med 71(3):227, Mar 1982

Katerndahl D: Obstetric and gynecologic application of ultrasound. Postgrad Med 71(4):177, Apr 1982

NR

X-Ray

JOURNALS

Bubb D: Teaching patients about ultrasound and CAT brain scans. RN 44(12):64, Dec 1981

Haughey G: CT/Scans. Nursing '81 11(12):72, Dec 1981

Imaging beyond imagination. Spirit, A Publication of the Pacific Medical Center, Winter 1983–1984

Paulfrey M: Upper gastrointestinal and small bowel series. Nursing '83 13(8):24N, Aug 1983

Powell D: "Will I glow in the dark?" Prof Med Assist 15(5):15, Sept/Oct 1982

Stiklorius C: When patient preparation is the key to success. RN 45(4):64, Apr 1982

BOOKS

Erlich R, McCloskey E: Patient Care in Radiography, 2nd ed. St Louis, CV Mosby, 1985

Fischbach F: A Manual of Laboratory Diagnostic Tests. Philadelphia JB Lippincott 1984.

4
Medical-Surgical Nursing (MSN)

GENERAL CONSIDERATIONS

ASSESSMENTS

NEUROLOGIC ASSESSMENT

Reliable and consistent assessments of consciousness levels are required, especially when brain damage is present. Good assessments can be obtained through the use of the Glasgow Coma Scale (GCS), which was developed at the University of Glasgow. It is widely used to grade changes in motor, verbal, and eye responses of patients with recent brain damage. The highest total score is 14; the lowest 3. A patient scoring below 8 should be in an ICU. Additionally, pupil size and reaction, along with vital signs, are recorded when "neuro checks" are indicated.

In the GCS pictured (Fig. 4-1), the patient went to the operating room at 2 PM after his previously stable condition began to deteriorate at 11 AM. Postoperatively, improvement was noted in the GCS.

*SYSTEMS ASSESSMENT**

(When recording a systems assessment, write heading on left of page and chart assessment information in narrative form to the right after each heading.)

- Central Nervous System (CNS)
  1. Level of consciousness; orientation to time, place, and person
  2. Pupil reaction, movement, and degree of strength or weakness of extremities
  3. Appropriateness of speech and behavior; sensitivity to pain.
- Skin
  1. Color
  2. Skin temperature and general condition (dryness, turgor, lesions)
  3. Condition of IV insertion site
- Cardiovascular System (CVS)
  1. Signs of congestive heart failure (CHF)
     a. Auscultate chest for quality of breath sounds and congestion.

*The systems assessment section was developed by Carolyn Smith Marker RN, MSN

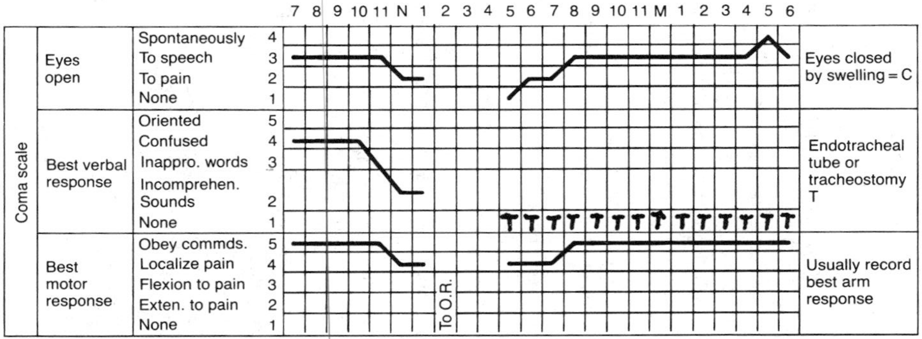

Fig. 4-1. *The Glasgow Coma Scale (GCS). The scale includes three parts—assessment of eye opening, verbal response, and motor response. Each can be assessed hourly, given a numerical value, and plotted graphically. A patient's neurologic status—unchanged, deteriorating, or improving—then can be monitored. In the GCS above, the patient remained stable until 10 AM, rapidly deteriorated between 10 AM and 1 PM at which time he went to the operating room. Postoperatively, his GCS improved.* (Jones C: The Glasgow coma scale. Am J Nurs 79 (9):1551, 1979. Copyright © 1979, American Journal of Nursing Company. Reproduced with permission.)

b. Presence of dyspnea at rest or with exertion
c. Appearance of neck veins at 45 degrees (flat or distended)
d. Presence of peripheral edema (hands, sacrum, lower extremities)

2. Heart tones (strong, regular, distant, muffled, murmurs, friction rub, and so forth)
3. Vital signs
   a. Quality of pulses; absence/presence of peripheral pulses
   b. Quality and numerical value of BP
   c. Apical/radial pulse (Document presence of deficit.)

- Pulmonary
  1. Respiratory rate and quality (labored, shallow, and so forth.)
  2. Chest auscultation (quality of breath sounds, retained secretions)
  3. Description of quality and quantity of secretions
  4. Mode of oxygenation (tracheostomy, mask, nasal prongs, and so forth)
  5. Type and frequency of chest physiotherapy
  6. Chest dressings/tubes (quality and quantity of drainage, amount of suction)
- Gastrointestinal (GI)
  1. Palpate and auscultate abdomen (bowel sounds, distention, tenderness, softness).
  2. Describe appetite or indicate if patient is not to eat (NPO).
  3. Nasogastric tubes (quality and quantity of drainage, type of tube, amount of suction)
  4. Abdominal dressings (dry, saturated, changed, reinforced)
  5. Wound (Describe appearance.)
- Genitourinary (GU)
  1. Foley catheter; voiding/not voiding
  2. Quality and quantity, and specific gravity if necessary
- Subjective Data

Document subjective data from patient interview/discussion. (State how your patient says he or she feels; *e.g.,* shortness of breath (SOB), tired, weak, and so forth)

Evaluation

Document effectiveness of your nursing approaches in relation to meeting present nursing-care goals. Notes should reflect evaluative statements, patient appearance (assessment), verbalization, or action that documents achievement or direction toward stated nursing-care goals. It should be understood that goals of care are incorporated into the nursing-care plan.

ELECTROLYTE IMBALANCES

Description

Electrolyte imbalance may be the result of insufficient or inappropriate fluid intake or of excessive loss of body fluids through perspiration, vomiting, diarrhea, gastrointestinal (GI) suctioning, and too frequent enemas (Table 4-1). Diuretic and steroid therapy, as well as severe trauma, chronic blood loss, and long-term immobilization cause losses and abnormal redistribution of electrolytes.

ONCOLOGY NURSING CONSIDERATIONS

Introduction

Cancer is a disease of uncontrolled cell proliferation resulting in the growth of malignant tumors capable of spread, or metastasis, to adjacent or distant tissues. It currently is treated with surgery, radiation, and chemotherapy. Additionally, immunotherapy, including substances such as interferon and BCG (Bacille Calmette-Guérin; vaccine for prevention of tuberculosis) may prove to be effective treatment, but this is still in the research and test phase. Surgery allows removal of as much of the tumor mass as possible, and therefore is most effective when the cancer is localized. Radiation must be focused on the cancerous area so that it directly kills the abnormal cells without causing excessive damage to healthy tissue. Deep focal penetration is now obtained with higher energy beam intensities, thereby providing safer treatment. Localized radiation is also achieved by implanting radioactive material at the cancerous site. In chemotherapy, drugs that are more toxic to the rapidly growing abnormal cells than to healthy tissue are used. All cells, whether malignant or normal, are affected adversely, and a balance must be maintained to kill the cancerous, faster-growing cells while not permanently harming the healthy cells. Even so, normal cells that proliferate at a fast rate, such as hair follicles, bone marrow, and the mucosa of the oral and gastrointestinal (GI) tract, are affected severely. This explains the well-known side effects such as hair loss, depressed bone marrow function, GI dysfunction, and stomatitis. Combinations of drugs, called drug protocols, are selected for the differing antineoplastic effects of the individual agents. Some of the drugs are "cycle specific" and have the greatest impact during certain phases of the cell life cycle; others are "nonspecific" and are capable of killing cells, regardless of the life cycle of the cell. Hormonal therapy, including corticosteroids and sex steroids, and surgery (oophorectomy, adrenalectomy) are used to treat tumors that are sensitive to alterations of the body's endocrine balance. Combined modality protocols that use the various modalities of surgery, radiation, chemotherapy, and hormonal therapy are called combined

TABLE 4-1 ELECTROLYTE IMBALANCE

Electrolyte	Causes	Symptoms
Sodium: hypernatremia (high sodium, above 145 mEq/L)	Renal impairment Diarrhea Decreased water intake Excessive sweating Fever	Increased temperature Flushed skin Oliguria Thirst Delirium
Sodium: hyponatremia (low sodium, below 135 mEq/L)	Water intoxication Repeated use of tap-water enemas Pancreatic fistulas Gastric suctioning Vomiting	Confusion Anorexia Diarrhea Seizures
Potassium: hyperkalemia (high potassium, above 5 mEq/L)	Renal failure High intake of potassium Massive tissue injury (*e.g.*, burns, trauma) Rapid transfusion of stored blood	Intestinal colic Nausea Diarrhea Muscle weakness Ventricular arrhythmias (cardiac arrest)
Potassium: hypokalemia (low potassium, below 3.4 mEq/L)	Loss from diuretics IV replacement fluids without potassium Vomiting and diarrhea, and prolonged gastric suctioning Excessive dieting	Muscle weakness Ventricular arrhythmias Paralytic ileus Hypotension

Calcium: hypercalcemia (high calcium, above 10.7 mg/dl)	Prolonged bedrest or confinement to a wheelchair Hyperparathyroidism Bone metastases/cancer of the bone that release calcium into the plasma	Calcium deposit in kidney that forms stones Muscle weakness Cardiac arrhythmias Intractable nausea and vomiting Confusion and lethargy Constipation
Calcium: hypocalcemia (low calcium, below 8.6 mg/dl)	Intestinal malabsorption Hypoparathyroidism Burns Chronic renal failure	Abdominal and muscle cramps Mental changes Tetany
Magnesium: hypermagnesemia (high magnesium, above 2.1 mEq/L)	Severe renal disease Overuse of magnesium-containing antacids or laxatives	Slowed heart conduction Hypotension CNS depression
Magnesium: hypomagnesemia (low magnesium, below 1.3 mEq/L)	Diuretics Malabsorption syndrome Chronic alcoholism Enterostomy drainage Vomiting and diarrhea Prolonged gastric suctioning	Disorientation Tremors Cardiac arrhythmias Hyperactive reflexes
Chloride: hyperchloremia (high chloride, above 109 mEq/L)	Severe dehydration Renal failure	Metabolic acidosis

(continued)

TABLE 4-1 ELECTROLYTE IMBALANCE

Electrolyte	Causes	Symptoms
Chloride: hypochloremia (low chloride, below 95 mEq/L)	Loss from prolonged nasogastric suctioning without chloride replacement	Metabolic alkalosis (*e.g.*, weakness, tetany and decreased respirations); hypokalemia accompanies metabolic alkalosis
High bicarbonate (above 33 mEq/L)	Loss of acid by vomiting, nasogastric suctioning, draining fistula Too much bicarbonate of soda or other antacids	Metabolic alkalosis with accompanying hypokalemia (*e.g.*, tetany, depressed respirations)
Low bicarbonate (below 20 mEq/L)	Diabetic acidosis Chronic kidney failure Diarrhea	Metabolic acidosis (*e.g.*, deep rapid breathing, weakness, stupor)

modality treatment protocols, and are designed to obtain a cure, remission, or relief of symptoms of cancer.

The National Cancer Institute (NCI) offers a public cancer information service (CIS), which answers questions regarding the medical facilities in the area of the caller, home-care assistance programs, and financial aid sources. Local phone numbers may be obtained by dialing 1-800-4-CANCER or by contacting the Office of Cancer Communications, NCI, Bethesda, Maryland 20014.

Basic Assessment

- Know the reason a patient is receiving a specific cancer therapy. Certain tumors can be cured in their early stages. Others can be placed in remission by shrinking their size and maintaining this state for a period of time.
- Always learn the specific side effects of the chemotherapy or radiologic therapy being used (e.g., color change in urine).
- Know the patient's history and be especially aware of his or her cardiac, respiratory, and renal status before chemotherapy is started.
- Check laboratory values daily; baseline blood counts should be done before starting treatment.

Chemotherapy

- It is important to save good veins for chemotherapy. Some routine lab work can be accomplished by finger sticks for blood. If indicated, write "bleeding tendency" on the lab slip to alert the person drawing the blood.
- IV chemotherapeutic drugs should be mixed in the pharmacy. Absorption of these drugs is possible through the skin and also by inhalation and ingestion; gloves should be worn and clothing protected when handling them. The containers, syringes, and needles should be discarded according to hospital policy for disposal of toxic material.
- Know the hospital policy concerning who is allowed to give IV chemotherapy. Be certain the IV needle is in the vein before any chemotherapy drugs are infused. *Severe* tissue necrosis can occur if some of these medications infiltrate. Know the procedure for treating any infiltration. Watch carefully during the infusion, and if it does occur, stop the infusion and treat *immediately*.
- Steroids often are included in chemotherapy drug combinations. The immunosuppressive effect of steroids often masks the signs of infection (*e.g.*, temperature elevation may not occur). Also, the skin as well as other tissue become very fragile, and GI bleeding, elevated blood pressure, and weight gain are possible. *Always* give this type of oral medication with milk or an antacid.
- The use of any over-the-counter medicine must be approved by the physician because of the possibility of drug interaction with

a chemotherapeutic agent. Aspirin (acetylsalicylic acid) or any medication containing it should be avoided because it inhibits platelet aggregation.

- In general, fluid intake should be increased to two liters a day, beginning the day before chemotherapy and continuing through one day following treatment. With children and adults, push fluids and worry about food and balanced diets later. *Caution:* with any greatly increased fluid intake, there is always the danger of congestive heart failure (CHF) (See MSN, Congestive Heart Failure).
- A high serum uric acid level frequently occurs because of massive cell destruction associated with chemotherapy. This is another reason for an increased fluid intake (2 liters/day). Allopurinol may be administered to prevent kidney damage that may result from increased uric acid.
- An extremely accurate fluid intake and output must be calculated and recorded. An excessive fluid loss requires replacement so that proper electrolyte balance may be maintained.

Pain and System Complications

- Bone metastases may cause pathologic fractures. Move these patients very carefully and never squeeze or pull on their body. Also, metastases or pressure of a tumor mass can cause superior vena cava syndrome, with symptoms similar to those of congestive heart failure; spinal cord compression, causing severe pain and neurologic dysfunction; and cardiac tamponade, leading to pump failure when fluid accumulates in the pericardial sac in response to inflammation accompanying tumor involvement or pressure on the pericardium. The release of calcium that accompanies bone destruction can result in hypercalcemia and serious electrolyte imbalance. Immobilization intensifies the release of calcium from the bone (See MSN, Pain Management).

Radiation

- Radiation may be given externally by machine, or internally with tissue implants or IV substances. Consult with the radiotherapist regarding necessary precautions in caring for patients with implants or IV substances; pregnant women should not care for these patients.
- Patients undergoing external radiation have the treatment area of their bodies identified with temporary skin markings or an indelible tattoo; do not wash off temporary markings. Friction from such things as shoulder straps or tight clothing as well as the use of perfumes, lotions, and heating pads on this area of the skin should be avoided.
- Skin reactions to external radiation in the treated area may occur, especially in friction areas, skin folds and creases, and the groin.

They appear as reddened or weeping patches, and may be itchy for the patient. They should be kept clean and dry; cornstarch is useful in relieving discomfort; healing is usually slow. Check with the radiotherapist before applying any ointment. There also may be an increased hypersensitivity to the sun following radiation or chemotherapy.

- Radiation to the abdomen and pelvis frequently causes diarrhea and sometimes a bladder irritation leading to cystitis.
- Radiation to the mouth and neck often causes an extermely dry mouth, mucositis, sore throat, difficulty in swallowing, and a loss of taste. Popsicles are soothing to a sore mouth and sucking citrus candy helps relieve the symptoms of a dry mouth. Encourage as much fluid intake as can be tolerated. Mouth care is especially important to eliminate foul taste, and odor, as well as to prevent the growth of bacteria and fungi in the mouth. A Water-Pik is useful for mouth care. Rinses should be used before and after each meal and before sleep. One commonly used solution consists of one part hydrogen peroxide to five parts of water. If this is too irritating, increase the amount of water. A mouthwash consisting of one tablespoon of bicarbonate of soda in a glass of warm water helps relieve a dry mouth. Dentures should be removed and rinsed several times a day.

- Radiation for the reduction of the tumor mass may be done before surgery to reduce the extent of tissue removal. Long-term effects of radiation therapy in children are on skeletal development and cause a disproportional bone growth.
- Relief from pain or pressure may be achieved with radiation that reduces the size of the tumor mass in certain areas. This is done frequently when there is bone or brain involvement.

Treatment Side-Effects

- Depressed white blood cell (WBC) production, as a result of either chemotherapy or radiation, predisposes the patient to infection. Anyone, including visitors and members of the hospital staff, with a cold or other infection should not come in contact with the patient. Strict aseptic technique must be observed for dressing changes, injection, IV administration, and urinary catheter insertion and care. Major sites of infection are the lung and urinary tract. Fungal infections are apt to occur in the mouth and perineal area. There is an increased susceptibility to viral infection (*e.g.,* herpes zoster, measles) when the patient is immunosuppressed.
- Anemia and thrombocytopenia (decreased platelets) may occur as side-effects of chemotherapy and radiation. Rest periods from treatment may be necessary, and blood and platelet transfusions may be given (See NR, Intravenous therapy).
- Petechiae are often the first sign of thrombocytopenia. If the platelets fall below 50,000 cells/mm^3, oozing and superficial

bleeding may occur; avoid intramuscular injections. Shaving should be done only with an electric razor to avoid cutting the skin.

- Alopecia (hair loss) occurs when the hair-follicle cells of the scalp are damaged. Radiation to the head always causes hair loss. The hair usually grows back within six months; some chemotherapy agents also cause alopecia.
- Ulcers of the mucosal lining of the GI tract often occur as a side-effect of some chemotherapeutic drugs. A daily oral assessment is necessary. Children tend to develop mouth ulcers with chemotherapy more frequently than adults. Avoid, when possible, rectal temperatures and suppositories because of irritation of the rectal mucosa. Rectal abscesses may occur.
- A dental examination and necessary work should be done before starting chemotherapy or radiation. Radiation involving the mouth, head, and neck is very damaging to the tooth enamel.
- Constipation may occur as an early symptom of CNS toxicity resulting from some chemotherapeutics. This, again, emphasizes the need to know side effects of drugs.
- Nausea, vomiting, and diarrhea may accompany chemotherapy or abdominal and pelvic radiation. Antiemetic and antidiarrheal medications (See PH) should be given at least one-half hour before a treatment and also before meals. Sometimes, they are given 24 hours prior to treatment. Observation of the patient's reaction to treatment is the best way to plan for control of these side-effects.
- Reasons given for not eating are fatigue, nausea and vomiting, mouth pain, bleeding gums, esophagitis causing strictures and decreased peristalsis, and altered food taste. Foods may taste bitter or excessively sweet; the use of plastic instead of metal eating utensils may lessen a bitter taste. Salty and very cold foods are often the most desired, while hot food, meat, coffee, and chocolate are rejected most frequently.
- Frequent small feedings usually are better tolerated, but meal planning must be individualized. When diarrhea is a problem, eliminate as much fat as possible from the diet.
- Fruits nectars, such as pear and apricot, are tolerated better than fruit juices when the mouth and throat are sore. Vitamin C needs to be supplemented with nectars.
- Physicians and nurses should know what dietary supplements, *e.g.*, ENSURE and SUSTACAL, taste like, and that they come in different flavors. They also must realize that the patient's taste and toleration must be considered. Instant breakfast mixes can also substitute for prepared diet supplements.
- Observe for signs of dehydration when vomiting and diarrhea occur. Record intake and output at least every 8 hours.

PAIN MANAGEMENT

Description

Tolerance to pain varies from individual to individual, and from time to time in the same person, depending upon many factors. Regardless of the cause, the pain as it is perceived by the patient is what must be treated. He or she is the judge of its severity and its relief.

Acute pain frequently is associated with anxiety, and chronic pain with depression. Anticipation of pain tends to magnify it. Lower doses of medication are required to relieve pain if they are given before pain is significant.

Removal of the primary cause is the definitive way to relieve pain.

Treatment

- Medication
  1. Analgesics, particularly narcotic analgesics in acute pain
  2. Antidepressants, especially for chronic pain
- Therapeutic nerve blocks by injection with lytic agents
- Surgical procedures used especially for relief of intractable pain, *e.g.*, cordotomy, commissural myelotomy, sacral neurectomy, sacral rhizotomy
- Steroid injections
- Transcutaneous electrical nerve stimulation (TENS) (See NR, TENS)
- Neuroaugmentation with peripheral nerve stimulators for selected patients
- Acupuncture
- Behavioral modification, for chronic pain
  1. Conditioning exercises
  2. Relaxation training
  3. Pacing activities of daily living
  4. Family counselling
  5. Biofeedback
- Hypnosis, usually as an adjunct to other therapy

Nursing Considerations

- Try to assess the cause of pain and provide appropriate relief.
- Recognize that individual needs for pain medication vary. When pain is expected, offer medication as often as it is ordered.
- Fear of addiction sometimes prompts patients to refuse pain medication, or nurses to hesitate to administer it. When there is acute pain (*e.g.*, in the first days following major surgery, in burn

cases and in advanced cancer) these fears are unfounded. As pain subsides, so will the patient's need for medication.

- The patient in acute pain may require medication around the clock to cover it. The goal is to prevent pain, rather than to relieve it. Narcotic analgesics, *e.g.,* meperidine (Demerol) or morphine sulfate (See PH) may be ordered to be given every 3 hours to 4 hours, as indicated. Orders may provide for flexible dosages that require nursing judgment. Ideally, medication should cover pain without producing untoward side-effects.
- As with all medications, watch for side-effects.
  1. Remember that respiratory depression, as well as signs and symptoms of shock, may be side-effects of most narcotics.
  2. Maximum respiratory depression will occur within 30 minutes after administration.
- Plan nursing care so that analgesics can be given a few minutes before any painful treatment, or before patient is asked to move, cough, deep breathe, or ambulate postoperatively.
- Extend the effects of pain-relieving medication with nursing measures.
  1. Teach the patient to splint a surgical incision when he or she coughs and deep breathes (See NR, Deep breathing techniques).
  2. Relaxation and breathing techniques used in childbirth have been found to be helpful in relieving other types of pain (See OB, Labor and delivery).
  3. A back rub may help the patient to relax.
  4. Diversion is believed to decrease pain's intensity. Such activities as watching television, reading, and visiting with friends may help.
  5. Provide a calm, restful environment.

POSTOPERATIVE CARE

IMMEDIATE CARE (WHEN PATIENT RETURNS FROM SURGERY)

Positioning

- The unconscious patient should always be positioned on his or her side to prevent aspiration of vomitus or obstruction of the airway by the tongue.
- The head should be to the side. The airway should remain in place until the patient coughs it out.
- Side rails of the bed should be up.

Providing Extra Warmth

There should be enough for comfort, but not enough to cause the patient to perspire profusely.

- The patient may require an extra thermal blanket. Remember that, to be effective, the thermal blanket should be covered with a bath blanket or some covering with a closer weave.
- Bath blankets next to the patient provide extra warmth.

Monitoring for Signs of Shock and Hemorrhage

(See below):

- Vital signs are monitored carefully, usually q 15 min, eight times; and then q 30 min, four times, or until stable. Use preoperative vital signs as a baseline.
- Changes in the level of consciousness (especially in the elderly) often are the first signs of impending problems, *e.g.,* shock, hemorrhage, fat and pulmonary embolism. Baseline data are essential.

Shock

Observations

- Using preoperative vital signs as a baseline, watch trends. The following may be indicators of shock.
- Falling blood pressure (BP): systolic reading dropping over 20 mm Hg, or drops in BP shown consistently when taken q 15 min
- Narrow pulse pressure (the difference between systolic and diastolic blood pressures)
- Rapid, weak pulse; rapid breathing
- Cold, moist, pale skin
- Failure of a compressed nail bed to fill within a fraction of a second after compression. In shock, capillary filling may take several seconds.
- Patient's level of consciousness. How does he or she feel?
- Fluid intake and output during surgery; estimated blood loss

Common Diagnostic Tests

- Arterial blood gases (ABGs)
- Serum lactate (the higher the elevation above normal, the greater the oxygen need)
- Hematocrit

Treatment

- Elevate the legs about 20°, leaving the rest of the body flat. *Caution:* In cases of possible increased intracranial pressure, keep the patient flat.
- If no IV infusion is running, start one with a #19 needle so that line is available (see NR, intravenous therapy).
- Blood volume will be restored according to need, with blood, electrolyte solutions, or volume expanders.
- Cover the patient with a light blanket to keep him or her warm, although not warm enough to make the patient perspire.
- Oxygen therapy may be required (see NR, Oxygen administration).
- Cardiovascular medications should be given as ordered.
- Indwelling catheter with urinometer, for accurate measurement of urinary output, should be used. Output under 30 ml/hr should be called to the attention of the physician (see NR, Urinary bladder catheterization).

Hemorrhage

Observations

- Apprehension, restlessness, and thirst. (Salivary glands, especially in shock from hemorrhage, are very sensitive to even slight decrease in circulating blood volume.)
- Tachycardia, deep rapid respirations, falling BP, and orthostatic hypotension (see NR, Postural hypotension). Using preoperative vital signs as a baseline, watch trends.
- Cool, moist, pale skin
- Symptoms of shock (see above, Shock: observations).
- Look for visible evidence of bleeding. Check under the patient with your hand. Blood or drainage may seep out of the dressing and pool underneath the patient and may be unseen on superficial inspection.
- Check the dressing. Mark the perimeters of any fresh spot on top of the dressing with a pen, and include the time. If the perimeter of the spot extends, you will have objective evidence that bleeding is continuing.

Treatment

- Start an IV infusion to replace blood volume with appropriate component.
- Treat shock if present.

Pain Control

Pain control is vital for the patient's comfort and postoperative recovery (see MSN, Pain management).

MANAGEMENT OF ABDOMINAL DISTENTION

- Auscultate (listen with a stethoscope) for bowel sounds. Nothing by mouth until peristalsis has returned—signaled by passing of flatus (gas), or stool or the return of bowel sounds. (See MSN, Postoperative complications, Paralytic ileus.)
- Nasogastric tube to low, intermittent suction may be ordered. Be sure tube is patent.
- Turn the patient q 2 hr. Have the patient move.
- Rectal tubes or enemas may be ordered.

MANAGEMENT OF NAUSEA AND VOMITING

- This is important not only for the patient's comfort, but also to prevent strain on the incision.
- Position patient on his or her side while recovering from anesthesia to prevent aspiration of vomitus.
- Describe symptoms and amount and character of vomitus.
- Administer antiemetic medications, as ordered.
- A nasogastric tube for suctioning may be ordered (see NR, Gastrointestinal intubation).
- Monitor for electrolyte imbalances. If they occur, correct with IV therapy as ordered (see MSN, Electrolyte imbalances, and NR, Intravenous therapy).

MANAGEMENT OF VOIDING PROBLEMS

- Most patients will urinate within the first 12 hours following surgery. Check the doctor's orders or hospital policy to find out when the physician should be notified if this has not occured.
- Try nursing measures to promote voiding (*e.g.,* allowing male patient to stand at the bedside—if permitted; running water within earshot of the patient; and providing privacy and a warm bedpan or urinal).
- Palpate for a distended bladder, especially if the patient frequently is voiding small amounts of urine. The patient may be experiencing retention with overflow.
- Catheterizaton should be avoided, if possible, but may be ordered if the problem persists (see NR, Catheterization—urinary).

PREVENTION OF ELECTROLYTE IMBALANCES

- See LAB and MSN, Electrolyte imbalances.
- Monitor for electrolyte imbalances, especially when nasogastric suction is in use, drainage is profuse, vomiting persists, or diarrhea is present.
- Measure intake and output accurately. Monitor weight.
- Imbalances are corrected with supplements ordered by the physician and usually administered in IV therapy (see NR, Intravenous therapy, Intravenous fluids).

PREVENTION OF RESPIRATORY COMPLICATIONS

- Identify patients who are at higher risk: those with existing respiratory problems, *e.g.*, chronic obstructive pulmonary disease (COPD) or upper respiratory infections; those with high abdominal incisions or chest incisions; those with congestive heart failure; those who are overweight, malnourished, anemic, or elderly; and those who have had a prolonged time in surgery, particularly if an endotracheal tube or oxygen was used.
- Watch for signs of atelectasis: elevated temperature, respirations that are labored or shallow and rigid, confusion (caused by anoxia), agitation (caused by hypoxia), diminished breath sounds on the affected side, and cyanosis.
- Watch for signs of pneumonia: elevated temperature, rusty-colored sputum, cough, chest pain, decreased chest movement on the affected side, and absence of chest sounds on the affected side (see MSN, Pneumonia).
- Assist the patient to ventilate completely (five to ten deep breaths every hour) by teaching him or her to splint the incision and to use one of the deep-breathing techniques (see NR, Deep breathing techniques). Encourage patient responsibility for this and for frequent position changes, if possible. Involve the family.
- Oxygen therapy sometimes is ordered (see NR, Oxygen administration).

PREVENTION OF VASCULAR COMPLICATIONS

(See MSN, Cardiovascular system, Thrombophlebitis)

- Reposition the postoperative patient every 2 hours. Teach him or her to use the side rail to help himself or herself, if appropriate.
- Range of motion exercise should first be passive, and then active (see NR, Range of motion exercises).
- Early ambulation, on surgeon's order

- Assessment for phlebothrombosis (clot formation in a vein)
    1. Homans' sign: pain in the calf upon dorsiflexion of the foot with the leg extended
    2. Pain in the calf at gentle pressure
- Elastic support stockings usually are applied preoperatively. They are changed daily, and are worn postoperatively until danger of thrombosis is minimal.

PROMOTION OF WOUND HEALING

- Identify patients who are at high risk for wound complications. Factors that increase risk are anemia, being overweight or undernourished, smoking, low serum albumin level, diabetes, radiation therapy at proposed operative site, certain cancers, stress, and certain medications (*e.g.,* aspirin, steroids, and prolonged use of antibiotics or cytoxic agents).
- The surgeon may prefer to do the first dressing change. Thereafter, if dressing changes are ordered, use scrupulous sterile technique. Remove soiled dressing down to the primary dressing or wound, and apply a sterile one. Never simply cover a wet dressing with a dry one.
- Inspect the wound during dressing changes for closure, drainage, and signs of infection (*e.g.,* redness or pus formation).
    1. A wound that is healing well looks pinkish, smooth, and firm, not yellow or macerated.
    2. Document the appearance of the wound.
- If there is copious drainage from the wound or a drain, protect the skin by keeping it dry. Apply a collecting bag, when appropriate (see NR, Ostomies, fistulas, and draining wounds).
    1. Montgomery straps may be used (see Fig. 3-12).
        a. Apply a protective skin preparation and let it dry before applying straps. The straps eliminate the changing of tape when frequent dressing changes are required.
        b. Ties should be tied in shoelace style for greater security.
- Dry wounds are now often being left open to the air (without a dressing). Inspect and palpate the wound frequently. Look for the following:
    1. Warmth along the wound should disappear approximately 72 hours postoperatively. Palpate the wound with the back of your hand.
    2. Thereafter, warmth in one area of the incision may indicate impending infection.
    3. A healing ridge is normal and healthy, and usually develops 5 days to 7 days postoperatively. If it is not easy to palpate, com-

plications (*e.g.*, hernia or wound dehiscence) may be anticipated.

- Surgical drains, tubes, and catheters may be used when there is an abscess cavity; insecure closure of the GI tract; anticipated leakage, as in gallbladder or pancreatic surgery; trauma; or radical surgery.
- The nurse should do the following:
  1. Understand why the drain is in place.
  2. Know what is expected if the tube is draining properly.
  3. Be sure that the tube is secured adequately.
  4. Observe and record the nature and volume of the drainage.
- Wound complications include infection, dehiscence, and evisceration (see MSN, Postoperative complications, Wound dehiscence and evisceration).

POSTOPERATIVE COMPLICATIONS

PARALYTIC ILEUS

Description

Paralytic (adynamic) ileus describes the condition in which intestinal peristalsis is absent or decreased. Some measure of ileus is common during the first two or three days following abdominal surgery and usually disappears spontaneously. It also is associated frequently with peritonitis, trauma, vertebral compression fracture, electrolyte deficiencies (especially hypokalemia), and mechanical obstruction.

Common Diagnostic Tests

- X-ray: A flat plate of the abdomen shows loops of the small bowel distended with gas.

Observations

- Abdominal distention and tenderness
- Persistent gas pains
- Vomiting after eating
- Absence of bowel sounds
- Failure to pass feces or gas

Prevention

- Nasointestinal tube to suction postoperatively, until peristalsis has returned. Most physicians withhold food and fluids until that time.

Treatment

- Nasointestinal tube to suction (See NR, Gastrointestinal intubation.)
- Intravenous fluids (See NR, Intravenous therapy.)
- Medications that stimulate intestinal activity occasionally are used, *e.g.*, vasopressin (Pitressin), bethanechol (Urecholine), and neostigmine (Prostigmin). *Caution:* If there is a possibility of mechanical obstruction, medications are used cautiously since they could precipitate perforation.
- Rectal tube for 30 minutes, tid, may be ordered.

Nursing Considerations

- Watch for return of normal function, signaled by the return of bowel sounds heard with a stethoscope and the passage of flatus. The patient should be instructed to tell the nurse when "gas" is first passed.
- Manage the nasointestinal tube to suction. Record the amount and describe the drainage (see NR, Gastrointestinal intubation).

SEPTIC SHOCK

Description

Septic shock is a complication of a complication, usually the result of a potentially avoidable nosocomial (hospital-acquired) infection. It is believed to be the result of the effects of cell damage caused by endotoxins produced by gram-negative bacteria, especially *Escherichia coli, Proteus,* and *Pseudomonas.* (Gram-positive bacteria rarely cause shock.) Patients at risk include those who are debilitated, those over 60 years of age, and those who have undergone urinary, gastrointestinal, or biliary tract instrumentation. The urinary tract is the portal of entry in more than 50% of the cases of these infections.

Common Diagnostic Tests

- Blood culture and sensitivity to identify offending organism (See LAB, Cultures.)
- Complete blood count (CBC), arterial blood gases (ABGs), electrolyte screen, and central venous pressure (CVP)

Observations

- Vital baseline clinical data include: vital signs, estimation of kidney function, and mental status. *Trends are important.*

- Early signs include the following:
  1. Chills and fever; warm, dry, flushed skin
  2. Increasing pulse and respiratory rates (The pulse may be full and often bounding.)
  3. Deteriorating mental status (confusion, restlessness, apprehension, lethargy)
  4. Blood pressure (BP) normal or slightly elevated, with widening pulse pressure (the difference between systolic and diastolic pressure)
- Untreated shock progresses rapidly.
- Late signs include:
  1. Elevated pulse and respiratory rates
  2. Cool, clammy, mottled, cyanotic skin
  3. Oliguria (markedly decreased urine output)
  4. Decreased BP

Treatment

- Identification and treatment of infections before they reach the shock stage
- When shock exists administer the following:
  1. Oxygen therapy (See NR, Oxygen administration.)
  2. Mechanical ventilation
  3. Intravenous fluids immediately (See NR, Intravenous therapy.)
  4. Specific antibiotics to treat infection

Nursing Considerations

- Hand washing, good catheter care (see NR, catheterization-urinary), and the use of aseptic technique when providing wound care are vital measures in the prevention of infection.
- Carefully observe all patients for signs of infection. Be aware of those who are at high risk for septic shock, especially those with long-term, indwelling catheters.

WOUND DEHISCENCE AND EVISCERATION

Description

Separation of the edges of a wound is called dehiscence. This complication is especially serious in abdominal wounds. It is more likely to occur in a long, vertical incision or following hasty, emergency surgery. In evisceration, intestinal contents protrude. Malignancy, prolonged paralytic ileus, malnutrition, and advanced age are predisposing factors.

Observations

- The patient may feel something "pop" as sutures give way and the wound opens—most often around the fifth to seventh post-operative day.
- This may be followed by the escape of large amounts of serous fluid.
- Evisceration usually occurs suddenly in the debilitated or obese patient after a sudden cough or strain.

Nursing Considerations

- Cover the wound and the evisceration with a sterile towel moistened with sterile normal saline. Do not try to return the intestines to their place.
- Keep the patient flat in bed with the knees slightly flexed.
- Notify the physician immediately. The operating room also must be notified.
- Stay with the patient.
- Treat for shock (see MSN, Postoperative care).

PREOPERATIVE CARE

The following are the highlights of general preoperative care. Nursing considerations in MNS sections deal with specific situations (*e.g.*, gastrointestinal (GI) surgery, thyroidectomy).

ADMISSION

- Confirm that the information on the patient's identification bracelet is correct.
- Obtain nursing history. Question patient as to his or her most recent use of aspirin. Some surgeons will not operate on a patient who has taken aspirin during the previous two weeks.
- Collect specimens and arrange for laboratory tests as needed.
- Orient patient to his or her environment, making sure that the call bell is within reach.
- Assessment of vital signs is essential to provide baseline data.
- Measure the patient's height and weight. Record.
- Provide emotional support.

BASIC PREOPERATIVE TEACHING

The goal of preoperative teaching is to prepare the patient for his postoperative situation. Inclusion of family members in the instruction is especially helpful if they will be at the patient's bedside after surgery. Both the patient and his or her family should have a realistic idea about what the postoperative condition is likely to be, and what therapies may be in progress (*e.g.*, oxygen administration, nasogastric suction, chest tubes, casts, traction). In addition:

- They need to understand why the patient will be turned frequently and encouraged to move both arms and legs.
- Foreknowledge that frequent monitoring of the patient's blood pressure postoperatively is one of the usual ways of following a patient's progress may allay unnecessary fears.
- They should know that the patient's postoperative pain will be controlled and that he or she should ask for medication when the pain begins.
- The patient will need "how to" instruction and an opportunity to practice deep-breathing techniques (see NR, Deep breathing techniques).

GENERAL PREOPERATIVE ORDERS

- If an enema is ordered, note results and how procedure was tolerated.
- Skin preparation of the operative site and the area around it usually will be ordered (see Fig. 4-2).
  1. The skin should be washed with soap and water or a bacterial skin cleanser.
  2. Shaving should be done carefully with a sharp razor. The skin must not be broken.
  3. Follow with a scrub or shower, using povidone-iodine solution (Betadine or Isodine) or other antibacterial solution, if ordered. In some cases, the area should be patted dry with a sterile towel and covered with another one. Check for hospital procedure or specific orders.
- A sedative usually is ordered for the patient on the evening before surgery. The patient should be encouraged to take it. Side rails should be up.
- The patient receives nothing by mouth (NPO) for at least 8 hours prior to surgery, and his or her cooperation should be enlisted. If the patient is scheduled for morning surgery, his or her chart and room will be marked "NPO after midnight," or with the appropriate directions. *Caution:* Check with the physician as to whether any medications are to be given in spite of the NPO instruction (*e.g.*, some cardiac medications and antithyroid medications are given right up to the time of surgery).
- Check to be sure that "consent for surgery" forms have been signed and that appropriate reports for laboratory work that has been ordered, or that is required by hospital policy, are in the chart. Variations from normal should be called to the surgeon's attention. If blood has been ordered, slips indicating that blood

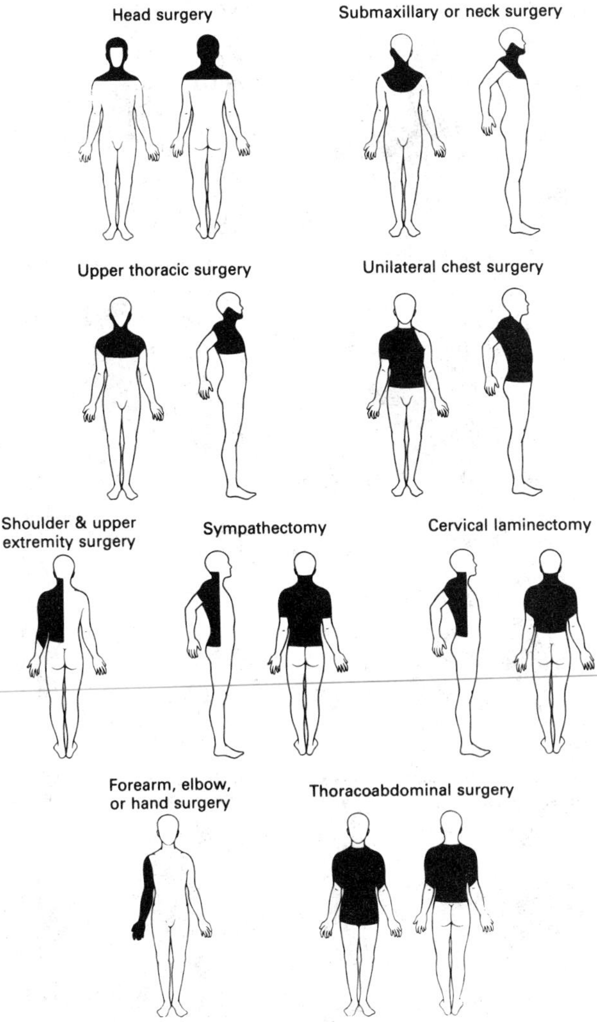

Fig. 4-2. *Preoperative preparation chart. The appropriate areas to be shaved and prepped for various types of surgery are shaded.*

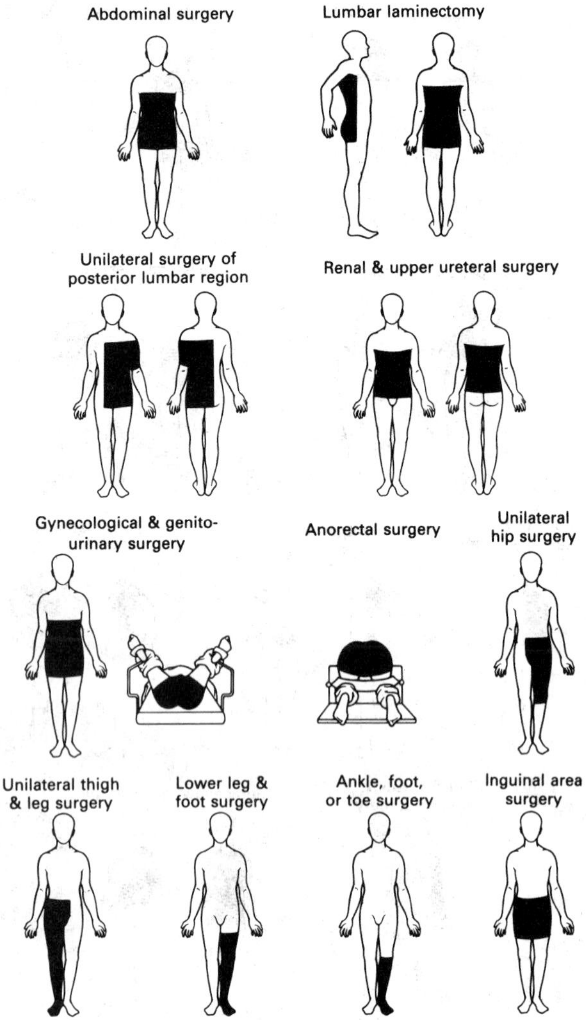
Abdominal surgery
Lumbar laminectomy
Unilateral surgery of posterior lumbar region
Renal & upper ureteral surgery
Gynecological & genito-urinary surgery
Anorectal surgery
Unilateral hip surgery
Unilateral thigh & leg surgery
Lower leg & foot surgery
Ankle, foot, or toe surgery
Inguinal area surgery

Fig. 4-2 *(continued)*

has been typed and crossmatched, and that it is available, should be in the chart.

IMMEDIATE PREOPERATIVE CARE

- Vital signs should be taken before preoperative medications are given. Any variation from normal should be reported.
- A shower usually is encouraged if the patient's condition, the procedure regarding preparation of the operative site, and time permit.
- Antiembolism stockings usually are ordered.
- The patient is asked to void.
- The patient is asked to remove jewelry, hair pins, contact lenses, dentures, and removable bridges, although some hospitals allow full dentures to be left in. Check hospital policy. Follow hospital policy regarding care of valuables.
- An intravenous infusion may be started in the patient's room with a needle of large enough gauge (#19) for administration of blood.
- A preoperative intramuscular injection usually is given 1 hour before anesthesia is scheduled. It usually contains a narcotic and an anticholinergic. Advise the patient that his or her mouth will feel dry, that he or she will feel drowsy, and that he or she must stay in bed. Side rails should be up.

BIBLIOGRAPHY • General Considerations

Oncology Nursing Considerations

BOOKS

A Cancer Source Book for Nurses. American Cancer Society Professional Education publication. Revised edition, 1981

Bakemeier R, Cooper R, Rubin P: The malignant lymphomas, multiple myelomas, and macroglobulinemia. In Rubin P (ed): Clinical Oncology for Medical Students and Physicians, 5th ed. New York, American Cancer Society, 1978

Berry C, Keeling J: Paediatric pathology. Embryonic Tumours of Children. Berlin, Springer-Verlag, 1981

Bouchard-Kurtz R, Speese-Owens N: Nursing Care of the Cancer Patient, 4th ed. St. Louis, CV Mosby, 1981

Carter S, Glatstein E, Livingston R: Principles of Cancer Treatment. New York, McGraw Hill, 1981

DeVita, V, Hellman S, Rosenberg S: Cancer: Principles and Practices of Oncology. Philadelphia, JB Lippincott, 1982

Dolan T: Female genital tract. In Rubin P (ed): Clinical Oncology for Medical Students and Physicians, 5th ed. New York, American Cancer Society, 1978

Donovan M, Girton S: Cancer Care Nursing. 2nd ed. Norwalk, Conn, Appleton-Century-Crofts, 1984

Frank I: Urologic and male genital cancers. In Rubin P (ed.): Clinical Oncology for Medical Students and Physicians, 5th ed. New York, American Cancer Society, 1978
Fochtman D, Foley G (eds): Nursing care of the child with cancer. Association of Pediatric Oncology Nurses. Boston Little Brown 1982
Lichtman M, Klemperer M: The leukemias. In Rubin P (ed): Clinical Oncology for Medical Students and Physicians, 5th ed. New York, American Cancer Society, 1978
Marino L: Cancer Nursing. St. Louis, CV Mosby, 1981
Salsbury K, Johnson E: The indispensable cancer handbook, 1st ed. New York, Wideview Books, 1981
Wallerstein R: Blood. In Krupp M, Chatton M (eds): Current Medical Diagnosis and Treatment. Lange Medical Publications. Los Altos, CA, 1983
Whaley L, Wong D: Nursing Care of Infants and Children, pp 1007–1023. St. Louis, CV Mosby, 1979
Ziai M: Bedside Pediatrics. Boston, Little, Brown, 1983

CONFERENCES

Cancer, Nutritional Implications and Therapy. Washington, DC, Walter Reed Army Medical Center, March 17, 1983.
Oncology Nursing Workshop. Washington, DC, Walter Reed Army Medical Center, February 16–17, 1983. Clinical Oncology. Clinico-Patho-Physiology Assoc. Workshop, August 27, 1982.
Oncology Update Issues. Washington, DC, Georgetown University, June 2, 1982.

AGENCIES

National Cancer Institute
National Institutes of Health
Bethesda, Maryland 20205

JOURNALS

Barrett W: Cancer of the bladder—A case history. Am J Nurs 81(12):2192, Dec 1981
Bersani G, William C: Oral care for cancer patients. Am J Nurs 83(4):533, April 1983
Bond A: New trends in endometrial cancer. Nurs Times 78(45): 1895, Nov 10, 1982
Do Santol L: The options in early laryngeal carcinoma. N Engl J Med 306(15):910, April 15, 1982
Doogan R: Hypercalcemia of malignancies. Cancer Nurs. 4(4):299, August 1981
Edlund B: Symposium on women's health issues. The needs of women with gynecological malignancies. Nurs Clin North Am 17(165):82, Mar 1982
Gaddy D: Nursing care in childhood cancer update. RN 82(3):415, March 1982

Gray S: Breast reconstruction. Nurs Mirror 152(7):40, Feb 12, 1981
Harder L: Primers assist patients in managing chemotherapy side effects. Oncology Nursing Forum 10(2)74 Spring 1983
Grunwald H, Rosner F: Acute leukemia associated with chemotherapy. Arch Intern Med 143(9):1322, Jul 1983
Henderson M: Pap smears. Consultant 22(1):77, Jan, 1982.
Houlihan N, Feeley A: Leukemia. The acute and chronic leukemias. Cancer Nurs 4(4):323, Aug 1981
Jones A, Koeft R: Cancer of the prostate. Am J Nurs: 82(5)826, May 1982
Kaplan B: Emergencies in the patient who has cancer. Emergency Med 14(1):192, Jan 1, 1982
Keddie G: Total Laryngectomy. Nurs Times 77(27):1155, Jul 1–7, 1981
Larsen G: Rehabilitation for the patient with head and neck cancer. Am J Nurs 82(1):119, Jan 1982
Levitt D: Multiple myeloma. Am J Nurs 81(7):1345, Jul 1981
McDevitt B, Standards of clinical nursing practice: The side effects of chemotherapy in the treatment of leukemia. Cancer Nurs 5(4):317, Aug 1982
Nicolson G: Cancer metastases. Sci Am 240:66, 1979
Oldani G, Grabstald H: Current management of benign and malignant bladder tumors. Consultant 21(2):238, Feb 1981
Patterson P: Experts stymied by mysteries of breast cancer. AORN J 33(4):770, Mar 1981
Reich S: Antineoplastic agents as potential carcinogens: Are nurses and pharmacists at risk? Cancer Nurs 4(6):500, Dec 1981
Rutledge D: Nurses knowledge of breast reconstruction. Cancer Nurs 5(6):469 Dec 1982
Savage K, Jones N: Carcinoma of the female reproductive system. Fam Commun Health 5(1):21, May 1982
Schmaier A: Oncologic emergencies. Med Times III(2):87, Feb 1983
Stromberg M: Screening for early detection. Am J Nurs 81(9):1652, Sept 1981
Tresler A: Nursing management of patients receiving cancer chemotherapy. Cancer Nurs 5(3):210, June 1982
U.S. Department of Health and Human Services. The Breast Cancer Digest. NIH Publication no. 81-1691, Dec. 1980
Valentine A, Stewart J: Oncologic emergencies. Am J Nurs 83(9)1282, Sept 1983.
Yergey L: Now an alternative to breast cancer surgery. RN 44(5):73, May 1981.

Pain Management

BOOKS

Chatton M: Current Medical Diagnosis and Treatment 1983, 22nd ed. Los Altos, Lange Medical Publications, 1983

JOURNALS

Alberico J: Breaking the chronic pain cycle. Am J Nurs 84(10):1222, Oct 1984

Cummings D: Stopping chronic pain before it starts. Nursing '81 11(1):60, Jan 1981

Fagerhaugh J, Shizuko Y, Strauss A: How to manage your patient's pain . . . and how not to. Nursing '80 8(2):44, Feb 1980

Jacox A: Assessing pain. Am J Nurs 79(5):895 May 1979

Long D: Surgical therapy for chronic pain. Neurosurgery 6:317, 1980

Long D: Relief of cancer pain by surgical and nerve blocking procedures. JAMA 244:2759, 1980

McCaffery M: Understanding your patient's pain. Nursing '80 10(9):26, Sept 1980

McCaffery M: Patients shouldn't have to suffer: How to relieve pain with injectable narcotics. Nursing '80 10(10):34, Oct 1980

McCaffery M: Relieve your patient's pain fast and effectively with oral analgesics. Nursing '80 10(11):58, Nov 1980

McCaffery M: Relieving pain with noninvasive techniques. Nursing '80 10(12):55, Dec 1980

Perry S, Heidrich G: Placebo response: myth and matter. Am J Nurs 81(6):720, Apr 1981

Porter J, Jick H: Addiction rate in patients treated with narcotics (letter). N Engl J Med 302:123, Jan 10, 1980

Steele B: Test your knowledge of post-operative pain management. Nursing '80 6(3):76, Mar 1980

West B, Green P, Bristol T: Understanding endorphins: Our natural pain relief system. Nursing '81 11(2):50, Feb 1981

Wilson R, Elmassian B: Endorphins. Am J Nurs 81(4):722, Apr 1981

Postoperative Care and Postoperative Complications

BOOKS

Brunner L, Suddarth D: The Lippincott Manual of Nursing Practice, 3rd ed. Philadelphia, JB Lippincott, 1982

LeMaitre G, Finnegan J: The Patient in Surgery: A Guide for Nurses, 4th ed. Philadelphia, WB Saunders, 1980

JOURNALS

Alberico J: Breaking the chronic pain cycle. Am J Nurs 84(10):1222, Oct 1984

Bobb J: What happens when your patient goes into shock? RN 47(3):26, Mar 1984

Burton F, Salminen C: Back to basics: controlling postoperative infection. Nursing '84 14(9):43, Sept 1984

Chang L: Abdominal wounds: A big payoff for painstaking care. RN 44(8):58, Aug 1981

Cohen S, Wells S: Nursing care of patients in shock. Part 1: Pharmacotherapy. Am J Nurs 82(6):943, June 1982

Cohen S, Well S: Nursing care of patients in shock. Part 2: Fluids,

oxygen, and the intra-aortic balloon pump. Am J Nurs 82(9):1401, Sept 1982
Cohen S, Well S: Nursing care of patients in shock. Part 3: Evaluating the patient. Am J Nurs 82(11):1723, 1982
Drain C: Managing postoperative pain: it's a matter of sighs. Nursing '84 14(8):52, Aug 1984
Flynn M. Rovee D: Promoting wound healing. Am J Nurs 82(10):1543, Oct 1982
Flynn M: Influencing repair and recovery. Am J Nurs 82(10): 1550, Oct 1982
Hall K: Detecting septic shock before it's too late. RN 44(9):29, Sept 1981
McConnell E: Toward complication-free recoveries for your surgical patients, Part I. RN 43(6):31, June 1980
McConnell E: Toward complication-free recoveries for your surgical patients, Part II. RN 43(7):35, July 1980
Podjasek J: Respiratory infection in the mechanically ventilated patient—an overview. Heart Lung 12(1):5, Jan 1983
Purcell J: Shock drugs, standardized guidelines. Am J Nurs 82(6):965, June 1982
Schumann D: How to help wound healing in your abdominal surgery patient. Nursing '80 10(4):34, Apr 1980

CARDIOVASCULAR SYSTEM

AORTIC ANEURYSM

Description

An aortic aneurysm is a sac-like distention at a weakened site on the arterial wall. If the distention occurs on only one side of an artery, it is called a saccular (sacciform) aneurysm. This type of aneurysm occurs most often in the ascending aorta. A fusiform aneurysm involves the entire circumference of an artery and generally is spindle shaped. This type predominates in the abdominal aorta, the most common site for an aneurysm. A dissecting aneurysm results from a tear in a vessel lining, permitting blood flow between the layers of the artery. Hypertension, the arteriosclerotic process, diabetes, and, in cases of thoracic aneurysms, direct trauma or injury to the chest wall are predisposing factors in the development of aortic aneurysms.

Common Diagnostic Tests

- Chest, abdominal, and lumbar-sacral spine x-rays
- Ultrasound and computed tomography CT scans (See NR, Scans.)
- Arteriogram, to plan operative procedure

Observations

- A thoracic aortic aneurysm usually is first detected on a chest x-ray. There are distended neck veins and edema in the arms and upper chest, because the size and position of the aneurysm causes pressure on blood vessels. Hoarseness, caused by pressure on the recurrent laryngeal nerve; dysphagia, resulting from pressure on the esophagus; inequality of the BP; and pulses in the arms all are late symptoms.
- With a dissecting aneurysm of the aorta, there is sudden, severe, retrosternal pain spreading to the abdominal area and the back; and hypertension coexisting with shock-like appearance of the patient.
- With an abdominal aortic aneurysm, a pulsing abdominal mass, often with mild tenderness on palpation, and a bruit (swishing sound) often can be heard over the aneurysm. Also, low back or flank pain because of pressure on lumbar nerves, and absence of one or both femoral pulses may occur. A ruptured abdominal aneurysm is evidenced by sudden, severe back pain and the signs and symptoms of hypovolemic shock.

Treatment

- Surgical repair, with the insertion of a synthetic graft, is the recommended therapy. Sonograms are done every 4 months to 6 months for patients with small aortic aneurysms to monitor almost inevitable growth. The size and site of the aneurysm and the physical condition of the patient are factors that determine whether or not elective surgery is recommended.
- Emergency surgery is done for ruptured aneurysms. The risk to the patient is increased greatly compared to that of elective surgery.
- Control of hypertension to lessen the possibility of rupture

Nursing Considerations

- The most common site of an aneurysm is the abdominal aorta, and although aneurysms are often asymptomatic, 80% are palpable.
- The farther the aneurysm is from the heart, the more successful will be the surgery.
- A partial or complete occlusion of a major branch of the aorta, caused by a dissecting aneurysm or following surgery on the aorta, produces symptoms related to ischemia. For example, oliguria, resulting from an occluded renal artery, or an ileus may occur with an occluded mesenteric artery.

Postoperative

- Ideally, the first 24 hours will be in an intensive care unit.
- A nasogastric tube will be in place to decompress the stomach.
- Pulmonary complications are common with abdominal surgery. It is especially important for the patient to cough, deep breathe, and use the incentive spirometer.
- Check the abdominal girth along with routine vital signs to detect bleeding into the peritoneal cavity from the graft site.
- Accurate intake and output must be measured. Notify the surgeon if the urine output is less than 30 ml per hour, or if hematuria develops.
- Vital signs must include the femoral, popliteal, and pedal pulses, as well as skin color and temperature on the legs. The Doppler pulse detector is very useful in detecting pulses that are difficult to palpate.
- After arterial grafts, be especially aware of any evidence of infection externally on the suture line or internally as evidenced by an elevation in temperature.

ARTERIAL OCCLUSIVE DISEASE OF THE LOWER EXTREMITIES

Description

This disease is the result of a decreased arterial blood flow to the lower extremities, generally caused by a gradual narrowing of the arteries. It manifests itself by pain, skin breakdown, and slow healing, often accompanied by infection and gangrene. This disease is seen often in diabetics. An acute arterial occlusion may occur as the result of an embolism that has traveled to the site or a thrombus formed at the site.

Common Diagnostic Tests

- Doppler measurement of the lower extremities (See NR, Ultrasound.)
- Arteriograms (angiograms)
- Tests to rule out or confirm diabetes (See LAB)

Observations

- Intermittent claudication, a muscle pain commonly in the calf of the leg or in the foot, occurs during exercise and is relieved by rest.
- Rest pain occurs in advanced cases, where the pain may awaken a sleeping person.

- Pedal pulses are absent or weak; there is hair loss on the leg and foot.
- Cyanosis and coolness of the legs and feet, frequently starting with just the toes, may be present.
- Taut and shiny skin and toenails that are thick and distorted are signs of poor circulation.
- There may be leg ulcers resulting from aortic insufficiency.
- Watch for sudden severe pain in the leg(s), and loss of sensation and function with cold and pale skin, which indicates an arterial occlusion. *Immediate medical attention is required.*

Treatment

- Anticoagulants, *e.g.,* heparin, warfarin
- Pain management (See MSN, Pain management.)
- Regulation of diabetes, including diabetic teaching (See MSN, Diabetes.)
- Leg ulcers are treated in a variety of ways, but the basic procedure is to medicate first for pain before beginning treatment. A wound culture is taken, and often oral or topical antibiotics are prescribed. The ulcer first is washed with sterile saline, patted dry, and then covered with sterile gauze, or one of various ointments may be applied. Do not put tape directly on the skin. When debridement is necessary, it often can be done with wet to dry dressings (dressing placed on wet and allowed to dry before removal) every 6 to 8 hours; in severe cases, surgical intervention may be required. Skin grafts may be necessary for ulcers that do not heal, provided there is adequate arterial circulation (see MSN, Decubitus care for more detail).
- A lumbar sympathectomy may be done to increase blood flow to the skin surface of the lower leg and foot.
- Surgical replacement or bypass of a severely occluded area of an artery using either a synthetic or venous graft may be done. An enarterectomy (incision and removal of an obstruction in an artery) also may be done. Amputation may be necessary in cases where gangrene develops.
- Percutaneous transluminal angioplasty (PTA) involves the dilatation of an arterial occlusion using a balloon catheter. It is done only on small lesions or for those patients who are operative risks. The care after the procedure is the same as that following an arterial puncture.

Nursing Considerations

The treatment of arterio-occlusive disease of the lower extremities is aimed at preventing skin breakdown, infection, and leg ulcers.

- In daily assessment, emphasize to the patient the necessity of keeping the feet clean and dry; wearing shoes that are well fitted; prompt medical attention to any cut or sore before it becomes infected or does not heal; of never wearing garters; of not crossing the knees or standing or sitting too long; of not smoking, which causes venous constriction; and the vulnerability to burns from heating pads because of decreased sensation to heat and cold.
- Several short walks a day often are suggested to develop collateral circulation. Patients should be instructed to walk up to the moment when they feel pain, rest a few moments, and then resume walking.
- Breakdown of the skin of the heel is common in the bedridden patient, especially with diabetic patients; do not allow the heels to rest directly on the mattress.
- Inspect the skin between the toes; this is often the first place that cracks in the skin occur.
- When the pedal, popliteal, and femoral pulses are located, mark these spots with a magic marker so they will be easy to locate for future palpation. Use of a Doppler pulse detector is often helpful.
- When an obstruction occurs in a major blood vessel and ischemia jeopardizes the survival of a limb, vascular surgery is necessary.

Postoperative

- Thrombosis and hemorrhage are the most common complications that occur during the postoperative period. Check the circulation in the feet every two hours. Skin temperature, color, and nail bed color also can be used to check circulatory status. Any changes or fresh bleeding must be reported to the surgeon *immediately*.
- Avoid flexing the knees to prevent pooling of blood and the formation of thrombi in the lower leg. While sitting in a chair, the patients should keep the legs extended and elevated on a foot rest.
- When the patient begins to ambulate, encourage walking, and avoidance of sitting, except on the toilet. This is especially important after arterial grafts have been done to prevent pressure on the graft site.
- Following arterial grafts, be especially aware of any evidence of infection externally on the suture line or internally as evidenced by an elevation in temperature. An infection in an arterial prosthesis is a serious complication.

BLOOD DISORDERS

LEUKEMIA

Description

Leukemia is a cancer involving blood cell production in the spleen, lymphatic system, and bone marrow. It causes a proliferation of immature white blood cells (WBCs) called blasts. It is classified by the type and origin of the immature WBCs that prevail, and as "acute" or "chronic." There are many cells in the acute form, and a mixture of mature and immature cells in chronic leukemia. The four major types of this disease are acute lymphatic leukemia (ALL), primarily occurring in patients under the age of 10 and the most common cancer in children; acute myelocytic (granulocytic) leukemia (AML or AGL), the most common adult acute leukemia, but it may occur at any age; chronic lymphatic leukemia (CLL), occurring primarily in older adults; and chronic myelocytic (granulocytic) leukemia (CML or CGL), usually found in young and middle-aged adults.

Common Diagnostic Tests

- Complete blood count (CBC) and platelet count (See LAB.)
- Bone marrow aspiration (See NR, Bone Marrow Aspiration and Biopsy).
- Lumbar puncture in ALL

Observations

- ALL and AML most often have a sudden onset, with flu-like symptoms or those of a chronic febrile illness. An enlarged spleen, liver, and lymph nodes usually are present in ALL, but not necessarily in AML. The WBC count may not be elevated, but there are many blast cells in the blood and bone marrow.
- CML develops more slowly, with symptoms of general malaise and an enlarged spleen. An elevated WBC count is found early in the disease. CML almost invariably becomes "acute" with a sudden increase in blast cells. This is called a "blast crisis," and usually does not respond to treatment.
- CLL also has a slow onset, with weakness and enlarged lymph nodes and spleen. The WBC count is usually very high.
- There is abnormal bleeding, especially in the skin and mucous membranes, because of decreased platelet production (thrombocytopenia).
- Susceptibility to infection is increased, because of increased numbers of immature WBCs that are ineffective in fighting infectious organisms.

- Weakness and fatigue caused by the abnormally rapid production of WBCs, and the resultant depletion of body reserves of amino acids and vitamins used in cell growth occur.
- Anemia develops because of displacement of red blood cells (RBCs) in the marrow by the increased WBC population. Shortness of breath, angina, and muscle pain occur because of the anemia and the resultant lack of oxygen to the tissues.
- Moderate-to-severe enlargement of the spleen, liver, and lymph glands may be seen in all types of leukemia. This is caused by the accumulation of large numbers of leukemic cells in these organs.
- Bone and joint pain is present in 25% of children with leukemia.
- Severe headache, vomiting, and irritability are symptoms of increased intracranial pressure (IICP), caused by leukemic cell invasion of the central nervous system (CNS), and are found most commonly with ALL in children. Meningeal infiltration will cause symptoms of meningitis from IICP, including a stiff neck and back. The seventh cranial nerve (the facial nerve) is especially susceptible to irritation and damage. The spinal nerves also may be affected.

Treatment

- Chemotherapy (See PH, Oncology nursing considerations.)
- Radiation (See Oncology nursing considerations.)
- Blood and platelet transfusions (See NR, Intravenous therapy.)
- Bone marrow transplants are done in some research centers.

Nursing Considerations

- Anemia, thrombocytopenia, and massive numbers of immature WBCs in the bone marrow occur jointly only in leukemia.
- Be particularly aware of a bleeding tendency; any drug containing aspirin should be avoided. Observe carefully for an increase in petechiae, hematuria, or gastrointestinal bleeding. When platelets fall below 20,000/mm^3, serious bleeding is possible. Intracranial hemorrhage can be fatal.
- Mark lab slips with "bleeding tendency" to alert those doing the venipunctures.
- Infection is the leading cause of death in these patients. Meticulous handwashing is a "must," and no one with the symptoms of any active infection should care for, or visit the patient. Childhood diseases are often fatal to leukemic children. They also may become infected from their own flora (*e.g., Staphylococcus, Escherichia coli*).

- Steroids "mask" infections, so symptoms such as a temperature elevation may not occur in a patient receiving steroids.
- A lumbar puncture is done after the diagnosis of acute leukemia in children to determine if there is CNS involvement. Intrathecal injection of chemotherapeutic agents and radiation is done to prevent and treat CNS involvement. Also, the CNS can harbor leukemic cells after remission occurs.
- Leukemic invasion of mucosa of the gastrointestinal tract may cause ulcers, mucositis, or bleeding. Chemotherapy also contributes to this problem. Therefore, avoid rectal temperatures and suppositories if possible.
- Allopurinol is given to decrease the amount of uric acid being formed from the increased cell breakdown. This breakdown is accentuated by radiation and chemotherapy treatments. A high fluid intake is needed to "flush" the kidneys to prevent renal failure.
- There is a 50% to 60% survival rate in children with ALL. Treatment is not as effective in adults who have this disease or AML. Chronic leukemia in adults carries a 3- to 5-year prognosis.

LYMPHOMA

Description

Lymphomas are cancers of lymphatic tissue. They are classified broadly by microscopic determination of the type of malignant cell as Hodgkin's lymphoma (HL) or non-Hodgkin's lymphoma (NHL). HL primarily involves lymph nodes, and usually is seen first in the neck. It spreads to adjacent nodes. NHL is more likely to involve other organs in addition to lymph nodes. Therefore, it is often widespread prior to detection. Staging is the term used to describe the extent of the disease.

Common Diagnostic Tests

- Biopsy of lymph nodes: The presence of Reed-Sternberg cells is diagnostic for HL; they are not found in NHL.
- Mediastinoscopy or laparoscopy enables viewing of mediastinal and peritoneal organs, and also is done to stage the disease. There may be a single node or organ involvement on one side of the diaphragm, or multiple nodes and organ involvement on both sides of the diaphragm.
- Lymphangiogram is done to visualize the lymphatic system with a radiographic contrast material in order to evaluate nodal involvement in the abdomen and pelvis.

- Liver, spleen, and abdominal CT scans (See NR, CT scan.)
- Bone marrow biopsy (See NR, Bone marrow aspiration and biopsy.)

Observations

- Increasing and painless enlargement of the lymph nodes primarily seen in the neck
- Weight loss of 10% or more in the past six months
- Recurring elevated temperature of 100° or more
- Night sweats
- Pruritus (severe itching) is a common symptom of HL. Herpes zoster occurs in 25% of these patients.
- Symptoms of organ or major vessel compression because of enlargement of the lymph nodes and tissue may be present. This may cause difficulty in breathing or swallowing, edema of the lower extremities, or obstruction of the intestines or ureters.
- In children, HL and NHL present essentially the same as in adults. There is, however, a higher incidence of bone marrow and CNS involvement in children.

Treatment

- Intestinal obstruction or other intra-abdominal complications may require surgery. Hypersplenism may require splenectomy (see MSN, Gastrointestinal surgery).
- Radiation is the primary treatment for localized HL and NHL.
- Chemotherapy may be administered along with radiation when systemic symptoms of HL are present and in generalized NHL.

Nursing Considerations

- Infection is the major cause of death in these patients.
- Lymphangiograms are done by injection of contrast material into the lymphatic system. The site of injection is between the first and second toe. The patients usually have sore feet and difficulty walking for several days. They should check their feet daily for signs of infection at the injection site. Urine and feces may be blue for a few weeks. Also, possible complications of lymphangiograms are oil embolisms to the brain, kidney, or lung.
- Following a splenectomy, watch carefully for atelectasis since it is high abdominal surgery. Also, these patients, especially children, are more susceptible to complications of bacterial infections, *e.g., Pneumococcus* pneumonia.
- See Oncology nursing considerations.

- The older names for NHL were lymphosarcoma, reticulum cell sarcoma, and giant follicular lymphoma. They are now classified by the make-up of the cell, *e.g.,* a small-cell, well-differentiated, nodular lymphocytic lymphoma.

MULTIPLE MYELOMA

Description

Multiple myeloma is a proliferation of malignant plasma cells in the bone marrow, which causes bone destruction. Normally, plasma cells produce immunoglobulins and normal antibodies. Malignant plasma cells alter this production, and decrease the body's immunity to infection.

Common Diagnostic Tests

- Bone marrow biopsy (See NR, Bone marrow aspiration and biopsy.)
- CBC (See LAB.)
- Serum and urine electrophoresis: The malignant plasma cells form high concentrations of abnormal protein.
- Urinalysis for Bence Jones protein, the abnormal protein found in the urine in multiple myeloma
- Serum calcium: Hypercalcemia is seen in advanced disease. (See LAB.)
- BUN, creatinine, and uric acid levels to determine kidney function (See LAB.)
- Bone x-rays: Lesions of this disease appear as punched-out lytic areas in the bone, or as osteoporosis without discrete lytic areas. They are found frequently in the ribs, vertebrae, pelvis, and skull.

Observations

- Bone pain, especially back pain. The pain often is associated with pathologic (caused by weakening of the bone) fractures.
- Anemia
- Anorexia, weight loss, and malaise
- Recurrent infections, especially pneumonia
- Renal failure can occur when there is a high level of Bence Jones protein or from hypercalcemia related to bone destruction.

Treatment

- Radiation for relief of bone pain
- Chemotherapy
- Hydration to enhance renal function

Nursing Considerations

- Localized pain, tenderness, and swelling, along with pathologic fractures, frequently are seen with bone tumors.
- Bone pain is *severe* pain. Try to set up a schedule for pain medication to provide relief before this pain becomes severe.
- Be certain the patient is medicated at least 30 minutes before any major physical movement, *e.g.,* movement to a stretcher. Have the patient direct body movement.
- Destruction of the bone frees bone calcium. When possible, ambulation should be encouraged to avoid hypercalcemia, which includes the following symptoms: nausea, vomiting, lethargy, and constipation.
- Avoid physical trauma because of the danger of pathologic fractures. Also, spinal cord compression can result from vertebral collapse.
- Patients must be protected from infection, and should not be exposed to anyone with symptoms of infection.
- A good urine output must be maintained to prevent kidney failure from hypercalcemia or protein blocking the renal tubules. Force fluids to maintain a urine output of at least 1,500 ml/day.
- These patients must never be NPO for any tests because of the danger of acute renal failure resulting from hypercalcemia or protein deposits in the kidneys.
- Bone scans are not helpful in diagnosing this disease because the lesions do not absorb the scan material.

PERNICIOUS ANEMIA

Description

Pernicious anemia (PA) results from a vitamin-B_{12} deficiency or its decreased absorption. This causes the RBCs to fail to mature in the bone marrow, and they are destroyed before entry into the circulation. The body cannot produce new cells fast enough to maintain an adequate RBC level. The nerve cells also require vitamin B_{12} for normal function; therefore, neurologic changes are often an indirect indication of PA. Assuming that there is an adequate dietary intake of vitamin B_{12}, two internal processes are necessary for its utilization by the body. Vitamin-B_{12} utilization requires the action of a protein (intrinsic factor) that is released by the gastric mucosal glands; thus, the stomach must be properly functioning. This vitamin-B_{12} intrinsic factor complex then must be absorbed by the mucosa of the small intestine. Malabsorption problems or parasites in this area may prevent absorption. The symptoms do not appear immediately because long-term supplies of vitamin B_{12} are stored in the liver.

Common Diagnostic Tests

- Bone marrow biopsy to confirm megaloblastic maturation (immature RBCs). (See NR, Bone marrow aspiration and biopsy.)
- Serum vitamin B_{12} and folic acid levels (Folic-acid deficiency is distinguished from PA by normal vitamin B_{12} levels and normal Schilling tests.)
- Schilling tests (See Hospital Lab manual.)
- Gastric analysis to determine presence of hydrochloric acid (See NR, Gastrointestinal intubation.)

Observations

- Anemia
- Sore, smooth tongue
- Mild jaundice
- Dyspnea
- Numbness, tingling, peripheral neuritis, and gait changes caused by spinal cord degeneration
- Fatigue
- Anorexia
- History of gastric or small bowel surgery, chronic pancreatitis, chronic gastritis, or alcoholism

Treatment

- Vitamin-B_{12} injections (IM) every month for life. They may be started on a weekly schedule for 1 month to 2 months.

Nursing Considerations

- Elderly people are the most susceptible to PA.
- Vegetarians who eat no animal products may develop PA. Plant foods do not contain vitamin B_{12}.
- Folic acid is never given to patients with PA because it increases the rate of neurologic involvement in PA.
- As in all anemias, there is a decrease in the oxygen-carrying capacity of the blood, and heart failure is a complication of longstanding PA.
- These patients are especially sensitive to cold.
- A family member or the patient can be taught to give the monthly injection.
- It must be stressed that lifetime, monthly vitamin-B_{12} injections are necessary.

CARDIAC PACEMAKERS

Definition

A pacemaker is an electronic device that delivers electrical stimulation to the heart and is used for individuals with impaired cardiac electrical impulses resulting in low cardiac output. It consists of a pulse generator attached to a catheter with an electrode tip. The pulse generator usually is implanted in a pocket of skin in the right upper chest. A fluoroscope aids in guiding the catheter through the cephalic or subclavian vein into the heart where the electrode tip usually rests on the apex of the right ventricle. The tip may, however, be positioned in the right atrium, or one electrode tip in the right atrium and one in the right ventricle. Occasionally, a thoracotomy is performed and the electrode is attached directly to the heart surface. The battery, which powers the pulse generator, used to last 3 years. The lithium batteries, currently in use, last 7 to 10 years. Demand pacemakers are the most commonly used. These are set at a rate consistent with the patient's need for cardiac output. They sense the heart's rate and only fire (called capture) when the heart rate falls below the set rate of the pacemaker.

Nursing Considerations

- Patients with new pacemaker insertions are cared for in units having cardiac monitoring equipment. However, they often enter regular hospital units because of unrelated illnesses.
- Know the rate set in the individual's pacemaker. Paste it in large numbers on the front of the chart, so that everyone knows that the patient has a pacemaker and its rate.
- Know that hiccups, fainting, and dizziness are often signs of pacemaker displacement, generally the catheter element or the electrode element.
- Pacemakers don't cure heart disease. The need for cardiac medications still exists. An individual with a pacemaker needs to take his pulse for one full minute daily, and report any changes. A decrease of as little as two beats per minute may be significant. Remember, even if a pacemaker patient goes into shock, the cardiac rate may not change.
- An identification bracelet should be worn signifying that the person has a pacemaker. Also, a pacemaker identification card should be kept with the patient at all times.
- Review with the patient what he or she knows, and be prepared to fill in the gaps. Note that specific cautions should be observed by avoiding interference from items such as microwave ovens, large motors or generators, and electrical substations. Such interference generally is not encountered unless the patient is

within close proximity to the radiation device. The standard home appliances, such as hair dryers and shavers, and new, well-sealed microwave ovens do not bother modern pacemakers.

CONGESTIVE HEART FAILURE

Description

Congestive heart failure (CHF) is a condition in which circulatory congestion exists as a result of the inability of the heart to pump an adequate supply of blood. This manifests itself as left-sided heart failure (LSF) or as right-sided heart failure (RSF), and can range from mild to life-threatening. Failure of either side generally is followed by some degree of failure in the other side. LSF results in lung congestion that may lead to pulmonary edema, an immediate life-threatening situation. RSF primarily affects the systemic system, with resulting liver congestion and peripheral edema. When CHF is caused solely by lung disease, it is called cor pulmonale. This is common in patients with chronic obstructive pulmonary disease (COPD).

Common Diagnostic Tests

- Chest x-ray
- Arterial blood gases (ABGs)

Observations

- Restlessness, irritability, and confusion, the symptoms of cerebral anoxia, are early symptoms of CHF.
- LSF can produce rales, cough (productive or nonproductive), and dyspnea. Paroxysmal nocturnal dyspnea (PND) and orthopnea are specific signs of LSF.
- Pulmonary edema is a common complication of LSF and may develop over a period of several hours or within minutes. *It must be treated as an extreme emergency.* Pallor, tachycardia, hypotension or hypertension, increased rales, and a cough with blood-tinged sputum are typical of pulmonary edema.
- Pitting edema of the extremities and sacral area generally indicates RSF. As the failure increases, the edema may progress bilaterally up the legs and extend into all body tissues. Generalized body edema is called anasarca. In a bedridden patient, leg edema may be absent, and sacral edema may be the only sign of RSF. Presence of jugular vein distention (JVD), most evident when the patient is at a 45° angle, is an indication of increased venous pressure resulting from RSF. Hepatic congestion causes abdominal pain and fluid congestion (ascites)

Treatment

- Oxygen therapy (See NR, Oxygen administration.)
- Rest and restful conditions constitute at least 50% of any treatment. Hot and humid conditions aggravate the problem. The diet must contain low sodium intake, and often includes a fluid restriction.
- Medication typically includes diuretics (*e.g.,* furosemide, Lasix) (see PH, Urinary system), digitalis preparations (see PH, Cardiovascular system), and potassium supplement (*e.g.,* Kaon) (see PH, Cardiovascular system).
- The patient or the family should have a clear understanding of diet, activity, and medication for effective, long-term management of the condition.
- Emergency treatment for pulmonary edema includes immediate vein access (see NR Intravenous therapy); morphine sulfate, furosemide (Lasix), and aminophyllin medications, *e.g.,* Theophylline ethylenediamine (see PH); rotating tourniquets (see NR, Rotating tourniquets); indwelling urinary catheter (see NR, Urinary bladder catheterization); and ABGs (see Lab). A pulmonary artery catheter (*e.g.,* Swan-Ganz) may be inserted through a large peripheral vein into the pulmonary artery to determine left ventricular function.

Nursing Considerations

- The nurse's skilled observations throughout a shift can provide an early detection of increasing CHF, especially lung congestion. Assess the lungs of all patients at the beginning of each shift to establish baselines. Any patient who suddenly develops a cough should be watched carefully.
- JVD should be assessed, and if present, reported and monitored frequently.
- Diuretics should be given early in the day. There is often a large fluid loss in a short period of time that causes weakness and affects electrolyte balances. Patients who are usually independent may need assistance getting out of bed. Postural hypotension is an early sign of hypovolemia.
- Weigh daily on the same scale after voiding and before breakfast.
- Patients with strict fluid limitations should not have water pitchers left at their bedsides, and the nurse caring for the patients should add the fluids to the meal trays.
- It is extremely important that a shift above or below the normal serum potassium level be reported to the physician at any hour of the day or night. Severe cardiac arrhythmias may develop from potassium imbalance. A low potassium level may cause digitalis toxicity.

- Measure ascites daily using a tape measure at the level of the umbilicus, and mark where the tape is placed with a magic marker.
- IV infusions should be monitored very closely to prevent a sudden rate increase causing a fluid overload. The tubing should be away from the grasp of a confused patient. It is good practice to hang the smallest possible container of IV fluid with a microdrip or pediatric drip. This ensures that if anything does increase the rate, the patient will receive the least amount of fluid. Heparin locks often are used for IV access instead of KVO (keep vein open) IVs.
- Cerebral anoxia often occurs, and restlessness and confusion are early symptoms. Be sure the patient is receiving oxygen. The brain is the organ most susceptible to hypoxia. Keep the lights on in the rooms of adults and children. The radio or TV often will allay the fear of being left alone.
- Sedatives may increase the level of restlessness because they are detoxified in the liver and its function may be compromised by CHF.

CORONARY ARTERY DISEASE

ANGINA PECTORIS

Description

Angina pectoris describes transient, insufficient coronary blood flow resulting from an obstruction or constriction of the coronary arteries. It does not cause cell death within the heart muscle. Stable angina refers to pain that occurs after physical or emotional exertion, thereby increasing the metabolic demand for oxygen. (The oxygen requirement of the myocardium is three times that of any other body tissue.) Stable angina tends to follow a consistent pattern of cause, intensity, and duration, and is relieved within 15 minutes by rest and vasodilators. As the disease progresses, as a result of further decrease in coronary blood flow, pain occurs with less provocation and lasts longer. This is called coronary insufficiency or pre-infarction angina. It is not relieved by medication and may wake the patient at night. Intractable angina causes chronic chest pain or discomfort that is incapacitating and does not respond to medical treatment. Prinzmetal's angina is an atypical angina caused by coronary artery spasm often unrelated to exercise or other stress.

Common Diagnostic Tests

- An electrocardiogram (ECG) should be done during any angina attack to rule out myocardial infarction (see NR, Electrocardiogram leads and how to place them).
- A CBC may indicate anemia as the cause of angina.

- A treadmill test is performed with the patient walking on a moving incline that slowly increases in speed. An ECG monitor, attached to the patient, records the heart's reaction to exercise.
- A cardiac catheterization is done by passing a catheter through the basilic or femoral vein and ultimately into the right side of the heart or through the femoral artery and ultimately into the coronary arteries. This procedure allows one to study blood flow in the heart as well as take blood samples for analysis.

Observations

- Chest pain may extend to the back, neck, jaws, and down one or both arms.
- Chest pains may be intense, as characterized by the fist drawn to the chest; symptoms may be described as a mild discomfort, indigestion, tightness, or a "funny feeling," rather than as pain.
- Extreme fear may be expressed or apparent during observation of the patient.
- Blood pressure (BP) may be elevated at the onset of pain as the body attempts to increase the blood flow to the coronary arteries, with a fall in BP after taking a vasodilator.
- A fall in BP at the onset of pain may indicate severe insufficiency or an impending infarction. This should be reported immediately to the physician.

Treatment

- Raise the head of the bed.
- Vasodilator, *e.g.*, nitroglycerin (NTG), taken immediately for pain as well as prophylactically (see PH).
- Oxygen should be administered to relieve ischemia. If a specific flow rate has not been ordered, 2 liters are safe as emergency administration (see NR, O_2 therapy).
- Prepare for an ECG. (See NR, Electrocardiogram leads and how to place them.)

Nursing Considerations

- At the onset of pain, take the patient's BP and give the prescribed medication. If the patient is allowed to keep the medication at his or her bedside, be sure that he or she understands that the nurse must be notified immediately when it is taken. NTG administration may be repeated at 5-minute intervals three times.
- A NTG tablet is not as effective if there is a decreased salivary flow as occurs with the aging process. If there is no relief, notify the physician. An ECG should be taken when there is any epi-

sode of chest pain. Explain this so the patient doesn't become apprehensive about the number of ECGs being done.

- Hypotension is a possible side-effect of calcium-channel blocker medications. Obtain baseline BP before giving any of these drugs. Check physicians orders for minimum BP, below which medication should NOT be given.
- Fear and apprehension are often severe during an angina attack, especially if the patient is awakened at night. Stay with the patient during the attack. Obtain a sedation order. Be especially aware at night of the patient's complaining of "indigestion" or of getting out of bed and moving about the room while denying pain. The nurse may be the only person to witness an attack. Document all observations. Later, ask the patient to describe the site, duration, radiation, and intensity of the pain or "feeling," and if there were precipitating factors. Document this carefully. When a patient understands what activities may bring on an attack, he or she will be able to take NTG prophylactically.
- Be prepared to explain any diagnostic tests to the patient. If cardiac surgery is contemplated, help the patient find out as much as he or she wants to know.
- Chest pain of an anginal nature may occur in children with aortic stenosis, pulmonic stenosis, or pulmonary vascular obstruction. The pain is usually substernal and nonradiating. It also occurs with exertion and is relieved by rest.

MYOCARDIAL INFARCTION

Description

A myocardial infarction (MI) is a localized area of cell death in the heart muscle. It results from a lack of blood supply to the area caused by a partial or complete occlusion of a coronary artery.

Common Diagnostic Tests

- Enzymes: increased serum glutamic oxaloacetic transaminase (SGOT), creatinine phosphokinase (CPK), and lactic dehydrogenase (LDH) myocardial-specific isoenzymes released into the blood from damaged heart tissue. The most important and specific test is the CPK with its isoenzymes, which will elevate in a few hours.
- The leukocyte count usually elevates within a few hours and soon returns to normal.
- ECG changes are frequently not immediately evident but most often do occur within three days (see NR, ECG).

Observations

- Pain is usually severe, but may be described as a heaviness or a burning sensation anywhere above the waistline, including the jaw, and may extend down the arms to the back and to the fingers of either hand. It is unchanged on inspiration or expiration, and it is not relieved by a change of position.
- Severe apprehension is present. Patients will often ask, "Am I going to die?"
- Diaphoresis is very common as cold sweat along with skin pallor.
- Nausea and vomiting are frequently present.
- Chest congestion is heard as rales and is indicative of heart failure.
- JVD is seen when the patient is sitting at a 45° angle, and is a sign of heart failure.

Treatment

- Patients usually are admitted to an intensive care unit (ICU). In the event this cannot be done the following are the immediate needs:
  1. Oxygen: Start with what is immediately available, usually a nasal cannula, and while the flow rate needs to be ordered by a physician, 2 liters are safe in an emergency while awaiting specific orders (see NR, O_2 therapy).
  2. Pain control is imperative, usually with IV morphine sulfate (see PH).
  3. Insert an IV line for immediate access for medications. Start with 5% dextrose in water at a very slow rate (10–20 ml/minute) with a microdrip or a pediatric drip, and preferably on a pump. Remember the high incidence of CHF with these patients.
  4. Medications include anti-arrhythmics, *e.g.,* lidocaine hydrochloride, procainamide hydrochloride (Pronestyl), quinidine; anticoagulants, *e.g.,* heparin; diuretics, *e.g.,* furosemide (Lasix); digitalis preparation; and NTG.
- Streptokinase and urokinase are clot-dissolving agents effective in reducing the damage of an MI when given within 4 to 6 hours of the onset of symptoms. They may be administered IV or injected directly into the thrombus by way of a catheter threaded through the femoral artery and into the occluded vessel in the heart. Side effects include decreased clotting capability of the blood, and the possibility of allergic reaction. A different and still experimental agent called tPA, a natural body protein, shows great promise of being even more effective than the kinases, and seems to have fewer adverse side effects.

- Daily weight and intake and output are used to determine how well the heart and kidneys are performing. If diuretics are being given, this also determines their effectiveness.

Nursing Considerations

- Life-threatening arrhythmias often develop in the first few hours of infarction, so establish vital sign baselines immediately, *e.g.,* BP, apical/radial pulse (ARP), and respirations (RESP). Take BP the first time in both arms, documenting any difference and the arm (RA, LA). Continue taking BP measurements in one arm every 15 minutes for one hour or until readings are stable. Be sure to use the same arm each time. Take ARP for one full minute, each time documenting irregularity, pulse deficit (difference between apical and radial rate), and quality (bounding or weak). Count RESP and note dyspnea and quality (shallow or labored).
- Pain relief is imperative. Continued uncontrollable pain is a poor prognostic sign.
- Anxiety levels in MI patients are very high. The constant attendance of calm and competent personnel is imperative. Talk to the patient as you work, explaining what you are doing. If the family is present, include them in your explanations. It is important that visitors do not upset the patient. Position the patient for his or her comfort. Clear the area around the bed for ease of movement for personnel and equipment.
- Observation of the patient is extremely important. Restlessness or confusion, resulting from cerebral anoxia, can be an early symptom of a failing heart.
- Patients with a MI should never use a bedpan or strain at stool. Provide a bedside commode, and be sure that stool softeners are ordered.
- Pulmonary embolism is a possible complication of bed rest. Check with the physician regarding orders for elastic stockings and range of motion (ROM) exercises. (See MSN, Pulmonary embolism.)
- Denial of having a MI is very common, especially when the pain disappears and there is no dyspnea.
- The cardiac teaching needs to start as early as possible, using the material used in each hospital or by contacting the American Heart Association.

HYPERTENSION

Description

Hypertension is a persistent elevation of arterial blood pressure (BP), primarily characterized by an increased diastolic pressure. This indicates increased resistance of the peripheral arterial vessels during the resting phase of the heart's pumping action. In adults, hypertension is defined as BP levels consistently above 140 mm Hg systolic and above 90 mm Hg diastolic. In children, a confirmed BP level above the 90th percentile for age is considered hypertension. Primary hypertension (also called essential hypertension) has no known cause. More than 90% of the adult cases fall into this category. Another type of hypertension is the result of a specific disease such as renal failure and endocrine dysfunction. Most cases of hypertension in very young children fall into this category. This is called secondary hypertension. Malignant hypertension is a sudden, severe increase in BP that quickly causes damage to vital organs. It generally is fatal if not treated immediately.

Common Diagnostic Tests

- Urinalysis and renal function tests, and 24-hour urine for vanillylmandelic acid (VMA) (See LAB.)
- CBC, creatinine, serum cholesterol, Triglycerides, BUN, electrolytes, uric acid, and glucose (See LAB.)
- ECG (See NR, ECG.)

Observations

- BP should be included in the routine examination of all individuals beginning at 3 years of age.
- BP measurements that remain elevated when taken at three 15-minute intervals should be taken in both arms three more times at one to two week intervals to confirm the elevation.
- A sudden onset of headaches, vertigo, nosebleeds, blurring of vision, and seeing spots before the eyes, along with nausea and vomiting, is indicative of a hypertensive crisis.
- Signs of hypertension in an infant or small child may include increased irritability, head banging, and awakening screaming at night, when the BP tends to be highest.

Treatment

- Adults with a diastolic pressure above 95 mm Hg are generally started on a stepped-care regimen of control beginning with weight control, reduced salt intake, and, if indicated, drug therapy.
- Infants and children with a sustained diastolic BP over 90 mm Hg need long-term follow-up. (See Pediatric BP tables)
- Immediate hospitalization is usually ordered for a diastolic BP over 130 mm Hg in adults; 100 mm Hg to 120 mm Hg in very young children. This can be a life-threatening situation called "hy-

pertensive crisis" with damage occurring to the brain, cardiovascular system, and kidneys.

- Treatment or correction of the underlying cause of secondary hypertension.

Nursing Considerations

- Take the BP with the cuff and the limb at the level of the heart. The inflatable bladder within the cuff must encircle at least 80 percent of the limb but not overlap it. The width of the inflatable bladder should cover two-thirds of the upper arm or thigh. A false high reading will be obtained if the cuff is too narrow. A false low reading will result if it is too wide. Oversize and narrow cuffs are available. A cuff of the proper size is especially important in taking a child's blood pressure. A Doppler pulse detector is useful in obtaining an infant's or young child's systolic BP.
- When a large BP cuff is not available for use on an obese patient, wrap a cuff of appropriate size on the forearm. Place the stethoscope on the radial artery at the wrist.
- When the BP in the thigh is being taken, the patient should be in the prone position, and the stethoscope should be placed over the popliteal artery.
- The BP in the thigh in an infant under 1 year is normally equal to the arm pressure. When the BP in the upper extremities is elevated, always palpate for femoral pulses. Measure the BP in the lower extremities to rule out coarctation of the aorta. This is an important cause of hypertension in early infancy. The femoral pulses will be weaker than the brachial pulses, or absent; the systolic BP will be lower in the legs than in the arms. After 1 year of age, the BP in the thigh is usually 15 to 20 mm Hg higher than the pressure in the arm.
- The first sound heard when the BP cuff is released is the systolic pressure (phase 1 Korotkoff sound). The disappearance of sound (phase 5 Korotkoff sound) is generally considered the diastolic pressure in adults. Phase 4, the muffling of sound just before it completely disappears, is considered the diastolic in infants and children.
- If no disappearance of sound is heard, record the BP at phase 1 Korotkoff sound, phase 4 and phase 5, e.g., 110/50/0.
- Potassium levels must be checked frequently when patients are on diuretics.
- When potent IV hypertensives are given, the patient's BP requires constant monitoring, either in the ICU or with one nurse assigned to the patient.
- A common side effect of the hypertensive medications is postural hypotension. In this condition, when patients stand, systolic pressure drops more than 20 mm Hg. Patients with this condition should be cautioned to stand up slowly.

- The nurse is in a unique position to help the patients with primary hypertension prepare themselves for a lifetime condition that, although not curable, is controllable. Sustained hypertension is the most important factor predisposing to strokes, myocardial infarctions, and renal disease.
- Weight control, elimination of smoking, and a restricted sodium diet go along with the medication as integral parts of the treatment in the lifelong control of hypertension. In some mildly hypertensive patients, loss of weight and a reduced sodium intake may lower the BP.
- It is estimated that as many as 80% of hypertensive patients stop taking their medication within 5 years. It must be emphasized that, while there may be no symptoms, medications must continue to be taken to prevent complications of stroke, heart disease, and renal failure.

PERIPHERAL VASCULAR INSUFFICIENCY

Parameter*	Chronic Arterial Insufficiency	Chronic Venous Insufficiency
Pulses	Decreased or absent distal to the occlusion	Normal (may be difficult to find because of edema)
Color	Pale when elevated; dusky red when dependent	Normal or cyanotic (especially when dependent)
Temperature	Cool	Normal
Edema	Little or none	Some to a large amount
Skin Changes	Shiny, thin, nails ridged, no hair on toes	Stasis dermatitis (brown)
Ulceration	Toes or places of trauma	Ankles
Gangrene	Yes	No

*Always compare the right to the left extremity.

THROMBOPHLEBITIS

Description

Thrombophlebitis is an inflammation of the veins in conjunction with a blood clot (thrombus). Usually the deep veins are involved. Any alterations or injury of a vein that restricts blood flow (venous stasis) tends to result in blood clots and thrombophlebitis. This is often a complication of prolonged bed rest. Phlebothrombosis refers to thrombosis not accompanied by symptoms of inflammation.

Common Diagnostic Tests

- The Doppler ultrasound blood flow detector can detect thrombosis in large veins in the extremities.

Observations

- Swelling, redness, warmth, and tenderness of a leg area commonly occur when superficial veins are involved. Sometimes the thrombus in such surface veins can be felt as a hard spot. A positive Homan's sign may be the only external evidence of thrombophlebitis in deep veins of the leg. This frequently is accompanied by a temperature elevation. Any evidence of a pulmonary embolism that may result from a dislodged thrombus must be reported to the physician at once (see MSN, Pulmonary embolism).

Treatment

- Bed rest, elevation of the leg on pillows, and warm moist packs to the leg are commonly prescribed, or elastic stockings are worn.
- Anticoagulants, *e.g.,* heparin, warfarin, are administered. Streptokinase, a plasminogen activator is occasionally used in cases of deep vein thrombosis. (See PH.)
- When the signs of inflammation subside, the patient is allowed out of bed to walk for increasing periods of time.
- Analgesics as necessary for pain.
- The insertion of a filter device in the vena cava is occasionally done in patients with frequently recurring thrombophlebitis or where anticoagulant therapy is contraindicated or ineffective. The filter is made of fine mesh that prevents emboli from traveling to the lung.

Nursing Considerations

- Read the Pharmacology Section on anticoagulants. There are many drugs that should not be taken together with anticoagulants. Be prepared to discuss this with the patient. Patients should consult with their physician about all medications, including over-the-counter products.
- Patients often are allowed to use a commode rather than a bedpan. Watch carefully while the patient is moving from and to bed

(and immediately afterward) for any signs of an embolus. Caution the patient not to strain.

- A special effort should be made to prevent thrombophlebitis in any hospitalized patient. Those on bed rest must have ROM exercises. Sitting in chairs for long periods should be avoided. Always elevate the legs when sitting and avoid crossed knees. Venous stasis occurs rapidly in anyone with impaired circulation.
- Check with the physician regarding the patient's use of elastic stockings when discharged. If required, they should be ordered before discharge.
- Patients often are discharged on a prophylactic anticoagulant regimen. Emphasize the importance of blood tests and prothrombin levels, as ordered by the physician. Emphasize to the patient that any unusual bleeding should be reported.
- An identification bracelet should be worn, noting that the patient is taking an anticoagulant.

VARICOSE VEINS

Description

Varicose veins are abnormally dilated veins that have an impaired valve function. They usually occur in the lower extremities, with the long saphenous vein most often affected. Varicose veins occur also as esophageal varices, which result from complications of liver diseases.

Observations

- Disfigurement in the lower extremities, with large discolored veins usually accompanied by edema, fiberosis, and pigmentation of the skin that may become very pruritic (an intense itching) is present. This is called stasis dermatitis. There is an increased susceptibility of this tissue to infection and trauma.
- Varicose ulcers often develop because of venous stasis, combined with the poor condition of the skin. The most common site is the ankle area.

Treatment

- Support stockings, prescribed by a physician's measurements and made to order
- Walking to improve venous flow
- Surgical: stripping or removal of the saphenous vein, provided the deep veins are able to supply collateral circulation. This is done with a general anesthetic.

- Injection of a caustic solution into the vein, which causes sclerosis of the vein. This usually is done with smaller veins or for patients unable to undergo surgery.

Nursing Considerations

- These patients are often allowed to walk the day of surgery. They need pain medication and assistance in walking. Sometimes bed rest is ordered for the first 24 hours.
- Check the dressings frequently for the first 24 hours for excessive bleeding.
- Check pedal pulses every 2 hours for the first 24 hours.
- Since it is a weakness of vessel walls that predisposes to varicose veins, the patient should know the problem may recur in the collateral veins.
- If elastic stockings are to be worn, arrangements should be made to have them fitted as soon after surgery as possible.
- Have the patient avoid excess weight, crossing of the legs, prolonged standing or sitting with legs not elevated, and constriction by garters or tight girdles.
- Varicose ulcers are often very painful. They are usually superficial and treated with systemic antibiotics and pressure dressings. Medicate for pain before beginning their care; use sterile technique.
- A care plan with step-by-step directions should be prepared and followed by everyone caring for the ulcer; this demonstrates to the patient the necessity for continuity of care. If a family member or a visiting nurse will be continuing care at home, have them observe and participate in the procedure in the hospital.
- When skin grafts are necessary, infection prevention measures become even more important during the healing period.

NORMAL AGING CHANGES IN THE CARDIOVASCULAR SYSTEM

- There is an increase in lipofuscin pigment, an insoluble and inert substance that causes the brown color in atrophic hearts.
- The percentage of muscle fiber in the heart decreases.
- Collagen, a major component of both the epicardium and endocardium, becomes increasingly stiff and insoluble.
- The concentration of amyloid (a protein complex having starch-like characteristics) increases. Deposits are found in both the epicardium and endocardium, in the valves, and in the walls of arteries, arterioles, and capillaries.
- Heart valves become fibrotic, and leaflets thicken.
- Atria become fibrotic and dilate. The fibrosis also affects the sinoatrial node.

- Large arteries tend to elongate and dilate.
- Elastin, a major component of arteries, becomes thin and fragmented.
- It is difficult to distinguish between normal aging changes and the process of atherosclerosis. Collagen and lipids do accumulate in the arteries, but metabolic and environmental factors also are involved.
- There is an increase in systemic vascular resistance.
- Baroreceptor reflex activity diminishes.
- Widened pulse pressure (difference between systolic and diastolic readings) occurs.

IMPLICATIONS

- A decline in cardiac efficiency occurs, but cardiac output is usually adequate to meet the oxygen needs of the body unless other stress is present (*e.g.,* illness, high activity level, surgery). The health-care personnel must consider that the elderly person's *reserve* capacity is diminished.
- Sluggish baroreceptor reflexes increase susceptibility to orthostatic hypotension, thus causing decreased cerebral perfusion and the possibility of fainting and falls.
- Aging changes can cause alterations in cardiac rhythm that are compatible with wellness and do not require treatment.
  1. Extrasystoles, such as premature atrial and ventricular contractions, occur.
  2. Wandering pacemakers are possible.
  3. Heart rate may increase with inspiration and decrease with expiration.
- Available evidence is not convincing that hypertension is an aging process (*e.g.,* progressive, irreversible, universal), but the risks of treatment to the elderly person must be considered. Side-effects of medications can pose as great a threat to the elderly person as the effects of the hypertension itself. Weight reduction and diet modification should be priorities of treatment.
- Aging changes throughout the body can mask symptoms of severe cardiovascular problems. An MI can occur without pain, and common symptoms of both MIs and CHF are tiredness, weakness, and mental confusion.

BIBLIOGRAPHY • Cardiovascular System

BOOKS

Andreoli KG, Fowkes VH, Zipes DP, Wallace AG: Comprehensive Cardiac Care, 3rd ed, pp 8–75. St. Louis, CV Mosby, 1983

Goldberger E: Textbook of Clinical Cardiology. St. Louis, CV Mosby, 1982

Hue M, McCombs N: Symposium on Hypertension. Nurs Clin North Am 16(4): 671–697, 1981

Melluzzo P, Nealon E: Living with Surgery, Before and After. Philadelphia, WB Saunders, 1981

Sanderson R, Kurth C: The Cardiac Patient, 2nd ed. Philadelphia, WB Saunders, 1983

Selzer A: Principals and Practice of Clinical Cardiology, 2nd ed. Philadelphia, JB Lippincott, 1983

Sokolow M, McIlroy M: Clinical Cardiology, 3rd ed. Los Altos, CA, Lange Medical Publications, 1981

Underhill S, Woods S, Sivarajan E, Halpenny C: Cardiac Nursing. Philadelphia, JB Lippincott, 1982

JOURNALS

Baum P: Abdominal aortic aneurysm? This patient takes AAA care. Nursing '82 12(12):34, 1982

Borhani NO: Mortality and morbidity associated with hypertension. Heart Lung 10(2):245, 1981

Bramoweth E: Acute aortic dissection. Am J Nurs 80(11):2010, 1980

Butler J, Harrison B: Keeping pace with calcium blockers. Nursing '83 13(7):38, 1983

Doyle J: All leg ulcers are not alike. Nursing '83 13(1):58, 1983

Gardy D: Hypertension. Discover 3(4):74, 1982

Grauer K: Early management of myocardial infarction. Am Fam Phys 28(2):162, 1983

Hammond B: Acute aortic dissection. J Emer Nurs 7(6):242, 1981

Hartshorn J: What to do when the patient's in hypertensive crisis. Nursing '80 10(7):36, 1980

Hill M, Fink J: In hypertensive emergencies, act quickly but also act cautiously. Nursing '83 13(2):34, 1983

Iveson–Iveson J: Varicose veins. Nursing Mirror, 153(10):37, 1981

Johansen K: Aneurysms. Scientific American 247(1):110, July 1982

Lee K: Aneurysm precautions: A physiologic basis for minimizing rebleeding. Heart Lung 9:336, 1980

Monohan R: What a patient must know to control hypertension. J Nurs Care 14(7):15, 1981

Moore MA: Hypertensive emergencies. Am Fam Phys 21(3):141 1980

Moore K: Coronary artery spasm. Nursing '83 13(8):49, 1983

Paskin L: Percutaneous transluminal angioplasty in peripheral vascular disease. Radiography 48(571):129, 1982

Satiani, B: Abdominal aortic aneurysms. Am Fam Phys 4:87, 1981

Sheahan S, Anderson L: The elusive disease, aortic aneurysm. Nurs Pract 6(4):31, 1981

Slusarczyke S, Hicks F: Helping your patient to live with a permanent pacemaker. Nursing '83 13(4):58, 1983

Urk F, Oakes A: Assessing the patient with acute aortic dissection. Focus Crit Care 10(2):15, 1983

Winston T, Henly W, Geis R: Surgery for peripheral vascular disease. AORN J 35(5):849, 1981

Young L: Streptokinase Therapy: Focus Crit Care 10(2):20, 1983
Proceedings of a Symposium: Coronary heart disease: Hypertension and other risk factors. Am J Med 76 (2A) 1, 1984

AGENCY

American Heart Association: Recommendations for Human Blood Pressure Determination by Sphygmomanometers. Pub. No. 70-019-B Dallas, American Heart Association, revised 1980
1980 Report of the Joint National Committee on Detection, Evaluation, and Treatment of High Blood Pressure. U.S. Department of Health and Human Services, Public Health Services NIH, June 27, 1980

Normal Aging Changes in the Cardiovascular System

Finch C. Hayflick L (eds): Handbook of the Biology of Aging. New York, Van Nostrand Reinhold, 1977
Reff M, Schneider E: Biological Markers of Aging. U.S. Department of Health and Human Services, NIH Publication No. 82-2221, 1982
Rockstein M, Sussman M: Biology of Aging. Belmont, Wadsworth Publishing, 1979

ENDOCRINE SYSTEM

The endocrine glands consist of highly specialized cells that secrete hormones that act as chemical messengers, creating an intricate chain of interactions between body systems. Hormones are released directly into the bloodstream, and when delivered to target organs, they elicit specific responses. In some cases, as with the thyroid, there is a more general effect on the entire body. In other cases, the effect is exceedingly specific; such is the case with the follicle-stimulating hormone (FSH), which influences the ovarian cycle. The adrenal medulla, the posterior pituitary, and, to a lesser extent, the pancreas are connected to the autonomic nervous system, secreting their hormones in response to electrical and chemical stimuli originating in the higher centers of the brain. The pituitary gland, formerly thought to be the master gland, is now believed to be under the influence of the hypothalamus. By controlling and integrating the body's functions, the endocrine glands help the body to interact with its environment.

In general, dysfunction of the endocrine system involves underproduction or overproduction of hormones or failure to secrete them according to the normal checks and balances of the body. Causes include congenital and genetic defects, surgery, atrophy, and neoplastic and nonneoplastic overactivity. Since the organs of the endocrine system are interdependent, dysfunction in one area can cause reciprocal dysfunction in another. Treatment involves correction of over- or underproduction.

Nursing Considerations

- Nursing care involves the following:
  1. Absolute accuracy in collecting specimens for sophisticated laboratory tests (check agency laboratory manual for specific instructions)
  2. Administration of hormones to patients with deficiencies
  3. Education and emotional support for patients who may face lifelong alterations in their bodies, activities, and lifestyle, and possibly a lifelong program of therapy

ADRENAL CORTEX

Description

The adrenal cortex produces hormones that control the body's adaptation to stress. They are essential to life. The gland acts principally, although not entirely, under the influence of the anterior lobe of the pituitary gland and its hormone messenger, the adrenocorticotropic hormone (ACTH).

- Glucocorticoids, such as cortisol, increase the catabolism of protein and fat, elevate the blood glucose level, inhibit protein synthesis, influence emotions, and suppress inflammation.
- Mineralocorticoids, principally aldosterone, regulate electrolytes and thereby influence fluid balance in the body by retaining sodium and excreting potassium.
- All corticoids are important for defense against stress or injury to body tissues.
- Adrenal androgens (weak male hormones found in both men and women) govern certain secondary sex characteristics in both males and females.

ADDISON'S DISEASE (PRIMARY ADRENOCORTICAL INSUFFICIENCY)

Description

Adrenocortical insufficiency may be caused by inadequate stimulation of the adrenals by the hypothalamus or pituitary, surgical removal of the adrenals, the inability of the adrenal cortex to resume function following abrupt withdrawal of steroid therapy, idiopathic atrophy, malignancy, possible autoimmune factors, or an infection such as tuberculosis.

Common Diagnostic Tests

- Plasma cortisol response to ACTH (corticotropin or cosyntropin) is measured.

- Low levels of adrenocortical hormones in plasma and urine, as reflected in plasma cortisol levels and in 24-hour urine tests for steroids (17-hydroxycorticosteroids), are common.
- Plasma ACTH levels are elevated in primary adrenal deficiency.
- Serum sodium, chloride, and blood glucose are often low.
- Serum potassium and BUN or creatinine usually are elevated.
- Complete blood count (CBC) may show eosinophilia and lymphocytosis.

Observations

- Muscular weakness, fatigue, emaciation, anorexia, nausea and vomiting, generalized and specific dark pigmentation of the skin, hypotension, emotional disturbances, and diminished resistance to even minor stress are commonly seen. Hypoglycemia may be seen in children.
- In *addisonian crisis,* there is a critical drop in corticosteroids leading to severe hypotension, hypoglycemia, hyperkalemia, and vascular collapse. It may be caused by stress, infection, surgery, severe perspiration and salt loss, or the inadequate replacement or sudden withdrawal of steroids.

Treatment

- Administration of replacement steroids, *e.g.,* hydrocortisone, fludrocortisone acetate, desoxycorticosterone acetate (See PH.)
- In addisonian crisis, reverse shock, restore circulation, replace steroids, treat hypoglycemia, and treat infection, if present. In crisis, fluid therapy provides more immediate benefit than does steroid replacement. Monitor ECG since hyperkalemia is usually present.
- Diet: high protein

Nursing Considerations

- Administer steroids, and instruct the patient concerning them (See PH). Emphasize that doses cannot be missed.
  1. Self-injection technique should be taught so that if the patient is unable to take medication by mouth, he or she can give himself or herself an injection of hydrocortisone.
  2. Injectable hydrocortisone should be carried by the patient at all times for emergency use.
- Monitor fluid and electrolytes carefully.
- Educate the patient as to the danger of infection, which could precipitate addisonian crisis. Infections, if they occur, should be treated promptly. Increased steroid doses often are required during the stress of infection, other illness, injury, surgery, or dental treatment.

- The patient should wear an identification tag or bracelet that indicates that he or she has adrenal insufficiency and requests that his or her physician be notified in case of an accident.

CUSHING'S SYNDROME

Description

Hypersecretion of the adrenal cortex may be caused by cortisol-secreting adrenal tumors or by hyperplasia of the adrenal cortex resulting from hypersecretion of ACTH by the pituitary or from ectopic hypersecretion of ACTH by malignancies in other areas, especially bronchogenic oat-cell carcinomas. Excessively high therapeutic dosages of steroids will produce the same effects as adrenocortical hypersecretion.

Common Diagnostic Tests

- Urinary 17-hydroxycorticosteroids and plasma cortisol levels are high, with the usual diurnal variation of cortisol absent. The urinary free cortisol level is elevated. Urinary 17-ketosteroids vary, depending on the cause of Cushing's syndrome.
- Dexamethasone suppression tests (high- and low-dose). Dexamethasone administration normally will suppress pituitary secretion of ACTH. In Cushing's syndrome, serum cortisol and urinary 17-hydroxycorticosteroids levels fail to drop.
- ACTH stimulation test
- Metyrapone (Metopirone) stimulation test
- Direct assay of plasma ACTH
- Abnormal glucose tolerance (hyperglycemia), hypernatremia and hypokalemia occur occasionally. Eosinophils and lymphocytes may be decreased.
- Other tests include CT scans; ultrasonography; adrenal angiography; intravenous urograms; and x-rays of the skull, spine, and ribs (often showing osteoporosis). CT scans of the sella turcica and examination of the visual fields should be done if pituitary dysfunction is suspected (see NR, X-ray preparations, Scans, and Ultrasound).
- Corticotropin-releasing factor (CRF) test with or without petrosal sinus sampling for suspected pituitary or Cushing's syndrome (still experimental)

Observations

- Edema, hypertension, and abnormal fat production and distribution, *e.g.*, "moon face," protruding abdomen, and fat pads on the back of the neck (buffalo hump); thin extremities are usually seen.

- Muscle weakness, osteoporosis, pathologic fractures, increased capillary fragility and bruising, emotional instability or frank psychosis, glucosuria, hyperglycemia, poor wound healing, increased susceptibility to infection, and impaired growth in children may be present. Thinning of scalp hair, the presence of facial hair, and acne are sometimes seen in female patients.

Treatment

- Removal of the cause, depending upon whether it originates in the pituitary, hypothalamus, or in an ACTH-like secreting tumor. It may be done by excision or irradiation of a pituitary tumor; removal of an adrenal tumor (or possibly one or both adrenal glands); or removal of an ectopic ACTH-secreting tumor. Partial or complete removal of one or both adrenal glands may be indicated.
- Reduce dosage of exogenous corticoids, if possible.

Nursing Considerations

- Give emotional support to the patient. Provide mental and physical rest. Depression is very common, and suicide is not rare in patients with Cushing's syndrome.
- Diet should be low in sodium and high in protein and potassium, with the amount of calories dependent upon weight and nutritional status of the patient.
- Test urine for glucose and acetone.
- Prevent or control infections.
- Give attention to safety factors because of the potential for easy bruising and pathologic fractures.

ADRENAL MEDULLA

Description

The adrenal medulla is under the control of the sympathetic nervous system and functions in conjunction with it. It is not essential to life. The effects of the catecholamines, epinephrine, and norepinephrine, hormones released by the adrenal medulla, are identical to those of the sympathetic nervous system.

Epinephrine elevates blood pressure (BP), converts glycogen to glucose when needed, increases heart rate, and dilates bronchioles. Norepinephrine constricts peripheral blood vessels, elevating BP. Underactivity or loss of the medullary function is rarely a problem. Replacement therapy for medullary hypofunction is not required.

PHEOCHROMOCYTOMA

Description

Overactivity of the adrenal medulla may be seen with a catecholamine-producing tumor called pheochromocytoma. It is usually benign, and also may be found outside the adrenal medulla (*e.g.*, in the urinary bladder, thorax, or brain).

Common Diagnostic Tests

- Assay of cathecholamines in a 24-hour urine specimen and assay of urinary vanillylmandelic acid (VMA)—the principal metabolite of catecholamines; usually show levels elevated above normal.
- Pheochromocytoma screen, including measurement for metanephrine on first AM voiding and on 24-hour urine specimen
- Assay of epinephrine and norepinephrine in the blood and urine during or following an attack
- CT scan, ultrasonography, and x-ray visualization of the tumor by intravenous urogram or angiography (see NR, Scans, Ultrasound, X-ray preparation.)
- The blood glucose level often is elevated, and glycosuria often is present.

Observations

- Hypertension may be persistent, fluctuating, intermittent, or paroxysmal.
- Pounding headache, sweating, apprehension, palpitations, nausea, and vomiting may be present.
- Symptoms may develop spontaneously or may be precipitated by emotional stress, physical exertion, or position change.

Treatment

- During paroxysmal episodes of hypertension
  1. Reduce all possible stimuli.
  2. Put the patient in a mid-Fowler's position to minimize intracranial pressure.
  3. Adrenolytic drugs, *e.g.*, phentolamine (Regitine), and hypotensive drugs, *e.g.*, phenoxybenzamine (Dibenzyline) and/or propranolol (Inderal), usually are ordered. *Caution:* Blood pressure must be checked at least q 30 min following administration of phentolamine.
- Surgical removal of pheochromocytoma, after preliminary control of hypertension

Nursing Considerations

Preoperative Care

- Promote rest and relief from emotional tension.
- Carefully monitor vital signs. Weigh the patient daily. Test urine for glucose and acetone, between meals and at bedtime.
- Omit stimulants from the diet, *e.g.,* coffee, tea, cola, and chocolate.
- Administer medications as ordered by the physician.

Postoperative Care

- Monitor BP carefully. Postoperative shock and hemorrhage are special dangers following this surgery. Report falling BP immediately.
- Measure and record hourly urinary output. If it is less than 30 ml/hr, report to the physician.
- Maintain IV therapy and administration of a vasopressor drug, usually norepinephrine, as ordered by the physician.
- Before discharge, instruct the patient regarding prescribed medications. If unilateral adrenalectomy has been performed, the remaining gland will produce adequate amounts of hormones to compensate for the loss of the other gland.

ADRENALECTOMY

Description

Adrenalectomy may be performed in cases of Cushing's syndrome, primary aldosteronism, adrenal tumors, and advanced carcinoma of the breast or prostate. Depending upon the indication, adrenalectomy can be bilateral, unilateral, and involving total or subtotal resection.

Nursing Considerations

- Carefully monitor vital signs; record BP up to q 5 min until readings are stable. Monitor for signs of shock, hypoglycemia, and infection.
- Urine output should be monitored each hour; if it drops below 30 ml/hr, notify the physician.
- Immediately postoperatively, stable BP is maintained by balancing rate of IV fluids and IV administration of a vasopressor drug.
- Replace hydrocortisone by IV drip intraoperatively and postoperatively. It also generally is given IM preoperatively.

- Hormone replacement will be ordered specifically for the patient, depending upon surgical procedure. The patient should be instructed regarding maintenance and immediate medication orders (See PH).
  1. Patients should be taught a self-injection technique and be furnished with a prefilled syringe of hydrocortisone for emergency use.
- At all times the patient should wear an identification bracelet stating that he or she is post-adrenalectomy and is taking oral steroids. The patient's and physician's names and phone numbers should be included with the information that the physician should be notified in case of an accident.

DIABETES MELLITUS

Description

Insulin normally is produced by the beta cells of the islets of Langerhans in the pancreas. In diabetes mellitus, there is inadequate production or inadequate utilization, or both, of insulin, causing disordered metabolism and inappropriate hyperglycemia. Genetic, viral, environmental, and autoimmune factors are believed to be interrelated causes of the disorder.

In 1979, the American Diabetes Association (ADA) endorsed a new, simpler classification for diabetes. Because the etiology of diabetes is still poorly understood, the disorder is classified along therapeutic lines. The two major types are Type I, or insulin-dependent diabetes mellitus (IDDM), and Type II, or non-insulin-dependent diabetes mellitus (NIDDM). Characteristics of these groups are summarized in Table 4-2.

Common Diagnostic Tests

- Elevated fasting blood sugar (FBS) on more than one occasion, greater than 120 mg/dl on either venous whole blood (WB) or capillary WB
- Oral glucose tolerance test (OGTT). This is not done if fasting levels are unequivocally high.
- Glycosylated hemoglobin (hemoglobin A_1) reflects metabolic control over preceding 8 weeks to 12 weeks, an increasingly popular and very useful means of evaluating long-term control.
- Self glucose monitoring on capillary blood glucose, done by the patient. A variety of kits are on the market, *e.g.*, Visidex-II or Chemstrips. They include reagent strips with or without a color-sensitive meter. Directions for use come with each kit and should be followed exactly. These systems are highly reliable and are recommended for all younger diabetics and many adult Type I diabetics for home monitoring of blood glucose.

TABLE 4-2 CHARACTERISTICS OF COMMON TYPES OF DIABETES MELLITUS

Type	Former Name	Description
Type I, insulin-dependent diabetes (IDDM)	Juvenile diabetes (JD) Juvenile-onset diabetes (JOD) Ketosis-prone diabetes Brittle diabetes	Patients produce little or no endogenous insulin. They require insulin by injection to prevent ketosis and to preserve life. Sudden onset most often occurs in children under 15 years, but may occur at any age. Onset frequently follows a viral infection. Chromosomal predisposition seems probable, although familial tendency is not as common as in Type II.
Type II, non-insulin-dependent mellitus (NIDDM)	Adult-onset diabetes (AOD) Maturity-onset diabetes (MOD) Ketosis-resistant diabetes Stable diabetes	Patients seem unable to utilize the insulin that their bodies are producing in seemingly normal or above-normal amounts. This group accounts for the great majority of diabetic patients. Onset is usually seen in patients who are over 40, obese, and have strong family history of diabetes. The risk of acquiring Type II diabetes increases with age. Women of all ages are at higher risk. Except in cases of stress or infection, persons with NIDDM rarely develop ketosis. Patients may have Type II diabetes for years, and then gradually become insulin dependent.

- Urinalysis for glucose and ketone is a second choice for self-monitoring by patients.

Observations

- Polydipsia (excessive thirst) and polyuria (excessive urination) is seen.
- Polyphagia (increased food intake) with weight loss is common in Type I (IDDM) diabetes. In Type II (NIDDM) patients, weight loss, even when desired, is difficult to attain.
- Weakness and fatigue may be present.
- Nocturnal enuresis is common among children.
- Blurred vision, vulvovaginitis, and pruritus are common, especially in NIDDM diabetics. Signs of peripheral neuropathy are seen more commonly in IDDM.
- Glucosuria (glucose in the urine) and/or ketonuria (ketones in the urine) may be shown in testing.
- NIDDM diabetics are frequently obese, but they may be asymptomatic.
- Diabetic complications may produce
  1. Diabetic acidosis (see below)
  2. Visual disturbances, which are evidence of retinopathy (Diabetes is the leading cause of blindness in the United States.)
  3. Hypertension and kidney failure (Kidney disease is 17 times more common in persons who are diabetic than in nondiabetics.)
  4. Evidence of occlusive vascular disease of the lower extremities (See MSN, Arterial occlusive disease of the lower extremities.)
  5. Lowered resistance to infections
  6. Male impotence
  7. Neuropathies primarily of the hands, legs, feet, and head
     Pain, numbness, lack of sensitivity to heat or cold, tingling sensation
  8. Complications of pregnancy (See OB, Coexisting medical conditions complicating pregnancy, diabetes mellitus)
  9. Cardiovascular disorders (Coronary heart disease and stroke are twice as likely to occur in persons with diabetes as those without.)

Treatment

- The goal of treatment is to prevent diabetic complications by maintaining blood glucose levels at as near normal as possible over the years.

- Control requires a balance between food intake, activity, and medication, if required. Stress management may diminish "brittleness" of control.
- Diet: A balanced diet will be prescribed by the physician to meet the individual needs of the patient. The single most important dietary principle is the attainment of ideal body weight.
  1. ADA diets are based on six groups, or exchange lists, of food. Each list consists of foods that, in the amounts specified, are nearly equal in calories, carbohydrates, proteins, and fats. The "exchanges," or groups, are milk, vegetables, fruits, bread, meat, and fats. Foods in the same exchange list are interchangeable. Substitutions may be made within groups but not between groups.
  2. The two food groups requiring significant restrictions are free sugars and animal fats.
  3. Foods with high-fiber content are recommended.
  4. Overall daily caloric intake must be maintained consistently.
  5. Adjustments must be made to compensate for illness, stress, or unplanned exercise.
  6. Diet and exercise alone may control hyperglycemia in the Type II diabetic patient.
- Exercise: A regular exercise program is an important part of the control of diabetes, but the program should be individualized for the patient.
- Medication
  1. Insulin by injection (see PH) is essential for Type I patients, and sometimes required for Type II patients if diet or oral hypoglycemic agents fail to provide control of hyperglycemia.
     a. Insulin pumps (open-loop) provide a continuous, subcutaneous infusion of insulin. Precalculated "bolus doses" are administered prior to each meal. Self monitoring of blood glucose provides the patient with information necessary to adjust insulin dosages, providing him or her more control and more flexibility in life-style.
     b. Still considered somewhat experimental, insulin pumps may offer advantages to the highly motivated, well-educated diabetic patient, who has been difficult to control with conventional methods. It may be especially valuable for pregnant patients. Fatal hypoglycemia is not rare with pumps, and the risk–benefit ratio of the device is still under study.
  2. Oral hypoglycemic agents, *e.g.,* tolbutamide (Orinase), tolazamide (Tolinase), may be ordered for Type II diabetics if weight reduction and diet do not control hyperglycemia (See PH).
- Islet transplantation is being done experimentally.

Nursing Considerations

- Administer medication: insulin and, infrequently, oral hypoglycemics (See PH.)
- Monitor fingerstick blood glucose levels or collection of double-voided urine specimens at specified times. Test urine for glucose and acetone (See LAB.)
- Fractional urines should be tested on all known hospitalized diabetic patients. The stress of surgery or infection may alter the control of diabetes.
- Be sure samples for fasting blood glucose tests, if ordered, are drawn before giving morning insulin or breakfast.
- Blood glucose levels should be monitored frequently when diabetic patients are receiving large amounts of intravenous glucose.
- Diabetic patients undergoing surgery require special consideration.
  1. The patient should be admitted at least one day prior to surgery for evaluation of diabetes control. Stress caused by anesthesia and surgery could cause hyperglycemia. Preoperative teaching, by relieving anxiety, may even decrease the amount of insulin required.
  2. Patients taking oral hypoglycemic agents usually are taken off them the day before surgery.
  3. Insulin dosages will be adjusted on the day of surgery and postoperatively.
  4. A fasting blood glucose test usually is ordered on the morning of surgery. Blood glucose levels are monitored carefully intraoperatively and postoperatively. Insulin is balanced with the glucose in IV fluids.
- General hygienic care includes meticulous attention to the skin, feet, and mouth.
- Patient should wear an identification bracelet at all times, showing that he or she is a diabetic patient.
- Education of the patient is directed toward self-care. His or her cooperation and active involvement in treatment are keys to staying well.
  1. Teach the patient that illness, decreased or increased intake of food, increased or decreased exercise, and certain medications may require adjustments to his diabetic control program. Under those circumstances, urine or blood should be tested several times a day.
  2. Recognize patients who require special help, *e.g.,* children, adolescents, the blind, and pregnant patients (see OB, Coexisting medical conditions complicating pregnancy).
  3. Many hospitals have on staff a diabetes educator who is available to help both patients and nursing staff.

4. Excellent informational materials are available through the following: American Diabetic Association, Inc., 2 Park Avenue, New York, New York 10016, or your local chapter; or the Juvenile Diabetes Foundation, 23 East 26th Street, New York, New York 10010, or your local chapter.

DIABETIC KETOACIDOSIS

Description

Diabetic ketoacidosis (DKA) usually develops as a result of marked insulin deficiency. Hyperglycemia results in severe glycosuria, causing profound water and electrolyte loss. Ketones appear in the blood and urine, as fat is metabolized faster than it can be used. Infection or omission of insulin is the most common cause. It is seen in insulin-dependent diabetic patients.

Myocardial infarction (MI) and stroke occasionally complicate diabetic acidosis in older patients.

Observations

- Symptoms usually come on over a period of days or weeks, but may develop in a period of hours if diabetes is not well controlled.
- Thirst
- Polyuria (excessive urination); bedwetting
- Sweet, fruity odor to the breath
- Weakness, fatigue
- Blurred vision
- Warm, flushed, and dry skin—symptoms of dehydration
- Later signs include deep, rapid respiration and "air hunger" (Kussmaul breathing).
- Hypotension
- Abdominal pain and tenderness, nausea, and vomiting
- Confusion and lethargy progressing to coma

Treatment

- Full-blown diabetic acidosis requires emergency medical care.
- Short-acting (regular) insulin should be administered intravenously or subcutaneously.
- A nasogastric tube may be ordered to drain stomach and prevent aspiration (see NR, Gastrointestinal intubation).
- Oxygen by face mask or nasal cannula may be ordered (see NR, Oxygen therapy).
- An IV infusion usually is started to correct hypovolemia and to provide IV access for medication (see NR, Intravenous therapy).

- Serum glucose, potassium, bicarbonate, and acetone levels must be monitored.
- Correct electrolyte and water imbalance.
- CVP line may be ordered, especially if patient is elderly or has cardiac problems.
- If infection is present, antibiotics will be ordered.

HYPEROSMOLAR HYPERGLYCEMIC NONKETOTIC COMA

Description

Hyperosmolar hyperglycemic nonketotic coma (HHNC) is a life-threatening emergency with a high mortality rate. Patients with this disorder produce enough insulin to prevent fat breakdown or ketosis, but not enough to avert mounting hyperglycemia, which leads to hyperosmolality and severe dehydration.

Seen most commonly in elderly, debilitated patients with mild or suspected diabetes, there frequently is a precipitating condition. Infection, pancreatitis, gastrointestinal hemorrhage, uremia, burns, hemodialysis, peritoneal dialysis, hyperalimentation therapy, surgery, and the ingestion of certain drugs known to aggravate diabetes control, *e.g.*, cortisone, phenytoin, and the thiazides, may precipitate HHNC.

Common Diagnostic Tests

- Serum glucose: 600 mg/dl, to as much as 2,800 mg/dl
- Serum osmolarity: 350–475 mOsm/kg
- Serum sodium level: frequently elevated
- Serum acetone: absent or mildly elevated

Observations

- Onset may be insidious, over a period of days or weeks.
- Polyuria and polydipsia may be present.
- Diminished sense of thirst may occur.
- Nausea, vomiting, and diarrhea may be seen.
- Signs of marked dehydration include decreased skin turgor, dryness of the mucous membranes, dry or shrunken tongue, and sunken eyeballs.
- Fever, tachycardia, and hypotension may be present.
- Lethargy or confusion may indicate hyperosmolar state.
- Stupor, seizures, and bizarre behavior may lead to coma.
- Kussmaul respiration is absent.

Treatment

- Replace fluids.
- If insulin is used, very small doses are given.
- Restore electrolyte balance.
- Correct underlying precipitating cause.

Nursing Considerations

- Try to prevent HHNC by identifying patients at risk.
  1. Maintain hydration and verify it by
     a. Carefully recording intake and output
     b. Recording daily weight
     c. Watching for signs of dehydration
- Watch for changes in sensorium.
- Protect high-risk patients by regularly monitoring urine from double-voided specimens for glucose and acetone, or by a fingerstick blood glucose test.
- During rehydration, carefully monitor vital signs and administration of IV fluids.

HYPOGLYCEMIC REACTION: INSULIN SHOCK

Description

Hypoglycemic reactions usually occur when the diabetic patient takes too much insulin, decreases food intake, or increases activity without increasing food intake. The blood glucose level drops below 60 mg/dl. Reactions occur less frequently with oral hypoglycemics, but are apt to be prolonged and severe, especially with chlorpropamide (Diabinese).

Observations

- Symptoms frequently have a rapid onset—sometimes minutes to hours. Patient may develop severe hypoglycemia with unconsciousness or seizures without experiencing any conscious symptoms.
- Hunger
- Weakness, nervousness, tremor
- Moist, clammy skin
- Blurred vision
- Changes in behavior, irritability, confusion
- Headaches

- Hypothermia, tachycardia
- Unconsciousness

Treatment

- Give a form of sugar, *e.g.*, one-half glass of any juice, ginger ale, cola (not diet), or 2 teaspoons of honey, sugar candy, or cake frosting (½ tube). Record time and the amount given.
- One protocol includes the following.
  1. One-half glass of juice is given initially.
  2. In 5 minutes to 10 minutes, if no response is seen, give another one-half glass. (It is important not to overtreat hypoglycemia since it may cause a rebound effect.)
  3. Follow with a long-acting carbohydrate and protein, *e.g.*, cheese and crackers.
- Fifty percent glucose IV. Viscosity makes it difficult to administer. Give over a period of 2 minutes to 5 minutes. While administering, aspirate blood frequently to counteract sclerosing effect of glucose.
- Glucagon stimulates the liver to release glucose from stored glycogen. It is sometimes ordered for very unstable diabetic patients, and may be injected at home by a member of the patient's family.
- *Caution:* If there is doubt as to whether the patient's blood glucose level is too high or too low, *always give glucose first.* If the patient is hypoglycemic, the response usually will be almost immediate.

PARATHYROID GLANDS

Description

The parathyroid glands are small bodies most typically located on the posterior aspect of the thyroid gland. They produce the parathyroid hormone, parathormone (PTH), that acts on bone, intestine, and kidney to maintain normal serum calcium levels. Parathormone maintains an inverse relationship between serum calcium and serum phosphate levels, thereby fostering normal excitability of nerves and muscles.

HYPERPARATHYROIDISM

Description

Primary hyperparathyroidism is caused by overactivity of one or more of the parathyroid glands caused most often by a single adenoma, hyperplasia of all the glands, or occasionally from a carcinoma of a single gland. Compensatory oversecretion of PTH in any clinical situation in which there is a tendency toward hypocalcemia, or ectopic secretion of parathormone by tumors elsewhere, is seen occasionally. Symptoms arise from the elevated blood calcium level, the increased resorption of calcium from bone, and the increased excretion of calcium in urine.

Common Diagnostic Tests

Diagnosis depends on demonstrating that hypercalcemia is not caused by one or another of a great many causes of hypercalcemia.

- Elevated serum calcium, depressed serum phosphate levels, hypercalciuria (elevated calcium in the urine) (See LAB.)
- Measurement of parathyroid hormone in the blood by immunoassay
- Skeletal changes detected by x-ray, showing diffuse demineralization of bones, subperiosteal resorption, bone cysts, or vertebral compression fracture
- ECG, slit-lamp examination of the eye may show corneal calcification (''band keratopathy'').
- Thermography, ultrasonography, CT scan

Observations

- Evidence of hypercalcemia, *e.g.*, apathy, fatigue, thirst, muscular weakness, nausea, vomiting, constipation, cardiac arrhythmias, emotional irritability, neurosis or psychosis, and increased excitement of nerves and muscles
- Evidence of demineralization of bones, such as backache, joint pain, and possible pathologic fractures
- Evidence of kidney damage, such as kidney stones or x-ray evidence of nephrocalcinosis (the precipitation of calcium phosphate at the renal tubules)

Treatment

- A high fluid intake to dilute urine and a low calcium diet are recommended.
- Severe hypercalcemia is an emergency that requires large volumes of fluid and vigorous therapy with furosemide (Lasix). *Caution:* Thiazides are contraindicated because they decrease the renal excretion of calcium, thereby increasing serum calcium levels.
- If renal function is impaired seriously, hemodialysis may be lifesaving during the time required to prepare patient for surgery.
- Surgical removal of hyperfunctioning gland or glands

Nursing Considerations

Preoperative Care

- Force fluids. Carefully monitor intake and output.
- Promote mobility of the patient (to minimize calcium resorption from bone) while protecting him or her from injury and falls.
- Strain all urine if stones are suspected.
- If the patient has heart disease, administer digitalis preparations cautiously. Interaction of calcium and digitalis can be hazardous. Watch for signs of digitalis toxicity (see PH).

Postoperative Care

- Same as for thyroidectomy
- Watch closely for signs of tetany, hyperirritability of nerves with spasms of hands and feet, generalized tremor, and incoordinated contractions.
- Monitor serum calcium and phosphorus frequently.

HYPOPARATHYROIDISM

Description

Hypoparathyroidism occurs when parathyroid tissue has been removed surgically, or as a result of idiopathic atrophy. It occasionally occurs spontaneously, particularly in childhood, but is seen most often following neck surgery with inadvertent loss of the parathyroids.

Common Diagnostic Tests

- Immunoassay measurement shows decreased parathyroid hormone.
- The serum calcium level is decreased, and the serum phosphate level is elevated (see LAB).
- Skull x-ray may show basal ganglia calcification in idiopathic hypoparathyroidism.

Observations

- Positive Chvostek's sign: Spasms of facial muscles occur when muscles or branches of facial nerves are tapped.
- Positive Trousseau's sign: Carpal spasm (flexion of the elbows and wrists and extension of the carpophalangeal joints) is induced by occluding the circulation in an arm with a blood pressure cuff.

- Numbness, tingling, and stiffness of hands and feet are seen in latent tetany.
- Bronchospasm, stridor, laryngeal spasm, carpal spasm, dysphagia, cardiac arrhythmias, and convulsions may be seen when overt tetany occurs.
- Lethargy, personality changes, anxiety, blurring of vision due to cataracts, and mental retardation may be seen in chronic hypoparathyroidism.

Treatment and Nursing Considerations

- In an acute attack, the goal is to elevate the serum calcium level enough to render the patient symptom free by IV administration of 10% calcium chloride or 10% calcium gluconate solution.
- If seizures continue, give anticonvulsants as ordered.
- Keep tracheostomy set, as well as calcium gluconate, ready for IV administration, at the bedside following parathyroid and thyroid surgery. *Caution:* Calcium gluconate and digitalis potentiate each other, so carefully monitor the cardiac patient (see PH).
- Dihydrotachysterol (Hytakerol, AT 10), a synthetic vitamin D, usually is started when oral calcium is begun after the acute attack subsides.
- Aluminum carbonate or aluminum hydroxide gel (Gelusil, Amphojel) after meals may be used to keep phosphate levels down (see PH).
- Provide a quiet environment for the patient.
- Mild hypoparathyroidism may prove to be transitory, and the patient may require only small amounts of calcium orally, or no therapy at all.
- Maintenance treatment includes
  1. A diet high in calcium and low in phosphorus. (Although milk products are high in calcium, they are also very high in phosphorus and therefore are restricted.)
  2. Calcium salts and vitamin D (calciferol or dihydrotachysterol) are continued.
  3. Chlorthalidone combined with low-sodium diet has been reported to be a regimen that controls hypoparathyroidism without the use of vitamin D.
  4. Instruct the patient about the need for lifelong, follow-up medical supervision. Frequent calcium level determinations are required. Hypercalcemia resulting from excess vitamin D and calcium intake is sometimes seen and may be quite dangerous.

PITUITARY

DIABETES INSIPIDUS

Description

Diabetes insipidus (DI) is a disorder that results from a deficiency of the antidiuretic hormone (ADH), vasopressin, and must be differentiated from nephrogenic and psychogenic DI. ADH normally is secreted by the posterior lobe of the pituitary gland. The deficiency may be caused by damage to the posterior pituitary itself from tumors (benign or malignant); partial or complete surgical ablation of the gland by hypophysectomy, trauma, or infectious processes; or the disorder may be caused by idiopathic deterioration of part of the hypothalamus.

Common Diagnostic Tests

- Serum and urine osmolality tests (Values will show an inappropriately dilute urine in the face of an elevated serum osmolality.)
- Urine specific gravity will be below 1.006, with a maximum of 1.014 on a concentration test (see LAB).
- No glycosuria will be present.
- X-ray films of the skull; CT scan of the sella turcica and the hypothalamus
- Fluid deprivation test. Normally urine will become more concentrated, but in DI, specific gravity will not go above 1.014.
- Vasopressin injection test, to see if urinary output will decrease and specific gravity will rise after injection of vasopressin.

Observations

- Polyuria and polydipsia are classic symptoms. Patient may drink and excrete up to 20 liters of fluid per day. Urine is dilute.
- Restriction of fluid intake causes dehydration, weight loss, headache, irritability, fatigue, muscular pains, tachycardia, and hypovolemic shock.

Treatment

- Give vasopressin tannate (Pitressin tannate) in oil in a deep IM injection immediately postoperatively following pituitary surgery (See PH).
- A synthetic substitute, *e.g.,* desmopressin (DDAVP) or lypressin, is now the treatment of choice in chronic DI (see PH).
- Chlorpropamide (Diabinese) has been found to be an effective antidiuretic. Warn patient about possible hypoglycemic reactions (see PH).

- Supplementary potassium may be ordered to prevent depletion (see PH).

Nursing Considerations

- Accurate measurements of fluid intake and output are essential.
- Check urine for specific gravity. Closely monitor patient's weight.
- Follow special instructions in administration of vasopressin, and prepare patient for lifelong therapy.
- Keep patient well hydrated. Replace the amount of fluid lost in urine. The patient is very susceptible to dehydration, hypovolemic shock, and collapse. (A patient with DI who is otherwise healthy, if allowed and able to drink and eat according to need, will maintain proper water balance without any therapy.)
- Excellent skin care is required.
- Emotional support is required for the patient dealing with the frustrating symptoms of urgent need to allay thirst and to void. Additional support will be required if patient is studied for possible cranial pathology.
- The patient should wear an identification bracelet describing his or her condition and treatment, and also providing the physician's name.

TRANSSPHENOIDAL HYPOPHYSECTOMY

Description

Transsphenoidal hypophysectomy, the surgical procedure of choice for partial or complete removal of the pituitary gland, may be performed to remove a pituitary tumor, control the progression of diabetic retinopathy, or control metastatic carcinoma of the breast or prostate. The operative approach is made by an incision in the inner aspect of the upper lip and gingiva and through the floor of the nose and sphenoid sinus into the sella turcica (the pituitary fossa). After the incision is closed, the nose is packed and a small sling is applied to prevent the packing from slipping out. A soft nasal airway may be inserted (see Fig. 4–3).

Common Diagnostic Tests

- Endocrinology work-up may include serum assays of pituitary hormones; adrenocorticotropic hormone (ACTH), follicle-stimulating hormone (FSH), human gonadotropin hormone (hGH), luteinizing hormone (LH), prolactin, thyroid-stimulating hormone (TSH), plus tests for adrenal function (see MSN, Adrenal cortex).
- Skull x-rays

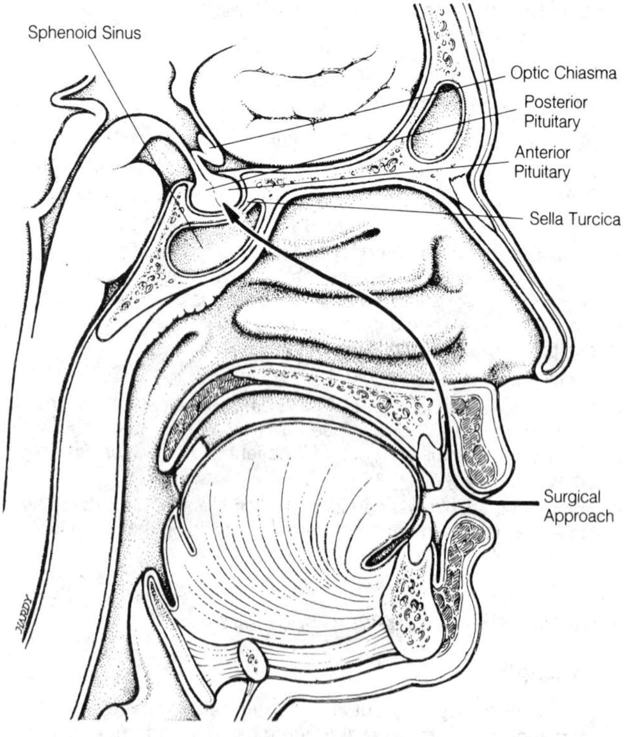

Fig. 4-3. *To remove the pituitary using a transsphenoidal approach, an incision is made in the inner aspect of the upper lip and gingiva, and the sella turcica is entered through the floor of the nose and sphenoid sinus.* (Camunas C: Transsphenoidal hypophysectomy. Am J Nurs 80(10):1821, Oct 1980)

- CT scan, tomograms, pneumoencephalograms, laminograms
- Angiography

Nursing Considerations

- Reassurance and emotional support for the patient both preoperatively and postoperatively are necessary

Postoperative Care

- The goal of care is to decrease pressure on the sella turcica, and to prevent stress on the area where sella turcica was entered, thereby preventing leaks of cerebrospinal fluid (CSF).

1. Elevate head of the bed approximately 30° at all times.
2. Vigorous coughing or sneezing should be avoided, but encourage the patient to deep breathe.
3. Any clear drainage from the nose, after packing has been removed, should be tested for glucose, which is found in cerebrospinal fluid (CSF). Most leaks heal spontaneously within 72 hours.

   If a leak occurs, antibiotics usually are ordered to prevent meningitis.

4. Patients should be advised to observe the following precautions for up to two months postoperatively.

   Avoid bending forward for any reason, *e.g.*, to tie a shoe, to pick up something on the floor, or to shampoo the hair in a sink.

   Avoid straining at stool. Increase fluids and fiber foods, and use stool softeners or laxatives, if necessary.

   Avoid tooth brushing for at least 10 days. Floss and rinse instead.

- Demerol or codeine may be ordered immediately postoperatively for pain. After that, aspirin and acetaminophen (Tylenol) will usually relieve headache. Sudden changes or severe pain should be reported.
- Diabetes insipidus is a common sequela (see MSN, Diabetes insipidus).
- If the entire gland has been removed, corticosteroids, sex hormones, and thyroid replacement probably will be required (see PH). (Surprisingly, very small residuals of pituitary tissue may provide adequate target gland support.) Patients will require education concerning these drugs, and counseling for both the patient and his or her partner regarding sexual problems that may arise from hormonal deficiencies.

THYROID

Description

Thyrotropin-releasing hormone (TRH), produced by the hypothalamus, stimulates the anterior pituitary gland to synthesize and release thyroid-stimulating hormone (TSH), thyrotropin. TSH, in turn, stimulates the thyroid gland to synthesize and secrete its two principal hormones, thyroxine (T_4) and triiodothyronine (T_3). These act to regulate body metabolism and energy production, to promote normal growth and cell reproduction, to influence fluid and electrolyte balance, and to control body use of fat, amino acids, and carbohydrates. The manufacture of thyroid hormones requires protein and iodine. Calcitonin, a third hormone, is secreted by the parafollicular cells of the thyroid. Its functions are to help maintain blood calcium balance by inhibiting calcium release from bone and to promote calcium deposit in bone, thereby preventing hypercalcemia. Parathyroid hormone is antagonistic to calcitonin.

Most thyroid disorders are more common in women than in men. Common abnormalities include

- Enlargement of the thyroid gland (goiter), caused primarily by adenomatous hyperplasia, inflammation (thyroiditis), benign or malignant tumors, or (rarely today) iodine deficiency
- Hypothyroidism (underactivity of the gland)
- Hyperthyroidism (overactivity of the gland)

Common Diagnostic Tests

Tests for thyroid function can determine whether hyper- or hypofunction is present, whether it is primary (*i.e.,* from dysfunction of the thyroid gland itself) or secondary to pituitary dysfunction, or whether some other malfunction is present. The tests are influenced greatly by the patient's sex hormone status, nutritional state, age, and exposure to drugs that alter the binding capacities of serum proteins, *e.g.,* oral contraceptives and phenytoin (Dilantin).

- Tests for evaluating thyroid function, none of which are influenced by exogenous iodides, are
  1. T_4 by radioimmunoassay (T_4-RIA)
  2. T_3 by radioimmunoassary (T_3-RIA)
  3. T_3 resin uptake (T_3 RU)
  4. Free thyroxine index (FTI): the calculated product of T_4 and T_3 resin uptake
- Tests that involve homeostatic controls from the pituitary and the hypothalamus
  1. Thyrotropin radioimmunoassay (TSH RIA)
  2. TRH stimulation test
- Thyroid scan (radioiodine or technetium scintiscan) for evaluating the anatomic "geography" of the gland, including "hot" or "cold" nodules (see NR, Scans, nuclear).
- Radioiodine uptake: helpful in diagnosis of hyperthyroidism and essential for calculating dose for those to be treated with radioiodine. It often is depressed in subacute thyroiditis (see NR, Scans, nuclear).
- Sonogram may help differentiate solid from cystic thyroid nodules (see NR, Ultrasound).
- Other tests: thyroid-binding globulin (TBG), thyroid antibodies (in thyroiditis), serum calcitonin (increased in medullary carcinoma of the thyroid).

Nursing Considerations

- A careful patient history regarding medication intake is essential for the correct evaluation of thyroid test results.
- Older tests, specifically protein-bound iodine (PBI), are influenced greatly by iodine-containing medications such as Lugol's solution, potassium iodide, x-ray contrast medium, antiseptics, cough syrups, and nail strengtheners. Radioactive iodine uptake also is affected.
- Many medications may alter T_4, T_3, or T_3 RU test results, *e.g.*, estrogens, progesterone, androgen, antithyroid drugs, probenecid, dilantin, salicylates, large doses of corticosteroids or ACTH, and heparin.

GOITER, SIMPLE

Description

The most common type of thyroid enlargement is caused most often by adenomatous hyperplasia of unknown origin. It is often familial. In the United States today, it rarely is caused by inadequate iodine intake. It may be caused by ingestion of large amounts of goitrogenic substances (goiter-producing agents that inhibit thyroxine production), such as propylthiouracil, iodine in large doses, lithium, cabbage, and soybeans. A goiter often begins at puberty, often begins or worsens with pregnancy, and may appear at menopause.

Observations

- An enlarged thyroid gland may cause difficulty in swallowing (dysphagia), respiratory difficulties (dyspnea), or voice changes.

Treatment and Nursing Considerations

- Thyroid hormone: Watch for symptoms of thyrotoxicosis (*e.g.*, rapid pulse, tremors, nervous symptoms, weight loss) (see PH).
- Subtotal thyroidectomy may be necessary if thyroid hormone therapy fails to shrink the goiter and symptoms or appearance require removal (see MSN, Thyroidectomy and subtotal thyroidectomy).

HYPERTHYROIDISM (GRAVES' DISEASE)

Description

Hyperthyroidism (Graves' disease) is caused by oversecretion of the two thyroid hormones. The phrase "exophthalmic goiter" describes two of the symptoms commonly seen: bulging of the eyeballs and enlargement of the thyroid gland. The condition is believed to have an autoimmune basis, and some evidence suggests an inherited factor.

Hyperthyroidism also may be caused by a thyroid adenoma, very rarely by a pituitary adenoma, and not infrequently by overtreatment with thyroid hormone.

Common Diagnostic Tests

- T_4 level and radioiodine and T_3 RU are increased.
- Radioiodine uptake cannot be suppressed by T_3 administration.
- The TSH level is low normal, or even below normal when very sensitive assay techniques are used.
- A thyroid scan may distinguish between diffuse and nodular goiter.

Observations

- Nervousness, weakness, tremor, tachycardia, sleeplessness are frequently seen.
- Poor toleration of heat; flushed hot skin; excessive perspiration are common.
- Exophthalmos (bulging eyes), stare, tremor may occur.
- Weight loss despite increased appetite, and diarrhea may be seen.
- Enlargement of the thyroid gland is usually seen.

Treatment

- Medications
  1. Antithyroid drugs, *e.g.,* propylthiouracil, methimazole (Tapazole) (See PH.)
  2. Iodide preparations, *e.g.,* Lugol's solution, saturated solution of potassium iodide (SSKI) (See PH.)

     These drugs also are used separately or in combination preoperatively to reduce the vascularity of the thyroid.

  3. Propranolol (Inderal), dexamethasone to alter the peripheral effects of the thyroid homrones

     Propranolol may be used alone for preoperative preparation.
- Thyroid ablation
  1. Radioactive iodine (^{131}I)—contraindicated in pregnant women; use in children is limited to very special situations.

2. Subtotal thyroidectomy—surgical removal of most of the thyroid tissue (see below) after the patient has been brought to the euthyroid (normal thyroid) state by antithyroid drugs.

- Supportive measures
  1. Rest
  2. A diet high in calories, proteins, vitamins, and fluids
  3. Sedation, if required
  4. Protections for the eyes, *e.g.*, dark glasses, methylcellulose solution (1%) eye-drops to prevent drying, elevation of the head of the bed at night

Nursing Considerations

- Administer medications, as ordered. Antithyroid drugs and propranolol (Inderal) must be given right up to the time of surgery (see PH).
- Provide a restful, cool environment. These patients are very intolerant of heat.
- Be accepting of the patient's behavior. These patients have poor control of their emotions and often fail to cooperate in their own care.
- Severe exophthalmos may require eye drops, dark glasses, eye exercises, and that eyelids be taped shut.
- Observe closely for arrhythmias, elevated blood pressure, and palpitations.

HYPOTHYROIDISM (MYXEDEMA, CRETINISM)

Description

Primary hypothyroidism refers to hypofunction originating with the thyroid gland itself. It often has an autoimmune basis. *Secondary hypothyroidism* involves disorders of the pituitary or hypothalamus that result in TSH deficiency.

Hypothyroidism may result from treatment of hyperthyroidism, *e.g.*, thyroidectomy or radioiodine therapy followed by too much destruction of thyroid tissue, or from too high a dose of antithyroid drugs being used to treat hyperthyroidism.

Myxedema refers to hypothyroidism seen in an adult that is so severe or has lasted so long, that profound metabolic and anatomic changes occur. In congenital hypothyroidism *(Cretinism)*, the thyroid gland is absent or rudimentary; or present but defective in hormone secretion; goitrous; or secondarily atrophied. Juvenile hypothyroidism is acquired during childhood and involves atrophy of the thyroid gland or defective function.

Common Diagnostic Tests

- FTI and T_4 are low. (Serum thyroxine-T_4 or TSH tests are part of routine neonatal screening in many states.)
- The TSH level is elevated in primary hypothyroidism but not in secondary hypothyroidism.
- A blood count frequently shows anemia (macrocytic) in adults.
- Serum cholesterol usually is elevated in primary but not secondary hypothyroidism.
- In children, delayed skeletal maturation, often with "stippling" of the epiphyses, is seen on x-ray.

Observations

Symptoms and findings caused by low metabolic rate generally come on slowly. All body systems eventually become involved.

- Apathy, fatigue, mental slow down, weight gain, and constipation
- Sensitivity to cold and diminished perspiration
- Menstrual irregularities (usually menorrhagia)
- Decreased sex drive
- Skin that becomes thickened, dry, flaky, and edematous; hair that thins and falls out; mask-like expression of the face
- Premature development of arteriosclerosis
- In children, in addition to the above, short stature is common; mental retardation, "pot belly" with umbilical hernia, and delayed development may be seen. Precocious puberty occasionally is present.

Treatment

- Correct deficiency by giving natural or synthetic thyroid hormones, *e.g.*, thyroid, U.S.P. (desiccated), levothyroxine sodium (T_4) (Synthroid) (see PH).
- If the hypothyroidism is of long duration, the dosage is increased gradually.
- Prognosis in congenital and juvenile hypothyroidism is dependent upon early diagnosis and faithful compliance with treatment. Mental development is at stake.

Nursing Considerations

- Instruct the patient about the lifelong need for daily hormone therapy. (For important nursing implications regarding administration of thyroid hormones, see PH.)
- *Caution:* The myxedematous patient has decreased ability to handle barbiturates, anesthesia, narcotics, and sedatives.

- Provide a warm environment. These patients have intolerance to cold.
- Do not overtire the patient.
- Give good skin care, range of motion exercises, foods with roughage, stool softeners, and fluids (but not enough to cause patient to go into congestive heart failure or water intoxication).
- Be aware of possible complications: cardiovascular (angina, myocardial infarction, congestive heart failure), psychosis, myxedema coma (when all body systems come to an almost standstill), grand mal seizures, or death.

THYROIDECTOMY AND SUBTOTAL THYROIDECTOMY

Nursing Considerations

Postoperative Care

- Care for the incision by maintaining semi-Fowler's position and support of the head, neck, and shoulders with sandbags and soft collar are necessary.
- Teach the patient to support his or her own head and neck.
- Provide humidification. Oxygen therapy may be required (see NR, Oxygen administration).
- Watch for, and be prepared for, complications.
  1. Hemorrhage (Check dressing and vital signs frequently.)
  2. Respiratory obstruction (Have tracheostomy set at bedside.)
  3. Laryngeal nerve damage (Ask the patient to speak every hour, but avoid unnecessary talking.)
  4. Tetany caused by inadvertent removal of parathyroid glands (Have calcium gluconate available for IV administration.)
  5. Thyroid crisis or storm, seen with patients inadequately prepared for surgery (Earliest manifestations are extreme tachycardia and hyperthermia.) (See MSN, Thyroid storm.)

THYROID STORM (THYROID CRISIS)

Description

Thyroid storm, or thyroid crisis, is a life-threatening condition of severe thyrotoxicosis precipitated by stress (*e.g.,* infection, injury, labor, or poor preparation for surgery). It rarely is seen today.

Observations

- Severe tachycardia, hyperthermia (high fever), dehydration, delirium, and disturbances of all major systems are frequently seen.

Treatment

- Hypothermia (reduce fever)
  1. Nursing measures (*e.g.*, cold packs or hypothermia blanket)
  2. Acetaminophen (Tylenol), preferred to salicylates
- Cardiac support, *e.g.*, propranolol (Inderal).
- Intravenous fluids containing dextrose; may include antithyroid medication
- Iodine preparations (*e.g.*, sodium iodide, IV initially; Lugol's solution PO after crisis has subsided).
- Corticosteroids (to treat shock or adrenal insufficiency).
- Oxygen therapy, if necessary
- Possible exchange transfusions or peritoneal dialysis

NORMAL AGING CHANGES IN THE ENDOCRINE SYSTEM

- Changes within the endocrine glands caused by aging tend to be subtle and less pronounced than those that occur in other organ systems.
- The pituitary gland demonstrates a decrease in weight and vascularity. There is an increase in the amount of connective tissue and an increase in the disorganization of the cellular components. Despite these changes, concentrations of pituitary hormones appear unaltered. Corticotropin (ACTH) levels, cortisol plasma levels, and circadian rhythms are similar to those of younger individuals.
- The thyroid gland experiences irreversible changes in the cells, and normal connective tissue fibers are replaced with dense collagenous fibers. There is a steady decrease in the accumulation of iodine in the thyroid and in thyroid hormone production. Both physical activity and basal metabolism are reduced. Therefore, thyroid function is adequate in most older people, and the thyroid maintains its reserve capacity.
- The parathyroid glands maintain their weight from middle adulthood into old age. Their secretions remain relatively constant but can be affected by aging changes in other endocrine glands and by plasma calcium levels.
- The adrenal glands exhibit an increase in connective tissue and pigmentation. Loss of lipids, vascular dilatation, and hemorrhage also are characteristic. The plasma levels of the glucocorticoids as well as their diurnal rhythms appear similar to those of younger individuals. The adrenal cortex may be less sensitive to ACTH stimulation. In healthy older persons, normal salt and water balance is maintained because aldosterone secretion shows little change with age. Corticoid androgen secretion is reduced, but it is not clear in what way, if any, the reduction affects the function of an older person.

- Normal aging changes in the pancreas are difficult to distinguish from the changes occurring in diabetes mellitus. Throughout adult life there is a progressive deterioration in glucose tolerance. The amount of insulin available for secretion does not appear to diminish with aging, but there is a delayed rise in insulin levels after oral glucose. The decreased, lean body mass and increased adiposity in elderly people may provide less tissue in which carbohydrates can be stored. Insulin antagonists may be present and there may be an increased production of proinsulin, a biologically less potent precursor of insulin.

IMPLICATIONS

- If the endocrine system could be considered in isolation, the changes occurring with aging probably would not cause significant problems in glandular function. But one must consider the role of multiple chronic illnesses, multiple medications, and stress in reducing the endocrine reserve capacity of the older individual.

MSN

BIBLIOGRAPHY • Endocrinology

BOOKS

Brunner L, Suddarth D: The Lippincott Manual of Nursing Practice, 3rd ed. Philadelphia, JB Lippincott, 1982

Dunphy J, Way L: Current Surgical Diagnosis and Treatment, 6th ed. Los Altos, CA, Lange Medical Publications, 1983

Krupp M, Chatton M: Current Medical Diagnosis & Treatment 1983, 22nd ed. Los Altos, CA, Lange Medical Publications, 1983

McClung M, Greer M: Treatment of hyperthyroidism. Annual Review of Medicine, 13th ed. p 385. Palo Alto, CA, Annual Reviews Inc, 1980

Phipps W, Long B, Woods N: Medical-Surgical Nursing: Concepts and Clinical Practice, 2nd ed. St Louis, CV Mosby, 1983

Williams R: Textbook of Endocrinology, 6th ed. Philadelphia, WB Saunders, 1981

JOURNALS

Adams C: Pulling your patient through an adrenal crisis. RN 46(10):36, Oct 1983

Arcangelo V: Simple goiter. Nursing '83 13(3):47, Mar 1983

Bergman M, Felig P: Newer approaches to the control of the insulin-dependent diabetic patient. Disease-a-Month, 29(7):1–65 Apr 1983

Bilezikan J: The medical management of primary hyperparathyroidism. Arch Intern Med 96:188, 1982

Burry M: ADH: Antidiuretic hormone and its inappropriate secretion. Can Nurse 76(2):41, Feb 1980

Camunas C: Pheochromocytoma. Am J Nurs 83(6):887, June 1983

Camunas C: Transsphenoidal hypophysectomy. Am J Nurs 80(10):1820, Oct 1980

Cavalier J: Crucial decisions in diabetic emergencies. RN 43(11):32, Nov 1980

Evangelisti J, Thorpe C: Thyroid storm—a nursing crisis. Heart Lung 12(2):184, Mar 1983

Fairchild R: Diabetes insipidus. Crit Care Q 3(2):111, Sept 1980

Finch C, Hayflick L (eds): Handbook of the Biology of Aging. New York, Van Nostrand Reinhold Co, 1977

Fode N, Laws E, Northcutt R: Pituitary tumors and hypertension: implications for neurosurgical nurses. J Neurosurg Nurs 15(1):33, Feb 1983

Forbes K, Stokes S: Saving the diabetic foot. Am J Nurs 84(7):884, July 1984

Fredholm N: The insulin pump: new method of insulin delivery. Am J Nurs 81(11):2024, Nov 1981

Fredholm N, Vignati L, Brown S: Insulin pumps: the patient's verdict Am J Nurs 84(1):36, Jan 1984

Graham S, Morley M: What 'foot care' really means. Am J Nurs, 84(7):889, July 1984

Gunter-Hunt G, Parker L, Spencer M: Adolescent diabetes clinic: a specialized treatment approach. Diabetes Educ 8(3):36, Fall 1982

Handy J: The transsphenoidal surgical approach to the pituitary. Hosp Pract 14(6):81, June 1979

Hoffman J, Newby T: Hypercalcemia in primary hyperparathyroidism. Nurs Clin North Am 15(3):469, Sept, 1980

Jones S: Adrenal patient, proceed with caution. RN 45(1):66, Jan 1982

Jones S: Kid-glove case in pheochromocytoma. RN 45(2):66, Feb 1982

Jones S: Bilateral adrenalectomy: dangers to watch for. RN 45(3):66, Mar 1982

Kiser D: The somogyi effect. Am J Nurs 80(2):236, Feb 1980

Lafferty F: Primary hyperparathyroidism. Arch Intern Med 141(13):1761, Dec 1981

Leshin M: Acute adrenal insufficiency, recognition, management, and prevention. Urol Clin North Am 9:229, June 1982

Marchesseault L: Diabetes mellitus and the elderly. Nurs Clin North Am 18(4):791, Dec 1983

Marecki M: Need priorities of adrenalectomy patients as perceived by patients, nurses, and physicians. JOGN 10(5):379, Sept/Oct 1981

McCarthy J: Diabetic nephropathy. Am J Nurs 81(11):2030, Nov 1981

McClung M, Greer M: Treatment of hyperthyroidism. Annu Rev Med 31:385, 1980

McNeil L: Self blood glucose monitoring: and update. Diabetes Educ 8(4):15, Winter 1983

Miller B, White N: Diabetes assessment guide. Am J Nurs 80(7):1314, July 1980
Nabarro J: Pituitary surgery for endocrine disorders. Clin Endocrinol 13:285, 1980
Nemchik R: Diabetes today: a startling new body of knowledge. RN 45(10):31, Oct 1982
Nemchik R: Diabetes today: a very different diet; a new generation of oral drugs. RN 45(11):41, Nov 1982
Nemchik R: Diabetes today: the news about insulin RN 45(12):49, Dec 1982
Nemchik R: Diabetes today: the new insulin pumps: tight control—at a price. RN 46(5):52, May 1983
Nemchik R: Diabetes today: facing up to the long-term complications. RN 46(7):38, Jul 1983
Nemeroff D: Transsphenoidal hypophysectomy. J Neurosurg Nurs 13:303, 1981
Nurs Mirror: Clinical insight, Cushing's syndrome 157(4):105, July 27, 1983.
Nyberg K: Diabetes today: when diabetes complicates your pre- and postop care. RN 46(1):42, Jan 1983
O'Daniel L: The adrenal gland and the use of cortisone in the management of patients with Addison's disease and Cushing's syndrome. American Ass'n of Nurse Anesthetists Journal 51(1):31, Feb 1983
Perkins M: Would you recognize pheochromocytoma? Nursing '85 15(5):64, May 1985
Podolsky S: Diagnosis and treatment of sexual dysfunction in the male diabetic. Med Clin North Am 66(6):1389, Nov 1982
Raskin P, Albin J, Christlieb A et al: Symposium on diabetes mellitus. Med Clin North Am 66(6):1188, Nov 1982
Reff M, Schneider E: Biological Markers of Aging. U.S. Department of Health and Human Services, 1982 (NIH Publication No. 82-2221)
Resler M, Bovington M: (eds): Symposium on diabetes mellitus. Nurs Clin North Am 19(4), Dec 1984
Riblett B: Insuring a safe pregnancy for your diabetic patient. RN 46(2):50, Feb 1983
Rockstein M, Sussman M: Biology of Aging. Belmont, Wadsworth Publishing, 1979
Sanford S: Dysfunction of the adrenal gland: physiological considerations and nursing problems. Nurs Clin North Am 15(3):481, Sept 1980
Schumann D: Appraisal of the diabetic patient. Diabetic Educ 8(1):24, Spring 1982
Solomon B: The hypothalamus and the pituitary gland: an overview, Nurs Clin North Am 15(3):435, Sept 1980
Stevens A: Monitoring blood glucose at home: who should do it. Am J Nurs 81(11):2026, Nov 1981

Surr C: Teaching patients to use the new blood-glucose monitoring products, Part 2. Nursing '83 13(2):58, Feb 1983
Sutherland D, Elick B, Goetz F et al: Pancreas transplantation—an historical overview and its current status. Diabetic Educ 8(1):11, Spring 1982
Wake M, Brensinger J: The nurses' role in hypothyroidism. Nurs Clin North Am 15(3):453, Sept 1980
Worth R: A comparative study of blood glucose tests. Diabetes Care 4:407, 1981

EYE, EAR, NOSE, AND THROAT

EYES

CATARACT

Description

A cataract is an increasing opaqueness of the lens of the eye. Eighty percent of people over 70 years of age have cataracts, and they frequently are seen in younger people. Cataracts are associated most commonly with the natural aging process, but congenital cataracts and those resulting from eye trauma, medications (steroids), or systemic disease such as diabetes also are not uncommon.

Common Diagnostic Tests

- Eye examination

Observations

- Gray or white opacity seen through the pupil
- Gradual blurring of vision
- Sensitivity to light and difficulty driving at night because of the glare of headlights

Treatment

- Surgical removal of the lens is the only cure. Two techniques of cataract surgery are performed. In intracapsular surgery, the lens and its membrane covering are removed with a cryoprobe (a freezing metal tip). In the extracapsular procedure, the membrane covering is cut open and the cloudy contents are aspirated.
- Ultrasonic fragmentation of the lens can be done when the lens is soft, as it is in young children. A very small incision is needed for this, and the cataract is broken up and aspirated.

Nursing Considerations

- Surgery is necessary when the lens opacity interferes with necessary vision.
- Many cataract patients have diabetes.
- Eye drops to dilate the eyes are given before surgery.
- Postoperative orders are written on an individual basis. Patients may be allowed to return home the day of surgery.
- Eye drops may be ordered for several days after surgery. Be sure the patient understands the procedure for instillation. An eye shield is worn at night over the operated eye for 4 weeks to 5 weeks to prevent eye injury. Hemorrhage and damage to the suture line are avoided by instructing the patient not to lift, bend over, squeeze the eye, or strain.
- Unless there are permanent intraocular implant lenses, hard or soft contact lenses are placed on the eye about 6 weeks after surgery. Extended wear soft lenses may be left in and removed every few weeks; eyeglasses also may be prescribed.
- It may be necessary to teach another family member to remove and clean the patient's contact lenses; or, the patient periodically may have to go to the physician's office for this purpose.

GLAUCOMA

Description

Glaucoma describes a condition of elevated intraocular pressure with resulting damage to the optic nerve. Normally, aqueous humor, which is produced within the eye, flows from the posterior chamber into the anterior chamber, and eventually drains into the venous system. When a blockage restricts this flow, increased pressure within the eye causes damage to the blood vessels supplying the optic nerve. Chronic or open-angle glaucoma is the most common form. Usually bilateral, it develops in middle-age to old-age groups. Congenital glaucoma, resulting from developmental defects, also occurs, but this is infrequent. Secondary glaucoma refers to an interference in the drainage system resulting from injury or inflammation of the eye. Acute or narrow-angle glaucoma occurs when a sudden increase of intraocular pressure takes place in an eye because of a complete obstruction of the drainage system.

Common Diagnostic Tests

- Tonometer test: A tonometer, placed directly on the anesthetized cornea, measures intraocular pressure. The normal pressure is in the range of 10 mm Hg to 21 mm Hg.
- Ophthalmoscopic examination: This provides a visual inspection of the inner eye and the optic nerve.

- Visual field test: This examination detects blind spots (scotomas), which are an indication of visual field loss.

Observations

- In chronic and secondary glaucoma, there are no symptoms until vision is decreased. This usually begins in the peripheral fields. In infants, eyes have excessive tearing, are sensitive to light, and hazy corneas develop.
- Acute glaucoma occurs suddenly with severe pain in the eye and often is accompanied by nausea and vomiting. The lens does not react to light. *This is a medical emergency and must be treated within hours to prevent blindness.*

Treatment

Chronic (open-angle) glaucoma

- Pilocarpine isomiotic eye drops are commonly used to constrict the pupil and the iris away from the drainage channels and lower the intraocular pressure.
- Epinephrine and timolol maleate (Timoptic) eye drops increase the outflow and decrease aqueous production.
- Acetazolamide (Diamox) may be given orally or intravenously to decrease the rate of aqueous production.
- Usually, chronic glaucoma can be controlled with medication. If this is not possible, then surgery (trabeculectomy) or a laser trabeculoplasty is required to open an artificial drainage channel in the eye.
- Congenital glaucoma is usually only treatable by surgery.

Acute (closed-angle) glaucoma

- Acute glaucoma is a *medical emergency,* and immediate treatment is necessary to reduce the high intraocular pressure. Intravenous medication, *e.g.,* acetazolamide (Diamox) or mannitol, often is used; miotic eye drops, *e.g.,* pilocarpine, also are given. A surgical or laser opening procedure in the iris usually is performed within a few hours.

Nursing Considerations

- The eye is anesthetized for tonometer examination. Instruct the patient *not* to rub the anesthetized eye for at least 15 minutes after the examination.
- Chronic glaucoma is bilateral, and often occurs in diabetic patients. There is a hereditary predisposition.
- Patients with glaucoma may be hospitalized for other reasons. They must *never* miss their daily administration of eye drops and

other medications for glaucoma. When possible, leave the medications with the patients so they can maintain their schedules. Be sure that medications, *e.g.*, atropine, propantheline bromide (Pro-Banthine), ordered for other conditions are not contraindicated for glaucoma patients.

- Acetazolamide (Diamox) is a diuretic and will increase urine output.
- Timolol maleate (Timoptic) is a beta-blocker drug and, therefore may decrease the heart rate. Press the inner corner of the eye for two minutes when administering these eye drops to prevent systemic absorption by occluding the lacrimal sac.
- Glaucoma cannot be cured by the use of drugs; even after surgery it may be necessary to continue medications. The aim of the therapy is to keep intraocular pressure within normal limits. Therefore, these patients must see their physicians for regular eye examinations and regulations of medication. When there is any indication of an eye infection, immediate medical attention is necessary.
- Following surgery the patient generally is kept flat for 24 hours, but may turn to the unoperated side. Anything that may increase pressure such as bending down, straining, or lifting should be avoided for several weeks.
- These patients must always wear an identification bracelet indicating that they have glaucoma. Also, they should always ask a pharmacist's advice before buying over-the-counter medications because of possible contraindications with glaucoma.

RETINAL DETACHMENT

Description

Retinal detachment is the separation of the neural retinal layer from the pigment epithelial layer of the eye. This usually is caused by a small tear or hole in the retina, which allows fluids within the eye to pass into the subretinal space, resulting in a detachment. A retinal detachment rarely is seen in infants and children; it is, however, frequently associated with myopia.

Common Diagnostic Tests

- Eye examination

Observations

- Patients will note floating spots before the eyes, flashes of light, and blocked peripheral vision appearing as shadows in the visual fields. These symptoms gradually increase with time as the detachment progresses.

Treatment

- Immediate bed rest with the head turned toward the area of detachment, in order to use gravity as a force to bring the retina back against the inner surface of the eyeball.
- Diathermy, photocoagulation, or cryosurgery are used to seal tears before a detachment occurs. These procedures cause a local inflammation that results in a scar sealing the hole.
- Scleral buckling is performed often after the fluid has been removed from the subretinal space. The sclera is shortened, resulting in renewed contact between the retina and the choroid.
- The success of the surgery depends upon the extent of the detachment, and how long it has existed before it was treated.

Nursing Considerations

- Sedation is often necessary to minimize head movements, while the patient is kept on bedrest awaiting surgery.
- Postoperative orders are written on an individual basis. The head usually is kept turned toward the detached area for a period of time immediately following surgery.
- Hemorrhage is a major potential complication.
- The eye may be inflamed for several weeks after surgery. Eye drops usually are given to decrease the inflammation.
- Warm eye compresses are used to relieve crusting on the eyelids.
- These patients usually must remain at home for several weeks after leaving the hospital, and reading, as well as heavy lifting, bending over, or any physical strain must be avoided during this postoperative period in order to decrease the possibility of a recurring detachment.

EYE PATIENT CARE

Frequently, patients with eye diseases are hospitalized for other problems. They must *never* omit their daily administration of eye medications. The physician treating their eyes should be contacted if any questions arise.

Preoperative

- Patients entering a hospital for eye surgery may have very limited vision. Orient them carefully to their physical surroundings as well as to hospital routine. The fact that hospital personnel will be entering the room at intervals during the day and night needs to be emphasized.
- Be familiar with the activity and position restrictions following the specific type of surgery and discuss these with the patient.

- One or both eyes may be covered for a few days following surgery to minimize eye movements. TV watching or reading may be restricted. It is important to prepare the patient for this situation.
- Demonstrate passive leg and breathing exercises during a period of bedrest. Have the patient return the demonstration. Assist the patient in flexing and extending each leg.
- Emphasize that following surgery, activities causing an increase in intraocular pressure need to be avoided. Such things as leaning over, hair combing and brushing, shaving, tooth brushing, and blowing the nose are often restricted. If it is necessary to cough, patients should keep their mouths open to decrease the intraocular pressure.
- When eyelashes must be cut off, coat the scissors with a sterile lubricant so that the lashes will adhere and not fall into the patient's eyes. If eye cosmetics normally are worn, caution that they must not be used after surgery until the surgeon approves of their use.

Postoperative

- See MSN, Postoperative care, for patients care following a general anesthetic.
- Be aware that hemorrhage and infection are the two major complications of eye surgery. Infection becomes obvious with increased drainage and fever.
- There may be moderate pain or discomfort following eye surgery. Notify the surgeon *immediately* if severe pain occurs.
- The patient should understand that if nausea occurs, the nurse should be notified because an antiemetic can be given. Vomiting needs to be prevented. Stool softeners and laxatives are necessary to prevent straining.
- While on bedrest, check every shift daily for signs and symptoms of thrombophlebitis (see MSN, Thrombophlebitis).
- Patients with patches over both eyes frequently become disoriented (see MNS, Disoriented patients). Always speak before touching these patients. Try to avoid the use of sleeping pills in elderly patients (especially when their eyes are covered) to avoid increased mental confusion. Family members or friends should be encouraged to stay with restless patients.
- If only one eye is covered with a patch, determine the vision in the other eye. Also, inform the patient that depth perception will be impaired.
- To enable patients with limited vision to feed themselves, place the food on the tray as the numbers of a clock and explain this system.
- Assist ambulating patient on the unpatched side.

- Metal eye shields often are applied over an eye pad to prevent injury to the eye when the patient sleeps. To hold shield in place, use several strips of tape, that are each approximately 5 inches long. Apply the tape diagonally across the shield, with the shield ends resting on the body prominences of the face. Be sure the patient or family members know how to do this.
- Discharge planning and teaching is critical to ensure understanding of necessary care and precautions following eye surgery.

EAR

MYRINGOTOMY AND MIDDLE-EAR VENTILATING TUBES

Description

A myringotomy is a small surgical incision in the eardrum (tympanic membrane). It is done to aspirate pus or mucoserous fluid from the middle ear; it also sometimes is accompanied by insertion of a middle-ear ventilating tube. This tube provides an artificial airway to the middle ear when the eustachian tube is obstructed, usually resulting from allergic inflammation or enlarged adenoids. Unless there is air in the middle ear and a patent eustachian tube, fluid collects in this space and hearing becomes impaired. Upon removal of the ventilating tube, the eardrum heals and no permanent hearing damage occurs.

Nursing Considerations

- A myringotomy may be performed with a local or general anesthetic; a general anesthetic usually is given to children.
- When a ventilating tube is in place, a discharge (otorrhea) frequently occurs. Antibiotic eardrops often are used to keep the tubes from becoming clogged.
- The patient must avoid getting water in the ear when a ventilating tube is in place. Well-fitting earplugs should be used when showering, shampooing hair, or swimming. Diving is not permissible.
- A ventilating tube is left in place until extruded spontaneously, usually in 9 months to 18 months. If this does not occur, it may need to be removed. Recurrence of hearing loss may signal fluid accumulation, and a tube may be reinserted.

OTOSCLEROSIS AND STAPEDECTOMY

Description

Otosclerosis is a form of deafness that results when the footplate of the stapes becomes fixed in the oval window of the middle ear. A stapedectomy is performed to restore hearing.

Normally, sound is conducted from the eardrum through the three ossicles (bones) of the middle ear—the malleus to the incus to the stapes. The footplate of the stapes transmits sound through the oval window into the inner ear. A stapedectomy removes the entire stapes and substitutes a prosthesis that recouples the incus to a graft of natural or synthetic material that covers, as well as creates, a patent oval window.

Nursing Considerations

- The position of the head for the first 24 hours following surgery is the surgeon's preference to ensure proper drainage and maintenance of the position of the prosthesis in the ear.
- Check for signs of facial paralysis developing anytime within the first few postoperative hours. This, increased bleeding, or excessive pain must be reported *immediately*.
- Vertigo may be present for the first few days and aggravated by sudden position changes. Antiemetics should be given to prevent vomiting.
- Bloody cotton pledgets in the ear canal may be replaced as necessary, but do not disturb the packing within the ear.
- Sneezing and blowing the nose should be avoided to prevent forcing air up the eustachian tube.
- Discharge teaching must emphasize that the patient should not allow water to enter the ear until permitted by the surgeon.

NOSE AND THROAT

CANCER OF THE LARYNX

Description

Cancer of the larynx occurs primarily in men, and is associated with a history of heavy smoking and alcoholism. Glottic or "intrinsic" cancer of the larynx is confined to the vocal cords. Cancer above the vocal cords is called supraglottic; cancer below the vocal cords is called infraglottic. These nonglottic cancers also are referred to as "extrinsic" cancers.

Common Diagnostic Tests

- Laryngoscopic examination is done to visualize and biopsy the lesion. Toluidine blue will stain cancer cells.
- Barium-swallow x-rays may be used to detect an esophageal lesion, there being a 5% to 10% chance that there will be a simultaneous primary lesion.

- PA and lateral x-rays will help assess vocal-cord paralysis.
- Tomograms will demonstrate involvement of bone or cartilage.

Observations

- Hoarseness is a symptom of glottic cancer.
- Painful or difficult swallowing is a symptom indicative of diseases other than vocal cord cancer.
- Stridor and tachypnea, signs of airway obstruction, are late and dangerous signs.

Treatment

- Removal at laryngoscopy is used for small and localized lesions, but only for diagnosis.
- Radiation, which will cause throat discomfort or dryness for several months.
- Surgery usually is reserved for larger or more advanced cases of cancer.
  1. Partial frontolateral laryngectomy usually is performed when the lesion is confined to only one cord. However, recent techniques demonstrate that this operation may sometimes be applied to more-extensive lesions involving both vocal cords. Removal of one cord leaves the patient's voice husky but recognizable, and there is no permanent tracheostomy.
  2. Supraglottic laryngectomy removes the epiglottis and adjacent bone and tissue, leaving a normal voice and airway. This surgery often is combined with radiation.
  3. Total laryngectomy results in a temporary loss of the voice and a permanent tracheostomy.
- A radical neck dissection may accompany a partial or total laryngectomy if there are cervical lymph node metastases.

Nursing Considerations

Preoperative

- Patients facing the loss of their larynx may be extremely depressed and fearful, thinking that they may lose their voice permanently. Encourage family and close friends to be with the patient, and emphasize that vocal rehabilitation will help in re-acquiring speech.
- A speech therapy consultation should be initiated prior to surgery to assist in vocal rehabilitation.
- Establish a method of communication to be used immediately after surgery, *e.g.*, magic slate, picture cards, paper and pencils.

- It is imperative that the physician and nurse confer regarding the planned surgery and the necessary patient education. The equipment that will be in use following surgery needs to be explained, *e.g.*, tracheostomy tube, feeding tube, and suctioning. Be sure the patient knows whether a tracheostomy is to be permanent or temporary.
- Plan to have the patient return after surgery to a room adjacent to the nurse's station.
- When there is a history of high alcohol use, be prepared for withdrawal symptoms.

Postoperative

- Answer call light *immediately* and check the patient every few minutes until the patient is competent in self care.
- Keep an extra tracheotomy or laryngectomy tube (with the obturator) taped to the head of the bed. A laryngectomy tube is shorter and wider than a tracheotomy tube, but the care is the same (see NR, Tracheostomy care). Be sure the tube is the proper size. After several days, the tube may not be needed since the stoma will heal and remain open.
- A humidified tracheostomy mask is necessary in the immediate postoperative period. Later, a humidifier in the room helps relieve tracheal dryness (see NR, Oxygen administration).
- The skin around the suture line may be very delicate from radiation therapy, so be very gentle in cleaning the area.
- Radiation also makes the skin more susceptible to infection and may delay healing.
- The danger of an airway obstruction always exists with these patients. If this happens, suction the tracheostomy, bag with oxygen, and call for help. If the tracheostomy tube has an inner cannula, remove it before bagging with oxygen.
- Do not deep suction through the nose or mouth without specific instructions because of the danger of penetrating suture lines.
- Tracheal suctioning can be taught to the patient. Have the patient sit in front of a mirror, and demonstrate while emphasizing the clean technique that will be used at home (see NR, Suctioning, Tracheostomy). A family member also should be taught the procedure.
- After a partial laryngectomy, there may be difficulty in swallowing, and a feeding tube always is used postoperatively until swallowing without aspiration is possible. The tube is inserted by the surgeon during the operation, and if reinsertion is necessary, it should be done by the surgeon because of the danger of penetrating suture lines. When food is taken by mouth, soft food is usually easier to swallow than liquids. These patients have temporary tracheostomies until tracheal edema subsides. They are able to speak by placing a finger over the tracheostomy opening.

- Following a supraglottic laryngectomy, there is a great deal of difficulty in swallowing, because without an epiglottis, food, especially liquids, easily slips directly into the trachea. Tube feeding may go on for several weeks, and the patient may go home after being taught the procedure. Mouth care should be done at least six times a day.
- After a total laryngectomy, there is no longer any internal connection between the mouth/nose, and the lungs. The sense of smell and taste is altered.
- The stoma will heal and a laryngectomy tube will not be necessary. Since the stoma forms a direct opening to the lungs, it should be kept clean and covered with a stoma cover. Be certain the call light is *always within reach* and that note pads and pencils are provided.
- Contact "Lost Chord" group through the American Cancer Society for a visit from a functioning laryngectomee. Frequently, severe depression occurs after surgery, after the full realization of loss of voice occurs. Again, emphasize that this loss is *temporary.*
- An identification bracelet should be worn noting that the person is a laryngectomee, as well as any other medical condition, and an emergency phone number.
- Discharge planning must include patient acquisition of a suctioning machine and humidifier. Also, emphasize *regular* follow-up visits to the surgeon.
- CPR for a person with neck stoma involves mouth-to-stoma resuscitation. There is no need to seal off the mouth and nose.

SUBMUCOUS RESECTION OR NASAL SEPTAL RECONSTRUCTION

Description

A submucous resection (SMR) or nasal septal reconstruction (NSR) is a surgical procedure commonly performed using local anesthesia. It is done to relieve a nasal obstruction to breathing. An incision is made internally on one side of the nasal septum, and bone or cartilage is removed.

Nursing Considerations

Postoperative

- Humidified air will make breathing more comfortable.
- Keep the head of the bed elevated.
- The patient will have nasal packing in place for two to three days. A drip pad taped under the nose is changed as necessary. Bloody drainage should decrease, not increase.

- Pain may be severe for the first few days.
- Frequent mouth care is necessary because of mouth breathing.
- The patients usually are hospitalized overnight.

NORMAL AGING CHANGES IN THE EYE, EAR, NOSE, AND THROAT

- Total mass of the eye shrinks and blood supply decreases.
- The cornea clouds and loses its transparency. It may be surrounded by a white or yellowish ring.
- The iris requires more light, and its accommodation to light changes decreases. Pupils may appear constricted.
- Lenses have less complete accommodation and cannot adjust to near work. Increased viscosity is common.
- Ciliary muscles are stiff and less functional.
- The vitreous shrinks and the collagen clumps, causing shadows (called floaters) on the retina.
- Age differences occur in color discrimination. Filtering of shorter wavelength colors occurs, and blue-green discrimination becomes difficult.
- The conjunctiva and optic disc appear pale.
- The efficiency of the mechanism for reabsorption of intraocular fluid decreases.
- Lacrimal secretions may decrease.
- Hearing becomes less acute, starting with the higher frequencies.
- There is a decrease in the sense of smell and an increase in amount of hair in nares.
- There is a decrease in the number of taste buds. Sweet and salty taste buds decline first; those for sour and bitter remain the longest.
- A decrease in salivary secretion occurs.
- The gag reflex may be sluggish.

IMPLICATIONS

- Loss of vision has a significant impact on lifestyle.
    1. Use of medication becomes hazardous.
    2. Cooking and shopping difficulties may decrease nutritional status; burns while cooking become an increased risk.
    3. Failure to observe objects in the environment or notice surface changes may increase the number of falls and bruises.
    4. Boredom occurs when the individual can no longer read, watch TV, write letters, or do crafts.

5. Because the iris cannot easily accommodate for changes in light, night driving may not be possible.
6. Isolation results from the failing ability to get about and socialize.

- Because pupils normally may appear constricted, monitoring changes from head injuries may be more difficult.
- Most equipment used to determine levels of glucose in the urine and blood require the ability to distinguish between shades of green. (Blue-green discrimination decreases with aging.)
- If high-frequency hearing loss has occurred, decrease the tone of your voice, but don't speak louder.
- Face the person when speaking because he or she may be able to read your lips.
- There is a high correlation between hearing loss and depression.
- Decreased hearing can lead to withdrawal and paranoia.
- Nutritional status may be affected adversely by the decrease in sense of smell, and the decrease in taste buds.
- Elderly persons may increase their use of seasonings, especially salt.
- Decrease in salivary secretions may increase halitosis. Mouth care is essential.
- A sluggish gag reflex may increase the risk of aspiration pneumonia, especially if the person is supine.

BIBLIOGRAPHY • Eye, Ear, Nose, and Throat

BOOKS

Boyd-Monk H (ed): Symposia on ophthalmic nursing. Nurs Clin North Am 16 (3), 1981

Brunner L, Suddarth D: Medical Surgical Nursing 4th ed. Philadelphia, J B Lippincott, 1980

Engelstein J (ed): Cataract Surgery. Orlando, FL, Grune and Stratton, 1984

Saunders W, Havener W, Keith O, Havener G: Nursing Care in Eye, Ear, Nose, and Throat Disorders, 4th ed. St. Louis, CV Mosby Co, 1979

Shin D: Glaucoma Surgery. International Ophthalmology Clinics, Spring 1981, vol 21, no. 1. Boston, Little Brown, 1981

Spaeth G (ed): Ophthalmic Surgery. Philadelphia, WB Saunders, 1982

JOURNALS

Boyd-Monk H: Screening for glaucoma. Nursing '79 9(8):42, 1979

Cataract Surgery. Nursing '83 13(4):65, 1983

Hallbrook P: On opening the airway. Emerg Med 14(1):137, 1982

Huber H: Draining the "fluid ear" with myringotomy and tube insertion. Nursing '78 8(7):78, 1978

Lindquist J, Franzen R, Ossoff R: Epiglottitis in adults. Ann Emerg Med 9(5):256, 1980
Luxford W, Sheey J: Myringotomy and ventilation tubes: A report of 1568 ears. Laryngoscope 92(11):1293, 1982
Marshakg NZ: Adenoidectomy versus tympanostomy in chronic secretory otitis media.Ann Otol Rhinol Laryngol 89 (suppl 68 (3) part 2):316, 1981
Meyerhoff W: Use of tympanostomy tube in otitis media. Ann Otol Rhinol Laryngol 90 (part 1):537, 1981
Naunton RF: Tympanostomy tubes: The conservative approach. Ann Otol Rhinol Laryngol 90(part 1):529, 1981

CONFERENCES

Eye Trauma, Georgetown University Emergency Medicine Update Series, June 18, 1980
Glaucoma and Cataracts, Sibley Hospital, Washington, DC, June 4, 1980

Normal Aging Changes in the Eye, Ear, Nose, and Throat

Finch C, Hayflick L (eds): Handbook of the Biology of Aging. New York, Van Nostrand Reinhold, 1977
Reff M, Schneider E: Biological Markers of Aging. US Department of Health and Human Services, 1982 (NIH Publication No. 82-2221)
Resler M, Tumulty G: Glaucoma update. Am J Nurs 83(5):752 1983
Rockstein M, Sussman M: Biology of Aging. Belmont, Wadsworth Publishing, 1979

GASTROINTESTINAL SYSTEM

ADENOMATOUS POLYPS

Description

Most often found in the colon and stomach, adenomatous polyps are the most common benign tumor in the gastrointestinal (GI) tract. They may be single or multiple, sessile (on a broad base) or pedunculated (on a stalk). Adenomas may become malignant.

- Polyps usually are asymptomatic; those in the distal bowel are diagnosed by visualization on a proctosigmoidoscopic examination.
- Bleeding may be gross or occult; obstruction occurs rarely, if the polyp is large.
- Polyps of the colon now frequently are removed without open abdominal surgery through the use of the flexible colonoscope (see NR, Endoscopic procedures).

- Familial polyposis, an inherited condition of multiple polyps, is associated with a high incidence of cancer development. Colectomy often is done to prevent malignancy, although meticulous, repeated, colonoscopic polypectomy may avoid such a drastic approach.

ANORECTAL CONDITIONS

Description

Hemorrhoids are spongy vascularities that lie both above (internal) and below (external) the anal sphincter. They are so common that they might be considered "normal" for adults. Treatment is indicated when they become symptomatic—inflamed, thrombosed, or bleeding.

Anal fissure (fissure in ano) is an ulcerated, elongated laceration of the lower anal canal, usually caused by injury during passage of a large hard stool. Defecation or rectal examination become extremely painful. Usually, the fissure will heal with conservative treatment.

Rectal fistulas (fistula in ano) are tracts that lead from the anorectal canal and open onto the skin near the anus. They are most commonly the result of neglect or unsuccessful treatment of anorectal abscesses, but are also complications of diseases of the large bowel, especially regional enteritis (Crohn's disease).

Common Diagnostic Tests

- Digital, anoscopic, and proctoscopic examinations of the rectum
- Examination of stool for occult blood
- For fistula in ano
  1. Probe of the fistulous tract
  2. Sigmoidoscopy to look for associated disease (See NR, Endoscopic procedures)
  3. Barium x-rays, if regional enteritis or ulcerative colitis is suspected (See NR, X-ray preparations.)

Observations

- Rectal bleeding that is bright red and usually on the outside of the stool or appears on toilet tissue is seen with hemorrhoids and anal fissure. (Other causes of rectal bleeding must be ruled out.)
- Pain, especially on defecation, is present in all three conditions.
- Pruritus (itching), mucoid discharge, and protrusion of hemorrhoids may be present.
- Purulent, irritating discharge near the anus occurs in rectal fistulas.

- Thrombosis of a hemorrhoid often is characterized by a fairly sudden onset of moderate-to-severe anal pain.

Treatment

- Hemorrhoids and anal fissure: conservative treatment
  1. Diet high in fiber and fluids
  2. Stool softeners to promote regular bowel movements without straining
  3. Anesthetic ointments, applied topically
  4. Witch hazel soaks (*e.g.,* Tucks)
  5. Sitz baths
  6. With edema and inflammation, cold and elevation may be indicated.
  7. Careful cleansing of the anal area after bowel movements
- If conservative treatment fails
  1. Hemorrhoids may be treated by sclerotherapy (injection with a sclerosing agent), rubber-band ligation, cryosurgery (not a widely accepted treatment in which hemorrhoids are necrosed by freezing with a cryoprobe), and hemorrhoidectomy (surgical removal of the hemorrhoids). A thrombosed hemorrhoid may require excision and evacuation.
  2. Surgical excision of anal fissure
- Wide excision of the fistulous tract and removal of the source of infection are required for rectal fistula. Temporary colostomy to provide for rest and healing of the area may be necessary for the patient with multiple fistulas. Some surgeons leave the excised areas open; others close them.

Nursing Considerations

Postoperative Care

USUAL PROBLEMS

- Pain: Expect anorectal surgery to cause pain the first day or two after surgery.
  1. Narcotic analgesics usually are ordered to be given generously the first 24 hours to 48 hours postoperatively, and immediately before or after the first postoperative bowel movement.
  2. Be with or near the patient when he has his first postoperative bowel movement. The pain may be severe enough to cause faintness.
  3. Sitz baths, three or four times a day are usually recommended. An ice bag to the head may prevent feelings of faintness.

- Urinary retention
  1. Fluids may be restricted drastically pre- and postoperatively, if ordered by surgeon.
  2. Check bladder for distention. Catheterize only if absolutely necessary. Some surgeons allow the patient to go 36 hours postoperatively without voiding, if fluids have been restricted and the bladder is not distended.
  3. Getting the patient out of bed to void usually is allowed.
  4. Try nursing measures to encourage patient to void (*e.g.*, providing a quiet, relaxed atmosphere, running water, blowing through a straw).
- Constipation
  1. Encourage the patient to develop good bowel habits by teaching him or her to avoid constipation by eating high-fiber foods, drinking plenty of fluids, and heeding the desire to have a bowel movement, at a regular time of the day, if possible.

COMPLICATION

- Hemorrhage
  1. Check the dressing or wound for signs of bleeding. Teach the patient to do so.
  2. Monitor vital signs. Evaluate restlessness, anxiety, or feelings of faintness.

APPENDICITIS

Description

Appendicitis is an infection of the vermiform appendix, a small, fingerlike blind pouch attached to the cecum just below the ileocecal valve. It may be caused by a fecalith (a stonelike mass of feces) or anything that occludes the lumen of the appendix (*e.g.*, adhesions, pinworms, or inflammation).

Common Diagnostic Tests

- Complete blood count usually shows leukocytosis (see Lab).

Observations

- Acute, generalized abdominal pain that localizes in the right lower quadrant (RLQ), also called McBurney's point; rebound tenderness (tenderness after the pressure is released) at this point
- Nausea and vomiting, constipation, anorexia, and low-grade fever
- Symptoms of ruptured appendix: severe abdominal pain, which may be relieved at the time of rupture, followed by generalized

intense pain, rigid abdomen, elevated white blood cell count, elevated temperature, and symptoms of shock

Treatment

- Rule out other causes of pain.
- If there is any doubt, a laparotomy is done rather than chance rupture of the appendix with resulting peritonitis.

Nursing Considerations

- Postoperative care for uncomplicated appendectomy is like that of any laparotomy.
- Appendectomy following rupture of the appendix requires the following additional elements of care:
  1. The incision is not always closed.
  2. A drain will remain in place. Observe and record amount of drainage.
  3. IV fluids are administered (see NR, IV therapy).
  4. A nasogastric tube is inserted (see NR, Gastrointestinal intubation).
  5. Large doses of IV antibiotics, often more than one are administered.
  6. The patient should be in a semi-Fowler's or Fowler's position to promote drainage into the pelvic cavity.
  7. Careful assessment for symptoms of paralytic ileus (absent bowel sounds, no passage of gas or feces by rectum) and peritonitis is necessary (see MSN, Postoperative care).

CANCER OF THE COLON

Description

Adenocarcinoma of the colon occurs most frequently in the descending colon and sigmoid. Metastasis is by direct extension to adjacent organs, or through the lymphatic or blood system to the liver and lungs. An increased incidence has been found in populations with high beef and fat consumptions, and among those individuals with a history of chronic colitis, intestinal polyps, and a familial history of cancer of the colon. A decreased incidence occurs in those with an increased transit time of fecal material, hence the recent interest in the high roughage diet.

Common Diagnostic Tests

- Rectal examination
- Stools for occult blood (See LAB.)

- Barium x-rays of GI tract (See NR, X-ray preparations.)
- Colonoscopy with biopsy (See NR, Endoscopic procedures.)
- Liver scan (See NR, Scans.)
- Chest x-ray
- Blood test for carcino-embryonic antigen (CEA). An increase of CEA frequently is observed in patients with colorectal cancer. It is *not* definitive, however, because it may be elevated in liver disease, pancreatitis, and in smokers.

Observations

- Rectal bleeding, often manifested by red blood and maroon-colored stools. Black stools may be seen when bleeding is from upper colon.
- Cancer in the right side of the colon frequently is associated with unexplained anemia, and less often with a vague feeling of abdominal fullness, or a palpable mass may occur.
- Cancer of the left side of the colon often is indicated by alternating constipation and diarrhea, and small-caliber stools. These symptoms are caused by a gradually increasing intestinal obstruction.

Treatment

- Surgery (See MSN, Intestinal surgery.)
- Radiation may be given before surgery to reduce the tumor size.
- Chemotherapy sometimes is used to treat metastatic disease.
- An implantable, refillable infusion pump sewn into the hepatic artery to provide continuous treatment with 5-fluorouracil may be used to treat hepatic metastases.

Nursing Considerations

- See MSN, Oncology nursing considerations.

DIVERTICULITIS AND DIVERTICULOSIS

Description

A diverticulum is an outpouching of the intestinal wall at a point of weakness. Usually found in the sigmoid colon, diverticula are now thought to be caused by lack of bulk in the diet and by increased intraluminal pressure. The presence of several of these herniations is called *diverticulosis*. Inflammation in one or more of the diverticula is called *diverticulitis*. Complications resulting from diverticulitis include perforation with resulting peritonitis, hemorrhage, abscess, and fistula formation.

Common Diagnostic Tests

- Barium enema (See NR, X-ray preparation.)
- Colonoscopy and sigmoidoscopy (fiberoptic) (See NR, Endoscopic procedures.)
- Elevated WBCs in diverticulitis
- Selective mesenteric arteriography, if there is bleeding

Observations

- Lower abdominal discomfort particularly localized to the left, lower quadrant; tenderness to palpation, and possibly a palpable mass
- Change in bowel habits: patient may have alternating diarrhea and constipation.
- Fever (in diverticulitis)
- Signs of complications (*e.g.*, perforation with peritonitis, obstruction, and massive bleeding evidenced by bright red blood or mahogany-colored stools and a drop in blood pressure) (See MSN, GI bleeding.)

Treatment

Medical

- Diverticulosis
  1. High-fiber diet, forced fluids, bulk laxatives (*e.g.*, Metamucil); no anticholinergic drugs
  2. Enemas shuld be avoided because they increase luminal pressure and could lead to perforation.
- Acute diverticulitis
  1. Antibiotics
  2. Bedrest
  3. Nothing by mouth; IV fluids; may go to hyperalimentation (See NR, IV therapy.)
  4. Nasogastric suction (See NR, Gastrointestinal System, intestinal intubation.)
  5. Meperidine (Demerol) usually is ordered for pain (see PH).
  6. Anticholinergic drugs may be ordered.

Surgical

- If possible, surgical treatment should be elective. It may be indicated in cases of intractability or in case of complications.
- Incision and drainage of abscesses
- Bowel resection of affected parts; may include temporary or permanent colostomy

Nursing Considerations

- See MSN, Surgery, intestinal, Nursing considerations.

MECKEL'S DIVERTICULUM

Description

Meckel's diverticulum is a congenital sacculation usually found near, but proximal to, the ileocecal valve. It is the most common congenital anomaly of the GI tract, and becomes symptomatic most often during childhood or early adulthood. When inflamed, it may lead to bowel obstruction.

Common Diagnostic Tests

- X-ray, barium
- Angiography
- Abdominal scan

Observations

- Bleeding, the most common cause of severe intestinal bleeding in children
- Signs of intestinal obstruction (See MSN, Obstruction of the GI tract.)
- Abdominal pain, anorexia, nausea and vomiting, abdominal tenderness, fever, leukocytosis (symptoms that mimic appendicitis)
- Chronic abdominal pain

Treatment

- Surgical removal of Meckel's diverticulum, performed electively, if possible

Nursing Considerations

- Postoperative care is similar to that of any laparotomy.

ESOPHAGEAL VARICES

Description

Esophageal varices (varicose veins of the esophagus) are most often caused by cirrhosis of the liver, with intrahepatic portal venous obstruction and portal hypertension. Because of the hepatocellular dysfunction caused by the underlying cirrhosis, these patients usually are poor surgical risks. Extrahepatic compression of the portal circulation by adjacent tumors, cysts, and aneurysms are rare causes of esophageal varices. Because liver function is normal in this latter group of patients, the underlying problem can be treated surgically.

Ruptured esophageal varices may result from any increase in intraabdominal pressure, such as coughing or vomiting, erosion of the esophageal mucosa caused by esophagitis, gastric acid reflux, alcohol use, and any drug that directly or indirectly injures the mucosal lining (*e.g.*, salicylates, and corticoids). Bleeding esophageal varices constitute a life-threatening emergency because blood loss under such pressure is rapid and great.

Common Diagnostic Tests

- Esophagogastroscopy (See NR, Endoscopic procedures.)
- Upper GI series—barium-swallow x-ray (See NR, X-ray preparation.)
- CT scan
- Portal venography and arteriography
- Complete blood count (CBC); serum alpha-fetoproteins; plasma ammonia; coagulation studies; serum electrolytes; type and cross-match; liver function studies (See LAB.)

Observations

- Bleeding tends to be sudden and unexpected, in large volume, and bright red in color (see MSN, GI bleeding)
- There usually is a history of alcoholism, or evidence of cirrhosis (see MSN, Liver, Cirrhosis).

Treatment

For bleeding esophageal varices (see MSN, GI bleeding)

- Blood and protein replacement.
- Vasopressin (Pitressin) given in an IV or intra-arterial infusion, or terlipressin.
- Balloon tamponade with either the Sengstaken-Blakemore or the newer Minnesota tube requires a highly skilled physician and highly specialized nursing care.
- An ice-water lavage.
- Vitamin K may be ordered.
- To prevent hepatic coma following massive bleeding, cathartics and enemas may be ordered to clear the GI tract of blood. Neomycin may be ordered to further reduce ammonia formation.

Surgical procedures, preferably done after the patient's condition has stabilized, include the following:

- Injection sclerotherapy—injection of the varices with a sclerosing agent (done through a flexible fiberoptic esophagoscope), with repeated injections
- Arterial embolization
- Portal shunt to reduce portal hypertension—several types are being done, each with specific advantages and disadvantages (see MSN Liver).

To reduce the risk of recurrence, patient must stop drinking alcohol.

Antacids may be ordered after the bleeding stops.

Nursing Considerations

- The patient and the family must understand that vomiting blood constitutes a medical emergency. Each member of the family should know, or have at hand, the telephone number of the local rescue squad.
- Both the patient and the family require emotional support. The patient faces a life-threatening situation.
- When in the hospital, blood that has been typed and cross-matched for these patients should be on hold at all times. Check on its availability.
- To reduce the chance of hemorrhage, the patient should avoid use of alcohol, aspirin, and other irritating substances. He or she should also avoid constipation, coughing, and heavy lifting—anything that increases intrathoracic pressure.

GALLBLADDER DISORDERS

Description

The gallbladder stores bile produced in the liver for later delivery to the duodenum for the digestion of dietary fats. Disorders of the gallbladder and the bile ducts usually are caused by inflammation, with or without the presence of stones. Symptoms usually are caused by inflammation of the gallbladder (cholecystitis), or by the attempt of the body to pass a stone down the bile duct.

Terms that define the location of either the pathology or the surgical procedure involved in the biliary tract include the following: chole (pertaining to bile); cyst (bladder); cholang (bile ducts); choledocho (common duct); and lith (stone). Cholelithiasis, for example, refers to biliary stones.

Common Diagnostic Tests

- Ultrasound scans (See NR, Ultrasound)
- Radionuclide excretion scan (*e.g.*, HIDA scan) (See NR, Scans.)
- Plain x-ray of the abdomen
- Contrast studies that visualize the biliary system on x-ray with a contrast dye (See NR, X-ray preparations.)
  1. Oral cholecystography
  2. Postoperative T-tube cholangiogram
  3. Endoscopic retrograde cholangiopancreatogram (ERCP) (See NR, Endoscopic procedures.)
- Laboratory studies may show moderately elevated WBCs, elevated bilirubin, mildly elevated alkaline phosphatase and serum amylase.

Observations

- Pain in the right upper quadrant of the abdomen; may radiate to the right shoulder; may be dull and achy, or usually severe and colicky following ingestion of fatty foods. There may be tenderness over the gallbladder region.
- Nausea and vomiting are common.
- Mild fever may be present.
- Jaundice may occur if the common bile duct is blocked by edema or a stone.
- History of digestive disturbances associated with ingestion of fatty foods may include nausea, vomiting, anorexia, belching, and flatulence.

Treatment

Medical

- Bedrest during the acute attack of cholecystitis or cholelithiasis
- IV fluids, especially when nausea and vomiting are present, maintenance of fluid and electrolyte balance (See NR, IV therapy.)
- Nasogastric tube for decompression (See NR, Gastrointestinal intubation.)
- Medications
  1. Analgesics for the relief of severe pain, usually meperidine (Demerol) (Morphine sulfate is avoided because it is believed to constrict the common duct sphincter.)
  2. Sedatives, antiemetics, antibiotics, vitamin K
  3. Chenodeoxycholic acid (CDCA or chenodiol) and ursodeoxy-

cholic acid (UDCA) may be prescribed for selected patients in an attempt to dissolve gallstones.

- A low-fat, high-protein, high-carbohydrate diet, if tolerated

Surgical

- *Cholecystectomy* is the operative procedure for 90% of patients with cholecystitis.
- Other procedures include *choledocholithotomy,* (incision of the common duct with removal of stone(s), and *cholecystostomy,* (drainage of the gallbladder). When there is evidence of gallstones, gallbladder and ducts are explored. Usually a Penrose drain is left in the gallbladder region. A T-tube may be inserted into the duct with drainage to the outside in an effort to keep the duct open.
- Nonoperative manipulation and extraction or crushing of retained stones may be done under fluoroscopy. A catheter and basket are inserted through a sinus tract left by a "T" tube that has been left in place for 6 weeks postoperatively.
- Endoscopic retrograde cholangiopancreatography (ERCP) may be done to retrieve a stone if it is lodged in the lower common bile duct.

Nursing Considerations

- Preoperative teaching should prepare patient for postoperative course (see MSN, Preoperative care).
- Postoperative nursing care is similar to that of any abdominal surgery, with these special points.
  1. Prevent respiratory complications by encouraging deep breathing and teaching incision splinting (see NR, Deep breathing techniques).
  2. Intake and output should be measured and recorded accurately.
  3. Drainage from the Penrose drain tends to be profuse and irritating to the skin, so keep it dry, clean, and protected. Montgomery straps (see Fig. 3-12) are practical for frequent dressing changes, or bagging the drainage may be required (see NR, Ostomies, draining wounds).
  4. Care of the T-tube (choledoschostomy tube). The "T" is inserted into the common duct, with the tube to the outside. It usually is sutured into place with the end of the tube attached to a gravity drainage bag. The drainage bag must be kept below the level of the gallbladder.
     a. Drainage is measured and recorded (200 ml to 500 ml is normal for the first day, with amounts decreasing each day

thereafter). Usually red or red-tinged at first, it soon becomes the color of bile. Record volume and color.

b. Patients must be cautioned against exerting tension on the tube or kinking it.
c. The physician may order that the T-tube be clamped at intervals before its removal. Observe how the patient tolerates this. Usually, the tube is removed around the seventh to tenth day, after cholangiogram indicates there is no obstruction.
d. Recycled bile may be taken from the drainage system and returned to the patient by giving it orally mixed with fruit juice and chilled, if drainage has been excessive over a period of time.

5. Watch for complications unique to biliary tract surgery.
   a. Signs of obstruction from either stones or edema include jaundice, failure of stools to return to normal color, or excessive T-tube drainage.
   b. Displacement of the T-tube may be indicated by a sudden change in the T-tube drainage or by leaking around it. Sudden chills, fever, or abdominal pain may indicate bile peritonitis.

GASTROINTESTINAL BLEEDING

Description

Bleeding may occur anywhere in the GI tract and may constitute a life-threatening emergency. Symptoms depend upon the location of the bleeding, site, and the rate of blood loss. Vomited blood nearly always indicates bleeding above the duodenojejunal juncture because blood that leaks into the GI tract below the duodenum rarely reenters the stomach. Common causes of upper GI bleeding include ulcer (either gastric or duodenal), esophageal varices, and gastritis, frequently secondary to the use of alcohol or certain drugs (*e.g.*, aspirin, steroids, and anticoagulants). Common causes of bleeding from the lower GI tract are diverticulitis, Meckel's diverticulum, ulcerative colitis, and Crohn's disease. Bleeding from the anorectal region may result from hemorrhoids, rectal polyps, anal fissure, and anal fistulas. Neoplasms anywhere along the intestinal tract may cause bleeding.

Common Diagnostic Tests

- Positive test for occult blood either in vomitus, aspirated gastric contents, or stool (See LAB.)
- Fiberoptic esophagogastroduodenoscopy and upper GI series to find the location of an upper GI bleed (See NR, endoscopic procedures.)

- Selective abdominal angiography (See NR, X-ray.)
- Sigmoidoscopy, colonoscopy, barium enema x-ray, radionuclide scan, and angiography, for lower GI bleeding
- CBC, serial determinations of hemoglobin and hematocrit, coagulation studies, arterial blood gases (ABGs), liver function tests, blood urea nitrogen (BUN), serum creatinine, blood ammonia levels (See LAB.)
- While not diagnostic, type and cross-match, ABGs, and screen electrolytes also may be done.

Observations

- History should include questions regarding amount and color of blood vomited or passed; when it occurred, how often; presence of hypertension, pain, bruising, or bleeding; drug or alcohol ingestion; loss of appetite or weight.
- Amount and character of vomitus or gastric aspirate
  1. Vomited bright red blood is fresh and usually from the upper GI tract; however, epistaxis (nose bleed) and hemoptysis (bleeding from the respiratory tract) must be ruled out. Sudden bright red hematemesis is characteristic of esophageal varices (see MSN, Esophageal varices).
  2. Vomitus with coffee ground appearance indicates that the blood has been in contact with gastric acid for perhaps several hours.
- Appearance of stools
  1. Melena (black tarry stools) usually are a sign of upper GI bleeding.
  2. Hematochezia (bright red blood in the stool) is usually a sign of bleeding from the colon or anorectal area, but may be seen in rapid, upper GI bleeding if intestinal transit is rapid.
- Weakness, irritability, fatigue, pallor, and anemia are seen in slow GI bleeding.
- Changes in daily weight may occur.

In Acute GI Bleeding

- Look for symptoms of shock: remember that it takes a 20% volume loss to change the vital signs.
  1. Restlessness, rapid pulse, fallen blood pressure, cold and clammy skin, hyperventilation, weakness, chills, confusion
  2. Syndromes resulting from diminished renal and liver function
  3. Accurate measurement of fluid intake and output. A urine meter for measurement of hourly output may be ordered.
  4. Shock and hemorrhage will be treated first. Efforts to discover the cause and the exact site of bleeding will follow.

- After the acute stage
  1. Check for postural hypotension (an early sign of sharply reduced blood volume and renewed bleeding) (see NR, Postural hypotension).
  2. Watch for pulmonary complications.

Treatment

In acute GI bleeding, depending upon the severity and the site, these elements of management are commonly used.

- Treat for shock. Keep the patient warm (see MSN, Postoperative care, Shock).
- Blood replacement.
  1. An IV should be started immediately with a #19-gauge needle, so that there will be access to the circulation both for taking samples for blood typing, cross-matching, hemoglobin, and hematocrit, and for administration of fluids and blood
  2. Until blood is available, albumin, plasmanate, and lactated Ringer's solutions may be ordered (see NR, IV therapy).
- Monitor pulse and blood pressure (BP) q 15 min.
- Keep central venous pressure >5 cm H_2O, hemoglobin over 10 g/dl, hematocrit >30%, and systolic BP >90 mmHg.
- A nasogastric tube (of large bore, 32F–36F) is usually passed for iced saline lavage (see NR, GI intubation). A lavage solution of norepinephrine injection (Levophed) may be used.
- Oxygen therapy is usually ordered (see NR, Oxygen therapy).
- Angiography may be done, to give vasopressin infusion into gastric arteries, to produce photocoagulation with laser, or to produce embolization.
- Balloon tamponade may be used in bleeding esophageal varices (see MSN, Esophageal varices).

After the bleeding has stopped:

- Continue to monitor the patient's vital signs, including checks for postural hypotension.
- Decompress the stomach with a GI tube to suction (see NR, Gastrointestinal intubation).
- Advance the diet slowly.
- Cimetidine (Tagamet), sucralfate (Carafate), or ranitidine (Zantac) may be ordered.
- Antacids frequently are given by nasogastric tube.

Surgical Intervention

- Surgical intervention may be required if the patient does not respond satisfactorily to vigorous medical therapy, or if complications develop (see MSN Esophageal varices, gastric surgery, intestinal surgery, anorectal conditions).

- Selective arterial embolization
- Endoscopic electrocoagulation of upper GI bleeding sites
- Laparoscopy, colectomy, or resection of bleeding sites may be required, depending upon the rate and duration of bleeding.

Nursing Considerations

- Psychological support
- Monitor carefully for signs of continued bleeding. Check vital signs q 15 min, or as frequently as the patient's condition indicates. Check for postural hypotension.
    1. Watch for signs of circulatory overload (rales or wheezing) caused by rapid infusion of IV fluid.
- Maintain the IV infusion.
- Keep an accurate record of intake and output, remembering that intake and output from the nasogastric tube are recorded separately.
- Be sure that blood has been typed and cross-matched, and that it is available and up to date.
- Special mouth care includes dilute hydrogen peroxide mouth washes, lozengers, lemon-swabs, gargles, and ice chips (if ordered). Water from ice chips equals half their volume in water (*e.g.*, 1 cup ice chips = ½ cup water).

HERNIA

ABDOMINAL HERNIA

Description

Hernia is a weakness in a wall of a cavity through which viscera may protrude.

- *Indirect inguinal hernia,* by far the most common hernia, occurs through the inguinal ring and extends down into the scrotum or labia. It is seen most often in men.
- *Direct inguinal hernia* passes through an area of muscular weakness in the abdominal wall (not through the inguinal canal).
- *Femoral hernia* descends through the femoral ring, and is more common in women.
- *Umbilical hernia* results from failure of the umbilical orifice to close. It is more common in obese women, in children, and in blacks.
- *Ventral or incisional hernias* occur in areas of weakness of the abdominal wall following surgery.

Hernias are described as *reducible* (when the contents can be returned to their original position), *incarcerated* or *irreducible* (when the contents cannot be returned to original position), and *strangulated* (when the hernia is irreducible and blood and intestinal flow through the intestine incarcerated in the hernia is stopped completely). Strangulation is a medical emergency, initially as an acute bowel obstruction. If the situation persists, gangrene of the strangulated loop of bowel can occur.

Observations

- Swelling or a soft outpouching, especially with increased intra-abdominal pressure (*e.g.,* coughing, lifting) is usually present.
- Pain may or may not be present.
- In a strangulated hernia, severe pain, tenderness, and symptoms of obstruction (ileus, distention, and absence of flatus or defecation) may be present.

Treatment

- Reduction of the hernia by applying gentle pressure in order to return contents of hernial pouch to original position.
- A truss (pad made with firm material and held in place over the hernia with a belt) may be used to keep the hernia from protruding. It does not correct the problem and is not recommended in most cases.
- *Herniorrhaphy* is the surgical repair of a hernia.
- *Hernioplasty* is the surgical repair of the hernia, with reinforcement of the area with synthetic sutures or mesh for additional support.

Nursing Considerations

Postoperatively (See MSN, Postoperative care)

- Teach the patient to splint the incision when he coughs and deep breathes. Coughing can damage the hernia repair. Cough depressants occasionally may be ordered.
- Urinary retention is not uncommon. It may be relieved if the patient is allowed to use the bathroom, or if the male patient is allowed to stand at the side of the bed to void.
- To relieve swelling of the scrotum following repair of an inguinal hernia, its elevation on a small rolled towel may be helpful. Intermittent use of a small ice bag (one that applies no pressure) may help. A scrotal support may be required.
- Following umbilical or incisional hernia repair, the patient may have a nasogastric tube in place to reduce intra-abdominal pressure (see NR, Gastrointestinal intubation).

HIATAL HERNIA

Description

In hiatal hernia, the stomach herniates into the thoracic cavity through the diaphragmatic esophageal opening. In a *sliding* hiatal hernia, the upper part of the stomach and the esophagogastric junction intermittently ride up into the chest cavity. In a *paraesophageal* or *rolling* hernia, some part of the greater curvature of the stomach extrudes through a diaphragmatic defect near the esophageal hiatus. In this type, there is danger of strangulation.

Loss of lower esophageal sphincter function permits reflux of stomach contents into the esophagus, leading to esophagitis, occasionally to esophageal ulceration or stricture, or to tracheal aspiration.

Common Diagnostic Tests

- Upper GI series with a barium swallow (See NR, X-ray.)
- Esophagoscopy (See NR, Endoscopic procedures.)
- Acid perfusion test (Bernstein test) is often positive when esophagitis is present.
- Manometric studies for evaluation of lower esophageal sphincter function, often with pH, motility, and acid-clearing studies

Observations

- There is a history of mild or intermittent indigestion aggravated by lying down or bending forward. Transitory relief is provided with antacids
- Substernal pain that sometimes mimics heart attack may occur.
- Dysphagia (difficulty in swallowing), regurgitation, and nocturnal respiratory distress may be present.
- Bleeding is seen occasionally (caused by erosions of the esophageal mucosa)
- Severe pain and shock occur if a large portion of the stomach becomes incarcerated above the diaphragm.

Treatment

Medical

- The recommended diet consists of small feedings of moderately bland food. Meals should be eaten slowly. Coffee, alcohol, smoking, and eating within two hours of bedtime should be avoided.
- Weight reduction for the obese patient is sometimes helpful.
- Antacids are usually ordered to be taken after meals, and occasionally may be ordered on a more frequent schedule.

- Silicone preparations (*e.g.*, polymethyl silicone) may be ordered.
- Metaclopramide and bethanechol may be ordered to increase the strength of the lower esophageal sphincter.
- The head of the bed should be elevated at least six inches. This is best done by putting the legs of the head of the bed on blocks.
- The patient should avoid constipation and straining at stool, corsets and girdles, heavy lifting, and leaning forward.

Surgical

- The stomach is put into its correct position, and the defect is repaired. The procedure may be done through the chest or through the abdomen, depending upon the surgeon's preference (see MSN, Pulmonary surgery and Gastric surgery for nursing considerations for appropriate postoperative care).
- Vagotomy is sometimes done in selected cases to reduce acid reflux.

LIVER

Description

A remarkable organ, sometimes called the body's chemical plant, the liver plays many roles, including those of synthesizer, detoxifier, and storehouse. The liver also has impressive powers of rejuvenation, a fact that has important implications for nursing care. Particularly in cases of liver failure, the patient who is carried through the crisis has a chance of recovering, for a time at least.

Table 4-3 highlights the effects of hepatic disfunctions that may have any one of a number of underlying causes.

Common Diagnostic Tests

- Liver function tests and common variations seen in hepatic disease (See Lab.)
  1. Serum and urine bilirubin levels are elevated.
  2. Urine urobilinogen is elevated in hepatocellular jaundice, and markedly decreased in complete obstruction.
  3. Fecal urobilinogen is unchanged or lowered in hepatocellular jaundice, and decreased in obstructive jaundice.
  4. Serum alkaline phosphatase (ALP) is elevated in obstructive jaundice and liver metastasis.
  5. Aspartate amino-transferase (AST), formerly serum glutamic-oxaloacetic transaminase (SGOT), and alanine amino-transferase (ALT), formerly serum glutamic-pyruvic transaminase (SGPT), are elevated in hepatocellular disease. ALT, found mainly in the liver, is especially significant.

TABLE 4-3 LIVER DISORDERS

Dysfunction	Consequences	Related Observations
Intrahepatic dysfunction: inflammation or disorder of hepatic cells (*e.g.*, hepatitis, cirrhosis, carcinoma)	Bilirubin accumulates in the bloodstream, staining tissues of the body, including skin, sclera, and mucous membranes	Jaundice (icterus) or yellowing of the skin, sclera, and mucous membranes is accompanied frequently by pruritus (itching).
Extrahepatic causes of jaundice: 1. Hemolytic jaundice caused by too rapid breakdown of RBCs 2. Mechanical obstruction in the flow of bile (*e.g.*, obstruction of the common bile duct by gallstones or tumors, or congenital portal vein abnormalities seen in children)	Same as above	Same as above
Changes in the liver that slow circulation and cause backup pressure in the portal venous system, seen especially in cases of cirrhosis	Portal hypertension	Esophageal varices (see MSN, Esophageal varices, GI bleeding), hemorrhoids, hepatomegaly, splenomegaly, distended abdominal veins,

		especially bluish varicose veins radiating from the navel (caput medusae), and telangiectasia (spider nevi) usually seen on upper chest
Interference with synthesis of blood-clotting factors	Bleeding tendencies	Petechiae, easy bruising, ecchymosis
Interference with protein and carbohydrate synthesis	Hypoalbuminemia, decreased glycogen reserves, decreased gluconeogenesis	Generalized edema, ascites, and hypoglycemia during fasting
Interference with the conversion of ammonia to urea.	Accumulation of ammonia in the blood, causing metabolic effects on the brain (hepatic encephalopathy)	Drowsiness, confusion, disorientation, flapping tremor (asterixis), behavioral and personality changes, convulsions, and gradual depression of level of consciousness developing into coma
Interference with the synthesis of some immunoglobulins	Reduced resistance to infections	Signs of infection
Interference with the liver's ability to detoxify toxic substances	Increased risk of toxicity from alcohol, and from drugs given in normal doses	Signs of alcohol or drug toxicity. Check which drugs are hepatotoxic, and which are detoxified by the liver.

(*continued*)

TABLE 4-3 LIVER DISORDERS

Dysfunction	Consequences	Related Observations
Decreases in adrenal and gonadal steroids		
1. Aldosterone decreases result in sodium and water retention and potassium excretion.	Fluid imbalances with sodium retention Decreased serum potassium levels	Thigh and leg edema. General weakness, shallow respirations, cardiac arrhythmias
2. Estrogen and testosterone imbalances.		Loss of axillary and pubic hair, impotence, testicular atrophy, gynecomastia in males, loss of libido, menstrual disorders, spider angiomas

6. Prothrombin time is prolonged. Administration of vitamin K will normalize prothrombin time in an obstructed liver, but will not in a cell-damaged liver.
7. Serum cholesterol is usually elevated in obstructive jaundice, but decreased in hepatocellular disease if damage is severe.
8. Serum ammonia levels are elevated in severe liver disease, especially following GI bleeding.

- Liver biopsy (See NR, Liver biopsy.)
- Ultrasonography, CT scan, radionuclide imaging, percutaneous transhepatic cholangiography, endoscopic retrograde cholangiopancreatography
- Radioimmunoassay for anti-hepatitis A virus (anti-HAV), hepatitis B surface antigen (HB_sAg), hepatitis B surface antibody (anti-HB_s)

Treatment and Nursing Considerations

- Bedrest in the acute phase of any liver disorder is required. Also, sympathetic support is important.
- Vital signs should be checked q 4 hours.
- For jaundice (icterus)
  1. Best seen in the sclera (white of the eye), especially in dark-skinned people
  2. Pruritus (itching)
     a. Avoid alkaline soaps.
     b. Keep nails trimmed to prevent scratching.
     c. Apply emollient lotions.
     d. Medications (such as benadryl) are of limited benefit.
- For ascites and fluid retention
  1. Evaluate the degree of abdominal distention.
     a. Weigh the patient daily, at the same time of day and under the same circumstances.
     b. Measure the patient's abdominal girth daily. Mark the abdomen at the level at which you are measuring, so that measurement can be taken consistently at the same place.
  2. Low semi-Fowler's position will relieve pressure on the diaphragm, diminishing dyspnea. Reposition frequently.
  3. Accurate measurement of intake and output is essential.
  4. A low sodium diet is necessary.
  5. Total fluid intake often is restricted.
  6. Diuretics may be introduced gradually. *Caution:* Hypokalemia is deadly to the damaged liver, so monitor potassium levels.
  7. Salt-poor albumin may be given IV (see NR, IV therapy).
  8. Special skin care is essential. Bathe with mild, nonalkaline

soap and water, rinse thoroughly, and use emollient lotions, especially to massage pressure points.

9. Paracentesis may be required to relieve pressure. Usually, no more than 1,000 ml of fluid are removed at one time.
10. LeVeen (peritoneovenous) shunt diverts fluid from the peritoneal cavity into a major vein (*e.g.,* the superior vena cava or the jugular) through a Silastic tube containing a one-way valve.

- For edema of the extremities
  1. Elevate extremities. Support stockings may be ordered.
  2. Provide comfort measures to relieve pressure on bony prominences (*e.g.,* sheepskin protectors and eggcrate mattress).
- For bleeding tendencies
  1. Monitor for bleeding: subcutaneous bleeding, petechiae, ecchymoses (bruises), nosebleeds, and bleeding gums.
  2. Test vomitus and stools for occult blood, as indicated (see Lab). Gastrointestinal bleeding is a frequent complication of cirrhosis (see MSN, Esophageal varices and Gastrointestinal bleeding).
- Check special cautions regarding all drugs prescribed for these patients.
  1. Check for hepatotoxicity. Some common offenders are acetaminophen (Tylenol), allopurinol (Zyloprim), isoniazid (INH), and methyldopa (Aldomet).
  2. Check for drugs detoxified by the liver (*e.g.,* sedatives, barbiturates, and some diuretics). These must be used cautiously. Many physicians avoid ordering sedatives for any patient with impaired liver function.
  3. Dosages of all drugs may have to be reduced.
- The diet is usually high in carbohydrates and proteins and low in fats in the early stages of liver disease. Protein is reduced in an effort to reduce ammonia formation in late-stage liver dysfunction.
- *Surgical shunts to relieve portal hypertension* are designed to provide variceal decompression and maintenance of optimal portal perfusion. Risk is reduced greatly if surgery is performed when the patient's condition is stable.
  1. End-to-side portacaval shunts divert all portal blood around the liver.
     a. Portacaval anastomosis joins the portal vein and inferior vena cava.
     b. Mesocaval anastomosis joins the superior mesenteric vein and inferior vena cava.
     c. Sphenorenal anastomosis joins the splenic vein and left renal vein; it also may be done side-to-side with possible splenectomy.

2. Side-to-side portacaval, mesocaval, and splenorenal shunts divert some blood but don't preserve liver perfusion.

- *Liver failure* may lead to *hepatic coma.* The patient may have all of the symptoms described in Table 4-3. Treatment and vital nursing care described previously will be required, as well as the following:
  1. Correction of fluid, acid-base, and electrolyte imbalances
  2. Protection of the patient from sources of infection
  3. Efforts to reduce the build-up of ammonia in the blood serum that leads to encephalopathy
     a. Restrict protein intake
     b. If GI bleeding exists, attempt to stop it (see MSN, Esophageal varices, Gastrointestinal bleeding). Remove blood from the GI tract with laxatives and enemas.
     c. Neomycin may be ordered in an effort to kill ammonia-producing bacteria.
     d. Lactulose (cephulac) may be ordered.
  4. Protect the patient from accidents caused by symptoms of encephalopathy (*e.g.,* confusion, daytime drowsiness, nighttime wandering) by carefully supervising his or her daily activities. Side rails should be up, especially at night. A restraining jacket may be required when the patient is sitting in a chair.
  5. Watch for signs of hypoglycemia. Correct it if it occurs.

CIRRHOSIS

Description

Laennec's cirrhosis is a chronic disease of the liver characterized by the destruction of normal liver tissue and the replacement of it by connective (scar) tissue that divides it into nodules. It is becoming a leading cause of death in the 25- to 65-year age group.

Portal system hypertension causing esophageal varices, hemorrhoids, hepatomegaly, splenomegaly, and other symptoms are common sequelae.

Cirrhosis usually results from the toxic effects of alcohol ingestion, but nutritional deficiencies, poisons, hepatitis, and biliary obstruction also may be causative factors.

Common Diagnostic Tests

- See MSN, Liver.

Observations

- See Table 4-3, Liver Disorders.

Treatment and Nursing Considerations

- See Treatment and nursing considerations under Liver section.
- Emphasize the importance of *no alcohol ingestion.*
- Surgical shunts can relieve portal hypertension (see MSN Liver).
- Treat esophageal varices and GI bleeding if present (see MSN Esophageal varices, Gastrointestinal bleeding).

HEPATIC TUMORS

Description

The liver is a common site of metastasis from malignancies originating elsewhere.

Primary liver carcinoma, while seldom seen in the United States, is common in parts of the Orient and Africa. Chronic hepatitis B virus (HBV) infection is believed to be a major etiologic factor.

Observations

- Anemia, weight loss, weakness, and jaundice (if the tumor obstructs the biliary system) are late symptoms that often appear too late for curative treatment.

Treatment

- Anticancer drugs infused directly into hepatic arteries may be palliative.
- Surgical resection of segments of the liver is the only treatment that offers a possibility of cure.
- See MSN, Oncology nursing considerations.

LIVER ABSCESS

Description

Liver abscesses may form as complications of infection elsewhere in the body. Offending organisms may be bacterial (usually enteric in origin, *e.g., Escherichia coli*), fungal, or parasitic. The amebiasis-causing protozoan *Entamoeba histolytica* is a common cause of liver abscess.

Observations

- High fever, jaundice, painful and enlarged liver, extreme toxicity
- History of travel to areas where endemic amebiasis is present

Treatment

- Antibiotics that are specific for the disease organism should be chosen.
- Metronidazole is the drug of choice for amebic abscess.
- Surgical drainage of the abscess often is required.

VIRAL HEPATITIS

Description

In viral hepatitis, inflammation of the liver with cell damage and necrosis is caused by a virus.

- *Hepatitis A* or infectious hepatitis, is caused by the hepatitis A virus (HAV) and usually is transmitted by the fecal-oral route, although it may be transmitted parenterally through serum and blood products. It is usually a milder disease than type B hepatitis.
- *Hepatitis B* or serum hepatitis, is caused by the hepatitis B virus (HBV) and is most commonly transmitted parenterally by exposure to blood or blood products of affected people, but it may be spread by exposure to any body secretion, including saliva and seminal fluid. It is a more severe infection and has a longer incubation period than HAV. People may be carriers without symptoms of the disease. Primary carcinoma of the liver is now associated with a history of HBV. People especially at risk to acquire hepatitis B include health personnel who handle blood products, especially those working in dialysis units; people receiving blood transfusions, especially hemophiliacs; drug addicts; male homosexuals; immigrants and refugees from areas where HBV is prevalent; persons in institutions for the developmentally disabled; household and sexual contacts of carriers; and newborns of HB_sAg-positive mothers.
- *Non-A, Non-B hepatitis* (NANB) designates any of the several, possible hepatitis-causing viruses that are neither type A nor type B. It is apparently bloodborne—seen in post-transfusion patients—but also can be spread through sexual contact.
- Inadequately cooked shellfish, when infected, is a source of infection for both HAV and HBV hepatitis.

Most patients recover from viral hepatitis with little residual damage. A few go on to develop chronic hepatitis or even fulminant hepatitis with fatal, massive liver necrosis.

Observations

- Clinical picture is extremely variable, ranging from no symptoms to a fulminating disease that may lead to death in a few days. The following signs and symptoms may be seen.

Before the jaundice appears

- General malaise, weakness, unusual fatigue, and muscle tenderness
- Upper respiratory symptoms, headache, and fever
- Severe anorexia, nausea and vomiting, diarrhea, or constipation
- In the smoker, distaste for cigarettes is typical.
- Mild, constant, abdominal pain in the upper right quadrant or right epigastrium
- Darkened urine and clay-colored stools just before jaundice appears

Jaundice phase

- Jaundice usually occurs after 5 days to 10 days, but may develop earlier, and in some cases, never.
- GI symptoms may decrease.
- Liver enlargement and tenderness may give the patient an uncomfortable feeling of fullness in the right upper quadrant.
- If hepatitis is severe, any of the symptoms listed in Table 4-3 under Liver disorders may be seen.

Recovery phase

- Gradual disappearance of symptoms may take several weeks to months.

Common Diagnostic Tests

- See Common diagnostic tests under MSN, Liver.
- Hepatitis screens include tests for various HAV and HBV antigens and antibodies in the serum.
  1. Hepatitis A
     a. Presence of hepatitis A virus antibodies (anti-HAV) of the IgM class of immunoglobulins is seen early. Anti-HAV of the IgG class indicates past infection.
  2. Hepatitis B
     a. Hepatitis B surface antigen (HB_sAg) is seen early, but its presence begins to decline during recovery. The patient is considered infectious as long as HB_sAg is detectable.
     b. Antibodies to HB_sAg (anti-HBs) appear following recovery and usually indicate immunity to hepatitis B.
     c. The antibody (anti-HBc) to the hepatitis B core antigen (HB_cAg) may be found in the serum during the phase of recovery when HB_sAg levels are too low to be detected in carriers or in those patients with chronic hepatitis.
  3. Hepatitis non-A, non-B (NANB)

     Rule out HAV and HBV.

Prevention

- Hepatitis A and NANB
  1. Immune globulin, formerly called immune serum globulin (ISG) or gamma globulin, is given
     a. Preexposure to travelers to high-risk areas
     b. Postexposure to household and sexual contacts, to residents and staff of custodial institutions; optional after accidental needle-stick inoculation if the patient is believed to have NANB hepatitis
- Hepatitis B
  1. Immune globulin is given
     a. Preexposure, for staff and patients of hemodialysis units and custodial institutions for the developmentally disabled, if other infection control measures fail.
     b. Postexposure immediately, if exposed to blood that is likely to be HB_sAg positive. (HBIG, described below, is recommended once the blood is proved to be HB_sAg-positive.)
  2. Hepatitis B Immune Globulin (HBIG)
     a. Given immediately and repeated for one month after exposure to HB_sAg-positive blood
     b. Given at birth to infants of HB_sAg-positive mothers. Repeat at 3 months and 6 months of age.
  3. Hepatitis B vaccine
     a. May be given to persons at high risk

Nursing Considerations

- All of the nursing considerations outlined in the treatment of liver disorders apply. (See MSN, Liver, Nursing Considerations.)
- Bedrest usually is ordered during the acute stage, with graduated activity during recovery.
- The diet is as tolerated, with alcohol restricted for at least 6 months.
- Hepatitis precautions, if hospitalization is required, focus on mode of transmission. (See NR, Isolation technique.)
  1. Scrupulous hand washing should be carried out by the patient, family, and the hospital staff before and after direct contact with the patient or items that are in contact with the patient's blood, feces, or other body secretions.
  2. Remember that hepatitis A is transmitted most commonly by the fecal-oral route.
  3. Although hepatitis B and non-A, non-B is transmitted primarily through blood and blood derivatives, it also may be spread through semen, saliva, or any body secretion. Nurses need to

be especially careful to avoid accidental needle-prick inoculation.

4. Avoid contaminating the outside of specimen containers. All specimens should be marked "HEPATITIS" in large letters before sending them to the laboratory.

- Prognosis generally is good in viral hepatitis, but the course and recovery period are discouragingly long. Emotional support for the patient is important.
- Drug rehabilitation programs should be strongly encouraged for the drug addict.

OBSTRUCTION OF THE INTESTINAL TRACT

Description

Obstruction occurs when there is partial or complete closing of a section of the lumen of the intestine. Strangulation, with resulting necrosis, occurs when the blood supply to a bowel segment is cut off.

Mechanical obstruction (dynamic) has a wide variety of possible causes, including tumors (malignant or benign, within or adjacent to the intestinal tract), adhesions, strangulated hernia, volvulus (twisting of the bowel on itself), intussusception (the telescoping of one segment of bowel into another; seen most often in children), polyps, impacted feces, and foreign bodies.

Paralytic (adynamic) ileus represents a failure of normal peristalsis and may result in obstruction. It may occur postoperatively following abdominal surgery; as a complication of peritonitis; and as a result of acute illness, of spinal cord lesions, or of embolism or thrombosis of one of the mesenteric arteries or their branches (see MSN, Postoperative care, Paralytic ileus).

Common Diagnostic Tests

- Flat plates (x-rays) of the abdomen
- X-rays using contrast media (See NR, X-ray preparations.)
- Hemoglobin and hematocrit, elevated with dehydration
- Leukocytosis (elevated WBCs)
- Serum sodium, potassium, chloride levels may be depressed because of continued vomiting (see LAB).
- Blood urea nitrogen (BUN) may be elevated
- Stools for occult blood

Observations

Symptoms will vary according to whether the obstruction is partial or complete; dynamic or adynamic; whether it is high or low in the GI tract; and whether there is interference with the blood supply to the affected part. In general, symptoms of obstruction high in the GI tract appear more suddenly and are more severe (See Small bowel obstruction, and Large bowel obstruction).

Careful assessment includes

- History and observation of character and amount of emesis; bowel sounds; passing of flatus or stool; and level of pain or discomfort
- Measurement of abdominal girth to assess distention: Mark level at which you are measuring on the abdomen with magic marker so that you can measure at the same place each day.
- Record daily weights before breakfast on the same scale to assess hydration.
- Vital signs must be checked every 4 hours. Watch for temperature elevation, a sign of peritonitis.

Small Bowel Obstruction

- Increased peristalsis and borborygmi (loud, gurgling bowel sounds heard on auscultation, or even without benefit of stethoscope)
- Cramping upper abdominal pain
- Frequent vomiting, may be projectile, starting with semi-digested food, next becoming watery, bile colored, and, finally dark and fecal in odor
- Signs of dehydration, increased respiratory rate, electrolyte imbalances, shock, and peritonitis
- Abdominal distention occurs later.
- Abdominal muscle guarding or rebound tenderness may indicate strangulation or perforation.

Large Bowel Obstruction

- Symptoms usually appear insidiously (except in the case of volvulus).
- Abdominal distention
- Vomiting and pain usually are less severe than in upper intestinal obstruction.
- Failure to pass gas or stool, if obstruction is complete. Irregular, small, or liquid stools are common if obstruction is partial.
- Absent bowel sound in paralytic ileus (See MSN, Postoperative complications, Ileus.)

Treatment

- Intestinal decompression with suction and GI intubation. A long tube such as the Miller-Abbot or Cantor may be required (see NR, Gastrointestinal intubation).

- Maintain fluid and electrolyte balance (see NR, Intravenous therapy).
- Antibiotics may be ordered.
- Surgical relief of mechanical obstruction is necessary if conservative measures fail. Surgery may involve lysis (cutting) of adhesions, bowel resection with re-anastomosis, or colostomy (possibly temporary), with further correction planned for a time when the patient is in better condition.

Nursing Considerations

- Maintain gastric or intestinal suction (see NR, Gastrointestinal intubation).
- Record accurate intake and output. Remember that vomitus and drainage from the GI tract are considered "output" and are recorded separately.
- Good skin care is required for the patient who may be both dehydrated and toxic.
- Good mouth care is necessary.
- Analgesics are used sparingly because of constipating side-effects and because they mask symptoms.
- Maintain the patient in Fowler's or low Fowler's position to relieve respiratory distress caused by distention.

PANCREAS

ACUTE PANCREATITIS

Description

Acute inflammation of the pancreas is associated most commonly with biliary tract disorders, alcoholism, trauma during surgery of adjacent organs, certain infections (*e.g.*, mumps), ingestion of some drugs, hyperparathyroidism, and hyperlipidemia. Progress from edema to hemorrhage to necrotic pathologic changes in the pancreas may occur. Seriousness of the symptoms and the incidence of mortality increase accordingly. The formation of pseudocysts and pancreatic abscesses and pulmonary edema with or without cardiac failure are serious complications. Approximately 10% of these cases go on to chronic pancreatitis.

Common Diagnostic Tests

- Serum amylase and serum lipase are elevated.
- Urinary amylase is elevated. Proteinuria, casts, and glycosuria may be seen.

- Serum bilirubin is elevated if the common bile duct is obstructed.
- Blood urea nitrogen (BUN) and serum alkaline phosphatase (ALP) levels are elevated.
- Elevated blood glucose levels may be seen, possibly to an insulin-requiring degree.
- Serum calcium levels may decrease, and tetany may occur.
- Complete blood count with differential may show leukocytosis. Hematocrit may be elevated.
- A CT scan is useful for detecting pseudocysts and pancreatic abscesses.
- X-ray—flat plate, upper GI series
- Cholangiography may be used to determine normalcy of biliary tract.

Observations

- History of recent, heavy alcohol intake or a high-fat meal
- Sudden onset of severe abdominal pain, usually across the upper abdomen, with radiation through the back
- Abdominal tenderness
- Nausea, vomiting, prostration, profuse perspiration
- Fever, developing during the first few days
- Symptoms of shock may develop in severe attacks. Condition may require vital signs to be checked up to q 15 minutes to 30 minutes in the acute phase.
- Jaundice, if the biliary tract is obstructed
- Stools may be pale, bulky, foul smelling, and high in fat content if chronic pancreatic insufficiency has developed.

Treatment

- Relief of pain, usually with meperidine (Demerol) (see PH). *Caution:* Morphine sulfate is contraindicated because it contracts the sphincter of Oddi.
- Bedrest is recommended during the acute phase.
- Nothing by mouth (NPO). Continuous nasogastric suction is usually used. (See NR, Gastrointestinal intubation.)
- Treat shock, if present. (See MSN, Postoperative care.)
- Maintain normal plasma volume and fluid and electrolyte balances. (See LAB, NR, Intravenous therapy, Fluid and electrolytes.)
- Calcium gluconate may be ordered. (See PH.)
- Hyperglycemia may be treated with insulin. (See PH.)
- Antibiotics may be ordered for specific reasons.

- The use of anticholinergic drugs, formerly an accepted part of treatment, is now under question.
- Diet, when resumed, should be low in fat and protein and high in carbohydrates. Intake of coffee should be limited. Alcohol should be avoided.
- Exploratory surgery may be required if the diagnosis is in doubt, or if stones are present in biliary tract.
- Cysts and abscesses usually are drained surgically.

Nursing Considerations

- Assume nursing responsibilities for treatment outlined above.
- Accurate measurement of intake and output is extremely important.
- Frequent, careful assessment of the patient's condition is essential.
- Provide all comfort measures, including back care, mouth care, and skin care. (If the patient is jaundiced, pruritus may be relieved by washing with water only, using emollient lotions.)
- The patient will be more comfortable sitting up, with some flexion at the waist. Bedrest in the most acute stage is required. Assistance may be needed for position changes.

CHRONIC PANCREATITIS

Description

Chronic pancreatitis consists of marked fibrous scarring of the pancreas, often associated with calcification. It is most commonly seen in chronic alcoholism. Repeated attacks of acute inflammation produce the scarring that eventually replaces the endocrine and exocrine cells. With progressive loss of the secretion of digestive enzymes, absorption of both fat and protein is impaired. Diabetes mellitus may result from destruction of the islets of Langerhans.

Common Diagnostic Tests

- Secretin and cholecystokinin stimulation tests for exocrine malfuction
- Serum carotene
- Fecal fat
- D-xylose absorption test
- X-ray—flat plate of the abdomen
- Endoscopic retrograde pancreatography
- Retrograde cholangiography

Observations

- Pain in the upper left quadrant of the abdomen, usually radiating to the back. It may be dull or severe; persistent or intermittent.
- Nausea and vomiting, anorexia, constipation, flatulence
- Fatty, foul-smelling stools (steatorrhea)
- Weight loss and malnutrition
- Evidence of diabetes mellitus (See MSN, Diabetes mellitus.)
- Narcotic addiction is common.

Treatment

- Control pain, although the need for analgesics frequently leads to drug addiction.
- Abstinence from alcohol and avoidance of caffeine are necessary.
- Diet should be low in fats. Small meals are recommended.
- Control diabetes mellitus, if it exists.
- Medications
    1. Pancreatic supplements, *e.g.,* pancreatin (Viokase, Elzyme), or pancrelipase (Cotazym, Pancrease, Ilozyme)
    2. Cimetidine decreases inactivation of lipase by gastric acid, thereby decreasing steatorrhea.
- Underlying gallbladder disease must be treated, if present.
- Surgical procedures may be necessary to ensure free flow of bile into duodenum, to eliminate obstruction of the pancreatic duct, to drain persistent pseudocysts, or to treat complications.

Nursing Considerations

- Provide emotional support for the patient who is frequently in great pain over a long period of time. Chronic pancreatitis is a debilitating disease that frequently is made more difficult by problems of underlying alcoholism and the problems of diabetes control.
- The patient and his or her family must be educated as to the absolute necessity of the patient's abstinence from alcohol.

PEPTIC ULCER

Description

Peptic ulcer is a sharply defined break in the mucosal lining of any part of the GI tract that is exposed to acid and pepsin. Most ulcers are found in the duodenum, just beyond the pylorus. They may penetrate the mucosa, submocosa, or muscle wall of the lower end of the esophagus, stomach, or duodenum; or stomal ulcers may form at the site of an anastomosis between the intestine and stomach.

While the pathogenesis is not fully understood, the following are contributing factors: stress and anxiety; familial predisposition; blood group 0; smoking; alcohol; caffeine; and usage of ulcerogenic drugs, *e.g.*, acetylsalicylic acid (aspirin), indomethacin (Indocin), other nonsteroidal anti-inflammatory drugs; and the steroids. Periods of exacerbation and remission are common. Personality type is believed, by some, to be a contributing factor.

Hemorrhage and perforation are complications caused by penetration of the ulcer through an arterial wall or fully through the intestinal wall. Pyloric obstruction may be caused by scarring or edema of the pylorus caused by the ulcer. Perforation, pyloric obstruction, and failure of the ulcer to heal after intensive medical treatment usually are indications for surgical treatment.

Symptoms of duodenal and gastric ulcers may be similar, and x-ray is useful in making a differential diagnosis. However, gastric ulcers, while usually benign, have a significant incidence of underlying cancer. They heal less quickly, and more often are treated surgically.

Common Diagnostic Tests

- X-ray: barium studies of the upper GI tract (See NR, X-ray preparations.)
- Endoscopic studies of the upper GI tract, often with biopsy or cytologic examination of washings to rule out malignancy (See NR, Endoscopic procedures.)
- Gastric analysis for the following
  1. Blood, either gross or occult (See LAB, Testing for occult blood.)
  2. Acid concentration (basic acid output, or BAO)
     a. Elevated in duodenal ulcer
     b. Normal or depressed in gastric ulcer or cancer

Observations

- A gnawing, boring epigastric pain that is relieved temporarily after ingestion of food or antacids, or after vomiting is a classic symptom.
- Epigastric tenderness also is common.
- Nausea and vomiting are frequent complaints.
- If bleeding is present the patient may vomit blood, that is often coffee ground in appearance, or pass tarry stools. Fatigue and symptoms of anemia may be signs of slow GI bleeding (see MSN, Gastrointestinal bleeding).
- With pyloric obstruction, vomiting that may or may not be preceded by feelings of nausea may be projectile. If persistent, it may lead to alkalosis. Anorexia also may result.

- Signs of perforation include a very sudden onset of severe, sharp abdominal pain with referred pain to shoulders, and a rigid and boardlike abdomen with decreased or absent bowel sounds, followed by symptoms of shock and peritonitis (see MSN, Peritonitis).

Treatment

Medical

About 85% of ulcers respond to conservative treatment.

- Drug therapy may be ordered.
  1. Antacids (*e.g.*, Maalox, Gelusil, Amphojel) frequently are given every hour while the patient is awake, then q 1 to 3 hr after eating, and at bedtime while the patient is hospitalized.
  2. Cimetidine (Tagamet), a synthetic hydrogen receptor antagonist, may be ordered.
  3. Sucralfate (Carafate), a mucosal protective agent that has anti-pepsin activity can be administered.
  4. Ranitidine (Zantoc) can be given.
  5. Anticholinergic drugs are now considered to be of questionable value.
- Diet: Small frequent feedings are recommended. Avoid acid-stimulating foods such as coffee, tea, cola, alcohol, and spices.
- Treat hemorrhage, if it occurs (see MSN, Gastrointestinal bleeding).

Surgical

- Emergency: closure of an area of perforation
- Elective: for recurrent ulcers, bleeding episodes, pyloric obstruction, or intractable ulcer
- Surgical procedures (See MSN, Gastric surgery.)

Nursing Considerations

- Try to provide mental and physical rest in the acute stage.
- Try to help patient find ways to reduce stress in his or her life.
- Patient teaching should include
  1. Information regarding prescribed drugs (See PH.)
  2. Cautions about ulcerogenic drugs and the need to be aware of their presence in over-the-counter preparations
  3. Emphasis on the importance of regular eating and living habits; the avoidance of alcohol, tobacco, and acid-stimulating foods; the avoidance of emotional stress and infections; and the return to ulcer regimen if symptoms recur.

Postoperative Care

- See MSN, Postoperative care, Gastric surgery

PERITONITIS

Description

Peritonitis is an inflammation of the lining (peritoneum) of the abdominal cavity. It is most often caused by bacterial invasion as a result of perforation or rupture of an organ into the abdominal cavity (*e.g.*, a perforated ulcer, or a ruptured diverticulum, appendix, or gallbladder). It also may be caused by leakage or contamination during abdominal surgery, or by an ascending infection through the female reproductive tract (*e.g.*, salpingitis).

Common Diagnostic Tests

- X-rays: Flat-plate x-rays of the abdomen may show free peritoneal fluid or air in the abdominal cavity if perforation has occurred.
- Elevated WBC (See LAB.)
- Blood and peritoneal cultures may identify the offending organism.

Observations

- Abdominal pain: diffuse at first, but becoming localized in the affected area; later becoming exquisitely tender with muscle guarding, abdominal rigidity, and abdominal distention
- Paralytic ileus and the absence of bowel sounds (See MSN, Postoperative complication, paralytic ileus.)
- Anorexia, nausea, and vomiting
- Elevated temperature, drop in blood pressure, tachycardia, and rapid, shallow breathing
- Effects of dehydration and electrolyte imbalance (See LAB, Electrolytes.)

Treatment

- Remove source of irritation; this may require surgical intervention.
- Control infection by using a broad-spectrum, antimicrobial drug until results of culture are available; then use specific antibiotic (see PH).
- Replace fluids and electrolytes. Monitor electrolytes daily.
- Relieve pain with minimum dose of medication to prevent masking of symptoms. Use nursing comfort measures.

- Oxygen therapy may be required.
- Keep the patient in a semi-Fowler's position to try to localize infection in lower abdominal cavity.
- A nasointestinal tube with suction to decompress bowel is usually ordered.

Nursing Considerations

- These patients are extremely ill. They require gentle, total nursing care including the following:
  1. Close assessment for change in symptoms
  2. Management of nasointestinal tubes, oxygen, IV, and drug therapy (See NR, Gastrointestinal intubation, oxygen administration, IV therapy.)
  3. Comfort measures, including mouth care, and fever reduction
  4. Nasogastric tubes are in place for a long time and cause sore nares and throat. Lubricating ointment helps the nares; anesthetic gargles are sometimes helpful for the throat.

PILONIDAL CYSTS AND SINUSES

Description

A pilonidal cyst is found in the sacrococcygeal region, usually at the upper part of the intergluteal fold. It is believed to be caused by a developmental defect in which epithelial tissue is trapped below the skin. Hair is often present and protrudes from the cyst. The cyst is usually asymptomatic until late adolescence or early adult life, when trauma may cause an inflammatory reaction, which results in swelling, abscess formation, and draining sinuses or fistulas.

Treatment

- Antibiotic therapy until inflammation is controlled
- Incision and drainage of an abscess
- Surgical excision of the cyst and sinuses

Nursing Considerations

- Surgical techniques vary as to how the wound is closed. Postoperative orders will vary accordingly.
- Analgesics usually are needed only during the first 24 hours.
- Early ambulation usually is encouraged, although patients are advised not to undertake strenuous activities until healing is complete.

REGIONAL ENTERITIS (CROHN'S DISEASE)

Description

Crohn's disease, also known as regional enteritis, granulomatous ileitis, or granuileocolitis, is an inflammatory process involving all layers of the intestinal wall, especially the submucosa. Areas of normal bowel lie between inflamed segments. Most often the disease affects the ileum alone, but it also may involve the colon; and infrequently only the colon is involved. Narrowing of the lumen of the intestine caused by thickening of the intestinal wall may lead to obstruction. Fistula formation and mesenteric abscesses are common late complications. There is a small but significant risk of cancer.

Common Diagnostic Tests

- X-rays of the small and large intestine (See NR, X-ray preparations.)
- Sigmoidoscopy (See NR, Endoscopic procedures.)

Observations

- There is a history of intermittent diarrhea, usually three or four semi-soft stools a day, some with fat. Usually, there is no blood or pus in the stools.
- Right lower quadrant pain in an acute attack may mimic appendicitis.
- Symptoms of obstruction (*e.g.*, severe abdominal pain, distention, constipation, and vomiting) may be present.
- Abdominal fistulas and abscesses, accompanied by fever, and painful abdominal masses may be present.
- General debilitation may occur if the disease has been present for a long time.

Treatment

Medical

- A diet that is low residue, bland, high caloric and high protein, with vitamin supplements (especially vitamin B_{12}) is usually ordered.
- Anticholinergics, diphenoxylate (Lomotil), tincture of opium (See PH.)
- Sulfasalazine (Azulfidine) may be given on a long-term basis. Other antibacterials may be given for specific complications (see PH).

- Corticosteroids may be administered during acute stages (see PH).
- Metronidazole (Flagyl) may be ordered.

Surgical

- Resection of involved bowel or bypass procedures have generally not been curative. Surgery may be required to deal with complications (*e.g.,* fistulas, recurrent obstruction, abscesses that do not respond to conservative treatment). Surgery is a last resort because postoperative healing is poor and interior fistula formation commonly occurs.

Nursing Considerations

- All of the nursing considerations outlined under "ulcerative colitis" would apply to the nursing care of the patient with Crohn's disease, except for the reference to ileostomy (see MSN, Ulcerative colitis).

SURGERY

GASTRIC SURGERY

Description

Most gastric surgery is performed to treat either carcinoma of the stomach or peptic ulcer. Presently, although other therapies are under investigation, surgical removal is the only cure for stomach cancer.

Partial gastrectomy, or removal of part of the stomach, may be attempted. Excision of nearby organs may be required, but an attempt is made to restore the GI tract to as near-normal functioning as possible. If metastases appears to be widespread, a bypass procedure may be attempted as a palliative measure. *Total gastrectomy* (the removal of the entire stomach with anastomosis of the esophagus to the jejunum) rarely is done, except in cases of Zollinger-Ellison syndrome (gastrin-producing tumors).

The goal of surgery for peptic ulcer is to reduce acid secretion, either by interference with the vagus nerve or by removal of the part of the stomach that contains the acid-producing parietal cells, or the antrum of the stomach, where gastrin (which stimulates acid production) is formed.

Gastric surgical procedures

- *Vagotomy* (resection of the vagus nerve) decreases acid secretion, but also may slow stomach emptying, thus causing symptoms of fullness, abdominal distention, and flatus. Therefore, *pyloroplasty* (increasing the pyloric opening) may be done at the same time to facilitate gastric emptying.

- In *selective parietal-cell vagotomy,* only the vagal supply to the body of the fundus is removed. Vagal denervation of just the parietal cell area of the stomach preserves vagal innervation of other visceral areas. Gastric emptying is relatively unimpaired.
- A *vagotomy plus antrectomy* is a vagotomy with removal of the distal part of the stomach (the antrum), where the acid-stimulating hormone gastrin is secreted.

Nursing Considerations

Preoperative Care

- If surgery is not being done on an emergency basis, general preparation of the patient will include attention to nutritional status and correction of anemia (with blood transfusions) and electrolyte imbalances, if present.
- A nasogastric tube connected to either low intermittent suction, or continuous low suction (when a gastric sump tube *e.g.,* Salem or Ventrol) is used (see NR, Gastrointestinal intubation).
- General preoperative teaching and preoperative care are important. (See MSN, Introduction.)

Postoperative Care

- General postoperative care (See MSN, Introduction, Postoperative care.)
- Nasogastric suction to remove gas and fluids (See NR, Gastrointestinal intubation.)
  1. A nasogastric tube connected to either low intermittent suction, or continuous low suction (if a gastric sump tube is used), for 3 days or 4 days after surgery.
  2. Irrigation or manipulation of the tube is done only with a specific order since disruption of the suture line is possible.

     If the tube's patency is in question, have the patient change his or her position and cough with the incision splinted. If this does not correct the situation, notify the surgeon.
  3. Drainage from the nasogastric tube will be bloody for the first 24 hours, and gradually will become dark red, then coffee ground-like, and finally, greenish yellow in color. Appearance of bright red blood after the first 12 hours should be called to the attention of the physician immediately.
  4. Accurate measurement of volume is essential. Intravenous replacement of fluids is often matched milliliter for milliliter with output.
  5. The nasogastric tube may be clamped at intervals to test for the amount of residual stomach contents as an indication of

when to remove it. After removal, look for signs of abdominal distention.

- Patient will have nothing by mouth (NPO) for the first few days and will require special mouth care with rinses, gargles, and lubricants.
- Intravenous fluids will be administered (see NR, Intravenous therapy).
- A semi-Fowler's position is maintained postoperatively to promote drainage.
- Attempt to prevent respiratory complications, possible because of high abdominal incision. Assist with deep-breathing techniques (see NR, Deep breathing techniques).
- Assess for bowel sounds.
  1. After peristalsis has returned, the patient will be allowed gradually increasing amounts of fluid, PO, even while the nasogastric tube still is in place.
  2. After the nasogastric tube is removed, the diet is advanced gradually. The patient should be cautioned to eat slowly.
- Following total gastrectomy
  1. There will be little nasogastric drainage because there are no stomach secretions and the stomach's storage function has been eliminated.
  2. Chest tubes are used often. (See NR, Chest tube drainage.)

Long-Term Postoperative Implications

- The patient who has had total gastrectomy will require injections of vitamin B_{12} (cyanocobalamin injection, USP) throughout the rest of his or her life since the intrinsic factor will be lacking. Those patients with partial gastrectomy may require some vitamin B_{12} supplements and should be checked for anemia. (See PH, Cardiovascular system.)
- *Dumping syndrome:* This vasomotor and GI disturbance is a fairly common sequela to subtotal gastrectomy with gastroduodenostomy. The patient may have a feeling of fullness and nausea 5 minutes to 40 minutes after eating, followed by sweating, pallor, headache, and dizziness. Two or three hours after a meal (particularly one high in carbohydrates), the patient may have a hypoglycemic reaction with weakness, sweating, anxiety, and tremor. Patient instruction includes
  1. Lie down immediately after eating.
  2. Meals should be small, frequent, and eaten slowly in a semi-recumbent position.
  3. Fluids should be taken between, *not with,* meals.
  4. Anticholinergic medications may help by slowing gastric emptying.

INTESTINAL SURGERY

Description

The goal of *bowel resection* is the removal of a section of diseased or obstructed bowel, with anastomosis (rejoining) of the two healthy ends, and the resumption of normal bowel function.

In a *colostomy,* an opening of some portion of the large bowel is made onto the skin. The consistency of the feces will depend upon the proximity of the stoma to the terminal ileum. Fecal material from a colostomy in the ascending colon will be quite liquid; feces from a colostomy in the descending or sigmoid colon (in the left lower quadrant of the abdomen) normally will be soft formed. Regulation of evacuation of a colostomy in the descending or sigmoid colon often is achieved by a regular diet, activity, and irrigation (see NR, Ostomies, fistulas, and draining wounds). If regulation is achieved, the patient will need to cover the stoma with a small dressing, but will not need to wear a pouch continuously. A *temporary colostomy* may be done if there is a possibility that the lower bowel will heal with rest (*e.g.,* in severe diverticulitis and rectovaginal or rectovesical fistula). There will be two openings. The surgeon will close the colostomy when deemed appropriate. A permanent diversion of fecal contents to the skin usually is done for carcinoma of the colon or rectum, or both (see MSN, Cancer of the colon).

- In a *cecostomy* (Fig. 4-4*A*), an opening is made into the lower right colon (the cecum), and a tube is introduced to decompress the bowel. Attention must be paid to the care of the skin around the tube because the drainage will be liquid and will include digestive enzymes.
- *Loop transverse colostomy* may be permanent or temporary. Because it can be done quickly with minimal trauma, it is done frequently in an emergency situation (*e.g.,* diverticulitis, bowel perforation, obstruction). A loop of transverse colon is brought up to the skin. A stomal support, such as a butterfly bridge, may be put in place until the bowel adheres to the abdominal wall (usually in 7 days to 10 days). A painless incision is made in the wall (usually 24 hours to 48 hours) later for fecal drainage. There will be two openings in a *loop colostomy:* the proximal opening (on the side closest to the small intestine), which will drain fecal material, and the distal opening which will drain mucus (Fig. 4-4*D*).
- In *Hartmann's colostomy,* a portion of the descending or sigmoid colon usually has been resected. The proximal end of the severed bowel is brought out onto the abdomen as a colostomy. The distal end may be brought out onto the abdomen as a mucous fistula, or oversewn and returned into the abdomen.
- *Abdominal perineal resection* with end sigmoid colostomy (Fig. 4-4*C*) usually is done for carcinoma near the anus (see MSN, Cancer of the bowel). A colostomy is formed, and the complete anus and rectum are resected, leaving a perineal wound.

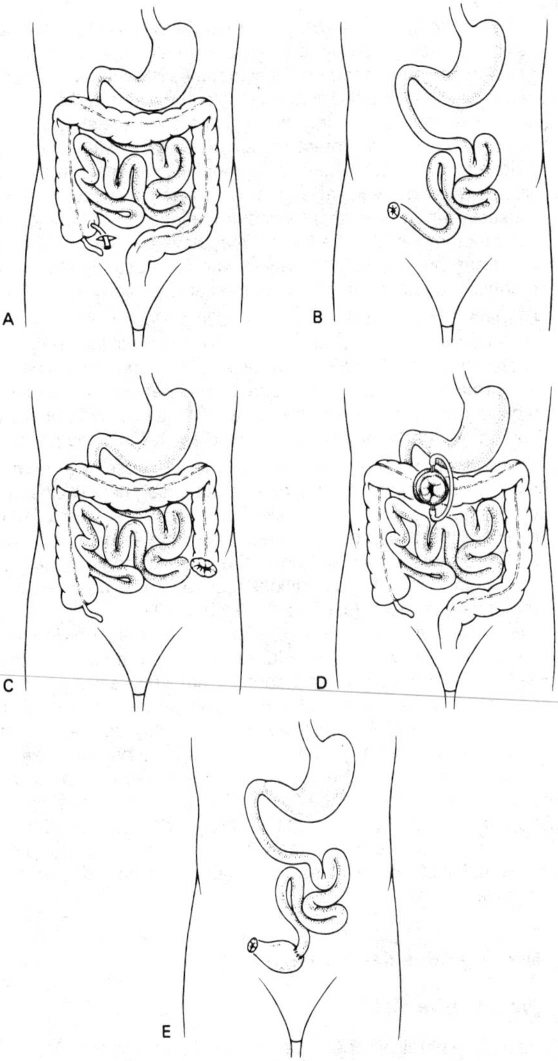

Fig. 4-4. *Types of ostomies. (A) Cecostomy. (B) Ileostomy with proctocolectomy. (C) Colostomy with abdominal perineal resection. (D) Loop colostomy. (E) Continent ileostomy (Kock pouch).*

In an *ileostomy* (Fig. 4-4*B*), the end of the ileum is brought out to the skin. Ileostomy usually is associated with total colectomy (removal of the colon and rectum). It sometimes is done as a temporary diversion of the feces. It differs from colostomy in that the feces are liquid and extremely irritating to the skin around the stoma. Special efforts are required to protect the skin (see NR, Ostomies, fistulas, and draining wounds). There is no regularity of evacuation, so an appliance must be worn at all times. It is emptied several times a day, usually when the patient voids. Irrigations are contraindicated. If a rectal stump is left, the patient may have periodic discharge of mucus from the rectum. The patient with an ileostomy should wear an identification bracelet with his or her name and physician's name.

- *Continent ileostomy* (Kock pouch): Using a loop of ileum, a pouch is devised to serve as a reservoir for fecal effluent before discharge from the ileostomy. A nipple valve is formed so that leakage from the stoma is prevented. The patient discharges the fecal contents of the pouch several times a day by temporary insertion of a catheter through the nipple valve into the pouch.
- *Ileal conduit or urinary diversion:* The ileum is resected and a segment is separated from it. One end of the segment is closed; the other end is brought to the skin to form an ileal stoma (anastomosis of the two ends of the resected ileum reinstates its continuity). Ureters are implanted in the ileal segment, forming a diversion for urine when conditions require bypassing or removal of the urinary bladder. (see Fig. 4-5*A*, page 303.)

Anorectal pull through procedure with or without a pelvic ileal reservoir is a relatively new procedure in which the mucosa of the affected part of the rectum and anus is removed, leaving the rectal wall, anal sphincter, and wall intact. The procedure frequently is done in two stages. A temporary ileostomy may be made to allow for healing of the rectal area, before the ileum is brought down and sutured to the anal muscle. A pelvic ileal reservoir may be devised, thereby reducing the number of stools. With proper postoperative management, continence is said to be good. The procedure may provide an alternative to ileostomy when there is a need for prophylactic removal of the colon, as in chronic ulcerative colitis or familial polyposis.

Nursing Considerations

Preoperative Care

- Review general preoperative care and teaching (see MSN, Preoperative care).
- General preparation of the patient is recommended, if time permits, with attention to nutritional status (hyperalimentation may be required), anemia (blood transfusions prn), and electrolyte balance.

- A high-calorie, low-residue, or clear-liquid diet for several days preoperative, may be ordered. NPO if there is a question of obstruction or perforation.
- Bowel preparation
  1. Enemas (may include a neomycin solution)
  2. Antibiotics are usually ordered to suppress flora in the bowel. Neomycin or sulfonamides (succinylsulfathiazole) are ordered most commonly (see PH).
- A nasogastric tube connected either to low intermittent suction, or to low continuous suction, (if a gastric sump tube is used) may be ordered (see NR, Gastrointestinal intubation).
- An indwelling catheter usually is ordered preoperatively for the patient undergoing lower abdominal surgery (see NR, urinary bladder catheterization and drainage).
- When the enterostomal therapist visits the patient who is to have an ostomy, at the request of the surgeon, he or she may mark an appropriate site for placement of the stoma.
- A visit from a member of the local ostomy association may be arranged.
- Provide emotional support.
- Preparation for the closure of a temporary colostomy usually includes a protocol similar to the following:
  1. The patient usually is admitted 2 days preoperatively.
  2. A clear-liquid diet is ordered.
  3. Antibiotics, systemically, and in irrigations of colostomy and distal stoma are given.
  4. Preparation of both stomas
     a. Colostomy irrigations b.i.d.
     b. Rectal enemas: Be sure to apply pouch to distal stoma to receive enema solution.
     c. Irrigations of distal stoma with patient sitting on the toilet (irrigation will be expelled through the rectum)

Postoperative Care

- General principles of postoperative care (See MSN, Postoperative care.)
  1. Auscultation for bowel sounds is particularly important. Their presence indicates the return of peristalsis.
- Management of nasogastric or nasointestinal suction (See NR, Gastrointestinal intubation.)
- Accurate intake and output measurements
- Progressive diet after the return of peristalsis
- Prevention of contamination of the abdominal wound by feces, when ostomy is present

- Care of the ostomy (see NR, ostomies, fistulas, and draining wounds). The color of the stoma should be dark pink to red. Blanching or deep red color could indicate interference with the blood supply and should be reported. If the patient complains of pain, check the pouch, open it, and release gas prn. Report unrelieved pain.
- Patients with ileostomy are advised to take oral medications in liquid form for quick absorption.
- Intelligent, thoughtful, emotional support will ease the ostomy patient's adjustment to the new body image. Emphasize the need for self-care and a return to normal living.
- The patient with Kock pouch will be taught how to evacuate the pouch into the toilet with a catheter. The patient should wear an identification bracelet that should read "Internal ileal pouch. Insert #28 catheter to drain. Do not irrigate."

Care Specific to Abdominal Perineal Resection with End Sigmoid Colostomy

- General care of the colostomy
- Drains may be left in the perineal wound. Packing, which the surgeon will remove after about 24 hours, may fill the cavity. Some surgeons leave the wound open.
    1. Expect copious, serosanguineous drainage from the perineal wound. Watch for signs of fresh hemorrhage, edema, and infection. The surgeon will do the first dressing.
- Medicate for pain, which may be especially severe in the first 24 hours.
- The patient may have the sensation of wanting to have a bowel movement because of the pressure from the packing.
- Cotton pants may be worn to hold the perineal dressing in place. A "T" binder, if used, should be snug enough so that it doesn't rub up and down.
- Position the patient on a foam rubber ring or turned on his or her side, so that there is no pressure on the perineal wound.
- After the packing is removed, the perineal wound may require the following:
    1. Perineal irrigations several times a day, using meticulous aseptic technique. Specifics, including type of irrigating solution, depth of insertion, and size of irrigating catheter, will be ordered.
    2. Sitz baths, ordered to stimulate circulation, promote healing, and cleanse. Be aware that the patient may feel faint. Protect and assist accordingly.

Management of Complications Associated with Colostomy

- Odor and gas
  1. Avoid gas-producing foods.
  2. For patients who do not have a lactose intolerance, one carton of yogurt each day is frequently helpful in reducing flatulence and fecal odor.
  3. Commercial pouch deodorants or a capful of mouthwash may be used in the pouch. Irrigation of the colostomy and cleanliness of the appliance help reduce odors. Gas may be passed by opening the pouch.
- A small amount of bleeding at the stoma site is rather common. Any appreciable amount should be reported to the surgeon.
- Cramping, abdominal pain, nausea and vomiting may be signs of obstruction. Notify the surgeon.
- Herniation around the colostomy may occur. Avoid forcing the irrigating tip into a herniated loop of bowel. It could cause perforation.
- Symptoms of perforation include acute onset of pain around the stoma, swelling and fever, and diffuse abdominal pain. Perforation constitutes a surgical emergency.
- Prolapse of the colostomy is seen most often in a loop colostomy.

Management of Complications of Ileostomy

The following are in addition to those associated with colostomy.

- Acute or chronic dehydration
  1. Fluid balance must be maintained.
  2. Measure and record intake and output accurately. Remember to count drainage from the ileostomy as output.
  3. A urine output of less than 30 ml/hr to 50 ml/hr should be reported to the physician.
- Breakdown of the parastomal (around the stoma) skin from contact with the irritating liquid feces from an ileostomy
  1. Careful shaving and preparation (no cuts) preoperatively is necessary.
  2. A well-fitting appliance is important. The stoma size will change during the first 6 weeks, so it should be measured every time the pouch is changed.
  3. The appliance should be changed every 3 days to 5 days, or often enough to avoid leakage. Leakage should be suspected if patient complains of burning or itching sensations around the stoma. Change the appliance immediately.
- A sharply diminished output or a more liquid output associated with nausea and abdominal cramps may indicate blockage of the

stoma. Note the type of discharge from the stoma. Notify the surgeon.

ULCERATIVE COLITIS

Description

Ulcerative colitis is a condition involving inflammation of the mucous membrane of the large bowel, which usually begins in the rectum and spreads to the entire colon. The disease is characterized by exacerbations and remissions. The cause is unknown, although it now is believed that there may be an autoimmune basis. Patients who have had the disease over a period of years are at greatly increased risk of colon cancer.

Common Diagnostic Tests

- Barium enema x-ray may show shortening, scarring, narrowing, and ulceration of the bowel (see NR, X-ray preparations).
- Proctoscopic and sigmoidoscopic examinations may include biopsy (see NR, Endoscopic procedures).
- Stool culture should be done to rule out amebic colitis and bacillary dysentery.
- Leukocytosis, anemia, and elevated sedimentation rate are common (see LAB).

Observations

- Diarrhea: In an acute attack, there may be 15 to 20 stools daily, containing blood, mucus, and pus. Document the frequency and character of stools.
- Abdominal cramps, sometimes with leakage of stool, are present.
- Anorexia (loss of appetite), occasional nausea and vomiting, low-grade fever, weakness, anemia, dehydration, weight loss, and hypoalbuminemia are common.
- Symptoms of complications that include hemorrhage, perforation, or toxic megacolon. A distended abdomen is symptomatic of toxic megacolon (massive colonic dilatation that may result in rupture of the colon).

Treatment

Medical

- Nutrition: A high-protein, high-caloric, high-vitamin, low-residue diet is recommended. Preparation for surgery may include hyperalimentation (see NR, Intravenous therapy).

- Medications (See PH for specific drugs.)
  1. Opium derivatives (*e.g.*, Paregoric) are for short-term use only (to decrease intestinal motility) (see *Caution* below).
  2. Kaolin or bismuth salts
  3. Antispasmodic drugs (*e.g.*, belladonna group), or diphenoxylate hydrochloride (Lomotil) in small doses *Caution:* These drugs may be very dangerous and may precipitate toxic megacolon. At any sign of abdominal distention, stop therapy and report this to a physician.
  4. Antibiotics are usually ordered to prevent secondary infections, *e.g.*, sulfasalazine (Azulfidine), which also is used frequently on a long-term basis to help prevent relapses.
  5. Corticotrophin (ACTH) or adrenal steroids are very effective in treatment of acute attacks. These drugs are started IV, then given PO. They also may be given rectally with great benefit, especially when disease is confined to the rectum.
- Azathioprine (Imuran) is being used, but it is still under study.
- Trials of S-aminosalicylic acid suppositories or enemas to reduce relapse rate seem promising.

Surgical

- Subtotal colectomy with ileostomy is done most frequently as emergency treatment for massive hemorrhage, toxic colitis, or perforation.
- Total colectomy with ileostomy is the procedure of choice in elective situations.
- Continent ileostomy (Kock pouch)
- Anorectal pull through
- See MSN, Intestinal surgery.

Nursing Considerations

- Rest is important
- Emotional support is imperative, especially in the acute phase, during preparation for and following surgery. The frustration and exhaustion associated with the patient's symptoms cannot be overemphasized.
- Relieve discomfort around anus by washing area frequently; use an anesthetic ointment, *e.g.*, dibucaine (Nupercaine), prn, if ordered. Sitz baths are also helpful.
- Have a bedpan within a patient's reach. Padding may add to comfort. Room deodorizers may be needed.

- The patient in the acute phase is very ill, and will require all comfort measures, including skin care, and decubitus prevention with protection of bony prominences.
- The patient, even when asymptomatic, will require medical supervision, including checks for colon cancer. If he is on long-term therapy with sulfasalazine (Azulfidine), give him information regarding this drug (see PH).
- Adjustment to and acceptance of an ileostomy can be eased by intelligent, sympathetic nursing care and patient education (see MSN, Intestinal surgery).

NORMAL AGING CHANGES IN THE GASTROINTESTINAL SYSTEM

- The teeth exhibit a number of changes with aging. The enamel darkens with age, and there is a slow formation of secondary dentine that reduces the size of the pulp cavity. The pulp decreases in size, fibrous tissue increases, and the number of blood vessels is reduced. The gums recede, and alveolar bone resorption (senile atrophy) occurs.
- There is a decrease in the amount of saliva secreted resulting from senile atrophy of the salivary glands. The secretions become more alkaline.
- The oral mucosa, including the covering of the tongue, loses its elasticity and becomes thin and dry. It is abraded easily and repairs itself more slowly. The superficial veins under the tongue enlarge and varicosities are a common finding ("caviar tongue").
- Peristalsis slows in the esophagus, and nonperistaltic waves are more common with aging. The cardiac sphincter often fails to relax, and emptying of the esophageal contents into the stomach is delayed. This pattern is referred to as presbyesophagus.
- Both the mucous glands and the peptic glands in the stomach atrophy with age. Secretion of digestive juices is reduced.
- Slowing of gastric motility and emptying has not been demonstrated conclusively, but may account for some nonspecific, upper GI symptoms in older persons.
- The mucosa, submucosa, and muscle tissue of the walls of the small intestine atrophy. Intestinal enzymes decrease. Diminished absorption of nutrients has not been demonstrated, possibly because of the enormous, reserve absorptive capacity of the small intestine mucosa.
- Atrophy of the mucosa and muscle of the wall of the large intestine also may occur with age.
- The liver gets smaller in relation to body weight and receives a decreased blood supply. Hepatic enzyme concentrations are re-

duced and may not respond as rapidly to external stimuli. However, the liver has a large reserve capacity, and the otherwise healthy elderly person will not demonstrate evidence of hypofunction.

- The walls of the gallbladder exhibit atrophic shrinking, sclerosis, and thickening. Bile is richer in cholesterol and more viscous. The incidence of gallstones increases with age.

Implications

- The aging changes in the teeth and gums increase the risk of infection and disease for the elderly person. Regular dental care is extremely important.
- Denture fitting is dependent upon the alveolar ridge. Both bone resorption and weight loss contribute to ill-fitting dentures.
- Poorly fitting dentures, lost teeth not replaced, and partial paralysis of the jaw (*e.g.,* from a stroke) may result in poor mastication. The elderly person may change to a soft, semisolid diet. If the diet is not balanced, vitamin and mineral deficiencies and malnutrition can occur.
- Gum tissue under dentures should be inspected for sores, yeast infections, and oral cancer.
- Older persons may experience a chronically dry mouth because of the decrease in saliva. Mouth breathing is common, especially among elderly with COPD, and contributes to the dryness. An adequate fluid intake and mouth care at intervals throughout the day can increase comfort and decrease halitosis.
- Malnutrition and low vitamin and mineral levels in the elderly appear to be a result of poor food intake rather than aging changes. Factors involved are low income, physical and mental deterioration, loneliness, and disease processes.
- Constipation is a common problem in the elderly. Many factors contribute to the problem and include decreased fluid intake and dietary bulk, decreased muscle tone of the colon, blunting or loss of defecation reflex, and the decreased physical activity of a sedentary life-style. Hemorrhoids and medication use (*e.g.,* sedatives, tranquillizers, antihypertensives, narcotics) also may be involved in the problem.
- Chronic constipation may lead to fecal impactions with overflow fecal incontinence. Laxative abuse is a common problem in the elderly that further aggravates the constipation and is the major cause of diarrhea in the elderly.
- The reduced hepatic blood supply and enzyme concentrations make it more difficult for the elderly person to metabolize drugs. Dosages require age adjustment.

BIBLIOGRAPHY • Gastrointestinal System

BOOKS

Brunner L, Suddarth D: The Lippincott Manual of Nursing Practice, 3rd ed. Philadelphia, JB Lippincott, 1982

Brunner L, Suddarth D: Textbook of Medical-Surgical Nursing, 5th ed. Philadelphia, JB Lippincott, 1984

Krupp M, Chatton M: Current Medical Diagnosis and Treatment, 22nd ed. Los Altos, CA, Lange Medical Publications, 1983

Given B, Simmons S: Gastroenterology in Clinical Nursing, 4th ed. St Louis, CV Mosby, 1984

Phipps W, Long B, Woods N: Medical-Surgical Nursing, Concepts and Clinical Practice, 7th ed. St Louis, CV Mosby, 1980

Way L: Current Surgical Diagnosis and Treatment, 6th ed. Los Altos, CA, Lange Medical Publications, 1983

JOURNALS

Bates M: Dissolving gallstones. Br Med J 284:1, Jan 2, 1982

Bauer D: Preventing the spread of hepatitis B in dialysis units. Am J Nurs 80(2):260, Feb 1980

Belliveau: Ileoanal anastomosis: improving functional results. Can J Surg 26(3):201, May, 1983

Byrne P: Inflammatory bowel disease: causing problems world wide. Nurs Mirror 151(5):30, July 1980

Campieri M, Lanfranchi G, Bazzocchi G et al: Treatment of ulcerative colitis with high dose 5-aminosalicylic acid enemas. Lancet 2:270, Aug 8, 1981

Cassell B: The new trend in ileostomy surgery. RN 47(1):48, Jan 1984

Dodd R: Ascites: when the liver can't cope. RN magazine 47(10):26, Oct 1984

Eisenstat T, Rubin T, Salvati E: Surgical management of diverticulitis: The role of the Hartmann procedure. Dis Colon Rectum 26(7):1429, Jul 1983

Frank-Stromborg M: Test your knowledge of caring for the patient with peptic ulcer. Nursing '81 11(5):66, May 1981

Fredette S: When the liver fails. Am J Nurs 84(1):64, Jan 1984

Gurevich I: Viral hepatitis. Am J Nurs 83(4):571, Apr 1983

Haas P, Haas G, Schmaltz S et al: The prevalence of hemorrhoids. Dis Colon Rectum 26(7):435, Jul 1983

Hartler C, Beghtol M, Adams J et al: Nursing grand rounds: What's a continent ileostomy? Nursing '81, 11(11):84, Nov 1981

Hiatus hernia. Nurs Mirror 153(14):32, Sept 30, 1981

Ito Y: Reappraisal of endorectal pull-through procedure. J Pediatr Surg 16(4):476, Aug 1981

Ivenson-Ivenson J: Abdominal hernia. Nurs Mirror 152:26, June 10, 1981

Ivenson-Ivenson J (ed): Background to congenital hypertrophic pyloric stenosis. Nurs Mirror 150(14):42, April 3, 1980

Ivenson-Ivenson J: Hiatus hernia. Nurs Mirror 153:32, Sept 30, 1981
Jackson M: Viral hepatitis. Nurs Clin North Am 15(4):729, Dec 1980
Keck J: Hepatitis B: An occupational risk. Can Nurse 76(11):33, Dec 1980
Kiely E, Deasy J, Harte P et al: Congenital hypertrophic pyloric stenosis: A review. Irish Med J 74(6):161, June 1981
Kirsner J: Observation on the medical treatment of inflammatory bowel disease. JAMA 242:557, 1980
Klotz V, Karlernst M, Fischer C et al: Therapeutic efficacy of sulfasalazine and its metabolites in patients with ulcerative colitis and Crohn's disease. N Engl J Med 303(26):1499, Dec 25, 1980
Kroner K: Are you prepared for your ulcerative colitis patient? Nursing '80 10(4):43, Apr 1980
Lamphier T, Lamphier R: Upper GI hemorrhage: Emergency evaluation and management. Am J Nurs 81(10):1814, Oct 1981
Leu M: Hepatitis B: You are at highest risk. RN 44(9):74, Sept 1981
Littlewood E, Ornstein M, McLean B et al: Doubts about diverticular disease. Br Med J 283:1524, Dec 5, 1981
MacClelland D: Kock pouch: A new type of ileostomy. AORN J 32(2):191, Aug 1980
Markowitz R, Wolfson B, Huff D et al: Infantile hypertrophic pyloric stenosis congenital or acquired. J Clin Gastroenterol 4(1):39, Feb 1982
McComas C: Congenital pyloric stenosis. J Nurs Care 13(4):8, Apr 1980
McConnell E: Curtailing a life-threatening crisis: GI bleeding. Nursing '81 11(4):70, Apr 1981
Meiner S: Diverticular disease. J Pract Nurs 31(8):27, Sept 1981
Mislovitz P: Peptic ulcers: On the front lines of research and treatment. J Pract Nurs 31(2):22, Mar 1981
Obstructive jaundice. Nurs Mirror 155(13):23, Sept 29, 1982
Penninger J, Moore S, Frager S: After the ostomy: helping the patient reclaim his sexuality. RN 48(4):46, Apr 1985
Petlin A, Carolan J: Getting your patient through a lower GI bleed. RN 45(2):42, Feb 1982
Petlin A, Carolan J: How to stop a GI bleed. RN 44(4):43, Apr 1981
Pescatori M, Manhire A, Bartram C: Evacuation pouchography in the evaluation of ileoanal reservoir function. Dis Colon Rectum 26(6):365, Jun 1983
Prognosis of Crohn's disease. Br Med J 282:1415, May 2, 1981
RN Master Care Plan: The patient with liver failure. RN 47(10):32, Oct 1984
Roplia M: Hiatal hernia. Nursing '82 12(4):126, Apr 1982
Rosenbert J, Kirchenbaum H: Cimetidine. RN 44(8):56, Aug 1981
Sagor G: Hiatus hernia: Slip sliding away. Nurs Mirror 154(13):38, Mar 31, 1982
Sanderson E: Henri Hartmann and the Hartmann operation. Arch Surg 115(6):792, June 1980

Schumman D: How to help wound healing in your abdominal surgery patient. Nursing '80 80(10):34, Apr 1980
Schwarz T: Life-threatening abdominal emergencies: Is it 'acute abdomen'? RN 45(7):28, Jul 1982
Shorter R: Risks of intestinal cancer in Crohn's disease. Dis Colon Rectum 26(10):686, Oct 1983
Stadl D, Tyler G, Fischer J: Inflammatory bowel disease: Relationship to carcinoma. Curr Prob Cancer 5(10):3-65, Apr 1981
Stark K: Nursing care of the Kock pouch patient. AORN J 32(2):202, Aug 1980
Stiklorius C: Getting ready for gallbladder studies. RN 45(7):64, Jul 1982
Sugar E: Hirschsprung's disease. Am J Nurs 81(11):2065, Nov 1981
Sutherland D: Nursing care study: Ulcerative colitis. Nurs Times 77(19):816, May 7, 1981
Symposium—Liver, gallbladder and pancreas. Practitioner 225:447, Apr 1981
Thompson H: Haemorrhoids and all that (others too). Practitioner 226:619, Apr 1982
Thompson J: Anorectal bleeding. Nurs Times 75(4):142, Jan 25, 1979
Thompson M: Managing the patient with liver dysfunction. Nursing '81 11(11):101, Nov 1981
Thorpe C, Caprini J: Gallbladder disease: Current trends and treatments. Am J Nurs 80(12):2181, Dec 1980
Vargo J: Viral hepatitis: how to protect patients and yourself. RN 47(7):22, July 1984
Venables C: Endoscopy and the ampulla of Vater. World Med 17(6):91, Dec 12, 1981
Wheeler P, Williams R: Liver diseases: A better outlook. Nurs Mirror 151:42, Jul 24, 1980
Williams M: Nursing care study: Ramstedt procedure for relief of pyloric stenosis. Nurs Times 78(33):1390, Aug 18–26, 1982
Wynne G: Bleeding on the inside. Nurs Mirror 153(2):42, July 8, 1981
Wyse M: Pyloric stenosis. Arizona Med 39(2):96, Feb 1982
Young S, Thomson T: Crohn's disease of the large bowel. Practitioner 226(1366):683, Apr 1982
Zimmerman C: Outpatient excision and primary closure of pilonidal cysts and sinuses. Am J Surg 136(5):640, Nov 1978

Normal Aging Changes in the Gastrointestinal System

Finch C, Hayflick L (eds): Handbook of the Biology of Aging. New York, Van Reinhold, 1977
Reff M, Schneider E: Biological Markers of Aging. U.S. Department of Health and Human Services, 1982. (NIH Publication No. 82-2221)
Rockstein M, Sussman M: Biology of Aging. Belmont, Wadsworth Publishing, 1979

GENITOURINARY SYSTEM

Description

The urinary system consists of the kidneys, the ureters, the bladder, and the urethra. Peristaltic waves propel the urine down the ureters from the kidneys, where urine is formed, to the urinary bladder, which provides temporary storage for it. (Bladder capacity in normal adults is 350 ml to 500 ml.) Urine then is expelled through the urethra. Reflux, or backward flow, of urine is abnormal at any stage of its excretion.

- Common disorders of the urinary system are usually the result of obstruction, neoplasms, calculi, or infection or interrelationships among them.
- In glomerulonephritis, the inflammatory process in the glomeruli has an autoimmune basis.
- Absorption of nephrotoxic substances (*e.g.,* gentamicin or the sulfonamides), vascular changes such as those in hypertension, and some systemic diseases (*e.g.,* diabetes, and systemic lupus erythematosus) may damage the kidneys.
- Any marked decrease in circulation of blood to the kidneys may cause renal shutdown.
- Injury to the kidneys and bladder also may be the result of trauma.
- Dialysis, both peritoneal dialysis and hemodialysis, and kidney transplant have revolutionized the treatment of end-stage renal disease in recent years (see NR, Dialysis).

Nursing Considerations

Nursing management of the patient with urinary tract disorders include the following:

- Careful assessment
- Accurate specimen collection
- Some urine testing
- Preoperative and postoperative care specific to the patient with genitourinary (GU) surgery
- Special attention to fluid management (particularly urinary drainage), comprehensive nursing care for the patient in renal failure, and awareness of the possibility of drug toxicity because of failing renal function

CANCER OF THE BLADDER

Description

The incidence of carcinoma of the bladder has increased rapidly in recent years, especially among men over 50 years of age. Some predisposing factors are exposure to carcinogens (*e.g.,* cigarette smoking and aniline dyes), chronic cystitis, bladder papillomas, and schistosomiasis.

Common Diagnostic Tests

- Cystoscopic examination, including bimanual examination of the bladder and biopsy of tumor or bladder wall
- Urinary cytology: Clean-catch specimen obtained about 3 hours after patient has voided or by bladder washing technique (The specimen must go directly to laboratory.)
- Intravenous pyelograms (IVP) (See NR, X-ray preparations.)
- Voiding cystourethrograms (VCUG) (See NR, X-ray.)
- Ultrasonic probe (see NR, Ultrasound.)
- Computerized tomography (CT scan; See NR, CT scan.)

Observations

- Painless hematuria
- History of recurring urinary tract infections (UTIs), with dysuria (pain), burning, and frequency of urination
- Pain in the back, hips, or legs may be signs of metastasis.

Treatment

- Transurethral resection with multiple biopsies and fulguration of superficial lesions or simple papillomas
- Cystoscopies with biopsies: repeated every 3 months to 6 months for 1 year to 2 years to check for recurrence
- Cystectomy (removal of part or all of the bladder) and lymphadenectomy: partial, total, or radical, depending upon stage (*i.e.,* invasiveness) of the disease. Total or radical cystectomy will require urinary diversion.
- Urinary diversion (Fig. 4-5) when required
    1. Cutaneous ureterostomy: The ureter(s) are brought to the abdominal wall.
    2. Ileal conduit (ureteroileostomy): The ureters are implanted into a loop of ileum, which is brought out to form an ileostomy. The two ends of ileum are anastomosed to reinstate normal contin-

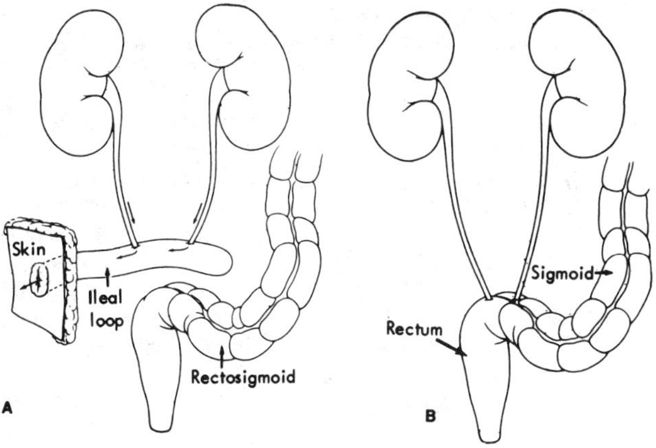

Fig. 4-5. *Types of urinary diversion. (A) Ileal conduit. (B) Ureterosigmoidostomy.* (Bloom J. Merrill JP: Review of methods uf urinary diversion. GP 23:94-97, 1961).

uity (see NR, Ostomies, fistulas, and draining wounds and MSN, Intestinal surgery). Sigmoid conduits also are performed.

3. Ureterosigmoidostomy: The ureters are implanted into the sigmoid colon, and urine is allowed to drain into it. Urine is expelled with feces through the rectum (see Fig. 4-5).

- Radiation may be complicated by very severe cystitis, rectal fistula, irritation of the rectum with accompanying diarrhea, or bladder spasms (see MSN, Oncology nursing considerations).
- Chemotherapy (topical and systemic): thiotepa bladder instillations for superficial lowgrade cancers or papillomas (See MSN, Oncology, nursing considerations.)
- Laser surgery

Nursing Considerations

- See MSN, Oncology nursing considerations.

For Partial Cystectomy (Segmental Resection)

- Adequate urinary drainage may require a cystostomy tube, as well as a urethral catheter, at first.
- Reduced bladder size may require patient to void every 20 minutes to 30 minutes. The bladder capacity will increase gradually.
- Fluids must be forced.

For Ureterosigmoidostomy

- Preoperative preparation usually includes: low-residue diet, bowel preparation with enemas; and a short course of oral neomycin.
- Immediately postoperative a sterile rectal tube will usually be in place to drain urine and prevent reflux or urine into ureters.
- In the postoperative period, watch for complications (*e.g.,* infection, electrolyte imbalance, and acidosis). Try to prevent them.
- Kegel exercises: should be taught preoperatively. Ask patient to practice frequently tightening the anus and perineum, as though to prevent urination or bowel movement (see NR, Kegel exercises).
- Postoperative orders usually include the following:
  1. Forced fluids
  2. Low-residue diet
  3. Stool softeners
  4. Medication, e.g., Lomotil, to decrease intestinal motility
  5. Antispasmodics that may relieve symptoms

For Thiotepa Bladder Instillation

- Medication is instilled into the bladder through a catheter. This usually is done by a physician in the operating room. In some centers, however, it is done by nurses.
- The patient must retain the medication in the bladder for 2 hours, so he or she may return to the floor with a clamped catheter.
- Reposition the patient every 15 minutes to help medication reach all areas of the bladder.
- Follow the physician's orders regarding the unclamping of the catheter or its removal.

For Ileal Conduit

- See MSN, Intestinal surgery; and NR, Ostomies, fistulas, and draining wounds.

INFLATABLE PENILE PROSTHESIS

Description

The inflatable penile prosthesis is one method of treating impotence—the inability of a man to have an erection firm enough, or to maintain it long enough, to have successful sexual intercourse.

Through either a suprapubic or a scrotal incision, this prosthesis is implanted surgically. It is designed to mimic a natural erection.

The patient can control whether the penis is firm for intercourse, or relaxed at other times. To inflate the prosthesis, the pump implanted into the scrotum is squeezed by hand several times. Fluid moves from the reservoir (implanted in the pelvis) into the cylinders, causing an erection. A release valve on the pump, when pressed, returns the fluid from the cylinders to the reservoir.

Another type of penile prosthesis, not under consideration here, consists of two semirigid silicone rubber rods that are inserted into the shaft of the penis.

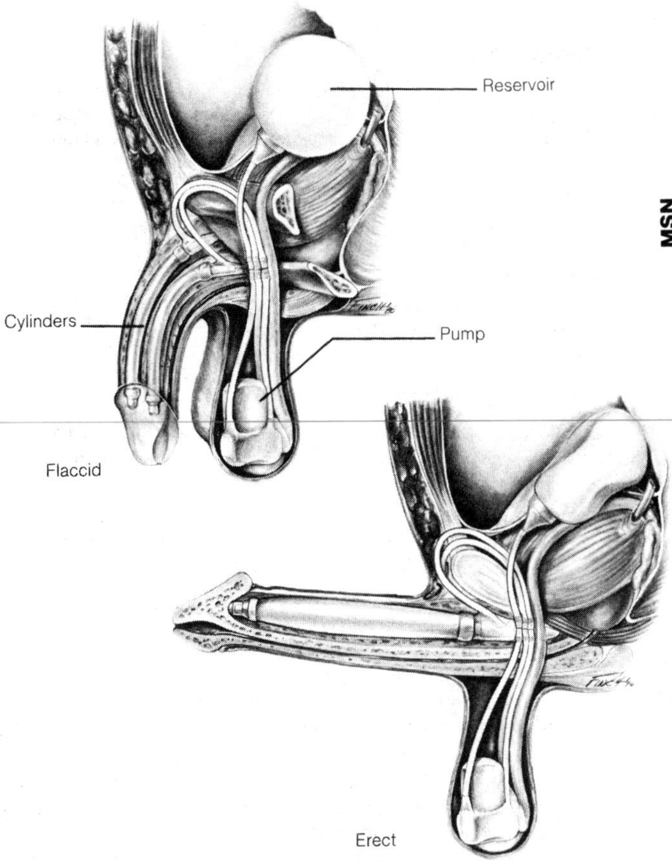

Fig. 4-6. *Inflatable penile prosthesis* (Courtesy of American Medical Systems, Inc., Minnetonka, Minnesota).

Common Diagnostic Tests

- Hormonal evaluation, especially for testosterone
- Tests for diabetes (See MSN, Endocrine, diabetes mellitus.)
- Non-invasive vascular testing—Doppler
- Phallogram: to measure nocturnal penile tumescence. It measures increases of circumference and height of the penis while the patient is sleeping.
- Arteriography—used rarely
- Psychological screening

Observations

- Look for the causes of impotence, such as a history of diabetes, use of antihypertensive drugs, radical pelvic surgery, vascular disease, trauma (including spinal cord injury), and psychogenic factors
- Postoperatively
  1. A moderate amount of pain is common, especially when the suprapubic approach has been used.
  2. Elevated temperature is a sign of infection.
  3. Bleeding into the scrotum, seen as enlargement or purple color of the scrotum, may occur.

Nursing Considerations

- Emotional support for the patient and his partner is necessary.
- IV antibiotics are started preoperatively and continued postoperatively.
- Postoperative care
  1. Empty Jackson-Pratt drains every shift. They will exit from the inguinal region. Use scrupulous clean technique.
  2. A Foley catheter usually is in place for the first 24 hours (see NR, Catheterization, urinary).
  3. Vitamin K may be ordered.
  4. A local anti-infective, *e.g.,* Cortisporin or Neosporin ointment, may be ordered to be applied to the tip of the penis, and at the exit of the Jackson-Pratt drain.
  5. Stool softeners may be ordered.
  6. No scrotol support is necessary, but a rubber donut may provide comfort. It is recommended that the patient wear loose-fitting shorts for the first month.
  7. Provide pain relief PRN, according to the surgeon's orders.
  8. Some surgeons order ice packs or local heat for relief of discomfort.

9. Some surgeons order that the patient be placed in the Trendelenburg position.
10. The patient should be taught that severe pain at the base of the penis, or inability to inflate or deflate the pump, are signs of possible hydraulic malfunctions of the device and should be reported to the physician immediately. Usually this problem, should it occur, can be corrected rather easily.
11. Be sure the patient understands the physician's instructions as to how and when to begin using the prosthesis. The patient may be hesitant to ask questions.

- Potency Restored is a self-help group of patients who are considering or have had implantation of an inflatable penile prosthesis. For more information, write Potency Restored, 8630 Fenton Street, Silver Spring, MD 20910.

KIDNEYS

MSN

Description

The kidneys, each one made up of approximately one million nephrons, receive about 25% of the blood volume circulated with each contraction of the heart. Each day, approximately 180 liters of filtrate are formed, of which only 1.5 liters normally are excreted as urine; the rest is reabsorbed by the tubules. The normal adult urinary output is therefore approximately 1,500 ml/24 hours, or 1 ml/minute.

The kidneys' functions include maintenance of homeostasis (the body's balance of fluids and electrolytes), excretion of the end-products of metabolism, regulation of arterial blood pressure through the renin-angiotensin system, and production of erythropoietin (a hormone), which stimulates bone marrow to increase red blood cell (RBC) production.

Common Diagnostic Tests

Urinalysis

- Glucose, ketones, albumin, bacteria, RBCs, white blood cells (WBCs), and casts are abnormal substances (see LAB).
- Specific gravity and osmolality: to measure concentrating and diluting functions of the kidney (See LAB.)
- pH
- Twenty-four-hour urine collections: to determine the volume of urine excreted, and to measure specific amounts of electrolytes and other substances, *e.g.,* creatinine and protein (See LAB.)
- Urine for culture and sensitivity (C and S): obtained by the "clean-catch" technique or catheterization (See LAB.)
- Urine cytology

Blood (Also See LAB)

- Serum creatinine: the most reliable index of renal and glomerular function
- Blood urea nitrogen (BUN): elevated in renal failure, obstructive uropathy, decreased blood flow to the kidneys, and increased protein catabolism (not as reliable an index of impaired renal function as serum creatinine)
- Serum osmolality
- Serum electrolytes: especially potassium, sodium, and calcium
- Creatinine clearance test
- Hemoglobin and hematocrit, complete blood count (CBC)
- Arterial blood gases (ABGs)

X-rays

- Flat plate of the abdomen or kidney, ureter, and bladder (KUB): for discovering location of calculi or abnormalities of renal contour that suggest tumors, hydronephrosis, and so forth (See NR, X-ray preparations.)
- Intravenous pyelogram (IVP) (See NR, X-ray preparations.) After preparation of the bowel and the use of a laxative or enema to clear the GI tract, the patient is given an IV dose of radiopaque organic iodide dye. Its excretion in the urine allows visualization of the urinary tract. *Caution:* before preparation begins, question the patient regarding possible sensitivity to iodine, *e.g.,* allergies to seafood, dyes used in previous x-ray examinations. Iodine sensitivity is a contraindication for doing the test.
- Retrograde pyelography: allows examination of the renal collecting system by introducing a contrast dye into the renal pelvis(s) by a catheter through the urethra, bladder, and one or both ureters (See NR, X-ray preparations).
- Nephrotomogram: combines techniques of IVP with tomography for more detailed visualization of the kidneys at different levels, and is useful if small tumors are suspected
- Digital subtraction angiography
- Renal arteriogram (aortogram or angiogram): outlines renal blood supply

Radioisotope Studies

- Renal scan: measures the percentage of renal function in each kidney as well as total renal function
- Renogram with radioisotope: evaluates renal blood flow, renal function, and ability to excrete urine

Ultrasound

- Ultrasound differentiates cystic disease, renal tumor, and hydronephrosis (see NR, Ultrasound).

Renal Biopsy

- Retrograde renal and ureteral brush biopsy
- Closed percutaneous needle biopsy performed with the aid of ultrasound equipment or CT scanner to position needle (See NR, Renal biopsy.)

Computed Tomography (CT scan)

- A CT scan (see NR, CT scan) may show outline of functioning renal tissue and the location and shape of kidneys, thereby differentiating renal masses or injury.

Concentration and Dilution Tests

(See hospital lab manuals for specifics.)

- Fishberg concentration test: after fluids have been restricted for a specific period of time, a urine specimen is collected to test the kidneys' ability to concentrate urine.
- Addis concentration test: fluids are restricted, and timed urine is analyzed for quantitative RBCs, WBCs, casts, and protein.
- Dilution test: fluids are forced up to a specified amount in a specified short time span. The urine's specific gravity and the osmolality is tested to evaluate urine-concentrating power of the kidneys. *Caution:* Prolonged dehydration or forced fluids may be hazardous to azotemic patients (those with elevated nitrogenous waste products, especially urea, in the blood).

Phenolsulfonphthalein (PSP) Excretion Tests

- These tests are rarely done today.

MSN

Source of Information for Patient Education

National Kidney Foundation, Inc.

2 Park Avenue, New York, New York 10016, Telephone (212)-683-8018, or local chapters.

CANCER OF THE KIDNEY

Description

Most tumors of the kidneys are malignant, the most common being renal cell carcinoma. The tumor is most often unilateral, encapsulated, solitary, and frequently silent. It tends to metastasize rapidly. Only a small percentage of patients with renal cancer have all three of the classic signs—hematuria, pain, and palpable mass.

Common Diagnostic Tests

- X-ray (IVP, retrograde pyelography, renal angiography), ultrasound, nephrotomography, and CT scan

- Urinary cytology and renal function tests (BUN, creatinine clearance)
- Routine blood work may show anemia, or occasionally polycythemia.

Observations

- Gross painless hematuria that may be intermittent is common.
- Back pain, enlarged palpable kidney, low-grade fever, and anemia may be seen.

Treatment

- Nephrectomy—radical lymphodenectomy
- Chemotherapy (See PH.)
- Radiation therapy

Nursing Considerations

- See MSN, Surgery of the kidneys and ureters, and MSN, Oncology nursing considerations.

POLYCYSTIC KIDNEY DISEASE

Description

Polycystic kidney disease is an inherited disorder that usually affects both kidneys. Multiple, enlarging cysts gradually destroy functional renal tissue by pressure. Complications include hypertension and progressive renal failure (see MSN, Renal failure).

Observations

- Usually the adult patient presents with hematuria, mild hypertension, flank pain, and recurring infection leading to uremia.

Common Diagnostic Tests

- X-ray, sonography, and scans

Treatment

- Treatment is symptomatic and similar to that of any kidney insufficiency, *e.g.,* chronic glomerulonephritis or chronic renal failure (see MSN, Glomerulonephritis and Chronic renal failure).
  1. A low-salt, low-protein diet is recommended
- These patients are sometimes candidates for dialysis and renal transplant.

PREOPERATIVE INFARCTION OF RENAL TUMORS

Description

Preoperative infarction of renal tumors is achieved by renal artery catheterization and occlusion of the renal artery supplying the tumor area. This technique is believed to encourage the development of the patient's own immune response and to limit the spread of tumor cells at the time of nephrectomy, which usually is scheduled a few days later. It also may be done as a palliative treatment for the patient with advanced cancer.

Observations

- Following this procedure, patients usually feel very ill.
- Symptoms include severe pain, high temperature elevations, nausea, and vomiting.

Nursing Considerations

- Elevated WBC count frequently is seen.
- Nursing care is supportive.

RENAL FAILURE

Description

Acute renal failure (ARF) is described as a rapid deterioration in renal function accompanied by azotemia (the build-up of nitrogenous waste in the blood) and, usually, oliguria (urinary output below 500 ml/24 hr).

- *Prerenal failure* may be precipitated by hypovolemia caused by cardiovascular failure, shock, hemorrhage, or burns, or by any factor outside the kidneys that decreases renal blood flow, and therefore reduces glomerular perfusion. Obstetric complications, such as separation of the placenta, severe preeclampsia, eclampsia, and septic abortion are other examples.
- *Intrarenal failure* is caused by disorders within the kidneys themselves, *e.g.,* primary renal diseases such as glomerulonephritis and pyelonephritis; systemic disease, *e.g.,* diabetes, and systemic lupus erythematosus (SLE); or acute tubular necrosis caused by transfusion reactions or the absorption of nephrotoxic substances, *e.g.,* the aminoglycosides—gentamycin, neomycin.
- *Postrenal failure* is caused by damage to the kidney from obstruction to the flow of urine as a result of calculi, neoplasms, or prostatic enlargement.

The clinical course of reversible failure is marked by an oliguric phase that may last 1 week to 2 weeks after the causative event, followed by a diuretic phase. Gradual recovery may require 3 months to 12 months.

- *Chronic renal failure,* or end-stage renal disease (ESRD), occurs in irreversible renal disease. Over an extended period of time, it progresses from renal insufficiency to uremia. The changes seen in uremia affect all systems of the body and are caused by retention of the end-products of metabolism, and disturbances in fluid, electrolyte, and acid-base balances.

Common Diagnostic Tests

- See MSN, Kidneys, common diagnostic tests.

Observations

In acute renal failure

- Urinary output suddenly is decreased markedly, although following burns and trauma, output may be up to 2 liters to 3 liters/day. A period of diuresis usually follows the oliguric phase.
- Signs of fluid retention—sacral, periorbital, or peripheral edema—and signs of congestive heart failure (CHF) (*e.g.,* moist rales and distended neck veins) may be present (See MSN, Congestive heart failure.)
- Pallor suggests anemia.
- Signs and symptoms of acidosis, hyperkalemia, and hyponatremia may occur. During diuresis, hypernatremia may be seen. (See NR, Intravenous therapy, electrolyte imbalances.)
- Signs and symptoms of uremia include acidosis, uremic frost on the skin with accompanying pruritus; headaches, visual disturbances, nausea and vomiting, and the odor of urine on the breath.

In chronic renal failure

- Anemia, a classic symptom; pallor and weakness
- Hypertension
- Edema or dehydration, depending upon status of renal function
- Symptoms of acidosis: hyperventilation, headache, lethargy, drowsiness, stupor, and coma
- Volume and character of urinary output may vary with progress of the disease.
- Cardiac problems
  1. Chest pain and pericardial friction rub, indicating pericarditis
  2. CHF (rales and distended neck veins) (see MSN, Congestive heart failure.)
- Electrolyte imbalances, particularly hyperkalemia (See LAB, and NR, Intravenous therapy, electrolytes imbalances.)
- Anorexia, weight loss, mucosal ulcerations of the mouth, stomatitis, urine odor to breath, nausea and vomiting, diarrhea, and ev-

idence of GI bleeding, further contributing to anemia and dehydration

- Pruritus (itching), area of ecchymosis, excoriations, uremic frost
- Neurologic manifestations (*e.g.,* headache, lethargy, confusion, convulsions, muscle weakness or irritability, and paresthesia)
- Amenorrhea, infertility, sexual dysfunction
- Signs of infection resulting from decreased resistance

Treatment

In acute renal failure

- The goal is to maintain good fluid and electrolyte balance until renal cells can recover.
- Fluid intake is restricted, usually to 400 ml/day, with possible increases to replace unusual losses.
- A low or nonprotein, restricted potassium, high-carbohydrate diet usually is ordered. (Hard candy and butterballs often are provided.)
- Intravenous glucose is administered, especially if nausea and vomiting are present.
- Correction of electrolyte imbalances
  1. Sodium polystyrene sulfonate (Kayexalate), a resin exchange, is mixed with water or sorbitol and given PO by nasogastric tube or rectally to treat hyperkalemia.
  2. IV glucose and insulin or calcium gluconate are temporary treatments for hyperkalemia (see PH).
  3. IV sodium bicarbonate is given to correct acidosis and to lower the serum potassium level.
  4. Aluminum hydroxide is given to bind phosphate (see PH).
- Dialysis: peritoneal dialysis or hemodialysis, if indicated (See NR, renal dialysis.)
- Prevent or control infection with good hand-washing technique. Antibiotics may be ordered.

In chronic renal failure

- The goal of conservative management is to preserve existing renal function; to treat symptoms of uremia; to maintain acid-base, fluid, and electrolyte balances; to prevent complications; and to provide maximal psychological and physical comfort.
- A diet low in protein, low in potassium, and high in carbohydrates usually is ordered.
- Fluids are replaced, usually 500 ml more than 24-hour output. (An amount of 500 ml represents insensible loss through respiration, perspiration, or stools.)
- Aluminum hydroxide antacids are given to bind phosphorus in GI tract (see PH).

- Hypertension is managed with medications, *e.g.,* methyldopa (Aldomet) and propranolol (Inderal).
- Diuretics may be ordered.
- Diazepam (Valium) and phenytoin (Dilantin) may be given IV to control seizures (see PH).
- Oxygen therapy may be required (see NR, Oxygen administration).
- Blood transfusions may be ordered.
- Iron and folic acid supplement may be ordered (see PH).
- Antiemetics may be required to relieve nausea and vomiting.
- Androgen therapy may stimulate RBC production.
- Dialysis, with efforts to minimize blood loss during treatments, may be required.
- A kidney transplant may be performed on selected patients.

Nursing Considerations

- Manage IV fluid and electrolyte administration.
- Monitor fluid intake and output carefully.
  1. Indwelling catheter with urometer may be needed to measure hourly urinary output, but will be avoided if possible. Frequent tests for specific gravity will be ordered.
- Take the patient's daily weights at the same time each day and under the same conditions.
  1. Fluctuations in body weight are probably the most accurate index of fluid retention: 1 lb/500 ml; 1 kg (2.2 lb) = 1,000 ml.
  2. During the oliguric stage, a 0.2-kg to 0.5-kg (0.5 lb to 1 lb) daily loss is expected.
- Severe fluid restrictions may be ordered during the anuria or oliguric stage. Obtain the patient's cooperation in meeting them. One approach is for the nursing staff to assume responsibility for offering all fluids; no fluids should come on the patient's tray. The daily allowance is divided. Even sips of water taken with oral medications must be counted.
- Monitor for physical signs and laboratory results that might indicate fluid overload, electrolyte imbalances, *e.g.,* acidosis, hypercalcemia, or hyponatremia (see NR, Intravenous therapy, electrolyte imbalances). Fluid imbalances are particularly dangerous in the diuretic phase of ARF.
- Monitor BUN and serum creatinine values.
- Monitor blood pressure and administer antihypertensives, as ordered in chronic renal failure.
- Good supportive care
  1. Oral hygiene to prevent stomatitis; pulmonary hygiene (turn, cough, and deep breathe); decubitus ulcer prevention (see MSN, Decubitus ulcer), and excellent skin care.

2. Relieve the itching or uremic dermatitis with dilute vinegar baths (2 tablespoons vinegar to 1 pint of water), antipruritic lotions, and antihistamines. Trim the patient's fingernails to prevent scratching.
3. Protect patient from injury; padded side rails and tongue blade may be required. (see MSN, Seizures).

- Safe drug administration: Drug toxicity is more likely with decreased renal function. Dosages must be adjusted.
- Awareness and prevention, where possible, of complications, such as cardiac failure and arrhythmias, convulsions, hemorrhage, and infection, are necessary. Reverse isolation may be required.
- Emotional support and reassurance are important.

TRAUMA OF THE KIDNEYS, URETERS, AND BLADDER

Description

Trauma to the lower thorax or upper abdomen may cause injury to the kidneys. When the pelvis is fractured, damage to the bladder or urethra may occur. Hematuria, a common sign of injury to the kidney, frequently subsides spontaneously.

Common Diagnostic Tests

- Gross and microscopic examination of the urine for blood
- Intravenous pyelogram (IVP)
- CT scan when renal injury is suspected
- Renal arteriogram
- Cystogram or cystourethrogram to rule out injury to bladder or urethra
- Establishment of function in uninjured kidney is a vital part of evaluation.
- Serial hematocrit and hemoglobin levels
- Racking the urine (see Nursing considerations) provides for visualization of gross hematuria.

Observations

- Blood in the urine
- Signs of shock, *e.g.,* falling blood pressure; rapid, weak pulse; rapid breathing; cold, moist, pale skin (See MSN, Postoperative care.)
- Signs of hemorrhage, *e.g.,* restlessness, thirst, rapid pulse, falling blood pressure, and cool, moist, pale skin (See MSN, Postoperative care.)

- Abdominal firmness and distention, increased pain, absence of bowel sounds are signs of peritonitis, a frequent complication of injuries to the ureters.
- Inability to void may indicate renal shutdown, rupture, or obstruction of the urinary tract. Oliguria or anuria usually occurs when the bladder or urethra is damaged.

Treatment

- Bedrest.
- Treat shock and hemorrhage, if present.
- Surgical repair of the kidney may be attempted after shock is under control and diagnostic studies are completed. (Whenever possible, the injured kidney is preserved.)
- Surgical repair of a traumatized bladder or urethra may be performed promptly. Some surgeons prefer to introduce a cystostomy tube and delay urethral repair. A cystostomy tube may be introduced.
- Broad-spectrum antibiotic therapy
- Medications for pain after diagnostic studies are completed

Nursing Considerations

- Provide bedrest.
- Monitor for signs of shock and hemorrhage by watching for changes in patient's condition. Provide treatment as indicated (see MSN, Postoperative care).
- Collect a specimen from each voiding. Put it in a test tube. Mark the tube with the time it was voided and put the tube in a test tube rack next to the specimen from the last voiding (racking the urine). Gross inspection gives an indication as to whether bleeding is increasing or decreasing. Microscopic examination for blood also may be done.
- See MSN, Postoperative care, and NR, Catheterization, urinary.

URINARY CALCULI (STONES)

Description

Urinary calculi (stones) may be found in the kidney pelvis, the ureters, and the bladder. Stasis of urine, especially when infection is present, predisposes to stone formation.

- Metabolic disorders (*e.g.,* hyperparathyroidism and gout), immobility, extended presence of an indwelling catheter, excessive intake of milk and vitamin D, deficiency of vitamin A, and familial tendencies all may be factors.

- Abnormal pH of the urine is associated with different types of stones, and prophylaxis may center around altering the pH through diet and medication.
- Straining urine and retrieving the stones for chemical analysis are essential. About 90% of calculi contain calcium, combined with phosphate or oxalate, and are radiopaque. Some stones cannot be visualized by x-ray.
- Ninety percent of stones pass spontaneously in a period of days to weeks, but if a calculus lodges in a ureter, causing complete obstruction, it can lead to severe hydronephrosis and constitutes a surgical emergency. Calculi, 1 cm or less, usually pass spontaneously.

Common Diagnostic Tests

- X-ray; intravenous urography; retrograde pyelography (See NR, X-ray preparations.)
- Urinalysis: high specific gravity, abnormal pH, RBCs indicative of injury caused by passage of stones, WBCs indicative of infection (see LAB for normal values).
  1. Twenty-four-hour specimen may show high levels of calcium, uric acid, oxalate, phosphorous, or cystine.
  2. Urine for culture and sensitivity
- Blood chemistry and electrolytes
- Examination of the stone for chemical composition
- Appropriate tests to try to find underlying cause of stone formation
- Percutaneous nephroscopy

Observations

- Excruciating intermittent flank pain may radiate to groin, testes, or labia. It may be accompanied by nausea, chills, and fever when the stone is being passed
- Gross or microscopic hematuria may be seen.
- Evidence of chronic urinary tract infection (UTI) also may be seen. (See MSN, Urinary tract infections.)

Treatment

Medical

- Force fluids, up to 4 liters (4,000 ml) daily.
- Ambulation usually is encouraged in an effort to move the stone. Some stones trapped in the kidney, and not causing obstruction, may be asymptomatic.

- Analgesics for the relief of renal colic (pain) are usually ordered (see PH).
- Hot baths may be helpful. Watch for feelings of faintness.
- Antibiotics can be given if there is evidence of infection (see PH).
- Treat underlying cause of stone formation.
- Recover and analyze the composition of the stone.

Prophylactic

- A high fluid intake, up to 4 liters (4000 ml) daily, is recommended.
- Diet should be modified to reduce the intake of the components of the stone. Medication and diet should be modified to acidify or alkalinize the urine, to maintain the recommended urinary pH.
    1. Ascorbic acid is given to acidify the urine (studies have shown that the amount of cranberry juice needed to acidify urine is too great to be practical).
    2. Sodium bicarbonate will alkalinize the urine.
- Allopurinol (Zyloprim) may be given to reduce uric acid excretion in patients with uric acid stones (see PH); or sodium cellulose phosphate may be given to patients who form calcium oxalate or calcium phosphate stones.
- Orthophosphates, *e.g.*, potassium acid phosphate (K-phos), acidifies urine and lowers calcium concentration.
- Aluminum hydroxide may be administered to bind with phosphorus and to increase the fecal phosphate excretion in the patient who develops phosphorus stones (see PH).
- Promote mobilization to prevent urinary stasis.
- Prevent UTIs.
- Thiazide diuretics may be ordered for patients with idiopathic hypercalciuria.

Surgical

- Percutaneous nephroscopy and stone extraction
- Surgical removal of an obstructive stone with as little trauma as possible
    1. Nephrolithotomy: incision into the kidney for removal of stone
    2. Pyelolithotomy: removal of stones in kidney pelvis
    3. Ureterolithotomy: removal of stone from ureter
    4. Nephrectomy: removal of kidney; performed only if the kidney is functionless and the other kidney is functional
    5. Cystolithotomy: removal of stone from bladder by incision through the abdomen
    6. Crushing the stone with an instrument introduced through the urethra into the bladder

- Percutaneous removal of kidney stones or fragments through a nephrostomy tube into the renal pelvis

Lithotripsy

In lithotripsy, stones are pulverized by high-energy shock waves generated by a device outside the body. The particles then can be passed spontaneously without pain to the patient.

Nursing Considerations

- All urine should be strained through a strainer or fine gauze, and stones should be saved for chemical analysis. Stones vary in size (some may be as small as a pin head), so rinse out the urinal or bedpan carefully, straining the water to be sure you have found stones that may have adhered to the sides. If the patient is discharged before the stone is passed, he or she must be taught how to do this.
- Large and frequent doses of analgesics should be administered for the relief of severe pain experienced as the stone passes through the ureter.
- Patient education is the key to preventing recurrence.
    1. The patient may be taught to test his or her urine pH with phenaphthazine (Nitrazine) paper daily, if ordered.
    2. Diet modification is essential; a visit from the dietitian is a must.
- See Postoperative care following surgery of the kidneys and ureters, for appropriate nursing considerations.

POSTOPERATIVE CARE FOLLOWING SURGERY OF THE KIDNEYS AND URETERS

Nursing Considerations

In addition to considerations of postoperative care in general (see MSN, Postoperative care), the following are special considerations in the management of patients who have undergone surgery of the kidneys or ureters, usually for the removal of urinary calculi.

- Hemorrhage is the greatest danger following renal surgery. Carefully monitor vital signs immediately postoperatively. Check dressings, catheters, tubes, and under the patient for signs of bleeding.
- High abdominal incision in renal surgery (sometimes with entrance into the chest cavity) increases the danger of pulmonary complications. Prevent them by planning administration of an analgesic 15 minutes before encouraging the patient to deep breathe and cough while splinting wound (see NR, Deep breathing techniques). The patient may have chest tubes (see NR, Chest tube drainage).

- Paralytic ileus is another common complication (see MSN, Paralytic ileus).
- Relieve pain with analgesics, and relieve discomfort resulting from the position during renal surgery with moist heat and massage.
- Accurate measurement of intake and output is essential.
  1. Differential output measurement may be required. Voided volume and wound drainage volume would be recorded separately.
- In cases of acute obstruction, in order to ensure adequate urinary drainage until corrective surgery can be done, the surgeon may place temporary tubes above the obstruction, *e.g.,* a nephrostomy tube opening into the kidney, or a pyelostomy tube opening into the renal pelvis. These tubes are always attached to closed gravity drainage.
- Management of catheters and tubes (See also NR, Catheterization, urinary)
  1. They are connected to closed drainage systems.
  2. Immediately postoperatively, check for patency of tube every hour by observing the urine in the tube and the amount collecting in the drainage bag. Mark the time on the bag with tape or a magic marker so that you can make an accurate comparison. Use a urometer for more accurate measurements. Notify the surgeon if less than 50 ml collects in 1 hour.
  3. Observe and note the color of urinary drainage. It is usually bloody the first days following renal surgery, except after nephrectomy, when there should be no blood. Urinary drainage bags should be emptied at the end of each shift and the amount recorded.
  4. Never clamp a urinary drainage tube unless there is a specific order to do so.
  5. A nephrostomy tube (by percutaneous or surgical placement) must be kept patent, and usually can be unclogged by periodically "milking" it by rolling it between your fingers. *Caution:* Never clamp a nephrostomy tube.

     The tube must be handled with the greatest care so that it is not dislodged.

     Sterile occlusive dressing should be placed around the tube. Use an antiseptic ointment, *e.g.,* Betadine ointment.

     Never irrigate without a physician's order. If ordered, always aspirate before irrigating, and never introduce more than 5 ml to 8 ml of sterile saline (the capacity of the kidney pelvis).

     Position the patient carefully so the tube is not kinked or obstructed.

6. Ureteral catheters usually exit from the urethra with a Foley catheter. They must be handled with great care. Catheters to either kidney should be appropriately marked "right" or "left" with tape or identified by color. Separate drainage collection with a urometer may be requested. Careful monitoring of amount of drainage is essential to confirm patency. The urologist will irrigate the ureteral catheter, if indicated.

- Management of drainage
  1. Copious amounts of drainage from drains placed in the operative area (pink at first, then becoming serous) immediately postoperatively require an ostomy appliance over the drain site or Montgomery straps (see Fig. 3-12) and frequent sterile dressing changes. Check under the patient for drainage. Patients should be informed that this amount of drainage is to be expected.
  2. Whenever there is surgical entry into the urinary tract, especially the ureters, the incision is never watertight. Tightening it too much could cause a stricture. Therefore, there is some urine drainage from the Penrose drain. It is irritating to the skin.
  3. If drainage is particularly heavy, a disposable colostomy pouch placed over the drain will collect the drainage and protect the skin. Remember that karaya rings are not practical because urine dissolves them, although karaya powder may be used on irritated skin (see NR, Ostomies, fistulas, and draining wounds).
  4. The drain will be withdrawn gradually by the surgeon. Drainage following ureterolithotomy or pyelolithotomy may last several days. The patient may be discharged with an ostomy pouch.
  5. For care of urostomy or ileal conduit, see NR, Ostomies, fistulas, and draining wounds.
- Fluid intake, usually intravenous, the first days after surgery is high enough to ensure adequate flushing of the kidneys. In most cases, oral fluid intake is encouraged thereafter, except in the case of repair of the kidney pelvis, where it may be restricted.

PROSTATIC ENLARGEMENT, PROSTATECTOMY

Description

Prostatic enlargement, whether benign prostatic hyperplasia (BPH) or malignant, is the most common cause of bladder-neck obstruction in older men. The symptoms caused by this obstruction are called prostatism. Carcinoma of the prostate frequently accompanies BPH but is not believed to be responsible for it. A differential diagnosis is essential. Since symptoms of carcinoma usually appear late, yearly rectal examinations, preferably done by the same examiner, of men over 40 years of age are the best method of early detection.

Common Diagnostic Tests

- Rectal examination
  1. An enlarged prostate with rubbery consistency indicates BPH.
  2. An enlarged, hard, and nodular prostate usually indicates carcinoma.
- Intravenous pyelograms (See NR, X-ray preparations.)
- Excretory urogram (See NR, X-ray preparations.)
- BUN and serum creatinine (See LAB.)
- Serum acid phosphatase level usually are elevated in prostatic carcinoma. (See LAB.)
- Serum alkaline phosphatase levels are elevated in bone metastasis. (See LAB.)
- Bone scan and x-ray of bones for confirmation of metastasis (See NR, Nuclear scans)
- Catheterization for residual urine, urinalysis, and culture
- Cystoscopy
- Biopsy, either by needle aspiration or by surgical incision through the perineum

Observations

- A history of slowing of the urinary stream, hesitancy, intermittency, frequency, nocturia, and dribbling usually is reported.
- Complete urinary retention may occur.
- Hematuria and signs of UTI may be present if the condition is long standing (see MSN, Urinary tract infections).
- Low back pain or pains in the hips or thighs may signal metastasis to the bones in prostatic carcinoma.

Treatment

- Relief of urinary obstruction: a Coude catheter (inserted by the physician) frequently is used. (It is stiffer, and the curved tip rides over obstruction.)
  1. Decompression of a distended bladder must be done slowly.

     Remove 300 ml of urine; clamp catheter; after 15 minutes, release another 300 ml; continue in this manner. Remove only 300 ml of urine at one time. Ordinarily, a catheter is never clamped.

Surgery

- Transurethral resection of the prostate (TURP): a resectoscope, introduced through the urethra, trims away the prostate. Prostatic fossa fills in with epithelial tissue to form a new urethra.
- Enucleation of the prostate gland: bilateral vasectomy may be done at the same time to decrease the incidence of epididymitis and orchitis postoperatively. Surgical approaches include the following:
  1. Suprapubic prostatectomy: enucleation of the prostate is done through the bladder; the incision is made through the lower abdomen and bladder wall.
  2. Retropubic prostatectomy: enucleation of the prostrate is achieved by making a lower abdominal incision, pulling the bladder forward, and then making an incision into the anterior prostatic capsule.
  3. Perineal prostatectomy: the approach is made through the perineum with care to avoid entering the rectum. (This procedure usually causes impotence; about 5% of perineal prostatectomies result in incontinence.)
- Radical resection of the prostate, either by the perineal or retropubic route, is done for carcinoma. This includes removal of the entire prostate gland (including capsule), seminal vesicles, and pelvic lymphodenectomy. The urethra is resected and reanastomosed. It may be followed by bilateral orchiectomy. If done before metastasis, prognosis is excellent, but carcinoma of the prostate can metastasize rapidly with few local symptoms. Sterility occurs in almost 100% of the patients who have had radical retropubic and perineal prostatectomy, but newer techniques have reduced the incidence of postoperative impotence. Treatment specific to radical resection of the prostate usually includes the following:
  1. Preoperative bowel preparation: enemas, and neomycin sulfate given p.o.
  2. Postoperative (after perineal prostatectomy): low-residue diet, medication to decrease bowel motility, and a urethral catheter secured with tape or suture that also acts as a splint for urethral anastomosis; no enemas
- Impotence and urinary incontinence, possible consequences of radical prostatectomy, are now being treated in some centers with some success, with penile prosthesis for impotence (see MSN, Penile prosthesis) and Teflon injection or surgically implanted devices to control incontinence.
- Other therapies may be used separately or in conjunction with surgery.
  1. Radiation preoperatively and postoperatively (external or interstitial) (See MSN, Oncology nursing considerations.)

2. Chemotherapy, including hormonal therapy (See MSN, Oncology nursing considerations.)
3. Symptomatic treatment may include transurethral resection to relieve obstructive symptoms.

Nursing Considerations

Preoperative

- If the patient is to have a vasectomy with the prostatectomy, be sure the surgeon has explained the reasons as well as consequences to him before the informed consent form is signed. (Following vasectomy, the patient will be sterile.)

Postoperative

- Watch for complications.
  1. *Hemorrhage* is a potential complication in all prostatic surgery. Check vital signs, urinary drainage, and dressings at least every 20 minutes immediately postoperatively.

     Following TURP, urine usually changes from reddish pink to light pink within 24 hours. Deepening red color may indicate renewed bleeding.

     Patients who have undergone TURP may have delayed bleeding 7 to 14 days postoperatively and should be forewarned.
  2. *Dilutional hyponatremia (TURP syndrome)*—a severe electrolyte imbalance

     Monitor the patient's electrolyte levels. Notify the surgeon immediately if blood chemistry results reflect hyponatremia.

     Symptoms include agitation, confusion, nausea, slow pulse, and elevated blood pressure, at first. If the disorder progresses, blood pressure falls, and pulmonary edema, renal failure, seizures, coma, and death may follow.

     Should you suspect TURP syndrome, slow down the IV infusion, notify the surgeon, and prepare to administer oxygen, and an IV of hypertonic saline solution, and osmotic diuretics.
  3. *Septic shock* (See MSN, Postoperative complications.)
- *Management of Catheters:* Catheters must be kept patent, and should be large enough (#22, #24, #26) to allow for passage of blood clots.
  1. Check for patency every 20 minutes for the first 2 hours postoperatively, every 30 minutes for the next 2 hours, and then every hour for 24 hours.
  2. Check the bladder for distention.
  3. If ordered, irrigate PRN by introducing 30 ml of sterile normal saline at room temperature with a Toomey or bulb (Asepto)

syringe, and aspirate gently. The bladder must be kept clear of clots. Irrigation is a sterile procedure (see NR, Catheterization, Intermittent bladder irrigation).

4. Continuous irrigation through a "Y" tube or a three-way catheter, or sometimes with the irrigant flowing into a suprapubic catheter and out a urethral one, requires checking for patency of the catheter, character of the drainage, and distention of the bladder. To calculate urinary output, subtract the amount of irrigant that has gone in from the amount in drainage bag (see NR, Catheterization, Continuous bladder irrigation).
5. Clots may be too large to be dislodged by the irrigant alone. If manual irrigation is required, obtain a physician's order. First stop the three-way irrigation, irrigate manually using sterile technique, and then restart the three-way irrigation.
6. *Traction* may be applied by the surgeon by the use of pressure to the Foley catheter. The catheter is pulled taut and taped to the patient's thigh. Its 30-ml balloon fits into the prostatic fossa and may control bleeding following TURP. Traction usually is released on the surgeon's order after 4 hours or 5 hours because of potential danger to the internal sphincter.
7. A *suprapubic cystostomy tube* (frequently a Malecot catheter) may be in place for decompression of the bladder. Excessive amounts of urinary drainage around the tube may indicate a clogged catheter. The skin must be protected.
8. Catheters usually are removed in about 4 days to 7 days following TURP, and in up to 2 weeks following perineal surgery.

- *Bladder spasms* are sudden, sharp, brief pains accompanied by the feeling of the need to move the bowels and urinate at the same time. Traction on the catheter may aggravate the spasms. They are relieved when the catheter is out. Anticholinergic drugs, *e.g.*, propantheline bromide (Pro-Banthine) and analgesics may be prescribed (see PH).
    1. Bloody drainage from the meatus (around catheter), usually caused by spasms, is seen often. Cleanse around the meatus with a povidone-iodine wipe. Leakage around the catheter, accompanied by an intense desire to void, may indicate a blocked catheter. Check for patency.
- *After catheter removal,* voiding problems such as frequency and incontinence are common, especially after TURP. Reassure the patient that these problems almost always are temporary, and encourage him to force fluids, usually up to 2,500 to 3,000 ml per day.
    1. Observe voiding patterns and measure intake and output.
    2. Note frequency and character of urine.
    3. Diuretics may be ordered (see PH).
    4. Watch for renewed bleeding, especially following TURP.

- *Dressings* in open prostatectomies frequently are saturated, so change them frequently. Keep wounds clean. Use Montgomery straps (see Fig. 3-12).
  1. *Tissue drains* near the incision must not be dislodged.
- A *perineal wound* must be kept clean. Heat lamp, Sitz baths, and irrigations with one-half hydrogen peroxide and one-half water may be ordered. Nothing (no enemas, rectal tubes, or suppositories) should be introduced into the rectum.
- Keep stools soft. The patient must avoid straining, which could cause hemorrhage.
- Kegel exercises may correct incontinence (see NR, Kegel exercises).
- Sexual activity may be resumed on the advice of the surgeon. Depending upon the type of surgery, erection or ejaculation may be impaired.
- For the patient receiving radiation or chemotherapy, see MSN, Oncology nursing considerations.

SEXUALLY TRANSMITTED DISEASES

Description

Sexually transmitted diseases (STD) are diseases that usually are, or can be, transmitted through intimate sexual activity, either heterosexual or homosexual.

The Sexually Transmitted Diseases Summary, 1982, published by the Centers for Disease Control (CDC), lists several diseases that were not commonly included in the older classification, veneral diseases. The summary includes gonorrhea, pelvic inflammatory disease (PID), syphilis, nongonococcal urethritis (NGU), vulvovaginitis, cytomegalovirus infections (CMV), hepatitis B, herpes genitalis, chancroid, granuloma inguinale (Donovanosis), lymphogranuloma vereneum (LGV), condylomata acuminata (genital warts), molluscum contagiosum, pediculosis pubis, scabies, and enteric infections. While it is believed that the agent causing acquired immune deficiency syndrome (AIDS) may be transmitted sexually, AIDS is treated separately by the CDC. The STD Summary is available as a wall chart from the US Department of Health and Human Services, Public Health Service, Centers for Disease Control, Technical Information Services, Atlanta, Georgia 30333.

For the purposes of this quick reference, the most common sexually transmitted diseases are summarized in Table 4-4. Because patients with PID may require hospital admission and extensive nursing care, PID is treated separately (see MSN, Gynecology-Female system). For hepatitis B, see MSN, Gastrointestinal system. For precautions required in the care of the AIDS patient, see NR, Infection Control.

TABLE 4-4 COMMON SEXUALLY TRANSMITTED DISEASES*

Diseases and Etiologic Agents	Symptoms	Common Diagnostic Tests	Treatment
Gonorrhea *Neisseria gonorrhoeae,* gram-negative diplococcus	When symptomatic, men usually have dysuria, frequency, and purulent urethral discharge. Women, when symptomatic, may have abnormal vaginal discharge, abnormal menses, and dysuria. Anorectal and pharyngeal infections are common.	Microscopic identification of *gonorrhoeae* on smear of urethral exudate (men) or endocervical material Culture on selective media	One of several antibiotic protocols will be ordered. Drugs that may be prescribed include tetracycline hydrochloride, doxycycline hyclate, ampicillin, aqueous procaine penicillin with probenecid, and spectinomycin (see PH).
Herpes genitalis Herpes simplex virus (HSV) types 1 and 2, DNA viruses that cannot be distinguished clinically	Single or multiple vesicles appear anywhere on the genitalia. Vesicles rupture to form shallow ulcers, which may be very painful. The initial infection may last 12 days. Subsequently, recurrent infections usually last 4 to 5 days. (Viral shedding occurs intermittently between clinical episodes.)	Microscopic identification of typical cells. Electron microscopy Radioisotope or enzyme assays for HSV antigens Serologic tests Annual Papanicolaou (Pap) smears are recommended.	There is no known cure. Acyclovir ointment applied to lesions and sitz baths may provide comfort, especially if initiated early. Involved areas should be kept clean and dry. A high-protein, high-fluid diet is recommended. It is vital that the clinician be aware if a pregnant patient has a history of herpes (see OB infections). Cesarean delivery may be required to prevent infection of the baby during vaginal delivery.

(*continued*)

TABLE 4-4 COMMON SEXUALLY TRANSMITTED DISEASES*

Diseases and Etiologic Agents	Symptoms	Common Diagnostic Tests	Treatment
Cytomegalovirus (CMV) A DNA virus of the herpes virus group	It is usually asymptomatic, but may present as nonspecific febrile illness, pneumonitis, hepatitis, mononucleosis, or a combination of these.	Identification is difficult because many healthy individuals shed CMV in body secretions.	Suggestive, nonspecific, and symptomatic Transplacental transmission can have devastating effects on fetal development; screening for CMV is a vital part of prenatal care.
Syphilis *Treponema pallidum* A spirochete	Primary: a painless, indurated chancre located at site of exposure Secondary: highly variable skin rash, mucous patches, condylomata lata (a broad, flat wartlike growth usually seen on genitalia), lymphadenopathy, or other signs Latent: The patient is asymptomatic.	Serologic tests for syphilis (STS), *e.g.*, the Venereal Disease Research Laboratory test (VDRL), or the Rapid Plasma Reagin card test (RPR) Fluorescent treponemal antibody absorption test (FTA-ABS) Return for follow-up serologic tests 3, 6, 12, and 24 months after therapy.	Antibiotic protocols include administration of benzathine penicillin; for those allergic to penicillin—tetracycline; and for penicillin-allergic, pregnant patients or tetracycline-intolerant patients only—erythromycin

	Late: neurosyphilis (general paresis, tabes dorsalis, and focal neurologic signs), cardiovascular syphilis, and localized gumma formation.		
Vulvovaginitis *Candida albicans,* a dimorphic fungus	Symptoms vary from none at all, to erythema, edema, pruritus of the external genitalia, and excessive or malodorous discharge. Male sexual partners may develop urethritis, balanitis, and lesions on the penis.	Microscopic identification of the yeast forms Positive cultures of *C. albicans* in symptomatic women. (Since yeasts normally are present in the vagina and on anogenital skin, a clinically insignificant infection may produce a positive culture.)	For candidiasis, nystatin vaginal suppositories, miconomitrate 2% vaginal cream, or clotrimazole vaginal suppositories may be ordered by the physician.
Gardnerella vaginalis (Formerly *Hemophilus vaginalis* or *Corynebacterium vaginale*), a small, gram-negative pheomorphic coccobacillus	See above.	Positive vaginal culture for *G. vaginalis* in a symptomatic woman	For *Gardnerella* vaginitis: metronidazole or ampicillin, as ordered (See PH.)
Trichomonas vaginalis	See above.	Positive vaginal culture for *T. vaginalis,* or identification of organism microscopically	For trichomoniasis, metronidazole, as ordered
Other infectious, chemical, allergenic, and physical agents cause vulvovaginitis.			

*Adapted from Sexually Transmitted Diseases Summary, 1982, Department of Health and Human Service.

Nursing Considerations

- Gloves should be worn when there is direct contact with genital lesions. Hand washing is imperative.
- General patient teaching
  1. Confirm that patient understands how to take any prescribed oral medications (See PH, particularly review special precautions regarding tetracycline.)
  2. Refer sexual partners for examination and treatment.
  3. Return for follow-up, as advised by the physician.
  4. Avoid sex until both the patient and partner(s) are cured.
  5. Use condoms to prevent future infections of gonorrhea, syphilis and vulvovaginitis.
- Information required in certain specific situations follows:
  1. Herpes genitalis
     a. Patients should abstain from sex while symptomatic. There is presumed to be a small risk of transmission during asymptomatic intervals. Condoms may offer some protection.
     b. A pregnant woman must make her obstetrician aware of a history of herpes.
  2. Candidiasis
     a. Patients should wear sanitary pad to protect clothing.
     b. Suppositories should be stored in the refrigerator.
     c. The patient must continue taking medicine even during a menstrual period.
  3. Trichomoniasis or *Gardnerella* vaginitis
     a. The patient must avoid taking alcohol until 3 days after completion of metronidazole therapy.

URETHROPEXY

Description

Urethropexy provides for lengthening of the urethra, reestablishment of the normal urethral-vesical angle, and placement of periurethral sutures in the periosteum of the pubic bone. Although others have made modifications, this operation, which treats stress incontinence in women, originally was devised by Drs. Marshall and Marchetti, and usually bears their names.

Endoscopic urethral suspension, another type of urethropexy, involves both small vaginal and small lower abdominal incisions, and suspension of the urethra with stitches. A suprapubic cystostomy tube is used instead of a urethral catheter.

Nursing Considerations

- When the patient returns from surgery, bedrest may be ordered.
- A catheter may be in place from 1 days to 3 days (either urethral or suprapubic cystostomy).
- Catheter time may be shortened and replaced by an intermittent catheterization regimen (see NR, Catheterization: intermittent catheterization).
- After the catheter is removed, observe for urinary frequency and the establishment of normal voiding patterns.

URETHROTOMY FOR URETHRAL STRICTURE

Description

Urethral strictures, one of the most common causes of urinary tract obstruction, traditionally have been treated by dilatation with sounds. Increasingly, however, internal urethrotomy (incision of the stricture) is becoming the treatment of choice.

Nursing Considerations

- The patient usually will return to the floor from the operating room with a catheter in place and some sort of compression dressing (*e.g.*, vaginal packing for a woman, or an external penile compression dressing for a man).
- After the catheter is removed (usually after 24 hours), observe for bleeding and the reestablishment of normal voiding patterns.

URINARY TRACT INFECTIONS

Description

Most urinary tract infections (UTI) ascend from the urethra, although some kidney infections are believed to be blood or lymphatic borne. UTIs are more common in females than in males.

Bacteria normally found in feces (*Escherichia coli, Klebsiella, Proteus,* and *Pseudomonas*) are the most common organisms found in UTIs (*E. coli* accounting for 85% of them). Bacteria inadvertently carried from the anus to the urethra, catheterization, cystoscopy, stasis of residual urine, and any type of obstruction to urinary flow are all potential causes of UTI.

Patients with diabetes mellitus, those on corticosteroids or other immunosuppressive agents, and those with neurologic disorders that interfere with bladder emptying also are more prone to UTIs.

UTIs are rather common during pregnancy, when they require particular attention and, frequently, modifications of drug therapy.

Urine is normally sterile. Infection is implied when the colony count of a clean-catch or catheterized urine specimen is over 100,000.

CYSTITIS

Description

Cystitis, an inflammation of the bladder wall, is seen most often in women in their sexually active years. It also is seen in young girls and elderly women. The short female urethra is traumatized easily and contaminated easily from the vagina or anus. Male cystitis most often arises from urethritis or prostatitis.

Common Diagnostic Tests

- Urine culture and sensitivity (a clean-catch specimen) (See LAB.)
- Stained urinary sediment
- Cystoscopy may be done to find the underlying cause for the patient who has recurrent infections.
- Intravenous pyelograms (IVP) and voiding cystourethrograms (See NR, X-ray preparations.)
- Cystometric and other urodynamic studies (No preoperative medications or anesthesia are given.)
- Suprapubic needle aspiration of the bladder contents is sometimes done.
- Multiple glass test to locate area of infection (*e.g.*, urethra, bladder, or prostate)
- Introital (the entrance to the vagina) culture (most frequent origin of infection)

Observations

- Colony count of over 100,000 in urine culture
- Patterns of urination: urgency, frequency, nocturia, pain and burning (dysuria), and bladder cramps and spasms
- Suprapubic pain and sometimes low-back pain
- Gross hematuria, especially at the end of the urinary stream, sometimes is seen.
- Fever usually is not present.
- Symptom of vaginitis include purulent vaginal discharge, irritation

and itching of the vulva and perineum, urinary frequency, and dysuria.

- Foul-smelling urine

Treatment

- Antibacterial therapy: sulfonamides, ampicillin, or tetracyclines, depending upon sensitivity of organism (See PH.)
- Urinary acidification with ascorbic acid to improve effectiveness of methenamine mandelate (Mandelamine) and tetracyclines (See PH.)
- Urinary tract germicides, *e.g.*, nitrofurantoin macrocystals (Macrodantin) or trimethoprim with sulfamethoxazole (Bactrim or Septra) (See PH.)
- Topical urinary analgesics: phenazopyridine hydrochloride (Pyridium) will turn urine orange; methylene blue will turn urine blue-green.
- Antispasmodics and barbiturates may be ordered (see PH).
- Force fluids.
- Sitz baths and heat may relieve discomfort.
- Prophylaxis for women who have several infections a year may include a low-dose antibacterial, *e.g.*, nitrofurantoin or trimethoprim with sulfamethoxazole (Bactrim or Septra), taken daily or after sexual intercourse.
- Introital antibiotic ointment
- Surgical correction of the underlying cause may be required.

Nursing Considerations

- To prevent recurrence, education of the female patient is essential.
  1. Wipe from front to back (urethra to anus) after each bowel movement.
  2. Void after sexual intercourse.
  3. Take prescribed medication following intercourse.
  4. Shower instead of tub bathing.
  5. Force fluids.
  6. Empty the bladder completely by pressing it with the heel of the hand. This should be done every 2 hours or 3 hours to prevent stasis.
  7. Take all of the medication prescribed, even if symptoms have subsided.
  8. Wear cotton underwear. Avoid wearing tight jeans or slacks. Keep perineal area dry.

PYELONEPHRITIS

Description

Pyelonephritis is an acute or chronic pyogenic infection of one or both kidneys, usually acquired by the ascending route, although sometimes it is bloodborne. It usually is associated with obstruction, stasis, and UTI. If uncontrolled, acute pyelonephritis may become chronic, with irreversible kidney damage leading to hypertension and uremia.

Common Diagnostic Tests

- Culture and sensitivity of multiple urine specimens: voided midstream clean-catch; or obtained by catheterization, or suprapubic aspiration (especially for infants)
- Urinalysis shows large quantities of bacteria, pus, and RBCs.
- Voiding cystourethrograms (VCUG)
- Intravenous pyelograms (IVP) (See NR, X-ray preparations.)

Observations

- Sudden onset of chills, fever, vomiting, flank pain, suprapubic tenderness, frequency and burning on urination, nocturia, and foul-smelling urine all may be seen in acute pyelonephritis.
- Fatigue, sallow complexion, and low-grade fever, with insidiously appearing signs of azotemia and chronic renal failure, may be seen in chronic pyelonephritis (see MSN, renal failure).

Treatment

- Bedrest in the acute stage
- Specific antibiotics (See PH.)
- Force fluids, if renal status permits.
- Relief of obstruction
- In chronic pyelonephritis
  1. Maintenance on low-dose antibiotics
  2. Control of hypertension
  3. Dialysis, if indicated

Nursing Considerations

- Nursing care should be directed at relief of symptoms.
- See sections dealing with patients with impaired renal function, especially acute glomerulonephritis, and chronic renal failure.

NORMAL AGING CHANGES IN THE GENITOURINARY SYSTEM

- The kidneys demonstrate a gradual decrease in weight with age, and also become darker in color as a result of an increasing accumulation of pigment.
- The nephrons decrease in number and size.
- Both the number of glomeruli within the nephrons and the total glomerular surface decrease. The number of abnormal glomeruli increases.
- The arteries that supply the kidney show increasing deposits of collagen and loss of muscle fiber.
- The glomerular filtration rate (the rate that plasma is filtered out of the blood passing through the kidneys) decreases steadily with age. Renal plasma flow declines, and proximal tubular function decreases.
- There is an increase in connective tissue in the kidneys, especially in the medulla.
- Urine is less concentrated, and specific gravity decreases with age.
- Diverticula are common in the bladder, and the bladder capacity decreases with age.
- The frequency and volume of residual urine increase after voiding. In an older person, the bladder must be nearly full before the sensation for the need to void occurs.
- Frequently, a mucosal prolapse at the external female urethral orifice is seen.
- In males, sperm production decreases with age but the percentage of viable spermatozoa remains quite high into the 70s.
- The circulating level of testosterone decreases, especially after age 60.
- The prostate gland demonstrates an increase in weight, degenerative cellular changes, and benign hypertrophy. The seminal vesicles and bulbo-urethral glands show regressive changes, and the amount of seminal fluid produced declines.
- Sclerosis of the arteries and veins of the penis occurs. The erectile tissue also demonstrates sclerotic changes.

Implications

- Because of aging changes occurring in the kidneys and bladder, there is an increased incidence of UTIs in older individuals.
- An elderly person may experience precipitancy because the urge to void does not occur until the bladder is nearly full. He or she may be hesitant to move far from a bathroom due to the fear of being incontinent.

- Older persons experience an increase in nocturnal frequency. In unfamiliar surroundings, such as a hospital room, falls are a definite risk.
- The ability of an older man to achieve and maintain an erection usually continues into old age. It may take an elderly man longer to achieve the erection (during the excitement phase), but the plateau is prolonged and he has a greater capacity to sustain erection without ejaculation for longer periods of time. In the orgasmic phase, climax is usually short and the ejaculate is scant and thin. Loss of erection and return to penile flaccidity in the resolution phase occurs very quickly.
- Sexual interest and activity in old age are frequently a reflection of the person's sexual habits in younger years. However, the presence of chronic illness, the use of multiple medications, and the absence of a suitable sexual partner can limit an older individual's sexual expression.

BIBLIOGRAPHY • Genitourinary System

BOOKS

Brunner L, Suddarth D: The Lippincott Manual of Nursing Practice, 3rd ed. Philadelphia, JB Lippincott, 1983
Krupp M, Chatton M: Current Medical Diagnosis and Treatment, 22nd ed. Los Altos, Lange Medical Publications, 1983
Lerner J, Khan Z: Mosby's Manual of Urologic Nursing. St Louis, CV Mosby, 1982
McConnell E, Zimmerman M: Care of Patients with Urologic Problems. Philadelphia, JB Lippincott, 1983
Nursing Photobook: Implementing urologic procedures. Horsham, Intermed Communications, 1981
Way L: Current Surgical Diagnosis and Treatment, 6th ed. Los Altos, Lange Medical Publications, 1983

JOURNALS

Alken P: Percutaneous ultrasonic destruction of renal calculi. Urol Clin North Am 9(1):145, Feb 1982
Barrett N: Cancer of the bladder. Am J Nurs 81(12):2192, Dec 1981
Bates P: Three post-op perils of prostate surgery. RN 47(2):40, Feb 1984
Benz C: Chronic renal failure and the common denominator: A practical application. Nephrol Nurs 4(4):4, Jul/Aug 1982
Bettoli E: Herpes: Facts and fallacies. Am J Nurs 82(6):924, June 1982

Campbell C, Herten RL: VD to STD: Redefining venereal disease. Am J Nurs 81(9):1629, Sept 1981

Castanedo-Zuniga W, Miller R et al: Percutaneous removal of kidney stones. Urol Clin of North Am 9(1):113, Feb 1982

Chaussy C: First clinical experience with extracorporeally induced destruction of kidney stones with shock waves. J Urol 127(3):417, Mar 1982

Champers J: Save your diabetic patient from early kidney damage. Nursing '83 13(5):58, May 1983

Chesmore G: Nursing management—the most common urological emergencies. Nurs Mirror 155(16):37, Oct 20, 1982

Cook L: Renal trauma: A challenging assessment, a cause for cautious care. RN 46 (2):58, Feb 1983

Cunha B: Nosocomial urinary tract infections—causes, diagnosis, control measures, treatment. Heart Lung 11(6):545, Nov/Dec 1982

Datta P: The post prostatectomy patient. Nurs Times 13(77):1759, Oct 7, 1981

Devore N, Jackson V, Piening S: TORCH infections. Am J Nurs 83(12):1660, Dec 1983

Furlow W: Use of the inflatable penile prosthesis in erectile dysfunction. Urol Clin North Am 8(1):181, Feb 1981

A gland for no reason? (A basic guide to prostate troubles). Harvard Medical School Health Letter 5(5):1, Mar 1980

Giuliani L, Carmignani G, Belgrano E et al: Usefulness of preoperative transcatheter embolization in kidney tumors. Urology 17:431, 1981

Googe M, Mook T: The inflatable penile prosthesis: New developments. Am J Nurs 83(7):1044, Jul 1983

Harwood A: Urologic emergencies. Emerg Med 15(6):112, Mar 30, 1983

Hodgson S: Anemia associated with chronic renal failure and chronic dialysis. Nephrol Nurse 2(3):43, May/June 1980

Hoover D: Genitourinary trauma. Top Emerg Med 1(3):55, Oct 1982

Kidd P: Trauma of the genitourinary system. Journal of Emergency Nursing 8(5):232, Sept/Oct 1982

Lang E, deKernion J: Transcatheter embolization of advanced renal cell carcinoma with radioactive seeds. J Urol 126:581, 1981

Lewis S (ed): Symposium on chronic renal failure. Nurs Clin North Am 16(3):487–597, Sept 1981

McCrony W: Acute renal failure: A guide to diagnosis during adolescence. Consultant 23(3):167, Mar 1983

Metheny N: Renal stones and urinary pH. Am J Nurs 82(9):1372, Sept 1982

More than one way to catch a stone—nephrostolithotomy—the percutaneous extraction of urinary calculi. Emerg Med 15(8):135, Apr 30, 1983

Orr M: Drugs and renal disease. Am J Nurs 81(5):969, May 1981

Polycystic kidney. Nurs Mirror 156(20):97 May 8, 1983
Poole K: A useful way to diagnose bladder disorders. RN 47(8):50, Aug 1984
Quinlan M: UTI: Helping your patient control it once and for all. RN 47(3):38, Mar 1984
Randolph G: Bringing them back out of renal failure. RN 44(5):34, May 1981
Satile W: The penile prosthesis and diabetic impotence: Some caveats. Diabetes Care 2(1):26, Jan/Feb 1979
Sexually transmitted diseases summary, 1982. Department of Health and Human Services, Public Health Service, Atlanta, Centers for Disease Control, 1982
Stark J: BUN/ creatinine: Your key to kidney function. Nursing '80 11(5):33, May 1980
Stark J, Hunt V: Helping your patient with chronic renal failure. Nursing '83 13(9):56, Sept 1983
Strauss J: Tips about renal diseases in children. Consultant 20:75, Apr 1980
Thompson P: Acute renal failure—a challenge for all nurses. Nephrol Nurse 3(5):4, Sept/Oct 1981
Tichy A: Renal failure. Crit Care Update 9:7, Aug 1982
Tobiason S: Benign prostatic hypertrophy. Am J Nurs 79(2):286, Feb 1979
Topur M: Symposium on chronic renal failure. Chronic renal disease in children. Nurs Cl of NA 16:587, Sept 1981
Tower M: Urinary obstruction: The hidden threats in treatment. RN 45(5):58, May 1982
Trimethoprim—now available alone—for initial treatment of acute symptomatic uncomplicated UTI. Nurses Drug Alert 6(10):75, Oct 1982
Tuffill S: Disorders of the male genitourinary tract. Nurs Mirror 155(16):26, Oct 20, 1982
Underwood M: Urinary tract infections. Crit Care Q 3(3):63, Dec 1980
Urich B: The physiological adaptation of end stage renal disease: A review and a proposed new model. Nephrol Nurse 2(3):48, May/June 1980

Normal Aging Changes in the Genitourinary System

Finch C, Hayflick L (eds): Handbook of the Biology of Aging. New York, Van Nostrand Reinhold, 1977
Reff M, Schneider E: Biological Markers of Aging. U.S. Department of Health and Human Services, 1982 (NIH Publication No. 82-2221)
Rockstein M, Sussman M: Biology of Aging. Belmont, Wadsworth Publishing, 1979

GYNECOLOGY

ABORTION, INDUCED

Since the legalization of induced abortion, this procedure has become increasingly common. *Therapeutic abortion* is done when the patient's health or well being is endangered by the pregnancy. Abortion in very early pregnancy may be performed in the doctor's office or family planning clinic. When the pregnancy is beyond 10 to 12 weeks' gestation, abortion generally is performed in the hospital.

Induced abortion for unwanted pregnancy is a controversial and emotional issue. The nurse who is uncomfortable with this practice should ask for a transfer to another clinical area. No matter what her personal feelings, the nurse's responsibility is to support the patient.

Types of induced abortions and reminders as to what to look for are described in Table 4-5.

Nursing Considerations

The following would apply to the patient undergoing either spontaneous or induced abortion.

- Upon admission, obtain a history and do a physical assessment (see OB Table 5-2, Bleeding during pregnancy—differential diagnosis and nursing considerations—for the care of a patient with bleeding during pregnancy).
- Explain to the patient and her support person what is happening, and what procedures will be used.
- Provide emotional support.
- Monitor contractions.
- Breathing techniques may be used when contractions occur (see OB, Labor and delivery, Nursing considerations).
- Administer analgesics and oxytocin, as ordered.
- Have the patient use the bedpan, so that it can be inspected for intrauterine material.
- Before induced abortion, the bladder should be empty, and an enema may be ordered.
- It is the position of the Roman Catholic church that all stillborns and aborted fetuses should be baptized.
- After abortion
  1. Check the following q 15 min for one hour and then as ordered:

     Vital signs

     Amount, color, and odor of vaginal discharge. Save all pads if bleeding seems unusual. Record the number of pads used during each shift, and the amount of blood on them.

     Uterine fundus for firmness.

TABLE 4-5 TYPES OF INDUCED ABORTIONS

Method	Description	Observations
First trimester		
Morning-after pill	Relatively high doses of synthetic estrogen are given the first three days after possible conception	Nausea and vomiting A menstrual period should follow about 3 days after the medication is taken.
Vacuum aspiration (menstrual extraction, mini-abortion)	The cervix is dilated by use of 1. Laminaria tent (a sterile, dried stem of a seaweed) that is inserted into the cervical canal and swells overnight, thus dilating the cervix 2. Increasingly larger sounds A cannula and suction remove the products of conception—dilation and evacuation (D&E). Curettage may complete the procedure. Paracervical block or supportive anesthesia may be used during this procedure.	The laminaria tent, usually inserted the evening before scheduled abortion, sometimes falls out. If it does, notify the physician. During the procedure, some cramping and discomfort may be experienced. Following the procedure, there normally is little or no discomfort. Bleeding should be minimal. High temperature, foul-smelling discharge, and general malaise should be recognized by the patient as signs of infection, and should be reported.
Dilatation and curettage (D&C), done prior to 12 weeks' gestation	The cervix is dilated with sounds. Products of conception are scraped from uterine wall with a curet. Regional or general anesthesia may be used. IV oxytocin may be ordered.	Some cramping with minimal vaginal bleeding following the procedure

Prostaglandin suppository or prostaglandin intra-amniotic injection may be used in late first trimester or early second trimester.	Prostaglandins cause smooth muscle to contract and have stimulating effects on the contractility of the myometrium.	
Sometimes as many as three suppositories given 4 to 6 hours apart may be required to stimulate labor.	A suppository is placed in the vaginal cul de sac by the physician.	Expulsion of uterine contents, usually within 24 hours, Retained placenta is not uncommon. Bleeding
Promethazine hydrochloride (Phenergan) may be given with the suppository to counteract nausea.	Intra-amniotic injection 1. A small dose is injected slowly to test for side-effects. If there are none, the remainder of the 20- to 40- mg dose of prostaglandin is given slowly. Curettage may be required to remove retained material.	Vomiting, diarrhea, and temperature elevation are common side-effects of prostaglandins. Symptoms are more apt to occur with the suppository than with intra-amniotic injection. Additional side-effects include chills and tissue reaction at the site of injection.
Second trimester Urea intra-amniotic injection Saline induction ("salting out"), used only after 16 weeks' gestation	Sedatives, analgesics, and tranquilizers are administered. The patient must be responsive. The patient empties her bladder, is given an enema, is shaved, and prepared for amniocentesis. Techniques vary, but amniotic fluid is withdrawn, and a small amount of hypertonic saline is injected into the amniotic sac as a test dose.	Symptoms of dehydration, alteration of coagulation factors may be present.

MSN

(*continued*)

TABLE 4-5 TYPES OF INDUCED ABORTIONS

Method	Description	Observations
	If severe side-effects occur, the procedure is discontinued, and an IV solution of 5% dextrose in water is started to prevent cerebral dehydration. If there are no side-effects, up to 250 ml of amniotic fluid is withdrawn and replaced with 20% saline.	Severe side-effects resulting from injection of saline into a blood vessel of the placenta may appear in the first hour. Severe shock-like symptoms, including abdominal pain, severe headache, backache, tachycardia, drowsiness, confusion, and seizures may occur. Hypernatremia—elevated temperature, flashed skin, oliguria, thirst, and delirium.
	Usually, fetal death occurs within an hour, and labor begins in about 24 hours. IV oxytocin may be started to hasten labor. Curettage may be necessary to remove retained placenta.	Signs and symptoms of labor (See OB, Labor and delivery); contractions Bleeding, especially if placenta is retained
Hysterotomy, now done infrequently	An incision is made through abdomen into the uterus to remove products of conception. The abortion of last choice: It is done sometimes in combination with tubal ligation. Cesarean section may be required in future pregnancies.	The postoperative course is like that of any abdominal surgery.

2. Perineal care is given immediately and patient may be instructed to continue it for 5 days–7 days. A kit containing plastic squeeze bottles and sterile towelettes may be sent home with her.
3. Monitor urinary output.
4. Administer analgesics and oxytocin, as ordered.
5. After the effects of anesthesia have worn off, a shower may be suggested. Frequently, showers only, up to 4 weeks, are ordered.
6. Provide emotional support and counseling. Depression following abortion is not uncommon.
7. An RH-negative mother with a negative indirect Coombs' test would receive RH_0 (D) immune human globulin (RH_0GAM) within 72 hours.

- Discharge planning usually includes the following patient education.
  1. Minimal vaginal bleeding or spotting should not last over 10 days. Bleeding beyond that time should be reported. Any excessive or bright-red bleeding should be reported immediately.
  2. Elevated temperature and foul-smelling vaginal discharge are signs of infection, and should be reported.
  3. Abstain from sexual intercourse for 2 weeks to 3 weeks.
  4. Avoid tampon use and douching for 2 weeks to 4 weeks.
  5. Counseling regarding contraceptive methods, especially following induced abortion, is usually appropriate. Most physicians advise patients to wait 2 months to 3 months following spontaneous abortion before becoming pregnant again.
  6. Return for a follow-up visit to clinician in 2 weeks to 4 weeks.

ATROPHIC VAGINITIS

Description

Atrophic, senile, or *postmenopausal vaginitis* is a common condition following menopause. Because of estrogen depletion, the vaginal mucosa atrophies, and then becomes more prone to infection.

Observations

- Complaints of dyspareunia (painful intercourse), itching, and burning
- A vaginal discharge, if infection is present

Treatment

- Estrogenic vaginal suppositories or vaginal creams
- Oral estrogen (premarin), as ordered
- Infection, if present, is treated appropriately.

Nursing Considerations

- FDA regulations require that female patients receive package insert describing possible side-effects before taking estrogen products.

CANCER OF THE BREAST

Description

Breast cancer is the most common cancer of women, 85% occurring in women over the age of 40. It generally is detected by manual examination of the breast, but only can be confirmed by tissue biopsy. It may metastasize initially to axillary or mediastinal lymph nodes, lung, and bones. Later, it may progress to the liver and brain.

Common Diagnostic Tests

- Breast examination: 85% to 90% of breast lumps are discovered by the patient.
- Mammograms: These are breast x-rays capable of detecting some breast cancers 1–2 years before they reach the palpable size of 1 cm. At the present time, a baseline mammogram is recommended for women between the ages of 35 and 50; all women over the age of 50 should have a yearly mammogram. Regardless of age, women with a family history of breast cancer in a mother or sister are often encouraged to have a yearly mammogram.
- Tissue examination is the only accurate method to determine the nature of the lesion. Biopsies may be done by aspiration, needle, incisional, or excisional methods.

Observations

- A solid, fixed, painless lump, most often in the upper outer quadrant of the breast, can be felt. The lump may be accompanied by a nipple discharge, nipple retraction, or elevation.
- Dimpling of the skin, resembling the skin of an orange, often develops as the disease progresses.

Treatment

Surgical

- Radical mastectomy is the removal of the breast, axillary nodes, lymphatic vessels draining the arm on the affected side, and pectoralis muscles.
- Modified radical mastectomy is the removal of the breast and most axillary lymph nodes.
- Simple mastectomy involves the removal of the breast, leaving axillary nodes intact.
- Partial or segmental mastectomy removes only the tumor mass and a small amount of surrounding breast tissue.
- Tylectomy (lumpectomy) is the removal of only the tumor mass.
- Less radical surgical procedures currently being done have made reconstructive mammoplasty more feasible. Silicone-gel-filled pouch implants, along with reconstruction of the nipple and areola, are possible. In order to match size and shape, reconstructive surgery often involves both breasts.

Chemotherapy

- Adjuvant chemotherapy is commonly used for women postoperatively when cancer involves the lymph nodes.

Hormone Therapy

- Tumors that are hormone dependent may be treated with various hormonal manipulations (surgery or medication).

Radiation

- Radioactive implant (See MSN, Oncology nursing considerations.)
- External radiation may be combined with surgery. It also may be used to decrease the size of the tumor mass before surgery. It sometimes is useful for pain relief in widespread metastases.

Nursing Considerations

- Mammography is not a substitute for breast palpation. Self-examination and physician consultation are essential.
- Radical mastectomies are not done as frequently as they once were. However, in this surgical procedure where the lymph nodes and vessels on the affected side are removed, infection of the arm is a possibility. Avoid injections or venipunctures in that arm. Blood pressures should not be taken in the affected arm to prevent trauma to the tissue. The patient should wear a bracelet on the arm identifying this problem. Any pain, redness, or swelling

in the affected arm should be reported immediately to the physician.

- Hemovacs are usually in the axilla after mastectomies. Be sure they drain well, are emptied during each shift, and are irrigated by order if necessary.
- Check the hand for circulatory impairment.
- Keep the arm elevated on a pillow.
- A progressive plan of arm exercises (Fig 4-7) should be ordered immediately postoperatively. This usually begins with flexion and extension of fingers in the first few hours, and progresses as ordered by the physician.
- Encourage the "Reach to Recovery" program available through the local Cancer Society. A physician's referral is necessary during the hospitalization. After discharge from the hospital, no referral is necessary.
- See MSN Oncology nursing considerations.

CANCER OF THE UTERUS

Description

Cancer of the uterus may occur in the lower part of the uterus (the cervix) or in the body (corpus), which is the upper part of the uterus. Cancer in the body of the uterus usually starts in the lining (endometrium); this is called endometrial cancer. Staging is the term used to describe the extent of the disease. Cancer of the cervix tends to spread by the lymphatic system; cancer of the body of the uterus tends to spread through the bloodstream.

Common Diagnostic Tests

- Pap smear: This is a test to detect cancer cells on the cervix. It is not a reliable indicator of endometrial cancer. Pap smear reports are by classes: I, normal; II, inflammation; III, IV, and V, abnormal cells. Class III and above are indicative of increasing dysplasia or malignant cells. When a report is other than normal, the following tests may be done:
    1. Colposcopy: This is the viewing of the vagina and cervix, as well as the endocervical canal, through a binocular microscope. Tissue samples are taken from suspicious-looking areas.
    2. Conization (cone biopsy): This is the surgical removal of a cone-shaped piece of tissue from the cervix or cervical canal for examination.
    3. Aspiration curettage of the uterus: Tissue specimens are obtained by intrauterine aspiration.

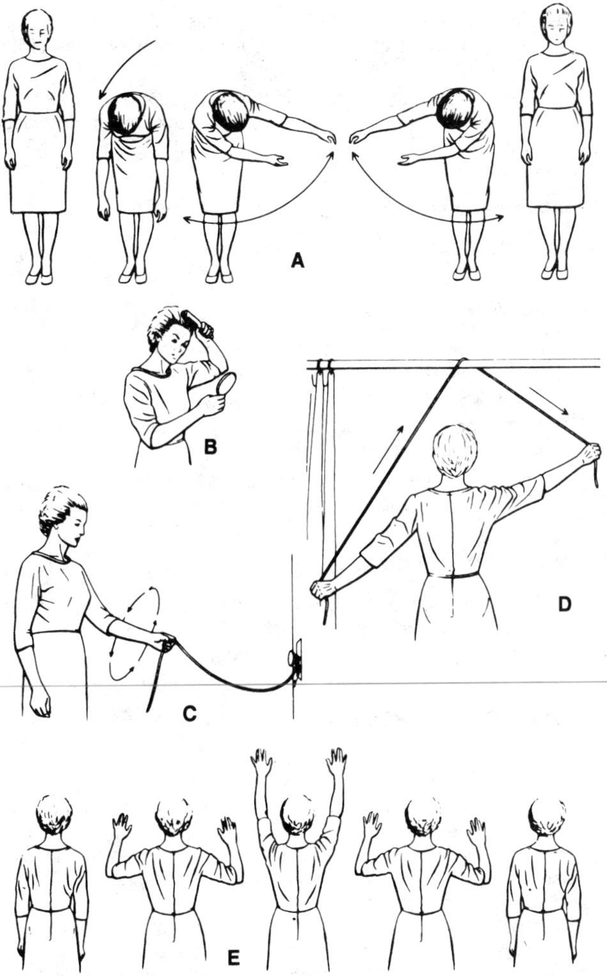

Fig. 4-7. *Exercises for the postmastectomy patient. (A) Pendulum-swinging exercise. (B) Hair-brushing exercise. (C) Rope-turning exercise. (D) Rope-sliding exercise. (E) Wall-climbing exercise.*

4. D and C (dilatation and curettage): This is the standard, classical, surgical procedure for obtaining tissue samples of the endometrium.
5. Gravelee test (or jet wash): In this procedure, fluid is injected into the uterus and the returned fluid is examined for cancer cells.

Observations

- Abnormal vaginal bleeding or discharge

Treatment

- The treatment is determined by the stage of the disease. Cryotherapy cauterization or laser surgery is done for the removal of localized lesions of the cervix.
- Surgery alone or combined with radiation is used in treating invasive cancer of the cervix or cancer of the uterus.
- Chemotherapy and hormonal therapy are primarily useful in promoting patient comfort in advanced disease.

Nursing Considerations

- Consult with the radiotherapist regarding necessary precautions in caring for patients with radioactive implants or IV substances.
- See MSN Oncology nursing considerations.

CYSTOCELE AND RECTOCELE

Description

Pelvic muscle weakness is usually the result of unrepaired lacerations or ill-advised bearing down during childbirth. Repeated, close pregnancies predispose to perineal muscle weakness that usually becomes evident later in life. In some cases, there apparently is congenital weakness of these muscles.

With pelvic muscle relaxation, the bladder may herniate into the vagina (cystocele), or the rectal wall may herniate into it (rectocele) or the intestine may push through into the posterior cul-de-sac (enterocele).

Common Diagnostic Tests

- For cystocele
  1. Residual urine will be left in the bladder after the patient voids.
  2. Cystography demonstrates bladder herniation.

- For rectocele and enterocele
  1. Barium enema shows rectocele by x-ray.

Observations

- For cystocele
  1. Complaints of vaginal fullness and inability to empty the bladder completely are common.
  2. There may be a soft, reducible mass in the anterior vagina. The patient may have found that she has to push it back in order to empty her bladder completely.
  3. Urinary frequency, dysuria, and stress incontinence may be present.
- For rectocele
  1. Complaints of constipation
  2. Hemorrhoids
  3. Incontinence of gas and liquid feces

Treatment

- For cystocele
  1. Surgical repair to tighten the vaginal wall—anterior colporrhaphy, perineorrhaphy, or anteriorcolpoplasty or posterior colpoperineoplasty.
  2. Transabdominal cystocele correction or obliterative vaginal operations (LeFort's operation or colpectomy) may be chosen in special instances.
  3. A pessary provides a supportive measure for the patient who refuses, or cannot withstand, surgery.
  4. Estrogen therapy and Kegel exercises may improve urinary control in postmenopausal women (see NR, Kegel exercises).
  5. Antibiotics for urinary tract infections (UTI) (See MSN, Urinary tract infections.)
- For rectocele and enterocele
  1. Surgical repair (posterior colporrhaphy or colpoperineorrhaphy
  2. Surgical repair of rectocele, cystocele, enterocele, uterine prolapse, and frequently hysterectomy, should be done concomitantly.

Nursing Considerations

For general preoperative care, see MSN, Preoperative care.

- In addition, for vaginal surgery, a cleansing douche frequently is ordered the morning of surgery.

Postoperative care after vaginal surgery includes

- General postoperative care (See MSN, Postoperative care.)
- Perineal care usually given at least twice a day and after each voiding or defecation
  1. With the patient on a bedpan, pour solution over the perineum. Normal saline or antiseptic solution (according to hospital protocol or the physician's orders) may be used.
  2. Cleansing is done away from the vagina toward the rectum.
- After perineal care, a heat lamp to the perineum may be used 15 minutes to 20 minutes, two to three times a day, to promote healing.
- An ice pack may provide local comfort and reduce swelling. It should not apply pressure to the sutures. Let it rest on the bed.
- After sutures are removed, Sitz baths usually are ordered.
- Vaginal douches using sterile normal saline or povidone-iodine solution (with dilution prescribed) and sterile equipment may be ordered immediately postoperatively, or started 5 days to 10 days later. The douche nozzle should be inserted gently and rotated carefully.
- Bladder care includes
  1. Keeping the bladder undistended, especially following repair of cystocele. No more than 150 ml of urine should be allowed to collect.
  2. An indwelling catheter is usually in place for at least 24 hours to 48 hours.
  3. Provide regular catheter care (see NR, Catheterization, urinary).
- Kegel exercises are encouraged (see NR, Kegel exercises).
- The patient should avoid jarring activities and heavy lifting for at least six weeks. Stair climbing should be limited.
- Following anterior colporrhaphy, a laxative may be ordered every night to prevent strain on the sutures.
- Following posterior colporrhaphy, many surgeons prefer to keep the bowels empty, in order to avoid bowel function and to prevent strain on the incision site until healing is established.
  1. Preoperative cathartic and enemas usually are ordered.
  2. Clear liquids (no *milk*) are given.
  3. Tincture of opium (Paregoric) (See PH.)
  4. After 5 days to 7 days, mineral oil is given at night, and followed in the morning by a small oil-retention enema (90–120 ml) given with a soft rectal tube.
  5. Stool softeners are ordered nightly thereafter during convalescence to avoid straining at stool.

- At the follow-up visit, the physician will advise when to discontinue douches and laxatives, and when it is safe to resume sexual intercourse.

DILATATION AND CURETTAGE (D & C)

Description

The cervical canal is enlarged with a dilator, and the uterine endometrium lining is scraped with a curette. D & C may be done for diagnostic purposes (to obtain endocervical and endometrial tissue samples for cytologic examination), to control abnormal uterine bleeding, or to remove all products of conception following incomplete abortion.

The procedure may be performed with general, or local anesthesia supplemented by Valium or Demerol.

Nursing Considerations

- The patient should understand the procedure, which usually is explained by the surgeon.
- Preoperatively, a small enema is ordered occasionally. The bladder is emptied.
- Postoperatively
  1. Packing may be in place for 24 hours.
  2. Perineal care is given immediately postoperatively, and usually continued for 5 days to 7 days.
  3. The perineal pad should be checked frequently for bleeding.
  4. Report excessive bleeding.
  5. Urge bedrest with bathroom privileges for the remainder of the day.
  6. Mild analgesics may be ordered for discomfort.

ENDOMETRIOSIS

Description

In endometriosis, cells from the endometrium are seeded throughout the pelvis, and occasionally to more distant locations. These cells, stimulated by ovarian hormones, menstruate along with the normal menstrual cycle. They bleed into the surrounding areas, causing inflammation, adhesions, and, when encased, tumor masses. Seen especially in the ovaries, these encased masses are known as chocolate cysts because the collected old blood is thick and dark, resembling chocolate.

When deprived of ovarian hormonal support the lesions regress, but they will recur if estrogen stimulation is reintroduced.

Endometriosis is seen most often in women between the ages of 25 and 40 years who have postponed childbearing. Women with this condition frequently also have fibroids. Endometriosis is a significant cause of infertility.

Common Diagnostic Tests

- X-ray contrast studies, when there is colonic involvement
- Laparoscopy

Treatment

- Analgesics for the relief of pain
- Suppression of ovulation
  1. Pregnancy has beneficial effects but is not curative.
  2. Progestins alone, or in combination with estrogen
  3. Danazol (Danocrine), a synthetic androgen
- Conservative surgery involves lysis of adhesions and removal of as many implants as possible, while maintaining reproductive function.
- Bilateral oophorectomy and salpingectomy, usually including hysterectomy, are the only definitive treatments.
- A diet high in iron, or iron supplements, may be ordered if anemia is present.

Observations

- Symptoms are variable, and sometimes absent.
- Dysmenorrhea (painful menstruation) that is progressive; dull, cramping lower abdominal pain, frequently accompanied by low-back pain
- Abnormal menstrual bleeding—excessive, prolonged, frequent, irregular
- Feeling of fullness in the lower abdomen
- Dyspareunia (painful sexual intercourse)
- History of infertility
- Weakness and fatigability caused by anemia from blood loss

Nursing Considerations

- Administer medications as ordered, instructing the patient regarding possible side-effects, and the importance of compliance in hormonal therapy.

- A heating pad to the abdomen may relieve abdominal pain.
- When counseling a patient with dyspareunia
  1. Ask her when the pain occurs.
  2. Suggest that she take pain medicine before beginning sexual activity.
  3. Urge clear communications between partners to promote maximum comfort.
- Teach what to expect with laparoscopy.
  1. Two ½-inch incisions will be made—one at the umbilicus and one at the midline of the lower abdomen. They will be covered with Band-aids after the procedure.
  2. Patient may belch or feel bloated afterward because of the introduction of CO_2 into the peritoneal cavity during the procedure.
  3. Minor vaginal bleeding is normal following this procedure.
- If surgery is performed, see MSN, Preoperative care and Postoperative care, and Hysterectomy (if appropriate).

HYSTERECTOMY

Description

Hysterectomy, or the removal of the uterus, has become one of the most commonly performed major surgical procedures. In *subtotal hysterectomy* all of the uterus except the cervix is removed. In *total hysterectomy* (or panhysterectomy) the entire uterus including the cervix is removed. The fallopian tubes and ovaries, in addition to the entire uterus, are removed in *total hysterectomy with salpingo-oophorectomy.*

Hysterectomy can be done from either an abdominal or a vaginal approach. Nursing observations and interventions vary slightly. (See Table 4-6 for a comparison of the two techniques.)

Indications for hysterectomy include removal of malignant and nonmalignant tumors of the uterus, cervix, or adjacent organs; severe pelvic infections, usually associated with childbirth, abortion, or intrauterine devices; control of severe uterine bleeding; problems associated with pelvic floor relaxation; intractable endometriosis; and for sterilization and prophylaxis when there is a strong history of disease.

Considerations made before a decision for hysterectomy is made include the patient's age, her wish to continue childbearing, her wish to retain her uterus, the probable effectiveness of alternative treatments, the degree of her dysfunction, and her willingness to tolerate it.

TABLE 4-6 COMPARISONS BETWEEN ABDOMINAL AND VAGINAL HYSTERECTOMY

Description	Abdominal Hysterectomy	Vaginal Hysterectomy
Indications	For removal of large tumors of the fallopian tubes and ovaries; usually also used when there is chronic pelvic inflammatory disease, irradiation, endometriosis, extensive adhesions, and when wider exploration or oophorectomy is indicated	To treat Stage O *in situ* cervical cancer when adjacent tissue is cancer free When there is pelvic relaxation, and hysterectomy is combined with plastic repair When patient is obese, and abdominal approach is not mandatory
Description	Midline incision through the abdomen Pfannensteil's incision (bikini line)—a lateral incision just above the symphysis	Using a vaginal approach, an incision is made above and around the cervix. Ovaries and fallopian tubes may be removed.
Advantages		Since there is no abdominal incision, patients are less likely to develop complications seen in abdominal surgery, *e.g.*, paralytic ileus, pulmonary problems, thrombophlebitis, wound dehiscence, but are more apt to run a febrile course. A shorter hospital stay is required

Observations Bleeding can occur because the abundant blood supply to pelvic organs increases this risk, especially during the first 24 hours postoperatively. Check q 2–4 hr. during that period. Bleeding may also occur during the first three postoperative weeks.	A small amount of pink, yellow, or brown serous drainage from the vagina may start and stop from day to day.	Same as abdominal hysterectomy
	A small amount of frank bleeding, no heavier than a light menstrual flow, may be normal. Saturated packing or perineal pad, or the appearance of clots should be reported to the physician. Save the pads so that the physician can estimate blood loss.	Same as abdominal hysterectomy
	Observe the abdominal incision for bleeding and drainage. Trace the outline of drainage on the dressing and mark the time, so you can recognize continued bleeding. Check the surgeon's notes to see whether a drain is in place.	Packing and/or a Penrose drain may be in place immediately postoperatively. They usually are removed by the surgeon within 24–48 hours.

(continued)

TABLE 4-6 COMPARISONS BETWEEN ABDOMINAL AND VAGINAL HYSTERECTOMY

Description	Abdominal Hysterectomy	Vaginal Hysterectomy
Signs of urinary tract complications 1. Bladder distention 2. Markedly decreased urinary output must be investigated to rule out damage to a ureter during surgery. Check patency of catheter and accurately observe urinary output. 3. Urgency, frequency, pain and burning on urination, signs of UTI	Check for the patency of the catheter, usually in place for the first 24 hr postoperatively. A suprapubic catheter may be used (see NR, Catheterization, urinary).	Same as for abdominal hysterectomy. If an anterior colporrhaphy (repair of a cystocele) has been done, the catheter may stay in place for 3 days. 1. Tiny clots and slightly blood-tinged urine may be normal, but grossly bloody urine should be reported.
Vaginal cuff infection—more common in vaginal hysterectomy		May include foul-smelling, purulent discharge, persistent temperature, or WBC elevation
Feelings of abdominal pressure may be caused by surgery itself or by complications, *e.g.*, distended bladder, UTI, intrasurgical bladder damage, or vaginal packing.		
Signs and symptoms of other postoperative complications (see MSN, Postoperative care, and postoperative complications)		

Nursing Considerations

- Preoperatively, prepare patient for her surgery. In addition to normal preoperative teaching (see MSN, Preoperative care), she probably will need education regarding what to expect in terms of changes in her body.
    1. If an ovary is left intact, the premenopausal patient will not have menopausal symptoms after hysterectomy, even though she will not menstruate. Hot flashes, believed to be due to manipulation of the ovaries, may occur for a few months.
    2. Other sensations that eventually disappear following hysterectomy include lower abdominal cramping and loss of vaginal sensation.
    3. The woman will continue to have orgasms, but the sensation may be different.
    4. Patient education booklets have been found useful in many institutions.
- A vaginal douche may be part of her preoperative preparation.
- Provide emotional support and an environment in which the patient can discuss her feelings.
- Postoperative care (See MSN, Postoperative care; and for vaginal hysterectomy, Nursing considerations for vaginal repair of cystocele, rectocele.)
- Following abdominal hysterectomy, the incision may be covered with thin gauze or Telfa, or a heavier pressure dressing. The latter may be an indication that bleeding was a problem during surgery, or that a drain is in place.
    1. Watch incision for bleeding, drainage, and signs of infection.
- Encourage changes in position and early ambulation, according to the physician's orders. Do not raise the foot of the bed or gatch the knees, which may cause pooling of blood in the pelvis.
- To prevent vaginal cuff infections, care should include meticulous perineal care after each voiding and bowel movement. Patient should wipe her perineum from front to back. Cephalosporin frequently is ordered pre- and postoperatively.
- Discharge instructions include avoidance of heavy lifting, fatigue, and sexual intercourse until her surgeon advises resumption of full activity. Stair climbing and driving also may be restricted. Swimming is considered beneficial.

PELVIC INFLAMMATORY DISEASE

Description

Pelvic inflammatory disease (PID) is any acute, subacute, recurrent, or chronic infection of the female reproductive organs. Inflammation of the fallopian tubes (salpingitis) is most common; but inflammation may be present in the cervix (cervicitis), uterus (endometritis), ovaries (oophoritis), or connective tissue lying between the broad ligaments (parametritis). Early treatment is essential to prevent infertility and potentially dangerous complications—septicemia, pulmonary emboli, and shock.

Neisseria gonorrhoeae, the microorganism that causes gonorrhea, is the most common cause of PID, but *Chlamydia trachomatis, Ureaplasma urealyticum,* and other organisms also may be involved. Infecting organisms may gain entry by ascending through the vagina and cervical canal (*e.g.,* by sexual contact, infected abortion, insertion of an intrauterine device, use of a biopsy curet, tubal insufflation, postpartum infection, hysterosalpingography), through pelvic surgery, or through the bloodstream.

Common Diagnostic Tests

- Smears and culture of vaginal discharge
- Complete blood count (CBC) shows elevated white blood cell count.
- Increased sedimentation rate
- Ultrasound—to identify masses in the uterus or adjoining organs
- X-ray may show tubal occlusion or ileus (a possible complication in the acute phase).

Observations

In the acute phase

- Severe, cramplike, lower abdominal (usually bilateral), nonradiating pain, chills and fever, menstrual disturbances, leukorrhea (white or yellowish discharge from the cervical canal or vagina)
- Complications, *e.g.,* paralytic ileus (see MSN, Postoperative complications), septicemia, pulmonary emboli, and shock

In the chronic phase

- Dysmenorrhea, dyspareunia (painful intercourse), infertility, recurrent low-grade fever, purulent vaginal discharge, tender pelvic masses

Treatment

In the acute phase

- Strict bedrest
- Restriction of oral feedings
- Administration of IV fluids (See NR Intravenous therapy.)
- Nasogastric suction may be necessary to treat ileus (see NR, Gastrointestinal intubation).
- Antibiotics, started immediately, and adjusted after culture results are available

1. Penicillin G, IV, and kanamycin, IM, usually are started (unless the patient has penicillin allergies). Cephalothin, erythromycin, metronidazole, or cefoxitin may be substituted. Oral antibiotics, ampicillin or tetracycline, complete the therapy.

- Analgesics for the control of pain
- Delay or prevent ovulation and menstruation for 2 months to 3 months by oral contraceptive hormone therapy

In the chronic phase

- Penicillin G, IM, with probenecid given orally, followed by ampicillin for 10 days
- Alternatively, in case of drug allergy, tetracycline for 10 days
- Rest, analgesics, and soft diet

Surgical measures, postponed until after the acute phase

- Drainage of a pelvic abscess, if one develops
- Hysterectomy with bilateral salpino-oophorectomy may be required in persistent PID that does not respond to treatment.

Nursing Considerations

- Prevent spread of infection by scrupulous hand washing and isolation technique, if there is a foul-smelling discharge or positive culture.
- A semi-Fowler position can promote dependent drainage.
- External heat may be applied to the abdomen.
- Warm douches may be ordered to improve circulation.
- Provide perineal care if vaginal drainage is present.
- Administer antibiotics and analgesics, as ordered, after ascertaining that there are no drug allergies.
- Stress the need for the patient's sexual partner to be treated.
- Following minor gynecologic procedures, proper patient advice may prevent development of major infections. The patient should report any fever, increased vaginal discharge, or pain (signs of inflammation). She should avoid sexual intercourse for at least 7 days.
- The patient should understand the seriousness of PID, the importance of compliance in treatment, and the avoidance of reinfection.

PROLAPSE OF THE UTERUS

Description

The uterus may be displaced when pelvic floor muscles are greatly weakened. Normally, the uterus lies with the cervix at right angles to the long axis of the vagina. Its body is inclined slightly forward.

Adhesions or weakening support may cause the uterus to be displaced backward (retroversion and retroflexion) or forward (anteflexion). Weakening support may permit marked displacement of the uterus downward through the vagina (prolapse). This occurs especially with retroposition. In first-degree prolapse, the cervix comes down to the introitus (opening of the vagina). In second-degree prolapse, it protrudes through the introitus. In third-degree prolapse, or total procidentia, the entire uterus protrudes.

Observations

- Chronic backache, pelvic pressure, easy fatigue, leukorrhea and dysmenorrhea (painful menstruation) are common symptoms.
- A firm mass may be found in the lower vagina, or the cervix and uterus may even protrude through the vaginal introitus.
- Incontinence and urinary retention may be caused by displacement of the bladder.

Treatment

- Treatment is dependent upon the degree of the problem, age of the patient, and her desire for menstruation, pregnancy, and coitus.
- Palliative treatment includes a well-fitted, vaginal pessary.
- Estrogen supplements can improve muscle tone in postmenopausal patients. Package literature must be given to the patient before the first dose (see PH).
- Kegel exercises (See NR, Kegel exercises.)
- Surgery for prolapse is usually a hysterectomy. Uterine suspension is done for displacements.
- Exercises using principles of gravity, *e.g.,* knee-chest, the "Monkey trot," or having the patient lie on her abdomen 2 hours a day, are recommended.

Nursing Considerations

- Knee-chest exercises: The woman assumes a knee-chest position with labia separated to allow air to enter the vagina. The position should be maintained for 5 minutes, two or three times a day.
- "Monkey trot" exercise: The woman walks about on her hands and feet, keeping the knees straight, for 5 minutes, two or three times a day.
- If a pessary is inserted, a string should be attached to it and the other end pinned to the patient's underclothing, so that if it becomes displaced, it will not cause embarrassment.
- Preoperatively, the patient may be kept in bed for two or three

days with a pessary or vaginal pack in place, to relieve tension on strained ligaments, thereby making the surgeon's work easier.

- Depending upon the surgery that is done, see MSN, Preoperative care; Postoperative care; Hysterectomy.

NORMAL AGING CHANGES IN THE FEMALE GENITOURINARY SYSTEM

- In women, the number of oocytes (immature ova) decreases with age, as well as the number of ova with the normal number of chromosomes.
- After menopause, the fallopian tubes and uterine wall atrophy. The size of the uterus, as well as its muscle tone, decreases.
- The cervical canal narrows and the cervix becomes fibrous.
- The vagina of postmenopausal women shortens and narrows. Changes occur in the elastic fibers of the wall and elasticity is reduced. Decreased estrogen levels cause the epithelium lining to become pale, thin, and dry. Rugae flatten, and secretions are reduced and become alkaline.
- Bartholin glands are less numerous and less effective, causing decreased vaginal lubrication.
- The size of the clitoris is moderately reduced.
- In the vulva (the external genitalia) both pubic hair and subcutaneous fat are lost. The skin appears thin, shiny, and pale, and the labial folds flatten.
- Mammary glandular tissue is replaced with fat and the breasts may sag and become less firm.
- Menopause occurs and is characterized by irregular menses, follicular exhaustion, failure of ova production, and the permanent ending of menstrual activity and estrogen production.
- Changes in the vagina and vulva with aging increase the susceptibility of women to inflammation and infection in these areas. Vulvitis and atrophic ("senile") vaginitis are common. Treatment with estrogen creams or suppositories can reduce the discomfort.
- Loss of tone of the muscles and ligaments supporting the bladder and uterus increases the risk of a prolapse (*e.g.,* cystocele, rectocele). Surgical correction may be indicated.
- Human female sexual activity is not limited by age. Women can experience the four phases of sexual response (excitement, plateau, orgasm, and resolution) despite aging changes. Limitations may occur because of poor physical health, attitude, and lack of an effective sexual partner.
- Occasionally, older women may experience discomfort during intercourse because of decreased vaginal lubrication. A lubricant such as K-Y jelly can relieve this problem.

BIBLIOGRAPHY • Gynecology

BOOKS

Brunner L, Suddarth D: Textbook of Medical-Surgical Nursing, 5th ed. Philadelphia, JB Lippincott, 1984

Brunner L, Suddarth D: The Lippincott Manual of Nursing Practice, 3rd ed. Philadelphia, JB Lippincott, 1982

Hawkins J, Higgins L: Maternity and Gynecological Nursing. Philadelphia, JB Lippincott, 1981

Krupp M, Chatton M: Current Medical Diagnosis and Treatment, 22nd ed. Los Altos, Lange Medical Publications, 1983

Phipps W, Long B, Woods N: Medical-Surgical Nursing: Concepts and Clinical Practice, 2nd ed. St Louis, Mosby, 1983

JOURNALS

Bernhard L; Endometriosis. JOGN Nurs 11(5):300, Sept/Oct 1982

Burchell R, Harris B, Marik J: Hysterectomy: For whom, when, how? Patient Care 14(11):16, June 15, 1980

Garline L, Stebauer C: What every nurse should know about vaginitis. Am J Nurs 82(2):1851, Dec 1982

Holden L: Helping your patient through her hysterectomy. RN 46(9):42, Sept 1983

Iveson-Iveson J: Background to acute salpingitis. Nurs Mirror 150(17):33, April 24, 1980

Patterson J: Colposcopy. JOGN Nurs 12(1):11, Jan/Feb 1983

Ritchie M: Total hysterectomy and bilateral salpingo-oophorectomy for endometriosis. Nurs Times 76(26):1133, June 26, 1980

Wheeler J, Malinak L: Recurrent endometriosis: Incidence, management and progress. JOGN/Nurs 146(2):247, June 1983

INTEGUMENTARY SYSTEM

BURNS

Description

Burns are produced by thermal, chemical, electrical, or radiation actions on the body that result in varying degrees of destruction at the points of contact. Electrical burns also cause internal damage resulting from the electrical current flow within the body. All chemical burns should be flooded with a hose or shower for 10 to 15 minutes to remove the chemical. If a chemical powder is present, brush it off before flooding the area with water. The severity of an external burn is described as first, second, or third degree.

First-degree burns are superficial but painful. A sunburn is a good example of this type of burn. There is no systemic reaction unless the burn is extensive, and then nausea, vomiting, and elevated temperature may be present.

Second-degree burns resemble a severe, painful sunburn accompanied by blisters and swelling. There are often areas of broken skin, and the underlying surface usually is wet. The epidermis (first layer of skin) and part of the dermis (second layer) are affected, making it a partial-thickness burn. These burns will blanche with pressure.

Third-degree burns appear as dry and leathery, white or charred, and painless areas involving the epidermis, dermis, and subcutaneous tissue. These full-thickness burns destroy the nerve endings, sweat glands, and hair follicles, and require skin grafts. These burns will not blanche with pressure.

Observations

- Hoarseness, inspiratory wheezing, stridor, and labored breathing indicating edema of the respiratory tract. This may occur anytime within 24 hours following smoke inhalation, and may require a tracheal intubation. Arterial blood gases are monitored carefully. (see NR, arterial blood gases). Change in the patient's level of consciousness is an indicator of hypoxia. In children, frantic behavior is often the response to hypoxia.
- Severe, generalized edema is caused by plasma shifting from capillaries to interstitial space after second- and third-degree burns. This is called "burn shock" and is seen during the first 48 hours following burn injury, but it is greatest in the first 8 hours to 12 hours.
- The amount and color of urine must be monitored. Output must be maintained at 30 ml to 60 ml per hour in adults and 0.5 ml to 1 ml/kg body weight in children. Red or hematuric urine may indicate hemochromogens in the urine, which may cause renal failure.
- Cardiac irregularities resulting from electrical burns with current passing through the heart or electrolyte imbalances may occur. Sodium and potassium levels should be monitored closely. Initial levels often reverse within the first 48 hours after injury. Digitalis toxicity may result if a patient is receiving digitalis.
- A tourniquet effect on the hands and feet, the result of circumferential, full-thickness burns of the arms and legs, may be seen. Peripheral pulses should be checked every hour with an ultrasonic doppler. Call the physician immediately if a pulse cannot be detected.
- Difficulty in breathing may result from restricted respiratory movement caused by circumferential burns of the chest. Call the physician immediately.
- There is extreme pain in partial-thickness burns, but often no

pain, at first, in full-thickness burns because the nerve endings are destroyed.

- Look for paralytic ileus when second- or third-degree burns cover more than 20% of the body surface. Check for bowel sounds every two hours.
- Gastrointestinal bleeding is a real possibility with burn patients because of Curling's ulcer, a duodenal ulcer specific to burn patients. All stools and nasogastric aspirant should be tested for occult blood.
- Burn wound sepsis is indicated by chills, change in level of consciousness, and a very high or abnormally low temperature. Report these findings to the physician immediately. After the first 72 hours, sepsis is the leading cause of death in burn patients.
- Wound infections become apparent by increased redness around the burn area, change in color or odor, increase of drainage, and temperature changes. Report these findings immediately.
- Bacterial pneumonia is a common cause of respiratory failure in pediatric burn patients.
- Electrical burns usually have two external sites, one entering and one leaving the body. The area of superficial injury is usually smaller than the internal injury. Internal hemorrhage and fractures are possible following electrical burns. The severity of damage to internal organs or to muscles may require an immediate operation (*e.g.,* fasciotomy, amputation, or colostomy).
- There may be increased blood and urine glucose levels without any history of diabetes. This is the body's response to stress, and the patient may require insulin for a short period of time. However, young children may develop hypoglycemia during their recovery if their body's high metabolic needs are not being met.
- The development of hypertension in pediatric burn patients is not unusual. It is controlled with appropriate antihypertension medication.

Treatment

- Intravenous fluids must be started immediately to replace circulating volume and electrolyte loss (see NR, Intravenous therapy). Initially, Lactated Ringer's solution is the solution of choice. A large vein and a large-bore needle suitable for high-volume fluid infusion is necessary. The amount, pH, and specific gravity of urine are major determinants for the type, amount, and rate of infusion of IV fluids. An indwelling catheter connected to a drainage bag equipped for hourly urine measurement is essential (see NR, Urinary Bladder catheterization and drainage). A central venous pressure line (see NR, Central venous pressure) or pulmonary artery catheter may be inserted to determine cardiac status and to avoid hypovolemia or fluid overload while delivering the high volumes of IV solutions needed by some patients with major burns.

- Oxygen is given by high-humidity face mask or tent to increase moisture in the respiratory tract, particularly in the presence of singed nasal hairs or mouth, which indicate smoke inhalation. (see NR, Oxygen administration).
- The upper extremities with a burn injury are elevated above the level of the heart to prevent severe edema from developing.
- Blood, urine, sputum, and the burn wound (after washing) are cultured on admission, and then usually every two days to three days to identify and treat pathogens. Surgical incision in burned tissue (escharotomy) may be performed to relieve constricton affecting circulation or respiration.
- A nasogastric tube may be inserted to prevent gastric distention because peristalsis often slows or stops after severe burns (see NR, Gastrointestinal intubation). Paralytic ileus is common. Antacids are commonly given every 1 hour to 2 hours to prevent Curling's ulcer, depending on the gastric pH, and the presence or absence of occult blood.
- The burn area is washed aseptically with warm, sterile saline or water mixed with any standard surgical soap or an antimicrobial agent, *e.g.*, povidone-iodine (Betadine), and then rinsed with warm sterile saline or water. Wearing sterile gloves, apply an antimicrobial ointment or cream, *e.g.*, silver sulfadiazine (Silvadene) to a one-eighth inch thickness. The ointment or cream also may be impregnated in gauze and then applied (see PH). Gauze soaked in a prescribed solution (*e.g.*, silver nitrate solution) and moistened frequently also may be used. Wet dressings are essential for burns that expose tendons, bones, or cartilage.
- Wet-to-dry dressings are used to aid in removing eschar (burned tissue) (see MSN Decubitus Ulcers, prevention and treatment).
- Know the possible systemic and local reactions to the topical medications.

Nursing Considerations

- It is crucial to determine the patient's pre-burn weight on admission and then daily thereafter (without dressings), because this is a factor in determining IV therapy.
- Burns of the face, neck, and head that have occurred in an enclosed area or have resulted in unconsciousness increase the probability of respiratory failure secondary to smoke inhalation. Look for singed nasal hairs, soot around the mouth or in the sputum, or respiratory distress. Pulmonary injury is a major cause of death after serious burns.
- Keep the patient in a supine position, suction as necessary, turn, have the patient cough, and reposition every hour.

- Dressing changes should be done as quickly and efficiently as possible. It is absolutely necessary that impeccable sterile technique be used. Gloves, gown, mask, and hair cap always are worn during dressing changes.
- The policy of individual institutions will determine whether burn wound care is to be carried out uncovered or covered with appropriate procedures. Uncovered burn wounds increase the risk of infection, increase fluid loss, decrease body temperature, and increase pain to patients. These patients are very sensitive to low room temperature. Conversely, when over 30% of the burn wounds are covered with dressings, impairment of heat loss and decreased mobility of the covered part occurs.
- Burn-wound care is directed toward maintaining a clean eschar (burned tissue), which gradually falls away or is surgically removed, allowing new skin to form or grafting to be done.
- Medicate for pain (usually IV) before starting wound care. Always access respiratory and neurologic status of the patient before giving narcotics.
- At least once each day, burn-wound care should be done when the physician is there to see the condition of the wound.
- Patients with circulatory problems and diabetes and those on steroids or chemotherapy have delayed healing ability.
- There is a very high demand for protein in the healing process of burns. When they are able to eat, patients require 2 to 2.5 times the normal intake of protein and calories. Keep a daily calorie count. Hyperalimentation and nasogastric tube feedings are used either in place of, or as a supplement to, oral intake.
- Partial-thickness burns that become infected can convert to full-thickness burns.
- Burns in the perineal area require special attention to maintain cleanliness.
- The position of the patient must be changed hourly to relieve pressure on burned areas. The limbs should be positioned to avoid contractures, and the hands and feet should be splinted in the position of function. Care must be taken not to inadvertently create a decubitus ulcer while using splints. Range of motion (ROM) exercises are extremely important. They are begun immediately and usually are done during dressing changes. (See NR, Range of motion exercises.)
- Newly healed, burned skin is easily injured and sunburned.
- The nurse is with the patient for long periods and should be a careful observer of changes. Each time the wound is redressed, the color, extent of granulation, sensation, tenderness, and odor should be documented, and changes should be reported to the physician.

- Burns do not cause the patient to become unconscious. Look for other reasons if this happens (*e.g.*, head injury).
- The extent of the burned area can be quickly estimated by the "rule of nines." (Fig. 4-8)
- Burns are considered to be major if more than 25% of the total body surface area in adults is involved and 20% in children. Patients under 2 years of age or over 60 of age, or those with an associated trauma, are considered poor-risk patients.
- Burns of the face, neck, hands, feet, and perineum always are considered major, as are electrical burns and those involving smoke inhalation.
- Burn patients are frequently in the hospital for long periods of time and require care that is very painful. Their personalities may change drastically, with periods of depression and apathy.
- A nursing-care plan that lists step-by-step care must be prepared and updated every 24 hours.

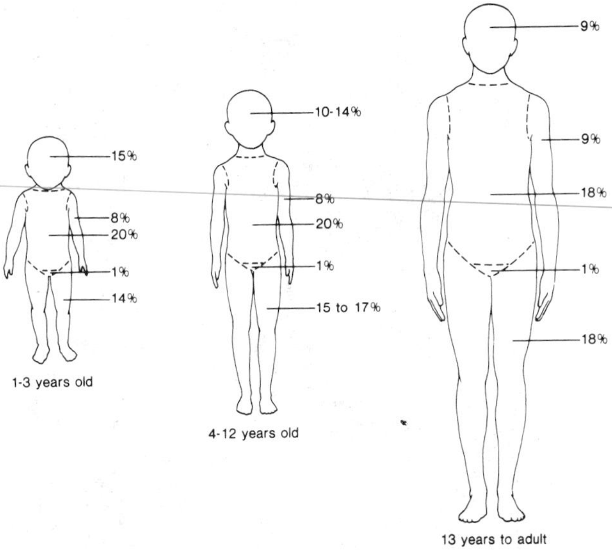

Fig. 4-8. *Method of estimating percentage of body surface covered by burns. Note that body propertions differ in infants and children. In adults, the method is known as the "Rule of Nines," since the percentages are all multiples of nine.*

DECUBITUS ULCERS

Description

A decubitus ulcer (pressure sore, bedsore) is the result of skin breakdown and subsequent necrosis of underlying tissue, fat, and muscle. The usual cause is a sustained pressure (two or more hours) on the skin surface, resulting in an interruption of the blood supply.

Observations

- Reddened area of skin that blanches with pressure
- Cyanotic area of skin that does not blanche with pressure
- Blistered area of skin, signifying necrosis of superficial layers of underlying tissue
- Open necrotic area of deep tissue, which is very susceptible to infection
- Casts or braces that rub and cause skin irritations
- Common sites are indicated in Figure 4-9.

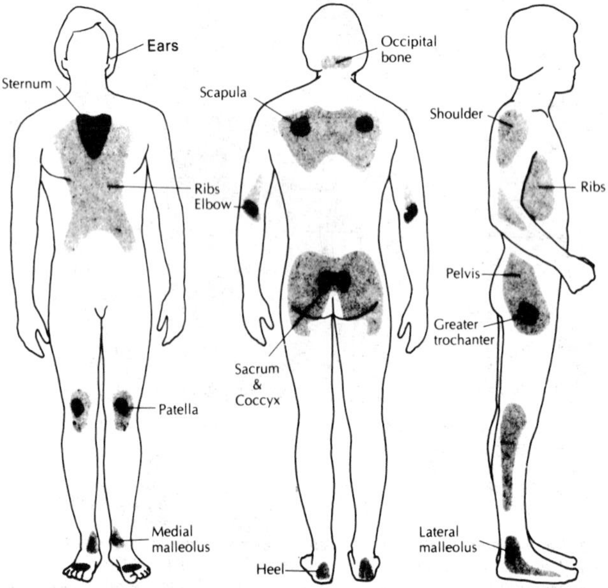

Fig. 4-9. *Sites of potential pressure sores.*

Prevention and Treatment

- Prevention is much easier than actual treatment. Also, treatment is very costly in terms of time, energy, and money.
- When possible, ensure frequent patient ambulation (10 minutes every 2 hours), and prevent sitting for more than 2 hours.
- Encourage strict adherence to a 2-hour turning schedule if the patient is bedridden. Once a reddened area is noted, turning should be done every hour followed by proper positioning

For Reddened or Cyanotic Unbroken Skin: The Pre-ulcer or Stage I

- Gently wash the area, pat thoroughly dry; do not use talcum powder.
- Gently massage around the area; do not use alcohol because it dries the skin, or lanolin, because of a possible allergic reaction. Some caution should be noted against massaging directly over the reddened area because injury to subcutaneous fat and muscle already has occurred.
- Use foam-rubber padding, cut to encircle the area. Several pieces of foam rubber may be stacked together to provide more relief from pressure. The wider the piece of cushioning material used, the more evenly the weight will be distributed.
- It is important to avoid pressure, friction, and moisture on the damaged area.
- Place a floatation or eggcrate mattress on the bed and reposition patient every hour.

For Broken Skin/Blister Without Necrosis: Stage II

- Continue treatment as described above for the surrounding, unbroken skin area; however, if drainage is present, absorption of drainage is necessary.
- Continue to relieve the pressure on the area.
- Use aseptic technique in tending broken skin areas.
- Consult with the physician on the advisability of flushing with an antiseptic cleaning agent, *e.g.*, providone-iodine (Betadine), followed with a saline irrigation to eliminate the possibility of irritation.
- At this stage, a patch, such as Duoderm, may be used to cover the cleaned and dried, nondraining abrasion and may be a totally effective treatment. This is a sterile dressing that provides a moist environment and does not displace new tissue when removed. It will also protect that area from contamination.
- One of the many healing agents that absorb drainage also may be used. They usually are applied every 8 hours after cleaning

and drying the area, and a light dressing is applied. Some of these agents are karaya powder, which also stimulates granulation tissue; Debrisan beads; and plain sugar, which is often mixed with betadine.

- An occlusive dressing, using polyurethane adhesive membrane (*e.g.,* Op-Site, Tegaderm) to form a second skin, may be used. This is applied over the decubitus ulcer after the area is cleaned and the surrounding area is dry. It serves as a permanent dressing until healing occurs. It is believed that healing occurs fastest in a moist environment. The serous exudate that collects is kept in place, thereby promoting healing. Ideally, the membrane should not be removed until healing occurs, but the accumulation of fluid may dislodge it. "Picture framing" the dressing with silk tape helps prevent the film from lifting up.
- In high drainage areas where a polyurethane adhesive membrane is inappropriate (*e.g.,* in areas where there is no healthy tissue to adhere to or too much drainage to keep intact), a product like Bard Absorption dressing is useful. It cleans the area while providing a moist environment.

For Broken Skin with Necrosis: Stage III with Extension of Necrosis into the Muscle: Stage IV, Destruction of Soft Tissue with Bone Exposure

- Continue treatment as described above for the surrounding, unbroken skin area, but surgical debridement is necessary for some necrotic decubitus ulcers. The wound will not heal until the eschar is either softened, sloughed, or removed. In some cases, debridement may be achieved using a Water Pik or whirlpool bath.
- Use aseptic technique in caring for the ulcer.
- Consult with an enterostomal therapist or the physician for specific treatment orders.
- A wound culture should be obtained to determine the appropriate antimicrobial agent, if infection is present. Watch for the warning signs of infection: redness of the surrounding tissue, increased drainage, and odor after cleaning.
- Wash the decubitus ulcer with normal saline, one-half strength hydrogen peroxide, or povidone-iodine (Betadine) to clean and debride necrotic tissue. Whenever these last two agents are used, flush them off with normal saline, and pat the area dry with sterile gauze.
- In some cases, special chemical debridement procedures may be adequate. Instructions for the use of enzymes (*e.g.,* Collagenase, Travase) for cleaning and debridement, must be read carefully. These medications should not come in contact with normal skin. Discontinue as soon as necrotic area is clean. They are applied once a day.

- Wet-to-dry dressings may be used for debridement and to eliminate infections. Aseptic technique always is used. Soak single layers of noncotton sterile gauze with a prescribed sterile solution and squeeze the excess out. Pack this gently into the wound, covering all exposed surfaces. Apply a thin layer of dry sterile gauze, and finish with a 4-inch × 8-inch full thickness of sterile gauze (do not use the thick ABD pads). Tape only around the edges so that the gauze will dry. With this treatment, the dressing should be dry in 6 hours to 8 hours. When the dry gauze is removed, necrotic tissue will be caught in the mesh and will be removed. The disadvantage is that newly formed skin also may be pulled away.
- If the area is infected, an appropriate antimicrobial agent often is applied after debridement.

Nursing Considerations

- Good nutrition is the first line of defense against skin breakdown, and is absolutely essential for healing. Protein loss from a weeping decubitus ulcer may be as high as 50 g/day. If the patient is not eating, other means of providing nutrition must be provided, *e.g.*, nasogastric feeding, hyperalimentation.
- A nursing-care plan, with step-by-step directions, is essential for continuity of care in the treatment of a decubitus ulcer. The care must be appropriately and consistently carried out by all nursing-care givers.
- Any immobilized, incontinent, or edematous patient is at high risk for decubitus ulcers. Additionally, patients receiving narcotics for pain or sleep medications are not sensitive to pressure discomfort. Diabetic patients and those who are immunosuppressed should be watched because of their increased susceptibility to skin breakdown.
- Pressure on any skin area for more than 2 hours will cause a loss of blood supply at the center of the pressure area and increase vulnerability to decubitus ulcers. The use of an alternating pressure or eggcrate mattress does not eliminate the need for turning and proper positioning.
- Turn any immobilized patient every 2 hours, or more frequently, depending on the skin condition. This should follow a sequence of right side, back, left side, abdomen. The patient often is not able to tolerate the abdominal position for 2 hours.
- Use pillows to position a patient in bed, relieving the pressure on bony prominences; maintain the feet in dorsiflexion and the wrists in a straight position.
- Look carefully at the patient's position before leaving the bedside. Place your hand under bony prominences. Do you feel pres-

sure? Ask yourself: Does the position achieve the desired effect? Is it comfortable? Is the position likely to be maintained?

- Post a chart at the patient's bedside with a turning rotation schedule (Fig. 4-10). Sometimes, a total change in position is impossible, but ROM exercises can be done, and pressure points can be relieved. Note this on the chart. Use the following for making notes: RS = right side; B = back; LS = left side; A = abdomen; and ROM = range of motion. Under comments, note the patient's intolerance to any position
- Do not schedule position changes at a change of shift.
- Lift, do not drag, the patient up in bed.
- Prolonged wheelchair sitting also causes pressure sores. Be sure a pad (*e.g.*, eggcrate or floatation) is placed on the seat. Patients must also shift their weight every 15 minutes to 20 minutes.
- Inflatable pressure mattresses must be semiinflated before placing the patient on them. Overinflation can cause increased pressure on the skin.
- Do not pull sheets tight over eggcrate mattresses.
- Cotton bath blankets can be used to cover plastic mattress covers and to absorb perspiration.
- Elderly patients do not require a daily bath. Their bath water may have an oil added to prevent dry skin if they are not allergic to

12^M Position, Comment	Initial
2	
4	
6	
8	
10	
12^N	
2	
4	
6	
8	
10	

Fig. 4-10. *Sample chart for turning rotation schedule to avoid pressure sores.*

these lubricants. Dry skin is conducive to skin breakdown. Vaseline is an excellent lubricant.

- Give a backrub at least once a day and include all the bony prominences. When a lotion is used, thoroughly rub it into the skin to avoid leaving a wet surface. Do not use talcum powder; however, cornstarch is acceptable. Remove crumbs and foreign objects from the bed, and tighten the bottom sheet.
- Some patients are allergic to chemical detergents used in washing linens, and this results in skin breakdown.
- Keep the patient's heels from rubbing on the mattress by placing a folded blanket under the lower leg, or by using heel protectors.
- Never allow the legs to rest on top of one another or on top of drainage tubing. Use a pillow or folded blanket to prevent pressure.
- Moisture is a major factor in causing skin breakdown. Be sure that urine and feces are completely washed off the skin of incontinent patients. Ideally, perianal care should be done every two hours. When the skin is excoriated, avoid using soap, and pat dry or use a hair dryer (set on cool setting) to completely dry the skin. A product such as Peri-wash is very useful in cleaning the skin of incontinent patients.
- When a 2-hour toileting routine is not possible, the only alternative is to keep the skin as clean and dry as possible. The prolonged use of indwelling catheters almost always leads to UTI.
- A Stryker frame, Circ-O-lectric, or Clinitron bed may be used when it is impossible to otherwise relieve pressure on skin areas.
- Enterostomal therapists often are referred to as "the skin-care specialists." Consult with them for skin-care problems.
- Physicians usually will follow the nurse's suggestions for effective decubital treatment.
- Read the package insert on any preparation specifically for decubitus ulcer care. Special wound-cleaning procedures may need to be followed.
- Topical applications of ointments containing debriding agents also are used in treating leg ulcers.

SHINGLES (HERPES ZOSTER)

Description

Shingles occurs most frequently in adults, and is caused by the same virus, VZ (varicella zoster) that causes chickenpox. It is a reactivation of a latent VZ virus. Skin eruptions appear in crops, spreading on one side of the body, following nerve pathways, most frequently on the trunk or the face.

Observations

- Localized pain and itching that exist for 3 days to 4 days, followed by the appearance of grouped vesicles on a reddened base. These eruptions change to crust-covered lesions within a few days. New eruptions may continue to appear for a period of 2 weeks, gradually healing in 2 weeks to 3 weeks. Swollen regional lymph nodes may be present.
- Herpetic skin eruptions on the face may indicate involvement of the fifth cranial nerve, which can cause permanent blindness; temporary facial paralysis may result from seventh cranial nerve involvement.
- Pain can persist for months and years along the affected nerve pathways, even though visual evidence of the disease has vanished. This is called post-herpetic neuralgia.
- Secondary bacterial infection of the lesions is not uncommon; pneumonia and encephalitis are rare complications.
- This disease can be fatal in immunosuppressed patients.

Treatment

- Cold, wet compresses may give temporary relief of the itching. Analgesics for pain control and antihistamines also are used.

Nursing Considerations

- There is usually moderate to severe pain with this disease. Often, these patients cannot tolerate any covering on the affected area, and any body movement is painful.
- Elderly patients with this disease may be very ill; hospitalization may be required in severe cases.
- This disease is considered infectious until all the lesions are dried (see NR, Infection Control); exposure may cause chickenpox in those not immune to it.

NORMAL AGING CHANGES IN THE INTEGUMENTARY SYSTEM

- When studying normal aging changes of the skin, the cumulative effects of wind, sun, and abrasion also must be considered.
- The skin characteristically becomes wrinkled, dry, and sagging.
- The epidermis, the outer layer of the skin, exhibits a decreased rate of cell division with aging. Replacement of damaged or dead cells is diminished. The melanocytes or pigment cells decrease in number and tend to be larger. They aggregate and form the pigment plaques that are seen in some older people.

- Age-related changes in the dermis are responsible for wrinkling and sagging. Elastin becomes coarse, cross-linked, and calcified. Fat and water content diminish, and collagen content changes. There is a decrease in the number of capillary loops and other blood vessels in the superficial dermis, as well as a decrease in nerve cells.
- Sweat glands atrophy, diminish in number, and experience an accumulation of lipofuscin pigment. Older persons experience a decreased output of sweat.
- The hair generally becomes sparser and turns gray. The reduction in pigment content usually begins in the late thirties or early forties and starts in the temple region. However, there is wide variation in the rate, onset, and extent of graying among individuals. The density of hair follicles decreases with age. Baldness is both genetically determined and age-related, and begins earlier in life. Baldness does progress with age, is rare in women, and proceeds with a slow recession of the anterior hair line.
- The nails become duller, more opaque, ridged, and yellowish to greenish or gray. Rate of growth decreases and the nails are more prone to splitting into layers.

Implications

- The aging changes in the epidermis will appear more pronounced in the areas most exposed to the environment (*e.g.*, face, neck, upper portion of chest, and dorsal surfaces of the hands and forearms).
- The skin, hair, and nails are the parts of the body most visible to others. Changes perceived as unattractive by the individual may lower self-esteem and cause the older person to avoid contact with other people.
- The pigment accumulations that occur most often on the face and the backs of the hands have no pathologic significance.
- The cosmetic implications of hair loss and color change may be of great concern to older people. Women also can experience an increase in facial hair, and men may have hair growth in their ears and nares.
- Dermal blood vessels become fragile and damage easily. Areas of bruising or purpura occur on the forearms and the backs of the hands from minimal pressure. Care must be taken when assisting an older individual with activities such as transfers and ambulation.
- Because of collagen changes in the dermal layer, tissue resiliency is decreased and the skin does not return to a normal position as quickly. This should be considered when assessing hydration and skin turgor.

- Older individuals frequently experience problems with dry skin. The skin is less efficient in retaining water, output from sweat glands is decreased, and protective lipids are washed away with soap and water. Skin dryness may be minimized by using soap only in the axillary and genital areas and rinsing well, using tepid rather than hot water for bathing, bathing less frequently, and applying a nonperfumed emollient that contains lanolin to the skin immediately following washing.
- Many lotions on the market contain alcohol and may contribute to skin dryness. Encourage individuals to read the labels and purchase products with minimal or no alcohol (*e.g.,* Kerilotion, Lubriderm).
- Cotton undergarments and increased moisture in the environment (*e.g.,* from humidifiers or pans of water over heating elements) also can decrease dryness problems.
- Increased variations in temperature regulation can occur because of skin changes. Hats, gloves, knit undergarments, and wool outer garments can help minimize heat loss in cold weather. Socks and sheet blankets add to comfort at night. High winds further stress adaptive mechanisms and should be avoided when possible. Hats and other protective clothing are useful on hot days, and outdoor work should be avoided during the hottest parts of the day.
- The older person may experience diminished sensitivity to touch, pressure, pain, and local temperature changes. Pressure areas must be watched carefully, and the use of heating pads, ice packs, and water bottles should be monitored.
- If touch is acceptable to the elderly person, it is an excellent way to reduce feelings of isolation and increase sensory input.

BIBLIOGRAPHY • Integumentary System

Burns

BOOKS

Hammond B, Lee G: Quick Reference to Emergency Nursing, pp 105-119. Philadelphia JB Lippincott, 1984

Wachtel T, Kahn V, Frank H: Current Topics in Burn Care. Rockville MD, Aspen Systems, 1983

JOURNALS

Braen GR: Minor Burns, Evaluation and Treatment. American College of Emergency Physicians, Marion Laboratories, Sept 1979

Dyer C: Burn care in the emergent period. J Emerg Nurs 6(1):9 Jan/Feb 1980

Head J: Inhalation injury in burns. Am J Surg 139(4):508. Apr 1980

Hurt R: More than skin deep: Guidelines on caring for the burn patient. Nursing '85, 15(6):52 1985

Kinzie V, Lau C: What to do for the severely burned. RN 43(4):47, Apr 1980
Lushbaugh M: Critical care of the child with burns. Nurs Clin North Am 16(4):635, Dec 1981
Martin M, Hanson A: Internal conductors: How to assess burn severity. Occup Health Saf 50(12):31, Dec 1981
Marvin J, Einfeld L: Infection control for the burn patient. Nurs Clin North Am 15(1):833, Dec 1980
Pruitt B: Early burn care. Consultant 21(11):192, Nov 1981
Schumann L, Gaston S: Commonsense guide to topical burn therapy. Nursing '79 9(3):34, Mar 1979
Van Oss S: Emergency burn care; Those crucial first minutes. RN 45(10):44, Oct 1982
Woolridge-King M: Nursing considerations of the burned patient during the emergent period. Heart Lung 11(4):356, July/Aug 1982

CONFERENCE

Treatment of Burns, Sibley Hospital Inservice, June 11, 1980 Wash DC

MSN

Decubitus Ulcers

BOOKS

Hebert P, Allerescu V: Pressure necrosis,. In Broadwell D, Jackson B (eds): Principles of Ostomy Care. St Louis, CV Mosby, 1982

JOURNALS

Ahmed M: Op site for decubitus care. Am J Nurs 82(1):61, Jan 1982
Arnell I: Treating decubitus ulcers: Two methods that work. Nursing 13(6):50, June 1983
Cameron G: Pressure sores: What to do when prevention fails. Nursing '79 9(1): 43, Jan 1979
Cooper-Smith F: Prevention of pressure sores. Nurs Times 75:1294, Aug 2, 1979
Cosman B, Freed M, Sparks S: Decubitus ulcers, where healing parallels preventions. Patient Care 16(15):58, Sept 15, 1982
Elliott T: Pressure ulcerations. Fam Physician 25(2):171, Feb 1982
Feustel D: Pressure sore prevention aye, there's the rub. Nursing '82 12(4):78, Apr 1982
Friedman F (ed): An innovation in decubitus treatment sparks debate. RN 45(2):46, Feb 1982
Mangieri D: Saving your elderly patients' skin. Nursing '82 12(10):44, Oct 1982
Snowden D: Decubitus ulcer. Nurs Mirror 148:26, Feb 1, 1979
Woodbine A: Pressure sores, a review of the problem. Nurs Times 75:1087, June 28, 1979

Normal Aging Changes in the Integumentary System

Finch C, Hayflick L (eds): Handbook of the Biology of Aging. New York, Van Nostrand Reinhold, 1977
Reff M, Schneider E: Biological Markers of Aging. U.S. Department of Health and Human Services, 1982 (NIH Publication No. 82-2221)
Rockstein M, Sussman M: Biology of Aging. Belmont, Wadsworth Publishing, 1979

MUSCULOSKELETAL SYSTEM

AMPUTATION

Description

Complications of peripheral vascular disorders and diabetes, trauma, malignant bone tumors, osteomyelitis, and congenital defects may be indications for amputation of all or part of an extremity.

The following are common abbreviations indicating the level of amputation: BK, below the knee; AK, above the knee; BE below the elbow; and AE, above the elbow. A Syme amputation removes the foot at the ankle joint, including the malleoli.

Long-range goals following amputation include proper fit of the prosthesis and rehabilitation of the patient both physically and psychologically.

Common Diagnostic Tests

- X-rays, bone scans (See NR, X-rays and scans.)
- Arteriography and oscillometric readings for evaluation of circulatory status
- Doppler (See NR, Ultrasound.)

Observations

Preoperative

- Changes in skin temperature, color, and pulses in both the affected and unaffected extremities must be checked. Assess when the limb is in both elevated and dependent position.
- Signs of gangrene: color changes (redness to black); skin may appear dry and wrinkled, especially in diabetes and peripheral vascular disease (see MSN, Diabetes, and MSN, Arterial occlusive diseases of the lower extremities).

Postoperative

- Watch for signs of hemorrhage, infection, and edema; later, watch for irritation on the stump (stumps of patients with diabetes or vascular problems are subject to wound separation and decubitus ulcer formation).

- Skin may break down on the heel of the normal foot because the patient uses it to push himself or herself up in bed.

Treatment

- Closed amputation (flap method): The skin flap covers the stump.
- Open amputation: The stump is left open to provide for drainage, especially when there is vascular impairment. Skin traction may be applied. The wound is closed days to weeks later.
- Immediate temporary prosthesis: A rigid dressing technique may be used.
  1. A plaster cast is applied to the stump in the operating room following the amputation. A pylon device (a prosthetic extension) with an artificial foot is incorporated into the cast (see Fig. 4-11).
  2. This technique allows for almost immediate mobility and early gait training, prevents edema, and reduces pain.
- The level of amputation is determined by adequacy of circulation, considerations regarding type of prosthesis that may be used, and future usefulness of the extremity.

MSN

Nursing Considerations

Preoperative

- Psychological preparation focusing on what the patient will be able to do, is important if there is time. Emotional support is needed.
- The prosthetist (the person who creates and supervises the use of the prosthesis) may visit the patient, if requested by the surgeon.
- Exercises initiated and supervised by physiotherapist
  1. Push-ups to strengthen the triceps in preparation for crutch walking
  2. Use of the trapeze
  3. Isometric abdominal-tightening exercises
  4. In an upper-extremity amputation, muscle-setting and joint-mobilizing exercises of both shoulders
  5. Practice in transferring (moving) from bed to chair

Postoperative

- Hemorrhage is the greatest danger.
  1. Assess frequently for oozing on the dressing. Mark it. A portable wound suction system, such as a Hemovac, may be used immediately postoperatively.

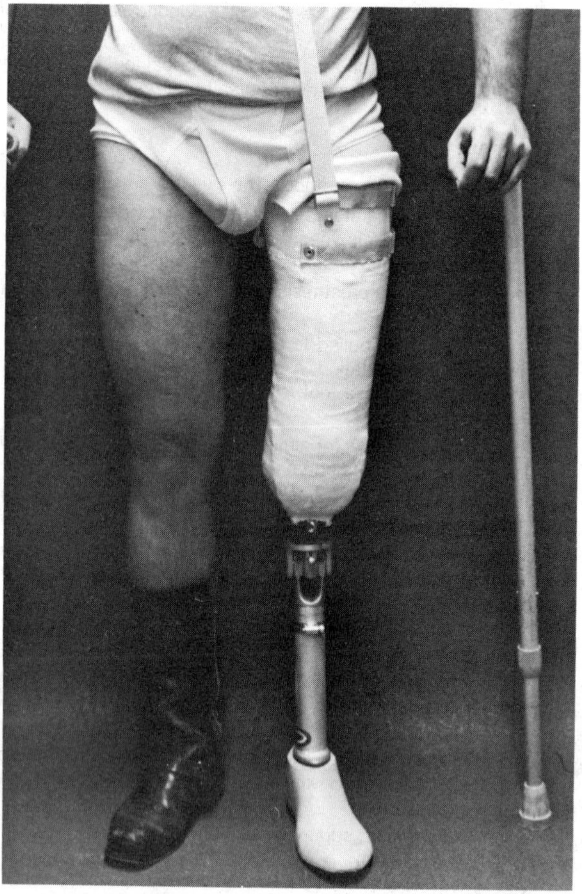

Fig. 4-11. Immediate, temporary prosthetic fitting (pylon) used following amputation. (Courtesy of the Prosthetic Research Study, Veterans Administration Contract V663P-784).

2. *Caution:* Bright red bleeding is not normal. Apply pressure dressing and elevate stump by raising foot of bed. Notify the surgeon immediately.
3. Keep large blood pressure cuff at bedside for emergency use as a tourniquet in case of sudden hemorrhage.
4. Check vital signs frequently, especially during the first 48

hours, for signs of shock and hemorrhage (see MSN, Postoperative care).

- Prevent edema, which occurs most during first 24 hours postoperatively. A heavy cast or pressure dressing is applied in surgery.
  1. Elevate the stump of the leg by elevating the foot of bed. (Avoid contractures. Pillows never are placed under an AK stump, and only if knee is extended for a BK one.)
  2. Ice bags can be applied to the part, only if ordered.
- Pain relief
  1. "Phantom limb sensation" is common; it lessens with activity, exercise, and weight-bearing.
  2. "Phantom limb pain" is uncommon; described as a burning, crushing kind of pain, it may be lessened by weight-bearing, if allowed. Other treatment may include whirlpool, massage, injection of the stump with a local anesthetic, sympathectomy, and transcutaneous electric nerve stimulation (TENS).
  3. Neuroma, in which there is scar formation on severed nerves, may cause great pain and require excision.
  4. Frequently, patients who have had gangrene feel surprisingly little pain after amputation.
- Infection
  1. Suspect infection if a bad odor comes from the stump dressing or cast, or if the patient's temperature elevates.
  2. Treatment may include antibiotics, elevation of the stump (by elevating the foot of bed in leg amputation), hot packs, incision and drainage, and possible reamputation at a higher level.
- Psychological support: Expect a grieving process, especially when amputation is the result of trauma. Referral to amputee support group may be indicated.
- An exercise program usually is initiated by a physiotherapist. It will commonly include the following objectives:
  1. Prevent contractures, particularly of hip, knee, and elbow.
     a. Prone position with head turned away from the affected side for 30 minutes, three or four times a day.
     b. Traction, trochanter rolls, and a firm mattress may keep the body in alignment while the patient is in bed. Avoid abduction of the hip.
     c. No prolonged sitting; no pillow under knee or under AK stump.
     d. Range of motion (ROM) exercise (See NR, ROM exercises.)
  2. Prepare for use of prosthesis, for crutch walking, and for transferring to a wheelchair, if the patient is not to get prosthesis.
  3. Assist in developing balance.

- Stump care
  1. Stump treatment will depend upon the patient's condition and the requirements of the anticipated prosthesis. Approaches include the following:
     a. Compression dressing with elastic bandage
     b. Skin traction for open amputation, with closure later
     c. Immediate temporary prosthesis: plaster cast with prosthetic extension and artificial foot (Fig. 4-11)
  2. The stump is bandaged after the wound has healed to shrink and shape the stump to a tapered, rounded, smooth end in preparation for the prosthesis (Fig. 4-12).
     a. A clean elastic bandage or stump shrinker should be used each day.
     b. While the joint above the amputation is extended, the bandage should be wrapped smoothly, applying even, moderate tension to all parts of the stump. Rewrap as needed to maintain continuous pressure. Avoid a tourniquet-like effect caused by too much pressure or circular turns. Use an oblique, modified, figure-eight pattern.
  3. Stump conditioning (ordered by the physician)
     a. Check the stump every day for minor irritations and edema, indications that the wrapping has been done incorrectly.
     b. Gently massage to increase the circulation; this may be started 5 days to 7 days postoperatively.
     c. Push the stump of a leg against increasingly harder surfaces to prepare for prosthesis.
  4. To maintain good condition of the stump, protocols vary slightly, but usually include patient instructions similar to the following:
     a. Wash stump with soap and water every night. Rinse and dry thoroughly. Use a mirror to observe incision and entire stump. Check for irritations and edema. Expose to air and sun when possible.
     b. Prosthetic socket for stump should be washed every night and left open to air.

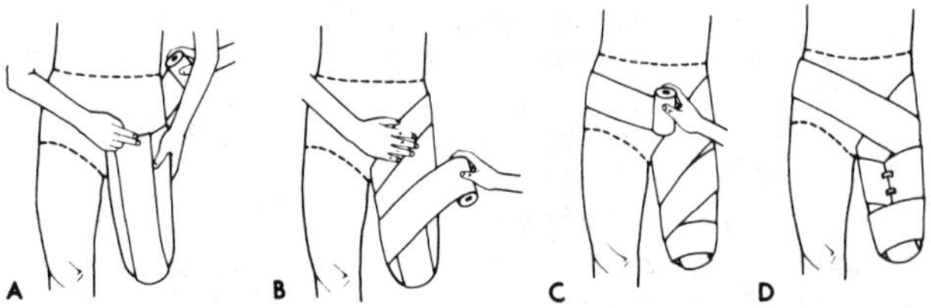

Fig. 4-12. *Method for bandaging an above-the-knee amputation stump.*

   c. Stump socks and stump wrapping should be clean every day. Wash and dry flat. Sock should be made of wool. Have several on hand so that there is time for thorough drying between washings. Never wear a mended sock.
   d. Avoid wearing shoes with unevenly worn heels.
   e. The stump may shrink for up to 2 years after surgery, so the prosthesis will need adjustment, as it will in growing children.
5. Immediate, temporary prosthesis with rigid dressing technique
   a. The cast will be changed at intervals two or three times before the stump is measured for a permanent prosthesis.
   b. Too much weight-bearing can disrupt healing, but controlled, progressive ambulation is allowed.
   c. *Caution:* If the cast comes off, wrap stump immediately with an elastic bandage and notify the surgeon. Edema could develop very rapidly.
   d. Pylon may be removed from the socket when the patient is in bed.
   e. Check skin condition around cast.
   f. Severe or increasing stump pain or odor coming from the cast should be reported.

ARTHRITIS

Description

Arthritis is defined as an inflammation of a joint, frequently the synovial membrane lining, in which there is usually pain and often eventual structural change. Its many causes include excessive joint use or trauma; autoimmune factors; and metabolic, vascular, infectious, or neoplastic disorders. Because of the wide variety of causes and presentation of symptoms, classification of arthritis and related rheumatic disorders is difficult. They are sometimes called connective or collagen diseases. In this reference, we will consider gouty arthritis, osteoarthritis, and rheumatoid arthritis, the most common types. Elements of nursing care of patients with inflamed joints have many common factors, regardless of the etiology of the arthritis.

GOUTY ARTHRITIS

Description

Gout or gouty arthritis occurs when there is an accumulation of urate deposits in the joint. Blood elevation of uric acid (hyperuricemia) usually occurs at the same time.

Primarily a genetic defect in purine metabolism, hyperuricemia also may occur secondarily in other situations in which there is an overproduction or underexcretion of uric acid, *e.g.*, in leukemia, multiple myeloma, and psoriasis, after prolonged use of diurectics (particularly the thiazides), and in certain cancer chemotherapies. The appearance of symptoms is directly related to the duration and degree of hyperuricemia.

It is characterized by acute inflammation of usually one joint with tophi (subcutaneous urate deposits) formation, and later by chronic deforming arthritis. Ninety percent of patients with gout are men, usually over 30 years old. Kidney stone formation leading to chronic renal disease may also occur.

Common Diagnostic Tests

- Urate crystals are found in synovial fluid aspirated from joint cavity.
- X-rays of affected joints, in the chronic disease, show tophi and destructive joint disease.
- Serum uric acid levels usually are elevated, unless the patient is taking uricosuric drugs.

Observations

- Sudden onset of acute extreme pain, accompanied by redness, warmth, swelling, and tenderness in one or more joints (most commonly the great toe or the knee), is characteristic. With treatment, it usually lasts a few days.
- Fever, headache, malaise, anorexia, and tachycardia during an acute attack are common, as is desquamation and pruritus after an attack.
- Asymptomatic periods commonly follow the initial acute attack.
- Tophi may be found in external ears, hands, feet, and prepatellar bursas, usually only after several attacks of acute arthritis.
- Permanent deformity with functional loss may be seen in patients with chronic gout.
- Signs and symptoms of renal stones (See MSN, Urinary calculi.)

Treatment

Acute Attacks

- Colchicine should be given IV or PO, at the first signs of impending attack and every 1 hour to 2 hours until the pain is relieved or until nausea, vomiting, and diarrhea appear.
- Nonsteroid anti-inflammatory drugs, *e.g.*, indomethacin (Indocin), phenylbutazone (Butazolidin), and ibuprofen (Motrin) may be given (see PH).
- Corticotropin (ACTH) and corticosteroids may be ordered.

- Narcotics and analgesics may be needed until other therapies provide relief.
- Bedrest should be continued for 24 hours after the acute attack has subsided.
  1. Provide a cradle to keep bedding off affected joint.
- Elevation of the joint and hot or cold compresses may provide comfort.
- Force fluids to promote urate excretion.

Prophylactic Treatment (Between Attacks)

- Uricosuric medications may increase excretion of uric acid, *e.g.*, probenecid (Benemid) and sulfinpyrazone (Anturane) (see PH).
  1. Salicylates antagonize the uricosuric effects of probenecid and sulfinpyrazone. They should not be used together. Acetaminophen (Tylenol) may be used.
  2. Force fluids to prevent high concentrations of urinary urates.
  3. Sodium bicarbonate may be ordered to maintain alkaline urine.
- Allopurinol (Zyloprim) inhibits uric acid synthesis (see PH).

MSN

Nursing Considerations

- During an acute attack, relieve pain, administer medications as ordered, monitor the effects of colchicine (if ordered), protect affected joint, and force fluids.
- Patient teaching to prevent recurrent attacks includes the following tips:
  1. Slow weight reduction is recommended for the obese patient to reduce strain on joints, but fasting should be avoided because it increases serum uric acid.
  2. The patient should avoid foods or situations that precipitate attacks. Foods high in purine (*e.g.,* organ meats, shellfish, anchovies, sardines, and meat extracts) usually are to be avoided.
  3. Alcohol usually is restricted to one or two cocktails a week.
  4. The patient should wear comfortable shoes with adequate toe room.
  5. The patient should understand the importance of taking medications as prescribed. He or she also should be aware of possible side-effects and special precautions associated with them.

OSTEOARTHRITIS

Description

Osteoarthritis is a degenerative joint disease (DJD), characterized by destruction of the joint cartilage and overgrowth of bone, causing impaired function. Sometimes called hypertrophic arthritis, it usually is associated with the aging process, but may be secondary to trauma or other arthropathies. DJD most commonly affects weight-bearing joints.

Common Diagnostic Tests

- X-ray shows characteristic narrowing of joint space and osteophyte or spur (bony outgrowth) formation.
- Sedimentation rate and aspirated synovial fluid usually are normal.

Observations

- Gradual onset of joint pain with motion; stiffness following inactivity, with gradual limits in motion
- Joint tenderness with gradual joint enlargement
- Crepitus (joint noise on motion caused by diseased cartilage, bone, or joint lining)
- Heberden's nodes (hard nodules and enlargement of the distal finger joints)
- Bouchard's nodes (nodules in the proximal interphalangeal joints)
- Joint involvement tends to be localized in one or a few joints. Most commonly affected are the distal finger joints, the hips, the knees, and the spine.

Treatment

- Rest the affected joints. This may involve use of cane, crutches, traction, or splints.
- Weight reduction in obese patients
- Moist heat to the affected joint; physiotherapy
- Progressive exercises, especially isometrics
- Nonsteroidal anti-inflammatory drugs (*e.g.*, salicylates)
- Mild analgesics for relief of pain.
- Interarticular corticosteroids: very effective for occasional use in acute inflammatory flare-ups
- Surgery, joint replacement (See MSN, Joint replacement.)
- Osteotomy or joint fusion may benefit an older patient whose joint damage is moderate.

Nursing Considerations

- Encourage activity and ROM exercises (see NR, Range of motion exercises). Urge the patient to avoid insults to joints or activities that precipitate flare-ups (*e.g.*, heavy lifting).

- Provide emotional support and measures that are ordered for the relief of chronic pain (see MSN, Pain Management).
- Encourage compliance with prescribed treatment.
- A bed cradle may provide comfort by keeping top covers off of the affected joint.
- Follow specifics of care following surgical treatment, such as joint replacement (see MSN, Joint replacement).

RHEUMATOID ARTHRITIS

Description

Rheumatoid arthritis (RA) is a chronic, systemic disease characterized by exacerbations and remissions. Thought by many to be an autoimmune disorder, it usually is manifested by symmetrical involvement of peripheral joints, starting with inflammation of the synovium (lining of the joint), and sometimes progressing to the destruction of the joint. Generalized symptoms may be present. A disease usually of moderately young adults (around 35 to 40 years of age), it is three times more common in women than in men.

When RA appears in young children, it is called Still's disease or juvenile rheumatoid arthritis.

Common Diagnostic Tests

- See LAB for normal values.
- Complete blood count (CBC)
- Hemoglobin depressed; usually below 10 g/dl
- Elevated white blood cell (WBC) count
- Elevated sedimentation rate
- Latex fixation test for the rheumatoid factor (RF): Presence of RFs helps confirm diagnosis if clinical picture is present.
- Synovial fluid aspirated from joint: viscosity poor, WBCs elevated
- Characteristic histological appearance of RA nodules from joints and subcutaneous areas
- X-rays of the joints
- Scans, especially with technetium; a gallium scan may be used for further study (see NR, Nuclear scans).

Observations

- There usually is a history of abrupt onset of inflammation in multiple joints or of gradual progressive joint involvement. This may be accompanied by low-grade fever, fatigue, anorexia, and weight loss. Family history of RA usually is present.
  1. Morning stiffness, gradually diminishing with activity

2. Pain and tenderness of joints, usually symmetrical involvement
3. Soft swelling of joint with redness, warmth, and subcutaneous nodules (rheumatic nodules), found especially over bony prominences
4. The hands often show involvement of proximal interphalangeal or metacarpophalangeal (knuckle) joints, or both, with swan neck deformities of the fingers, muscle wasting, and ulnar deviation of fingers (fingers drift away from thumb).
5. Involvement of wrists, feet, ankles, and elbows also is typical, although other joints may be involved.

- If the disease process continues, the end-result may be instability and subluxation (partial or incomplete dislocation) of joints.
- Systemic changes may include pulmonary changes that must be differentiated from carcinoma (*e.g.,* pleural effusion, fibrosis, nodules), pericarditis, leg ulcers caused by vasculitis, enlargement of the spleen, and carpal tunnel syndrome.
  1. Sjögren's syndrome (dry eyes because of insufficient tearing, dry mouth) may appear in advanced RA.

Treatment

The goal is to prevent deformity and disability.

Drug Therapy

- Nonsteroidal anti-inflammatory drugs (See PH.)
  1. Acetylsalicylic acid (aspirin) in high doses must be continued even during periods of remission. Enteric-coated aspirin (Ecotrin) may be ordered for h.s.
  2. Ibuprofen (Motrin), naproxen (Naprosyn), indomethacin (Indocin), phenylbutazone (Butazolidin), or others may be tried (see PH).
- Specific drugs (See PH.)
  1. Gold salts, *e.g.,* gold sodium thiomalate (Myochrysine)
  2. Penicillamine (Cuprimine)
  3. Antimalarial agents, *e.g.,* hydroxychloroquine (Plaquenil) and chloroquine phosphate (Aralen)
  4. Immunosuppressant drugs, *e.g.,* Azathioprine (Imuran)
  5. Cytotoxic agents: cyclophosphamide (Cytoxan) or methotrexate, which is sometimes tried as a last resort
  6. Corticosteroids

     These are used systemically only in acute flare-ups, and are not for long-term use.

     Intra-articular injections may relieve pain and improve mobility in selected joints.

Physiotherapy

- An exercise program is devised by the physiotherapist based on patient's condition. The program will avoid strain on joints and may emphasize isometrics and hydrotherapy.
- Joints should be put through a full ROM several times every day (see NR, Range of motion exercises).
- Heat treatment: Moist heat preferred. It may include moist hot packs, warm tub baths, and warm paraffin applications (usually done before exercises).
- Cold applications may be tried when heat increases pain.

Rest for Inflamed Joints; General Bodyrest

- Bedrest may be indicated in acute stages, although exercises should be continued. Avoid flexion contractures by not placing any pillows under the patient's knees or large pillows under the head. Have the patient lie prone several times a day.
- Splints or traction may rest inflamed joints and provide proper alignment.
- Orthopedic shoes may help decrease metatarsophalangeal joint pain on weight-bearing.

Surgery

- Synovectomy may produce pain relief and prevent tissue destruction.
- Arthrodesis: fusion of a joint to provide stability
- Joint replacements (*e.g.*, total hip replacement) (See MSN, Orthopedics, Joint replacement.)

Nursing Considerations

- Provide emotional support for the patient who is experiencing pain and potential body changes that may be deforming and disabling. Use a positive approach, working with the patient's hope to live as normal a life as possible.
- Stress faithful adherence to the individualized rehabilitation program.
- Help the patient develop a plan to avoid stress and to rest before he or she becomes tired. Joint pain for longer than one hour following an activity indicates that the activity should be restricted or eliminated.
- An occupational therapist may provide specific tips regarding ways to protect joints while performing activities of daily living, including use of self-help devices.
- Provide patient education regarding prescribed medications and their potential side-effects.

- Local arthritis associations may be sources of both information and support.

Sources of Patient Information

- National Institute of Arthritis, Metabolism and Digestive Diseases, National Institutes of Health, Bethesda, Maryland 20205
- Arthritis Foundation, 1314 Spring Street, NE, Atlanta, Georgia 30309. Telephone (404) 872-7100 or local chapters. Excellent booklets and pamphlets for patients are available.

CHEMONUCLEOLYSIS

Description

In chemonucleolysis, chymopapain (Chymodiactin), a purified enzyme of the papaya plant, is injected into a herniated disk. The enzyme causes hydrolysis of the proteins, decreasing their water-binding capacity in the nucleus pulposus (inner disk material), thus decreasing its size, and therefore the intradiscal pressure. The treatment is being used as an alternative to laminectomy in patients with herniated discs who do not respond to conservative treatment. It is done with a fluoroscope in the operating room. Improvement in symptoms is seen in approximately 75% of these patients.

Chemonucleolysis is contraindicated in children or when there is a rapidly increasing neurologic deficit, any bladder or bowel dysfunction, pregnancy, a sedimentation rate greater than 20 in women, a history of allergy to papaya derivatives (*e.g.*, meat tenderizer), previous treatment with chymopapain, extensive lumbar spondylosis or stenosis, or previous surgery in that area.

Common Diagnostic Tests

- X-ray, sometimes with contrast myelography
- CT scan
- Electromyography
- Chemofast antigen test—a blood test to detect possible allergic reaction to the enzyme

Observations

- A history of allergy to any papaya derivative (*e.g.*, meat tenderizer), is a contraindication for this treatment.

Pre-injection

- The patient has the following signs and symptoms of a herniated disc.

1. Severe unrelieved leg pain (sciatica)
2. Backache that is exacerbated by increased intra-abdominal pressure with coughing, sneezing, and movement
3. No response to conservative treatment—bedrest, traction, analgesics, physiotherapy, and a firm mattress
4. Continued signs of nerve-root irritation, *e.g.*, positive straight leg raising test

Postinjection

- Although back spasms usually improve 10 days to 3 weeks postinjection, back pain and stiffness often take several weeks to subside.
- Signs of allergic reaction to chymopapain ranging from rash, urticaria, edema, and nausea, vomiting, and diarrhea, to anaphylaxis with respiratory distress and vascular collapse (profound hypotension, arrhythmias, loss of consciousness,and cardiac arrest) may occur. The first 2.5 hours are considered most critical, but symptoms may occur up until 24 hours postinjection.
- Neurologic deficits, especially the inability to void, loss of bowel or bladder control, or numbness or tingling in the extremities may be present.

Nursing Considerations

Preoperative

- Anticipate that cimetidine (Tagamet), benadryl, and solucortef may be ordered to minimize or prevent anaphylactic reaction to the enzyme.

Postoperative

- Expect wide variations in response to chemonucleolysis. Stiffness and soreness may continue for several weeks.
- Bedrest usually is ordered from 4 hours to 48 hours, depending upon the physician's preference and the patient's comfort and ability to void.
- A semi-Fowler's or side-lying position is usually most comfortable immediately postinjection.
- Narcotic analgesics for pain usually are required.
- Muscle relaxants may be ordered.
- Ambulation may be delayed until severe pain and muscle spasms pass.
- Heat, warm showers, or ice massage may relieve discomfort.
- Occasionally, physiotherapy or therapy in Hubbard tank may be ordered.

- Good body mechanics
  1. Patients should be taught to get out of bed from a side-lying position with their knees together.
  2. When standing, the patient should rest the affected leg as much as possible.
  3. Sitting should be limited to 20 minutes to 30 minutes at a time in a firm, straight-backed chair.
  4. Bending and lifting should be avoided for several weeks.
  5. A back brace or corset may be ordered.
  6. Exercises may be prescribed after 3 weeks.
- Discharge is usually 48 hours to 72 hours after injection.

FAT EMBOLISM

Description

Following injury, particularly of the long bones and the pelvis, fat cells leave the bone and go into the bloodstream, causing occlusion of small blood vessels in distant organs, especially the lungs, brain, and kidneys. Most common in young adults, the onset of this syndrome may appear 12 hours to 36 hours after trauma, or up to two weeks later.

Common Diagnostic Tests

- Arterial blood gases (ABGs) (See LAB.)
- Chest x-ray
- Urinalysis for fat; decreased hemoglobin and platelets
- Elevated serum lipase
- ECG changes (See NR, ECG.)

Observations

- Sudden, steady rise in pulse, respiratory rate, and temperature
- Respiratory distress and dyspnea
- Bizarre mental symptoms: confusion, disorientation, mild agitation, and coma (related to reduced oxygen to brain)
- Petechiae over the anterior aspect of the chest, shoulders, conjunctival sacs, and buccal membranes
- Increased weakness

Treatment

- Oxygen therapy (See NR, Oxygen administration.)
- Elevation of the head of bed if no signs of shock are present

- Controlled volume ventilation with positive end-expiratory pressure (PEEP)
- Steroids
- Low-molecular-weight dextran (See NR, Intravenous therapy.)
- Heparin (See PH.)
- Antihyperlipemics
- IV fluids; blood transfusions (See NR, Intravenous therapy.)

Nursing Considerations

- Try to prevent fat embolism by gentle, proper handling of the injured part.
- Never massage the affected limb.

FRACTURES

Description

A fracture is a break in a bone. An open or compound fracture is one in which there is direct continuity between the fracture and a break in the skin. It is always considered infected (see MSN, Open fracture).

Common Diagnostic Tests

- X-ray
- Scan (see NR, Scans)
- Routine urine and blood work preoperatively may include typing and cross-matching.
- Hemoglobin and hematocrit usually are repeated 3 days or 4 days postoperatively.
- Serum calcium may be ordered (see LAB).

Observations

- Pain or tenderness at the site, which increases with pressure or movement
- Deformity of the part
    1. Muscle spasm may cause shortening of a limb.
    2. Changes in contour or alignment.
- Swelling: usually rapid over the fracture; possibility of some bruising
- Numbness, tingling, and, occasionally, paralysis
- Abnormal mobility

- Crepitation: grating sound when ends of bones move against each other
- Signs of visceral (internal) injury
  1. Hemoptysis (bloody sputum) may result from injury to the lungs caused by fractured ribs
  2. Oliguria or anuria or blood in the urine may result from injury to the urethra or bladder by fractured pelvis. (Oliguria or anuria also is seen in shock.)
- Sign and symptoms of complications

Treatment

- Reduction: replacement of bone fragments into normal position
  1. Traction: may be temporary before internal fixation of fracture, or may be the definitive treatment (Skeletal traction requires surgical placement of a pin.)
  2. Closed reduction (without surgery)
  3. Open reduction: surgical reduction with use of plates, nails, screws, wires, and rods for stabilization
- Immobilization (to maintain reduction)
  1. Splints
  2. Cast or cast brace (See NR, Cast brace; Cast care.)
  3. Continuous traction (See NR, Traction.)
  4. Internal fixation with plates, nails, screws, and so forth
  5. External fixation device (See NR, External fixation device.)
  6. Bandages of muslin or elastic (*e.g,* Velpeau's bandage for fracture of scapula, clavicle, and humerus)
- Rehabilitation, including physiotherapy, and training to resume activities of daily living
- Non-union or delayed union (a complication seen after months or even years) may be treated by
  1. Bone grafts
  2. Electronic bone stimulator
     a. Bone formation is stimulated by directing electricity at the non-union site and by placing negative electrodes (cathodes) near it.
     b. Present devices may be noninvasive, semi-invasive, or totally invasive (surgically implanted).
     c. The limb is immobilized with a cast.
     d. An anode pad is placed on the patient's skin near the cast.
     e. Physician's orders should specify nursing responsibilities for the care of the patient and the specific type of stimulator being used.

3. Magnetic stimulator
   a. A total immobilizing cast is applied.
   b. A piece of plastic on the cast marks the location for removable magnetic coils used for a specific total time per day, usually 10 hours.
   c. With evidence of healing over months, weight-bearing or function is increased.

- A replacement head of the femur may be required for avascular necrosis, (death of a tissue resulting from a decreased blood supply). This is rather common, in capsular fractures of the femur.

Nursing Considerations

See also NR, Traction; Casts; Cast brace; External fixation device; and MSN, Fat embolism; Open fractures.

Preoperative

- A preparation with antibacterial scrub may be ordered. Shaving usually is done in the operating room.
- Acquaint the patient with traction equipment.
- Have the patient practice voiding while in a recumbent position so that he or she will know how to do this postoperatively.

Postoperative

- See MSN, Postoperative care.
- Turn the patient to the unaffected side, unless otherwise ordered.
- Early ambulation is desirable when possible. However, this must be ordered by a physician.
- Watch for urinary retention.
- Be alert for the following complications; try to prevent them.
  1. Shock and hemorrhage (See MSN, Postoperative care.)
     a. Assess vital signs frequently until they are stable.
     b. Check the dressing or cast for evidence of bleeding. Run your hand underneath to be sure that the blood is not pooling there.
     c. Look for changes in the circumference of the limb (*e.g.*, swelling).
     d. Blood loss may be high, especially in cases of fracture of the femur. Blood volume should be replaced appropriately.
  2. Circulatory impairment, if present, may be due to arterial blockage or to swelling in a confined space *(compartment syndrome).* It constitutes a medical emergency because, if unrelieved, it can lead to permanent disability, *Volkmann's contracture,* within a few hours.

a. Check every digit of the affected limb for color, pulses, and skin temperature every 2 hours or as ordered, especially during the first 24 hours post-trauma or postoperatively. If there is any doubt about the presence of pulses, use a Doppler.

b. Pain usually decreases after reduction. Any increase should be reported immediately. Pain, paresthesia (tingling, numbness, difference in sensation), pallor (blanching, usually indicating arterial impairment; cyanosis, indicating venous impairment), peripheral pulselessness, abnormal coolness, or paralysis (difficulty in movement) should be reported immediately.

c. The cascade of events in *compartment syndrome* must be recognized before permanent damage occurs:

Increasing pain, with motor function intact

Severe pain with decreased motor function

Severe pain with no motor function, but sensation and pulses in extremities may still be intact (passive stretching, such as flexion/extension of fingers or toes, is very painful)

Sensation disappears

Loss of pulse (by now the muscle is probably already dead, unless the onset was within 4 hours)

3. Neurologic impairment

   a. Check for sensory disturbances and loss of motion.

   b. The area over the peroneal nerve (3 inches below the knee on its outer aspect) must be kept free from pressure.

4. Muscle spasm

   a. Prevent spasm by changing the patient's position frequently and by keeping pressure off the limb.

   b. Skeletal muscle relaxants, *e.g.*, carisoprodol (Soma), chlorzoxazone (Paraflex), and methocarbamol (Roboxin), may be ordered.

   c. Benedryl at bedtime also may be helpful (see PH).

5. Anemia

   a. Hemoglobin and hematocrit tests usually are ordered 3 days or 4 days postoperatively. Blood transfusions or iron supplements may be ordered.

6. Fat embolism (See MSN, Fat embolism.)

7. Infection (especially common following open fractures)

   a. Maintain sterile technique when dressing wounds.

   b. Provide regular pin care, as ordered or according to hospital policy, when the patient has skeletal traction or external fixation.

8. Thrombophlebitis (See MSN, Postoperative care.)
   a. Any respiratory distress in patients with injuries to the lower extremities should be considered pulmonary embolism until proven otherwise.
9. Disseminated intravascular coagulation (DIC)
10. Problems of immobilization
    a. Renal calculi and urinary tract infections are possible (see MSN, Urinary calculi and urinary tract infections).
    b. Respiratory problems (*e.g.,* hypostatic pneumonia) may occur (see MSN, Pneumonia and NR, Deep breathing techniques).
    c. Decubitus ulcers must be prevented. Inspect all pressure areas, especially the heels and coccyx. Keep the patient's heels from resting on the bed (see MSN, Decubitus ulcer prevention and treatment).
    d. Contractures may occur.

    For hip fractures, lower the head of the bed several times a day to permit extension of the hip.

    The knee tends to flex when there is pain in the hip. Do not support the knee with a pillow.

HIP FRACTURES

Description

Intracapsular hip fractures occur within the hip joint or capsule, near the head or through the neck of the femur. Extracapsular fractures are those occurring outside the joint and capsule in the area of the greater or lesser trochanter. They may be referred to as trochanteric fractures.

These hip fractures, which occur most often in the elderly, require special management because of frequently concurring medical, physical, and age-related problems. Early ambulation and restoration of daily living activities, when possible, are high priorities in treatment.

Common Diagnostic Tests

- See Fractures, common diagnostic tests.
- Type and cross-match blood. Usually, reservation of packed cells is ordered.

Observations

- The affected leg usually is shortened and externally rotated.
- Pain and inability to move the leg are present.

- Slight pain in the groin or the inner side of the knee may be the only symptoms of an impacted fracture.

Treatment

Preoperative

(To reduce pain and muscle spasm)

- Buck's extension traction, especially for subcapital fractures (See NR, Traction.)
- Russell's traction, for intertrochanteric or subtrochanteric fractures (See NR, Traction.)
- Trochanter rolls to maintain alignment of leg (Fig. 4-13)
- Anticoagulant therapy may be initiated.

Surgical

- Internal fixation of the reduced fracture with nails, screws, plates, and pins
- Replacement of the femoral head with a prosthesis; used frequently in intracapsular fractures where nonunion and avascular necrosis are frequent complications of internal fixation techniques
- Total hip replacement on occasion (See MSN, Total hip replacement.)

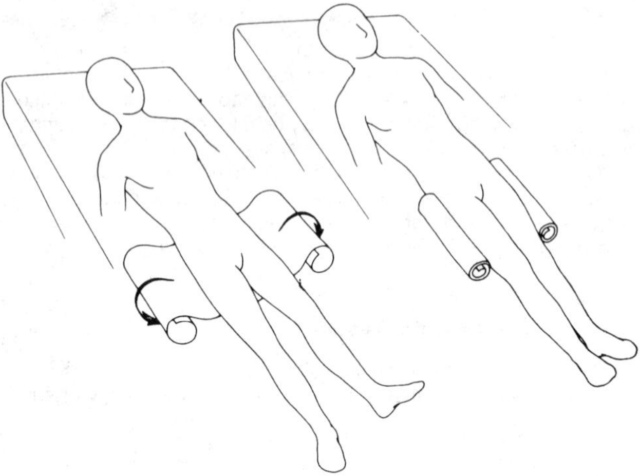

Fig. 4-13. *Method of making trochanter rolls to support the patient's legs and prevent them from rotating outward.*

Nursing Considerations

- See MSN, Fractures; Nursing considerations, and NR, Traction.
- Specifics of patient care must be ordered by the surgeon, but the following are general principles for care of patient who has had internal fixation of a hip fracture:
  1. Antiembolism stockings
  2. Turning
     a. Initially, the patient usually may be turned gently to the unaffected side with a pillow between the legs to maintain abduction of the affected leg. Turning to the affected side eventually will be permitted.
  3. Positioning of affected leg as ordered
     a. Use a trochanter roll (Fig. 4-13) or sandbags to maintain alignment. Prevent hip and knee flexion deformities by lowering the head of the bed several times a day; no pillow shound be under the knees. Generally, avoid flexing the affected hip immediately postoperatively.
  4. Exercise
     a. Quadriceps setting, arm and shoulder strengthening (use of overhead trapeze), range of motion, and isometric muscle exercises of the abdomen and gluteal muscles usually are encouraged.
  5. Early transfer to chair with weight on unaffected leg
     a. The knee should be flexed at a 90° angle while the patient is in the chair.
  6. Early ambulation with a walker, usually with no or partial weight-bearing.
  7. See Nursing considerations under Total Hip Replacement for the patient with a prosthesis.
- Watch for complications (see Fractures, Nursing considerations).
  1. Bleeding is rather common.
     a. Closed drainage suction (*e.g.*, Hemovac) may be in place for the first 24 hours to 48 hours.
     b. Hemoglobin and hematocrit measurements will be repeated.
     c. Packed cells usually are kept on reserve.
  2. Confusion, particularly in elderly injured patients, is common.
     a. Preoperatively, assess mental awareness and orientation of the patient.
     b. Increased confusion may indicate stress reaction, but may also indicate blood loss, embolism, stroke, or medication reaction (see MSN, Disoriented patients).

OPEN (COMPOUND) FRACTURES

Description

In an open fracture there is an open wound directly contiguous to the fracture, through which a fragment of bone may protrude. The wound always is considered infected, and there are additional dangers of osteomyelitis, gas gangrene and tetanus.

Common Diagnostic Tests

- X-ray and scans (See NR, Nuclear scans.)
- Routine urine and blood work, preoperatively; may include typing and cross-matching
- Wound culture for bacteria and sensitivity (See LAB.)

Treatment

- The wound is cleaned and debrided in the operating room.
- For reduction and stabilization of the fracture, external fixation is being used with increasing frequency. (See NR, External fixation device).
- The wound may be left open until there is no sign of infection.
  1. Frequent sterile dressing changes will be required.
  2. Wound and skin precautions must be followed (see NR, Infection control).
  3. The wound will be closed later by suture or grafts.
- Tetanus prophylaxis is recommended.
- IV antibiotics may be ordered

Nursing Considerations

- Check distal pulses. Observe for circulatory and neurologic impairment (see Fractures, Nursing considerations).
- Check vital signs every 4 hours. Watch for temperature elevation, which is a sign of infection.
- See Nursing considerations under MSN, Fractures, NR, Traction, and NR, External fixation device.

JOINT REPLACEMENT

TOTAL HIP REPLACEMENT

Description

In total hip replacement (THR) two component parts bound firmly in place, usually with bone cement, are implanted in place of the acetabulum and the femoral head and neck. Performed primarily to relieve pain, THR also may restore function to patients with diseased or injured hip joints (*e.g.,* from arthritis or aseptic necrosis of the femoral head). Infection and dislocation of the affected hip are serious complications of THR.

Common Diagnostic Tests

- X-rays
- Preoperative urine and blood work, include typing, cross-matching, and prothrombin time.
- ECG

Treatment

- The surgery involves replacement of hip joint with synthetic components.
- Intravenous antibiotics may be started 24 hours before surgery, and continued several days postoperatively.
- Anticoagulants may be ordered prophylactically to prevent pulmonary embolism.

Nursing Considerations

Preoperative

- Infection is a dreaded complication; report any sign of any infection, *e.g.,* upper respiratory or urinary tract. Should infection occur, surgery may be postponed.
- The skin must be clean and in perfect condition. Antibacterial scrubs of the operative area and antibacterial showers with shampoo usually are ordered. Shaving usually is done in the operating room, unless otherwise ordered.
- Specific preparation regarding what is to be expected postoperatively with THR should accompany general preoperative teaching (see MSN, Preoperative care).

Postoperative

- Provide general postoperative care (see MSN, Postoperative care).
- Blood loss is usually relatively large; replacement may be expected. Be sure blood is on reserve, if ordered. Hemoglobin and hematocrit are frequently ordered for the postoperative evening and the following morning.
- A closed-wound suction drainage unit is frequently in place (*e.g.,* Hemovac). This must be monitored carefully. Report if drainage exceeds 100 ml in 4 hours.

- Check dressings frequently for the amount of drainage. In order to have a basis for comparison, outline the area of visible drainage and record the time on the dressing with a marking pen.
- Ice bags may be ordered for immediate postoperative use.
- Analgesics may be administered for pain the first day or two postoperatively. *Severe pain thereafter indicates that there is a problem.*
- Full-length antiembolic stockings, an overhead frame, and a trapeze usually are ordered.
- The heel of the affected leg must be protected with either a heel protector or a device such as the "leg cradle" (by Zimmer or Spandaid) that keeps the leg in position as well as the heel off of the bed.
- Positioning and limitations of movement are prescribed specifically for the patient by the surgeon. The goal is to prevent dislocation of the affected hip by maintaining it in a position of abduction (outward from the midline), thus avoiding rotation and acute hip flexion. The following tips usually will apply:
  1. An abduction splint or wedge (triangle pillow) is placed between the patient's legs (Fig. 4-14). Straps should be applied loosely enough so that there is no pressure over the peroneal nerve (3 inches below the knee on outer aspect). Traction and pillows between the legs are additional ways of maintaining abduction (see NR, Traction).
  2. Use a trochanter roll (see Fig. 4-13) to prevent too much external rotation of the femur. Toes should point upward.

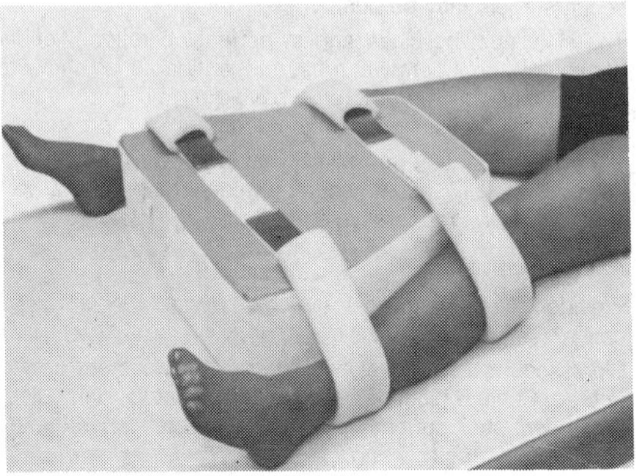

Fig. 4-14. *Abductor pillow.*

3. Flexion of the hip should always be less than 90° to avoid strain on the joint.
   a. At first, the bed may be kept flat most of the time; the head can be raised 45° at mealtime.
   b. When sitting is permitted (for a brief time at first), the seat of the chair or wheelchair should be raised with a pillow. Another pillow should be placed between the patient's legs. The legs must not be crossed.
   c. Provide an elevated toilet seat.
4. When placing the patient on the bed pan, assist him or her, have him or her use the trapeze, and keep the hip in partial flexion. Hyperextension is a common cause of prosthesis dislocation.
5. To prevent adduction of the operated hip when transferring the patient from the bed to a chair, assist the patient to exit with the operative side leading. Do not allow the patient to pivot toward the surgical side. When returning to bed, the operative side leads.
6. Turning toward the affected side (while controversial) seems to be common practice now. The over-riding consideration is that abduction must be maintained. Two nurses are required, because one must support the entire length of the leg in an abducted position. An abductor splint or two pillows should be used.
7. Having the patient lie prone with feet over the end of the bed several times a day or night (to prevent hip flexor tightness) may be ordered by the surgeon 4 days or 5 days postoperatively.

- Exercise programs during the pre- and postoperative period usually are supervised by a physiotherapist. Emphasis is on quadriceps and hamstring setting, ankle pumping (dorsiflexion and plantar flexion), transferring techniques, and walking.
  1. The amount of weight-bearing is prescribed on an individual basis. The patient should wear well-fitting shoes or slippers with nonskid soles.
- Reminders for the patient on discharge usually include the following for the first six weeks:
  1. Roll to the operative side.
  2. No abducting of the hip beyond midline of the body should occur.
     a. Legs should not be crossed.
     b. Sleep with a pillow between the legs.
  3. No hip flexion beyond 90° is allowed.
     a. Continue to raise the seat of the chair, toilet, and car.

b. Driving a car is not allowed until the physician gives permission.

4. Ask the physician for specific advice about sexual intercourse.
5. Notify the orthopedic surgeon of any planned surgical procedures or dental extractions.

Postoperative Complications

- In addition to signs of general postoperative complications (see MSN, Postoperative care and Postoperative complications), watch for the following:
  1. Temperature elevation, and redness or discharge at the wound site, all common indications of infection
  2. Inability to rotate the hip internally or externally, inability to bear weight, shortening of the affected leg, and increased pain, all symptoms of prosthesis dislocation
- Source of patient information
  Arthritis Foundation, 1314 Spring Street, N.E., Atlanta, Georgia 30309, Telephone (404) 872-7100, or local chapters

TOTAL KNEE REPLACEMENT

Description

Total knee replacement is indicated when chronic pain and deformity limit joint function, usually as a result of degenerative joint disease or rheumatoid arthritis (see MSN, Arthritis).

Nursing Considerations

Preoperative

- See MSN, Preoperative care.
- A preoperative program, frequently under the supervision of the physical therapist, usually will include the following:
  1. Isometric quadricep setting, hamstring setting, and straight leg raising
  2. Ankle pumping (dorsiflexion and plantar flexion) and circumduction (right and left)
  3. Instruction in the care and use of the walker, crutches, and cane

Postoperative

- See MSN, Postoperative care.
- Protocols vary with regard to postoperative treatment of the knee itself. Any of the following approaches may be used:
  1. A light cast, which may be split and further spread prn to relieve pressure may be applied (see NR, Cast care).

2. A knee immobilizer, made of heavy canvas material, heavy metal stays, and Velcro straps and buckles that may be adjusted, may be used. There may be prescribed periods of removal.
3. A continuous passive motion (CPM) machine may be applied after surgery to flex and extend the new knee joint automatically.
   a. The leg must be in correct alignment with the machine.
   b. Avoid compromising circulation with the Velcro straps that secure the knee in position.
   c. Be alert for signs of skin breakdown, and report if it is seen.

- Elevate the knee to reduce swelling by elevating the foot of bed. The foot should be level with or higher than the knee. The knee should be higher than the heart. Protect the heel from pressure.
- Closed-wound suction (*e.g.*, Hemovac) may collect up to 500 ml drainage in the first 24 hours, but it usually is removed after approximately 48 hours or when drainage has ceased.
- Ice bags to be propped against the sides of the knee frequently are ordered.
- An elastic stocking for the uninvolved leg usually is ordered routinely.
- Guidelines for ambulation and exercise should be followed as ordered. An exercise program such as the one begun preoperatively is vital to maximum success.
- Urge patients to avoid obesity and overactivity, both factors that contribute to prosthesis failure.

MSN

LAMINECTOMY, DISC EXCISION, SPINAL FUSION

Description

Laminectomy, or surgical removal of the lamina (the flattened part on either side of the arch of a vertebra), may be done in any case where exploration of the nerves or spinal cord is indicated, including cases of trauma, suspected tumor, hematoma, or herniated intervertebral disc.

Spinal fusion may be done with laminectomy to stabilize the spine by fusing the remaining posterior spinal elements with a bone graft that usually is taken from the iliac crest, but sometimes from the tibia.

A *ruptured or herniated lumbar intervetebral disc* is frequently the cause of pressure on a spinal nerve or nerves, and may be removed. In the cervical spine, the disc often is removed by an anterior approach so that no laminectomy is required.

Observations

Preoperative

- Pain, paresthesia, and muscle spasm may be present. Record the history so that there is a baseline for postoperative evaluation.
- Function and movement of extremities, bladder, and bowels should be watched.

Postoperative

- Following cervical disc excision, hoarseness and inability to cough effectively may be the result of recurrent laryngeal nerve damage. Slight hoarseness is normal, but any increase should be reported. A sore throat and difficulty in swallowing are fairly common. A sudden return of pain may mean that the spine has become unstable.
- Following lumbar disc excision, check vital signs frequently. Check dressing for signs of hemorrhage. Check lower extremities for sensation, movement, color, and temperature. Check for urinary retention, bowel control, or sensation. Changes in bowel and bladder control represent a surgical emergency, and must be reported immediately.

Nursing Considerations

Cervical Disc Excision with or without Cervical Laminectomy

- A cool, mist vaporizer frequently is ordered.
- Support the patient's head when he or she gets up. Apply a cervical brace or soft collar to support the head and neck, if ordered.

Lumbar Laminectomy with or without Spinal Fusion

PREOPERATIVE

- Teach "log rolling" (turning body as a unit), deep breathing (see NR, Deep breathing techniques), and muscle-setting exercises.

POSTOPERATIVE

- Two people turn the patient as a unit (log rolling). The patient's knees should be flexed with a pillow between them. A turn sheet may be used.
- Position the patient according to the surgeon's orders, usually with a pillow under the head and with slight knee flexion, while the patient is on his or her back. The back must be kept in alignment in all positions.
- Relieve pain and anxiety with analgesics, as ordered.
- Early ambulation usually is encouraged in patients with laminectomy. The patient will require assistance in keeping the back

straight and in rising smoothly. Keep the bed elevated. Patients with spinal fusions should not bear weight until ordered.

- Watch the dressing for signs of hemorrhage or leakage of cerebrospinal fluid (CSF) which is more common after spinal fusion. Check any clear drainage for glucose with a Dextrostix reagent strip. CSF contains glucose and normal urine does not. Report apparent leakage of CSF immediately. Keep the patient at bedrest.
- A lumbar brace frequently is ordered.
- Recovery following spinal fusion takes longer than recovery from laminectomy or disc excision, and requires the following additional elements of care:
  1. Monitor vital signs frequently postoperatively.
  2. Closed drainage suction (*e.g.*, Hemovac) is frequently in place. Notify the surgeon if drainage exceeds 100 ml every 3 hours to 4 hours.
  3. Care for the site of graft removal.
  4. Bedrest 2 days or 3 days postoperatively usually is ordered. Prolonged sitting should be avoided.

MENISCECTOMY AND LIGAMENTOUS REPAIR OF THE KNEE

Description

The meniscus, a crescent-shaped cartilage, attaches to the capsule of the knee and provides for wider weight distribution between the tibia and femur. Total or partial removal of the meniscus is done to treat tears that causes pain, locking (limitation of motion), or persistent swelling. Repair of torn ligaments may or may not accompany meniscectomy.

If ligamentous or meniscal repair is not required, the meniscectomy often is done arthroscopically. The arthroscope, therefore, is both a diagnostic and surgical tool.

Common Diagnostic Tests

For Internal Derangements of the Knee Joint

- Arthroscopy
- Arthrography using single or double-contrast media

Observations

In Injuries to the Menisci

- Pain and swelling, usually severe at onset, are present following injury.

- Atrophy of the quadriceps may develop if the condition persists.
- True locking, or inability to fully flex or extend the knee, may occur.

Nursing Considerations

- Orders concerning the amount of flexion and weight-bearing vary according to the type of surgery. The following tips usually apply.
  1. Compression dressing usually is used. Only elastic wrap should be redone. Any sign of drainage should be reported to the surgeon immediately.
  2. An immobilization splint or cast may be applied (see NR, Cast care).
  3. Elevate the limb postoperatively.
  4. Quadriceps strengthening exercises may be ordered. Straight leg raising with weights often is prescribed.
  5. Pain resulting from postoperative exercise is not uncommon.
  6. Watch for complications (*e.g.,* thromboembolism, infection, decreased muscle strength, and recurrent effusions).

OSTEOMYELITIS

Description

Osteomyelitis is an inflammation of the bone, particularly the marrow, often caused by *Staphylococcus aureus,* although other organisms may be causative agents. Infection-causing organisms may enter the bone directly from an open wound or from an adjacent infection; or they may be bloodborne.

Chronic osteomyelitis describes the disease process that continues and fails to respond to normal defense mechanisms or antibiotic therapy. A localized area of pus in the bone (bone abscess) may form. A local area of devitalized bone, a *sequestrum,* often will become apparent. The reactive new bone surrounding the infected one is called *involucrum.*

Common Diagnostic Tests

- See LAB for normal values.
- An elevated WBC count almost always is present.
- The sedimentation rate will be elevated.
- Blood cultures occasionally are positive.
- Specimens are taken of aspirated material from bone or nearby joint for culture and sensitivity (C and S).
- X-rays may or may not show bone involvement.

- Bone scans reveal marked increase in uptake of radionuclear material.

Observations

Acute Osteomyelitis

- Fever and sudden pain in affected bone
- Swelling and tenderness over the bone and painful movement of the adjacent joint
- Later development of swelling over the bone and joint

Chronic Osteomyelitis

- Persisting or recurring bone abscesses that "point" and rupture to produce a sinus tract that drains, at least periodically
- Sudden rises in temperature and new painful areas on bones or joints, indicating extension or formation of secondary abscesses

Treatment

- Complete bedrest may be ordered for patients with acute osteomyelitis.
- Immediate and long-term antibiotic therapy directed against the causative organism may be ordered. It usually is given IV or IM before bone necrosis has taken place, but also may be instilled directly into the wound.
- Sensitivity of the organism to the antibiotic must be tested periodically.
- In addition, chronic osteomyelitis may require the following treatment:
  1. A sequestrectomy, or removal of sequestrum and surrounding new bone (involucrum), sometimes in sufficient amounts to form a saucerlike cavity, may be done. Grafting with bone, skin, or muscle may be done to fill the cavity.
  2. Tubes from closed suction irrigation (*e.g.*, the Jergesen tube system) may be left in the wound after incision and drainage for periodic delivery of antibiotics directly to the infected area of the bone.
  3. Immobilization may be necessary to decrease the pain and muscle spasms.

Nursing Considerations

- Bones and joints require gentle handling. They may be very painful.

- Dressing changes may be frequent. Scrupulous sterile technique is required.
- Wound and skin isolation precautions often are required.

NORMAL AGING CHANGES IN THE MUSCULOSKELETAL SYSTEM

- Aging bone is characterized by demineralization and loss of supporting bone matrix. Calcium leaves the bones and moves into the bloodstream. Total bone mass is less, and the bone becomes increasingly porous and brittle. Bone loss is much greater in women than in men.
- Some degree of collapse of the bones of the spine occurs, thus causing a decrease in height in older individuals. Curvature of the spine (kyphosis) is possible, and there may be a change in the person's center of gravity. Arms and legs may appear longer in relation to the shortened or curved trunk.
- There is a progressive loss of muscle mass with age because muscle fibers are postmitotic and cannot replace themselves.
- Both the diameter and the number of muscle fibers decrease.
- Muscle fibers are replaced by fat and collagen.
- Most enzymes demonstrate a decline in activity with age, especially those involved with the release of energy during contraction.
- The cartilage in joints becomes more yellow, brittle, and may wear away, allowing bone to rub on bone. Extra bone forms and may chip.
- The synovium becomes more rigid as a result of calcium and collagen deposits, and nutrition to the area is reduced. The synovial fluid becomes less viscous and more watery.
- Ligaments lose elasticity and joints become less stable. Slight knee and elbow flexion may occur from the ligament relaxation.

IMPLICATIONS

- The changes with age in the bone structure of an elderly person predispose the individual to a fracture, even following a seemingly "minor" fall. The implications of the immobility resulting from the fracture are very serious. Other systems of the body (*e.g.*, circulatory and respiratory) may have minimal reserve capacity to tolerate the limitations necessary during rehabilitation. Sensory deprivation and isolation may lead to changes in mental alertness and behavior. The loss of functional independence can be devastating to the elderly person, and may necessitate a temporary or permanent change of residence to the home of a relative or to a nursing home.

- There is a progressive loss of muscle strength and speed of movement in aging individuals. There is an increase in reaction time (also resulting from aging changes in the nervous system), and the elderly person may experience muscle fatigue and flaccidity. Impaired muscle coordination also can increase the risk of accidents and injury.
- Exercise is important for people of any age, but can be crucial for the elderly person. Regular, safe exercise can help maintain joint mobility and delay muscle atrophy. Many communities have group exercise programs for the elderly that provide valuable social interaction as well as needed exercise.
- An elderly person may accept or minimize aches and pains as normal and age-related problems because the complaints are common among his cohorts and have developed insidiously. However, the discomforts may indicate a treatable, pathologic problem that should be evaluated. Regular health examinations should be encouraged.

BIBLIOGRAPHY • Musculoskeletal System

BOOKS

Farrell J: Illustrated Guide to Orthopedic Nursing, 2nd ed. Philadelphia, JB Lippincott, 1982

Ferguson A: Orthopaedic Surgery in Infancy and Childhood, Chapter 6. Baltimore, Williams & Wilkins, 1981

Hughes J: Synopsis of Pediatrics, 5th ed. St Louis, CV Mosby, 1980

Larson C, Gould M: Orthopedic Nursing, 9th ed. St Louis, CV Mosby, 1978

Nursing photobook: Nursing skillbook. Working with Orthopedic Patients. Springhouse, PA, Intermed Communications, 1982

Mourad L: Nursing Care of Adults with Orthopedic Conditions. New York, John Wiley & Sons, 1980

Way L: Current Surgical Diagnosis and Treatment, 6th ed. Los Altos, Lange Medical Publications, 1983

JOURNALS

Acute Osteomyelitis. Nurs Mirros 155(15):17, Oct 13, 1982

Blechman W: Rheumatoid arthritis: Tips on improving diagnostic accuracy and avoiding pitfalls. Consultant 22(8):181, Aug 1982

Brown R: Electrical bone growth stimulator (EBGS). J Operating Room Res Inst 2(4):26, Apr 1982

Brown R: External fixation. J Operating Room Res Inst 2(3):17, Mar 1982

Brown R: Immobilization: putting on a cast. JORRI 2(5):16, May 1982

Brown S: Avoiding postoperative pitfalls with hip fracture patients. RN 45(5):48, May 1982

Cast bracing of femoral shaft fractures. Nurs Times 76:700, Apr 17, 1980

Calabro J: Relieving the aches of osteoarthritis. Emer Med 15(4):110, Feb 28, 1983

Diagnostic overview: Osteoarthritis—a new look at an old disease. The National Arthritis News. The Arthritis Foundation, Spring 1983

Farrell J: Helping the new amputee. Orthop Nurse 1(3):18, May/June 1982

Farrell J: Orienting the float team to orthopedic patient care. Orthop Nurse 1(5):42, Sept/Oct 1982

Fuller E: Rheumatoid arthritis: devising a treatment plan. Patient Care 16(20):81, Nov 30, 1982

Hart F: Rheumatology: osteoarthritis and rheumatoid arthritis, Clin Forum #11. Nurs Mirror 153: Nov 11, 1981

Helt N: Orthopaedic scientific update. Orthop Nurs 1 (2):41, Mar/Apr 1982

Hensinger R: Congenital dislocation of the hip. Clinical Symp CIBA Pharmaceutical Co. 31(1):79, 1979

Hilt N: Musculoskeletal assessment: Screening for congenital dislocation of the hip. Orthop Nurs 1(2):22, Mar/Apr 1982

Howard M, Corbo-Pelaia S: Psychological after effects of halo traction. Am J Nurs 82(12):1839, Dec 1982

Howard M, Corbo-Pelaia S: A review of acute care (halo traction). Am J Nurs 82(12):1841, Dec 1982

Jabos R: Musculoskeletal assessment. Cranial nerve assessment with halo traction. Orthop Nurse 1(4):11, July/Aug 1982

Javid M: Treatment of herniated lumbar disc syndrome with chymopapain. JAMA 243(20):2043, May 23/30, 1980

Johnson C (ed): Symposium on orthopedic nursing. Nurs Clin North Am 16(4) 707–766, Dec 1981

Kahn J: Transcutaneous electrical nerve stimulation for nonunited fractures. Phys Ther 62(6):840, June 1982

Kawashima M: The treatment of pyogenic bone and joint infections by closed irrigation-suction. Clin Orthop 148:240, May 1980

Koerner M: Adult arthritis: A look at some of its forms. Am J Nurs 83(2):253, Feb 1983

Kryschyshen P, Fischer D: External fixation for complicated fractures. Am J Nurs 80(2):256, Feb 1980

Kutcher J: Amputation: helping a patient face loss of a limb. RN 48(2):38, Feb 1985

Lane P: New synthetic casts: What nurses need to know. Orthop Nurs 1(6):13, Nov/Dec 1982

Manning D: Unstable hip in the newborn. Ir Med J 75(12):463, Dec 1982

Meredith S: Those formidable external fixation devices. RN 42(12)18, Dec 1979

Miller M: Nursing care of the patient with external fixation therapy. Orthop Nurs 2(1):11, Jan/Feb 1983

Moye C: Nursing care of the amputee: An overview. Orthop Nurs 1(3):11, May/Jun 1982

Musolf J: Chemonucleolysis: A new approach to patients with herniated intervertebral disks. Am J Nurs 83(6):882, June 1983

Needle surgery of the back—an update. Harvard Med School Health Lett 8(5):5, Mar 1983

Nowatny M: If your patient's joints hurt, the reason may be osteoarthritis. Nursing '80 10(9):39, Sept 1980

Orthopaedic scientific update: A special report of the scientific sessions of the 49th annual meeting of the American Academy of Orthopaedic Surgeons. Orthop Nurse 1(2):41, Mar/Apr 1982

Orthopedic unit . . . refreshers as you start out on your float assignment. Nursing '82 12(6):72, June 1982

Patterson P: Awareness is the key to rheumatoid arthritis. AORN J 32(4):614, Oct 1980

Pellino T: Chymopapain: Alternative to laminectomy for herniated lumbar discs. Orthop Nurs 2(2):14, Mar/Apr 1983

Perdue P: Abdominal injuries and dangerous fractures. RN 44(7):34, Jul 1981

Phillips K: The use of gold therapy with rheumatoid arthritis. Orthop Nurse 2(4):31, Jul/Aug 1983

RN Master Care Plan: Postop needs of the amputee. RN 48(2):46, Feb 1985

Robinson J, Marx L: Nail-safe method. Am J Nurs, 85(2):158, Feb 1985

Rodts M: An orthopedic assessment you can do in 15 minutes. Nursing '83 13(5): 65, May 1983

Rutechki B: Caring for a patient in a halo apparatus. Nursing '80 10(10):73, Oct 1980

Ruton F: Preprosthetic program for the amputee. Orthop Nurse 1(2):14, May/June 1982

Shelton M, Guise E: Variation on the pylon for the below knee amputee. Phys Ther 62(11):1601, Nov 1982

Walters J: Coping with a leg amputation. Am J Nurs 81(7):1349, Jul 1981

Weiss T; Osteoarthritis protective measures that work. Consultant 22(7):213, Jul 1982

Normal Aging Changes in the Musculoskeletal System

Finch C, Hayflick L (eds): Handbook of the Biology of Aging. New York, Van Nostrand Reinhold, 1977

Reff M, Schneider E: Biological Markers of Aging. U.S. Department of Health and Human Services, 1982 (NIH Publication No. 82-2221)

Rockstein M, Sussman M: Biology of Aging. Belmont, Wadsworth Publishing, 1979

NEUROLOGIC SYSTEM

CEREBROVASCULAR ACCIDENT

Definition

A cerebrovascular accident (CVA), or stroke, occurs when the blood supply to a part of the brain tissue is cut off, and the nerve cells in that part of the brain can then no longer function. A CVA may be described as extracranial or intracranial in origin. Extracranial CVA's are most commonly the result of a thrombus forming on plaque at the bifurcation of the carotid artery. Occasionally, an embolus, which is carried in the bloodstream from a diseased heart, will lodge in a cerebral vessel. These are called cerebral embolisms. Intracranial CVAs may be hemorrhagic, and the result of a diseased artery. This type of CVA is most likely to occur in patients who have both hypertension and diabetes. The most common CVA is intracranial and results from thrombus formation within the lumen of cerebral vessels that have become progressively occluded with plaque.

A stroke in evolution refers to continuing neurologic changes over a period of 24 hours to 48 hours or more. When the patient ceases to exhibit further progression in neurologic impairment, a completed stroke has taken place.

A transient ischemic attack (TIA) is caused by momentary impairment of cerebral blood flow. It usually lasts 5 minutes to 30 minutes, and is accompanied by fleeting neurologic signs, fainting, or a brief dizzy spell. About 30% to 50% of patients experiencing TIAs suffer a full CVA within 5 years if untreated.

Common Diagnostic Tests

- Neurologic examination
- Brain scan (See NR, Scans.)
- CT scan (See NR, Scans.)
- Cerebral arteriogram

Observations

- Stroke victims who show some stability or improvement within 24 hours have a good prognosis.
- The most visible sign of a stroke is paralysis of one side of the body. Watch to be sure that the patient can swallow, and that the eye on the affected side has a blink reflex. When one cheek puffs out with each expiration, it indicates paralysis of that side of the face.
- Patients with occlusive disease rarely lose consciousness. They typically display focal neurologic signs (see MSN, Neurologic System, Increased intracranial pressure.)

- When a hemorrhage is the cause of a CVA, the patient often will have lost consciousness.
- Right-sided hemiplegia (paralysis) indicates injury to the left side of the brain. Symptoms of this type of injury are aphasia, or trouble in speaking and understanding; use of inappropriate words; inability to see of the far right; and slowness and caution in movement.
- Left-sided hemiplegia indicates injury to the right side of the brain. Symptoms of this type of injury are spacial and perceptual difficulty, such as trouble in steering a wheelchair and inability to keep place while reading or feeding oneself; impulsive movements; and inability to see on far left.
- These symptoms may be very mild and gradually disappear, or be severe and lasting, depending on the location and pervasiveness of the CVA.

Treatment

- IV line for vein access (See NR, Intravenous therapy.)
- Anticoagulants, *e.g.*, heparin, warfarin
- Nasogastric tube feedings (See MSN, Gastrointestinal intubation.)

Nursing Considerations

- Place the patient, both in and out of bed, so that the unimpaired side is toward the movement in the room. Left hemiplegics often have left-field cuts, meaning that they have difficulty seeing objects that are to the left of the center in the field of vision. The opposite often is true of right hemiplegics.
- A patient who needs to be fed should never be left unattended with a tray of hot food. An uncoordinated hand movement can result in burns.
- An unconscious or otherwise disabled patient must be turned from side to side at least every 2 hours and maintained in a semi-prone position.
- Check unconscious patients for contact lenses, and if present, remove them. (see MSN, Eye care).
- When the eyelids do not close, they must be taped closed. Check with the physician for lubricating drops.
- Airway obstruction caused by the tongue falling backward leads to atelectasis and pneumonia, and may be the result of leaving a helpless patient on his or her back.
- In dealing with an aphasic patient, remember that speechlessness does not mean deafness or a loss of understanding. Don't shout. Test the patient by asking him or her to perform a simple

task such as "Wink an eye," or a nonsense question such as "Am I green?"

- A speech therapist should start therapy as soon as practical, and also is able to help with swallowing difficulties. The nurse must be sure that there is a system of communication. A communication board is useful, or alphabet cards are good for the patient who is unable to write. Be sure that the nurse call-light system is one that the patient is able to use.
- There are often some memory and personality changes in CVA patients. These may be manifested by difficulty in remembering new information or in carryover learning from one situation to another. Some patients may laugh or cry inappropriately. It is possible to interrupt this by abruptly changing the subject or snapping the fingers, if it is a result of emotional lability and not depression or euphoria. The patient's family needs to be aware of these potential memory and personality changes.
- Mouth care is an absolute requirement after each feeding to check for food that may left in the mouth.
- Soft foods are often easier to swallow than liquids. Milk and milk products thicken saliva and mucous secretions and make swallowing more difficult.
- Nighttime darkness is disturbing, and increased restlessness and confusion often occur. Keeping the lights, radio, or TV on is helpful (see MSN, Disoriented patients).
- Physiotherapy should be started at the bedside with range of motion (ROM) exercises as early as possible. The physiotherapist should come to evaluate the patient within 24 hours after a completed stroke. Remind the physician to order this.
- The voiding reflex is diminished when a Foley catheter is used for a long time. Also, the incidence of urinary tract infection increases. Within a week after a completed stroke, a toileting schedule every 2 hours to 3 hours should begin for relearning bladder control.
- A CVA is a possible major complication in children with sickle cell anemia (see MSN, Sickle cell anemia).

DEMENTIA

Description

Dementia describes a group of symptoms relating to a loss or impairment of mental functioning. Problems common to all dementias include mental confusion, memory loss, disorientation, and intellectual impairment. Dementias are slow, steady, progressive in nature, and irreversible. In the past, dementia was referred to as chronic organic brain syndrome or senility.

Delirium (also called acute organic brain syndrome) is easily confused with dementia because a delirious person can exhibit many of the same symptoms. However, delirium usually has a sudden onset and the person has a fluctuating level of awareness (drowsy at times and then very restless and agitated). It is extremely important to distinguish between delirium and dementia because the delirium is reversible. Common causes of delirium are illnesses (*e.g.*, pneumonia, kidney infection), malnutrition, and reactions to medications.

Dementias can be classified in four categories. The largest (more than 50% of autopsied cases) is senile dementia, Alzheimer's type (SDAT), or Alzheimer's disease. Brain atrophy occurs and specific brain changes can be seen on autopsy (senile plaques and neurofibrillary tangles). At present, the cause in unknown, but many factors have been implicated in the disease (*e.g.*, toxic factors such as aluminum, Down's syndrome, old age, viruses, hereditofamilial factors, chromosomal breakage, and transcriptional error).

Multi-infarct dementia (MID) is secondary to repeated strokes that destroy small areas of the brain. These dementias (approximately 15% of autopsied cases) usually progress in a step-like way, with further deterioration following each new stroke. This is contrasted to the gradual and progressive decline seen in SDAT.

Mixed dementias include individuals with both SDAT and MID (approximately 24% of autopsied cases). The final category is referred to as "pseudodementia," and frequently is secondary to depression.

Common Diagnostic Tests

- CT scan (See NR, Scans.)
- PET scan: detects areas of increased metabolism in the brain
- Tests of mental status
- Differential diagnosis is *extremely* important. Because Alzheimer's disease is presently untreatable and irreversible, all other possible causes of the dementia symptoms must be ruled out.

Observations

- Symptoms frequently occur in order:
  1. Memory impairment, especially for recent memory
  2. Mild personality changes such as withdrawal and apathy
  3. Intellectual deterioration (*e.g.*, the person can not balance a checkbook, shop, or learn recent material)
  4. Disorientation
  5. Decline in social habits
  6. Decline in judgment
  7. Physical decline accompanies the intellectual decline. Failure to eat, falling, and improper body hygiene occur. The person

gradually progresses to the point where all of his or her needs must be met by others.

Treatment

- There is no known cure for Alzheimer's disease.
- Management of symptoms assists the patient's caretaker. Haloperidol (Haldol) given at regular intervals (to maintain a constant blood level) is effective in calming agitation (see PH).
- Some MIDs may be stopped by preventing further strokes. Drugs such as aspirin and antihypertensives are used. The progression of other MIDs can not be stopped.

Nursing Considerations

- In the early stages of a dementing illness, the person is aware of the changes that are occurring. Depression is common, and if treated, may improve the person's functioning. Usually the more educated and intellectual the person, the greater is the depression.
- The individual may develop mechanisms for hiding symptoms, such as lies, repetition, humor, and social graces.
- Denial is common.
- The family may be so supportive that symptoms are not obvious. When the person is deprived of that support, he or she can no longer function adequately. Symptoms may appear to have a sudden onset during a crisis situation. *Hospitalization* often precipitates such a crisis!
- Dusk and darkness frequently increase anxiety and restlessness. Restraints often make it worse. A familiar family member or friend may be needed to stay with the patient. Keeping the patient near the nurses' station also may have a calming affect.
- Barbiturates and hypnotics frequently increase the confusion and agitation.
- Acute reactions (*e.g.,* from drugs or infection) do occur in persons with dementia. Treatment of the acute problem can improve functioning.
- Family members need a great deal of support and encouragement. Disrupted sleeping patterns are common in dementia, and the caregivers may be exhausted from the constant responsibility.
- The family may have developed very effective ways of managing the demented individual. Include the family when planning care.
- Discharge planning is crucial. The family may need help in determining home-care needs or nursing-home planning.

- For practical suggestions in the day-to-day management of individuals with Alzheimer's disease, consider *The 36-Hour Day* by Mace and Rabins. This is a good resource for the caregivers also.
- Support groups for family members are forming all over the country. For further information and locations of the groups contact:

  Alzheimer's Disease and Related Disorders Association, Inc.,
  360 North Michigan Avenue,
  Chicago, Illinois 60601.

GUILLAIN-BARRÉ SYNDROME (LANDRY-GUILLAIN-BARRÉ SYNDROME: INFECTIOUS POLYNEURITIS)

Description

Guillain-Barré syndrome describes symptoms caused by inflammatory and degenerative changes affecting peripheral and cranial nerve roots. The exact cause in unknown. However, if often is preceded by a viral infection with flu-like symptoms, and has followed immunizations. It usually begins with muscle weakness of the legs and, within days or hours, may extend upward to produce a partial or total paralysis. When the cranial nerves are involved, swallowing is often affected and respiratory failure may occur. The prognosis depends on the severity of the symptoms. Since peripheral nerves have the capacity to regenerate, recovery can occur, but it may take many months before the paralysis disappears, commonly in the reverse order of appearance.

Common Diagnostic Tests

- A lumbar puncture is done to obtain cerebrospinal fluid (CSF). In this disease, the fluid will have a greatly increased protein content but a normal cell count and normal glucose content.
- The nerve conduction velocity (NCV) test, a test of nerve conduction, will invariably be slowed in this disease.
- The electromyograph, a test that records electrical activity in a muscle, will record abnormalities in the affected muscles at rest and during activity.
- Serial vital capacity measurements are recommended.

Observations

- Acute weakness and transient tingling and numbness, usually first noted in the feet and legs, and subsequently progressing upward will be present
- Any changes in breathing, swallowing, or speaking must be called to the attention of the physician immediately.

- Excessive sweating, flushed face, and fluctuations in blood pressure often are present because of direct effects on the autonomic nervous system.

Treatment

- There is no known cure for this disease.
- Heparin may be given to prevent thrombosis resulting from immobilization.
- If respiratory muscle failure occurs, tracheostomy or intubation and mechanical ventilation are necessary.
- After the acute phase, long-term physiotherapy is useful to facilitate muscle recovery.
- A high-caloric, high-protein diet is helpful in preventing muscle atrophy.

Nursing Considerations

- These patients usually are very frightened because of their rapidly developing paralysis. They have a real need for someone to stay with them.
- Be certain a call system that the patient is able to use is always available.
- Careful observation, documentation, and reporting is imperative so that nurses following on each shift are aware of the exact neurologic and respiratory status of the patient. Note the strength and ability to move the feet, legs, hands, arms, and shoulders in the neurologic assessment. Changes are important; this can be a very fast moving disease.
- Respiratory failure is the most life-threatening complication of this disease.
- Respiratory assessment and measurement of vital capacity, along with a neurologic assessment, must be done at least every 2 hours, and more often if indicated. These must continue until the disease has reached its peak. Respiratory assessment must include observation of chest movement and whether diaphragmatic movement is needed for breathing. Listen for breath sounds in the chest. Have the patient count to ten. If breathlessness occurs while counting, then there is respiratory difficulty.
- There is usually an increase in bronchial secretions and a decreased ability to clear them. Always have suction available.
- Nasogastric tube feedings are necessary when swallowing is affected.
- Urinary incontinence, retention, and constipation may occur.
- When the orbicularis muscles are affected, the eyes will not close properly. Eye care is necessary to prevent infection and injury; tape eyelids closed while the patient is sleeping.

- These patients may be immobile for many weeks. Pressure sores, deep vein thrombosis, and pulmonary embolism are possible complications. Frequent position changes and ROM exercises are absolutely necessary.
- This is a very disabling disease with possible life-threatening complications. Recovery is slow and involves retraining of muscles for such things as walking and speech. Depression, anger, and frustration all may accompany this prolonged recovery period.

INCREASED INTRACRANIAL PRESSURE

Description

Increased intracranial pressure (IICP) results from increases in any of the three components within the skull: brain, blood, and cerebrospinal fluid (CSF). The skull, being nonflexible, cannot accommodate such internal expansions.

Space-occupying lesions, such as brain tumors, abscesses, or hematomas, are common causes of IICP. Head injuries, brain surgery, hemorrhage, or hydrocephalus also may result in IICP. If such pressure is not treated, the patient may die from cerebral anoxia (lack of oxygen reaching brain tissue resulting from compressed arteries) or heart or respiratory failure resulting from the pressure on the vital center controlling these functions.

MSN

Common Diagnostic Tests

- Neurologic examination—to identify neurologic impairments that help locate the affected brain area
- Skull x-rays—especially in head trauma
- CT scan—the preferred technique in diagnosing intracranial clots, tumors, cerebral edema, and aneurysms (See NR, Scans.)
- Angiography—to detect aneurysms and to study blood supply of brain and tumors
- EEG—to reflect seizure activity (See NR, Electroencephalogram.)
- Lumbar puncture—primarily to obtain specimens of CSF (contraindicated when IICP is known to exist because of possible brain shift, leading to herniation and death)

Observations

- Restlessness: This often is the first sign of IICP, and is followed by a decrease in the level of consciousness.
- In infants, bulging fontanels along with a high-pitched cry usually occur.
- An unusual increase in head circumference is seen in young children.

- Pupil reactions: Changes in the pupils, especially if unilateral, are significant. The ocular motor (cranial nerve III) is the first nerve to be affected by IICP. The development of a unilateral fixed dilated pupil is an emergency situation. Use of a flashlight is helpful to see that the patient has coordinated eye movements and that the pupils:
  1. Are equal in size
  2. Constrict when exposed to light
  3. React equally to light
  4. Dilate after covering the eyes for a few minutes
- Changes in rate and depth of respirations: These often begin as slight irregularities. Thus, it is important to observe respirations for at least a minute.
- Any sudden weakness or paralysis or difficulties with verbal responses should be noted.
- Seizures may take place (see MSN, Seizures).
- Stiff necks usually are associated with subarachnoid hemorrhages and with meningitis.
- Malignant tumors of the breast and lung frequently metastasize to the brain.
- Metastatic tumors comprise 50% of all brain tumors.

Treatment

- No narcotics, occasionally sedatives (phenobarbitol)
- IV access for medication
- ABGs to determine respiratory efficiency
- Steroids and osmotic diuretics, which reduce cerebral edema
- Fluid restriction including IV *and* PO fluids.
- Antifibrinolytics, *e.g.,* aminocaptoic acid (Amicar), to prevent rebleeding in case of an aneurysm
- Anticonvulsants, *e.g.,* phenytoin (dilantin)
- Antihypertensives
- Surgery for tumors, clots, and repair of aneurysms
- Chemotherapy and radiation for tumors (See MSN, oncology nursing considerations.)

Nursing Considerations

- Keep an open airway. Position an unconscious patient on his or her side, or semiprone, but never fully prone. Keep suction equipment immediately available. Suctioning increases IICP by 15 mm Hg to 20 mm Hg. Hyperventilate before and after suctioning. Tracheostomy or endotracheal tube may be required.

- The head of the bed should be at a 30° to 45° angle, unless contraindicated by vertebral fractures. This aids the venous return from the head, which decreases cerebral volume.
- Always check unconscious patients for the possibility that they may be wearing contact lenses (see MSN, Eye patient care).
- Neurologic assessment, blood pressure, pulse and respiration should be taken every 15 minutes, four times; every 30 minutes, four times; and then every hour, or as frequently as needed, depending upon the patient's condition (see MSN, Assessment). During the 24 hours following even mild head injuries, the patient should be awakened every 1 hour to 2 hours for neurologic check. This assessment, to be valid, requires that everyone use the same criteria (see MSN, Neurologic assessment).
- Patients who are rendered unconscious by head injuries later have increased incidences of headaches, vertigo, irritability, impaired mental abilities, and seizures.
- Take seizure precautions. Tape a padded tongue blade or soft airway to the head of the bed or bedside stand. Pad side rails the full length of the bed, and have suction and oxygen equipment immediately available.
- Take the patient's temperature every 4 hours. Continuing changes in temperature signify that the temperature regulating center of the brain is affected. Hypothermia blankets are useful in lowering body temperature, which decreases cerebral edema (see NR, Hypothermia blanket). A temperature of 105° can increase blood in head by 62%. Ice applied to the groin and axilla will bring the fastest decrease in temperature.
- Patients with IICP should be in a quiet environment. Avoid bright lights, and strictly limit visitors.
- Coughing, vomiting, or straining of any type should be prevented.
- Avoid use of restraints, if possible, since restraints often will increase agitation.
- Monitor IV therapy carefully to avoid fluid overload.
- Carefully observe and record intake and output every hour, and specific gravity of the urine every shift.

INFECTIONS

BACTERIAL MENINGITIS

Description

Bacterial meningitis is an inflammation of the meninges covering the brain and spinal cord. If left untreated, death or permanent nerve damage from increased intracranial pressure (ICPP) may result. (see MSN, Increased intracranial pressure). Bacterial infections in the brain or spinal cord are usually secondary to an infection originating elsewhere in the body and spread through the bloodstream. Bacterial meningitis also may be secondary to an ear or sinus infection, craniotomy, or open head injury. Spina bifida and ventricular shunts (see Hydrocephalus) also provide entry for bacteria. Meningococcal meningitis is the contagious form of bacterial meningitis and may occur in epidemics. It is transmitted by droplets sprayed from the nose and mouth of infected individuals.

Common Diagnostic Tests (See LAB)

- Lumbar puncture for cerebrospinal fluid analysis and culture
- Blood cultures to identify bacteria
- Nose and throat cultures to identify bacteria

Observations

- In infants, irritability, loss of appetite or vomiting, a high-pitched cry, and bulging fontanels may be present. Seizures are common, and a fever or hypothermia may be present.
- In older infants, children, and adults, severe headache, fever, vomiting without nausea, photophobia (sensitivity to light), drowsiness, and a stiff neck that prevents pressing the chin into the chest may be seen.
- Kernig's sign, or difficulty in extending the lower leg when the thigh is flexed onto the abdomen, also may be present.
- Brudzinski's sign, or involuntary flexion of the legs when the neck is bent forward, may be noted.
- Note changes in the level of consciousness leading to coma (see MSN, Increased intracranial pressure). This is most often seen in young children and in the elderly.
- Dehydration and hyponatremia may occur.
- A skin and mucous membrane rash is characteristic in meningococcal meningitis, as are symptoms of shock.

Treatment

- IV antibiotics specific for causative organisms
- Anti-convulsants, *e.g.,* phenytoin sodium (Dilantin) (see PH.)
- Adequate fluid intake, which requires careful monitoring of intake and output.
- Isolation in accordance with communicable disease regulations (Refer to the infection control manual of the institution, or contact the local public health agency.)

Nursing Considerations

- Problems that may arise include septic shock, acute cerebral edema, and seizures.
- Provide a quiet and dark room because of increased sensitivity to light and noise.
- A hypothermia blanket is useful in controlling body temperature (see NR, Hypothermia blanket). However, for a rapid decrease in temperature ice applied to the axilla and groin is most effective.
- All secretions from the mouth, nose, and ears should be disposed of promptly and carefully.
- Seizure precautions should be observed because of the possibility of convulsions.
- Accurate intake and output and daily weights need to be watched. There is the possibility of an inappropriate secretion of the antidiuretic hormone, which may result in retention of fluid and worsening of cerebral edema.
- Vital signs should be taken at least every 2 hours during the acute stage.
- The highest incidence of meningitis occurs in children between 6 and 12 months of age. Therefore, any infant or child with an upper respiratory infection and a change in level of consciousness or behavior should be examined by a physician.
- Meningococcal meningitis progresses rapidly to shock. It is fatal within hours if untreated.
- Meningococcal meningitis is a reportable disease and contacts may warrant prophylactic treatment, *e.g.,* rifampin. There is also a vaccine effective against some strains of meningococci.
- There is a high incidence of deafness in children who recover from meningitis.

VIRAL ENCEPHALITIS

Description

Viral encephalitis generally results from direct viral invasion of the brain and often the spinal cord. It results in inflammation, edema, and tissue destruction in the brain or spinal cord. The herpes simplex virus and arboviruses are common causes of this disease. A neonate acquires the herpes virus during passage through the birth canal from an active infection in the mother's genital tract. The arboviruses are athropod-borne (mosquitoes, ticks) viruses, and the disease is acquired through a bite from the infective agent.

Postinfectious encephalitis is the result of a toxic reaction to a viral disease elsewhere in the body, such as measles or mumps, or a vaccination or other immunization.

Common Diagnostic Tests

- Lumbar puncture for CSF analysis and possible identification of the virus
- Blood examination for antibody titers
- CT scan to detect area of brain damage

Observations

- The most significant finding in encephalitis is an altered mental state and some degree of prostration.
- Encephalitis symptoms usually resemble a severe case of meningitis with high fever, seizures (both focal and generalized), and muscle weakness. Neurologic signs and symptoms depend on the area of the central nervous system that is affected.
- Herpes encephalitis progresses rapidly and has a poor prognosis.

Treatment

- Care depends on the symptoms. It is directed toward reducing fever, providing adequate nutrition, and increased hydration.
- Respiratory problems may require a tracheostomy and a mechanical ventilator,

Nursing Considerations

- Monitor temperature, respirations, and neurochecks as frequently as indicated by the patient's condition.
- Cerebral edema is often a serious complication of encephalitis.
- Seizures are always a possibility because of inflammation of brain tissue, especially in infants.
- Disorientation may cause combative behavior.
- Hypothermia blankets are useful in the control of temperature elevations. However, for a rapid decrease in temperature, ice applied to the axilla and groin is most effective.
- Mental retardation may result from the residual brain damage from encephalitis.

MULTIPLE SCLEROSIS

Description

Multiple sclerosis is a disease characterized by sclerotic areas that form in random patterns in the brain and spinal cord. The symptoms vary depending on the location of the sclerotic areas. It is a chronic disease with unpredictable exacerbations and remissions. Emotional upsets and any illness tend to intensify the symptoms. The cause is unknown, but a viral agent or a disorder involving the body's immune system is suspect.

Common Diagnostic Tests

- Lumbar puncture: CSF often has increased immunoglobulin.
- Tests are conducted to rule out other possible causes of symptoms, *e.g.*, pernicious anemia or brain tumor.
- Classic symptoms increase with time and are considered sufficiently distinctive to permit confirmation of the disease.

Observations

- Unusual fatigue, weakness, and clumsiness, affecting arms or legs, and often resulting in gait disturbances
- Double vision and other ocular problems
- Numbness, particularly on one side of the face, sometimes with mild pain
- Impaired bladder control; possible incontinence in advanced cases
- Speech disturbances

Treatment

- No specific curative treatment is known.
- Steroids are given in acute exacerbations to shorten the length of time of the acute attack.
- Exercise, especially swimming, and daily physiotherapy to improve muscle tone are beneficial.
- A fever or exposure to heat tends to accentuate symptoms.

Nursing Considerations

- No two patients exhibit identical symptoms, and symptoms often shift from one body area to another. However, usually one side of the body is more affected than the other.
- The symptoms may subside and then recur in a more severe form.
- These patients are very easily fatigued, and just eating may be an exhausting experience. Bedrest often relieves symptoms.
- Bladder and respiratory infections are often a recurring problem.
- The Multiple Sclerosis Society, 205 E. 42nd Street, New York, New York 10017, offers helpful supportive information, which is available to patients.

MYASTHENIA GRAVIS

Description

Myasthenia gravis (MG) is a chronic disease causing variable weakness, which ranges from mild to life-threatening and is often progressive. The ocular and facial muscles are commonly affected, but any voluntary muscle may become involved. The cause is unknown, but it is thought to be an autoimmune disease. There is also an association with tumors or enlargements of the thymus gland; a thymectomy is sometimes done with beneficial results. Infants of mothers with MG may have signs of the disease at birth that usually disappear within a few weeks. The term "myasthenic crisis" refers to a sudden increase in the severity of symptoms caused by stress, an infection, or too little anticholinesterase medication, or the lack of response to the medication. A "cholinergic crisis," also implies an increase in the severity of symptoms, but is caused by overmedication with anticholinesterase drugs.

Common Diagnostic Tests

- Neostigmine bromide (Prostigmin) is given subcutaneously (SC) or intramuscularly (IM). If the patient has MG, weak muscles become stronger within 45 minutes, and this effect lasts for several hours (see PH).
- Edrophonium chloride (Tensilon) is given intravenously (IV). If the patient has MG, weak muscles become stronger almost immediately, but this effect only lasts for 5 minutes to 10 minutes (see PH).
- The Tensilon IV test can be used to differentiate between a myasthenic crisis and a cholinergic crisis. Symptoms of the disease will improve in a myasthenic crisis and worsen in a cholinergic crisis. Atropine sulfate is given to counteract a cholinergic reaction.

Observations

- Ptosis (drooping of the upper eyelid) or diplopia (double vision) may occur. This is often most evident late in the day.
- Limb weakness and abnormal exhaustion of voluntary muscle strength occurring with normal exercise may be noted. After a short rest, such weakness subsides.
- Chewing, swallowing, and breathing difficulties as well as weakness of the voice may be evident.
- Both myasthenic crisis and a cholinergic crisis result in increased severity of basic symptoms, especially a marked inability to swallow or breathe. This may necessitate an intubation and mechanical ventilation. These patients should be cared for in an intensive care unit. In any case, they must not be left unattended during a crisis.

- Anticholinesterase drugs, *e.g.*, pyridostigmine bromide (Mestinon), treat symptoms by acting as a temporary muscle stimulant (see PH).
- Corticosteroids, *e.g.*, prednisone, are often effective as a long-term treatment for autoimmune diseases since steroids block immune mechanisms.

Nursing Considerations

- A tracheostomy set and suction equipment must be readily available at or near the bedside. Its location should be known to all of the staff.
- Patients should fully understand the action of their medications and the consequences of improper dosage.
- Anticholinesterase medications must be taken on a schedule that is individualized for each person. Thus, a hospitalized patient with MG should keep to his or her own medication schedule and, if able, should have the medicine at the bedside for self-administration.
- When dysphagia (difficulty in swallowing) is a problem, the medication should be taken about 30 minutes before a meal.
- Any patient with muscle weakness should have a call light adapted to this problem and be in a room near the nurses' station.
- Neomycin, quinidine, pronestyl, quinine, phenobarbital, and phenothiazides precipitate crises (see PH). Patients should also check with their physicians before using any over-the-counter medication.
- Upper respiratory infections are dangerous because muscle weakness limits the coughing ability to clear the airway of secretion.
- Fatigue and physical or emotional stress should be avoided, because these aggravate the symptoms.
- A medical identification bracelet should be worn signifying that the person has MG.
- The Myasthenia Gravis Foundation, 230 Park Avenue, New York, New York 20017, offers current information that may be helpful to patients.

PARKINSON'S DISEASE

Description

Parkinson's disease is a chronic progressive disorder associated with a deficient neurochemical process in the brain and results in a lack of dopamine. Dopamine is used in nuclei near the center of the brain that regulate voluntary movements of the body. Physical stability is affected, and as the condition worsens, the patient becomes bedridden and unable to speak or eat.

Common Diagnostic Tests

- Parkinson's disease is determined by observing classic symptoms of involuntary tremors (often the first symptom), rigidity, and slowness of movement.

Observations

- Stooped posture, slow voluntary movements, stiff passive movements, and resting tremors
- Fixed facial expression and nodding of the head
- Slurred and monotonous speech
- Mental processes not usually affected; depression is common

Treatment

- Levodopa (See PH.)
- Sinemet (a levodopa compound) (See PH.)
- Anticholinesterase drugs, *e.g.,* tetrihexyphenidyl (Artane) (See PH.)
- Physiotherapy
- Although it is not a cure, levodopa is extremely effective in controlling the symptoms of Parkinson's disease. There are serious side-effects that can be debilitating. Nausea and vomiting often occur for periods up to several months after the medication is started. An antiemetic drug, *e.g.,* trimethobenzamide hydrochloride (Tigan), may be ordered to control this (see PH). It is helpful to give levodopa after a meal or with an antacid.
- Orthostatic hypotension may occur as a side-effect in the first few months of treatment. Be sure the patient wears elastic stockings to help control this, and that he or she changes position slowly to prevent vertigo.
- An anticholinesterase drug (*e.g.,* trihexyphenidyl [Artane]), often is used in conjunction with levodopa. Under no circumstances should anticholinergic drugs be stopped suddenly, because severe tremors and rigidity may occur.
- Mental confusion may occur as a side-effect of medications used to control Parkinson's disease.
- Constipation is a common problem; a bowel regimen is necessary. A diet high in fibers and liquids should be encouraged.
- A daily schedule of exercise is extremely important to prevent muscle rigidity. A physiotherapy referral is very helpful for specific exercises that improve balance and walking.

SEIZURES (CONVULSIONS)

Description

Seizures are the result of a functional brain disorder that causes changes in the level of consciousness with involuntary motor and sensory responses. The effect may vary from minor to severe dysfunctions. A metabolic or toxic abnormality, such as hypoglycemia, uremia, cerebral anoxia, drug overdose, or alcohol withdrawal, may cause transient seizures that disappear when the underlying condition is corrected. Generalized seizures are more likely caused by meningitis or electrolyte imbalance.

Idiopathic epilepsy is the name given recurrent seizures that occur spontaneously, and that have no readily identifiable cause. Frequently, lesions in the brain are associated with epilepsy. There are four common types of seizures:

- *Grand mal* (also called tonic–clonic) seizures are characterized by loss of consciousness with severe generalized motor dysfunction that involves the entire body.
- *Jacksonian seizures* have an initial localized motor dysfunction that tends to spread in a regular progression to adjacent areas of the body. Changes in consciousness may occur.
- *Petit mal* seizures are momentary changes in level of consciousness, rarely seen after the age of 20 years.
- *Psychomotor* (also called Temporal lobe) *seizures* are periods of altered behavior that the patient is unable to control, *e.g.*, repetitive hand movements or lip smacking. They are characterized afterward by amnesia.

Febrile seizures are the initial symptoms of an acute febrile illness seen primarily in the 6-month to 3-year-old child. These seizures accompany a rapid temperature rise, and are generalized grand-mal, lasting less than 20 minutes.

Status epilepticus describes continuous grand mal seizures that occur in rapid succession without the patient regaining consciousness; this *requires immediate medical attention.* Such seizures are frequently the result of abruptly discontinuing anticonvulsant medication or sudden alcohol withdrawal.

Posttraumatic epilepsy frequently follows severe head injuries and may occur within the first few days or several months later. The prognosis for remission is good in cases appearing in the first few days or weeks.

Common Diagnostic Tests (After Seizures Are Controlled)

- Neurologic examination is necessary.
- An EEG may be ordered.
- A CT scan may be ordered.

- An angiogram, or x-ray visualization of the blood supply to the brain, may be done.
- Blood glucose abnormalities may cause or be the result of seizures.
- Arterial blood gases: Hypoxia may be the cause or the result of seizures.
- Electrolyte abnormalities may precipitate or be the result of prolonged seizures.
- Lumbar puncture is contraindicated when there is increased intracranial pressure.

Observations

Observation and recording of seizure activity are extremely important. You may be the only witness. Be sure to describe any injuries that are the result of the seizure. Document as accurately as possible, recording the following information:

- *Duration:* Note how long the seizure lasted and any activity or specific sensation (aura) that preceded it.
- *Level of Consciousness (LOC):* If the patient was unconscious, record the length of time and the mental state when consciousness returned. Did sleep follow, and if so, for how long?
- *Motor activity:* Describe as tonic movements (contraction of muscles causing rigidity) and clonic movements (alternating contraction and relaxation of muscles, producing jerking spasms). Did muscle activity start in one area of the body and move to another? Was it unilateral or bilateral? Were the teeth clenched? Was there frothing at the mouth? Describe the respirations and whether there was cyanosis. Were the eyes open or closed or in an unusual position?

Treatment

- Maintain an airway and prevent aspiration of secretions. If the teeth are not clenched insert a bite stick. *Never force entry.* Try to keep the patient on his or her side. When the seizure is over, mouth suctioning may be necessary if the level of consciousness is depressed.
- Never leave the patient alone during a seizure.
- Protect the patient from self-injury, but restrain movements as little as is necessary. Pay particular attention to the prevention of head injury. It may be possible to put a blanket under the patient's head or cradle it in your lap. If the patient has fallen onto the floor don't try to get him or her into bed until the seizure is over.
- Start an IV infusion as soon as possible.

- Anticonvulsants, *e.g.*, phenytoin sodium (Dilantin), diazepam (Valium), phenobarbitol, may be ordered (see PH).

Nursing Considerations

- Be familiar with the patient's history and laboratory results so that you are alert to the possibility of seizures.
- Seizures associated with alcohol withdrawal usually appear within 48 hours after the cessation of drinking.
- Those patients with a history of seizures or a predisposing condition must have seizure precautions. These include a padded tongue blade or soft airway taped to the bedside stand or the head of the bed, and suction equipment immediately available. If warranted by the frequency and severity of seizures, padded side rails should be used around the full length of the bed. Temperatures should be taken rectally to avoid thermometer breakage in the mouth. Place the patient in a room that is visible from the nurses station.
- The highest incidence of seizures occur at night and in the early morning.
- Once a patient has a seizure, chances are increased that others will occur.
- Anticonvulsant medication must be given on schedule. If the patient is NPO for any reason, the physician must be aware of this so that medications can be given parenterally or orally with a sip of water.
- When a seizure occurs, the patient's roommate, if there is one, may be the only witness. Ask the roommate for information about the seizure.
- If possible, try to provide some privacy for the patient during a seizure. This can be an extremely upsetting experience for other patients.
- Patients who have epilepsy should wear bracelets that identify this problem.

SPINAL CORD TRAUMA

Description

Spinal cord trauma may be caused by fracture of the vertebrae with direct damage to the cord, or by indirect damage from compression, primarily caused by a tumor or a ruptured intervertebral disc. Fractured vertebrae are a major cause of spinal cord injury. The effects of the injury may be apparent in parts of the body below the point of the spinal cord damage. This may be only a brief loss of neurologic function, such as that which occurs from spinal cord concussion. Varying degrees of paralysis result from compression and laceration. Initially, cord damage generally results in flaccid paralysis and areflexia (loss of reflexes). Later there may be spastic paralysis and some return of reflexes. Additionally, cervical cord damage affects respiratory function. Permanent loss of voluntary and involuntary movement results from transection of the cord. (See Table 4-7.)

Common Diagnostic Tests

- Neurologic examination
- Myelogram (to outline spinal cord)
- Skull and vertebrae x-rays
- CT scan

Observations

- Spinal shock occurs, which results in an immediate loss of all functions below the level of injury. This happens within minutes and is the result of direct injury or edema of the spinal cord. It is usually transient, but may last weeks to months. There is no voluntary or involuntary elimination of urine or stool. A major risk is the possibility of overdistention of the bladder, which may cause it to rupture. Also, hypotension, bradycardia, and lack of tissue perfusion, indicated by a decrease in urine output, are complications of spinal shock. Impactions, abdominal distention, and paralytic ileus are the effects of spinal shock on the bowel.
- Respiratory failure occurs when injury is above the fifth cervical vertebra. The patient can only live with the aid of a respirator, and a tracheostomy is necessary. These patients are very susceptible to pneumonia, a major complication of spinal cord injuries.
- Thrombophlebitis and pulmonary emboli are complications that result from immobility; therefore, prophylactic heparin therapy is often given (see NR, Thrombophlebitis; Pulmonary embolus).
- Stress ulcers are frequently associated with spinal cord injuries.
- Bladder dysfunction occurs because of the high incidence of urine retention after spinal cord trauma. A flaccid or areflexic bladder results, with dribbling incontinence because of overdistention. There is an increased incidence of infection because of stagnant urine. A spastic or reflex bladder empties spontaneously with no controlling influence to regulate it.
- A flaccid bowel has no sphincter control. A reflex bowel has sphincter control.
- Autonomic hyperreflexia causes a sudden, severe increase in blood pressure accompanied by headache and profuse sweating, resulting from damage of the sympathetic nerves. It is seen most frequently in patients with injury to the T6 level or higher. It is usually the result of a distended bladder or impacted rectum. This is a *medical emergency. Notify the physician immediately!* If

possible, sit the patient up after relieving the distention or impaction.

- Pressure sores are an entirely preventable complication. They are difficult to heal and slow down rehabilitation.
- Muscle spasms, which are involuntary contractions of muscles, develop after cord shock has subsided. They occur most often following high cord injury, and frequently are severe.
- Neurologic function and vital signs must be monitored and recorded carefully. Significant changes should be reported to the physician immediately.

Treatment

- Mechanical ventilation in the event of respiratory failure
- Steroids to reduce spinal cord edema
- Analgesics for pain, often occurring at the site of injury or disease
- Crutchfield tongs for cervical fractures, or halo traction (See NR, Traction.)
- Laminectomy for decompression, especially with increased neurologic deficit, or to remove bone or disc fragments (See MSN, Orthopedics.)
- Surgical stabilization of vertebral column, *e.g.,* fusion or stabilizing rods (See MSN, Orthopedics.)
- Nasogastric suction until peristalsis returns (See NR, Gastrointestinal intubation.)

Nursing Considerations

- In cervical injuries, aspiration resulting from a decreased ability to cough must be anticipated. Suction equipment should always be immediately available. An emergency tracheotomy set should be at the bedside whether or not there is a tracheostomy.
- The severity of signs and symptoms immediately following an injury is not always a reliable indicator of the eventual extent of permanent damage. Spinal shock may increase the severity of the symptoms at the onset.
- A return of function within a few days after an initial loss of all function indicates the patient was in spinal shock. There also may be a return of involuntary movements; if they do not return after several months, permanent damage is indicated.
- Turning every 2 hours is a necessity. This should be accomplished by log rolling with a pull sheet. Use three people to do this properly. Patients with a spinal cord injury need to avoid all movement and flexion of the spinal column. Movement of the head also must be avoided.

TABLE 4-7 FUNCTIONAL EXPECTATIONS FOLLOWING SPINAL CORD INJURY

Level of Injury	Functional Expectations
Sacral (S2 to S4)	Only bowel and bladder function initially impaired. Bowel evacuation via strain or manual removal; bladder satisfactorily emptied by strain and crede. Incontinence a possible problem if bladder neck surgery required. External appliance possibly necessary for male. Normal ambulation.
Lumbosacral (L4 to S1)	Bowel and bladder controlled as above. Independence in walking possible with two canes or crutches and often with short leg braces (ankle-foot orthoses). Prolonged standing possibly impaired, but wheelchair unnecessary.
Lumbar (L1 to L3)	Bowel evacuation via suppository and rectal stimulation. Bladder evacuation assisted by stimulating sacral reflexes if present (tapping or anal stretch). Sphincterotomy possibly required or long-term intermittent catheterization used. Walking in long leg braces (knee-ankle-foot orthoses) and with crutches possible for short distances. Complete independence in wheelchair possible.
Thoracic (T7 to T12)	Bowel and bladder (almost always upper motor neuron-type dysfunction) controlled as for L1 to L3 patients, with complete independence in function possible. Unless lower extremities deformed, independent walking in long leg braces possible but too strenuous to be very functional. Complete independence in wheelchair always expected, including dressing, driving, and transfer out of wheelchair.
Thoracic (T2 to T6)	Bowel and bladder controlled as for L1 to L3 patients. Wheelchair is required as main means of transportation. With extensive training, complete independence possible. Ambulation with orthoses never functional.

Cervical (C7 to T1)	Bowel and bladder controlled as for L1 to L3 patients. Reflex voiding often too frequent for patient to remain dry between catheterizations. If so, external collection device for male and indwelling catheter for female necessary for injury at this level and above. Self-catheterization difficult for C7 patients because of poor hand dexterity. A wheelchair primary means of transportation. Complete independence possible except in patients with deformities, weakness, obesity, or other medical problems.
Cervical (C6)	Long-term intermittent catheterization usually not practical since most patients lack dexterity, even with orthotic hand devices. External collectors and often bladder outlet surgery required in males. Manual wheelchair with modified hand rims operated with difficulty; electric wheelchair possibly required for ramps and grades. Self-care skills facilitated by othotic equipment. Complete independence in very few patients. Driving sometimes possible.
Cervical (C5)	Some assistance required in all activities; living alone not practical. Independent electric wheelchair ambulation possible.
Cervical (above C5)	Patient totally dependent. Ventilation compromised and special respiratory equipment required in C4 impairment. For some patients, ambulation possible in electric wheelchair fitted with appropriate chin or mouthpiece.

- Skin care, proper body alignment, and range of motion exercises are immediate needs from the onset of injury. Also, footboards and wrist splints should be used to prevent contractions. Heels should never rest directly on the mattress. Circulation is decreased and, with no sense of feeling, pressure sores may develop. It is just as important to relieve pressure points when the patient is sitting in a chair as it is when he or she is lying in a bed. Teach the patient to raise the buttocks off the seat for 20 seconds every 15 minutes. If the patient's arms are too weak to do this, assistance is necessary.
- There is often pain at the level of injury. Occasionally, patients experience acute pain in paralyzed areas, although physiologically it should not be possible to feel it.
- Be sure the patient has a usable nurse's call signal (such as a whistle for those not able to move their hands) available. All nursing personnel must know what it is. The more helpless the patient is, the greater is his or her fear of being left unattended.
- Intake and output recording is extremely important.
- Flaccid bladders lack the stimulus to empty and will continue to distend. Never catheterize more than 300 ml from a distended bladder. Wait 15 minutes and remove the remainder in amounts of 300 ml at 15-minute intervals. Sudden decompression of a distended bladder in a patient with injury to nerve tracts may cause sudden, severe hypotension. Permanent indwelling catheters are often necessary, or ileo-conduit surgery may be performed.
- In reflex bladders there is a loss of sensation of a full bladder. The bladder will empty by reflex activity, which the patient will be unable to control consciously. Catheterization should be done every 4 hours to 6 hours. (see NR, Urinary bladder catheterization and drainage). Intake is monitored carefully, with less fluid allowed in the evening. Total daily intake should not exceed 2000 ml.
- Self-catheterization should be taught if the patient is capable of managing this procedure. It is hoped that the individual will begin to recognize secondary symptoms of a full bladder, such as headache or sweating. Pressing down on the abdomen or tapping on it at this time (the Crede maneuver) may initiate urine flow. Bethanechol chloride (Urecholine), PO, may help stimulate voiding. Catheterization for residual urine must be done after each reflex voiding, until there is a regular pattern of less than 100 ml. When this is accomplished, catheterization for urine residual is only done once or twice a week.
- Urinary tract infection (UTI) must be treated immediately. Renal failure is the most common cause of death in the patient with impaired bladder function. The urine specific gravity must be determined daily, and the urine must be kept acidic to decrease the possibility of UTI. Urine cultures are done weekly, and colony counts of 50,000 and above are treated. The patient must know

the signs and symptoms of UTI (foul smelling urine, flu-like symptoms, and an elevated temperature).

- Demineralization of bones occurs after long periods of immobilization and may result in urinary stone formation. Fluid intake of 1800 ml to 2000 ml should be maintained to prevent this occurrence.
- Bowel training for those with a reflex bowel and sphincter control problem begins with a diet high in fiber and daily stool softeners. A regular time of day is selected, and a bowel movement is stimulated with gentle manual evacuation of the rectal vault. Suppositories or enemas should be used only when absolutely necessary.
- In both bowel and bladder training, a nursing-care plan is imperative; an inflexible routine and schedule must be maintained.

NORMAL AGING CHANGES IN THE NEUROLOGIC SYSTEM

- Nerve cells die each day and cannot be replaced. The cell loss differs throughout the nervous system, but is especially marked in certain parts of the cerebral cortex.
- Definite loss in brain mass occurs. A small but consistent weight loss is evident from maximum maturity to advanced old age (partially from a decrease in water content).
- Cells demonstrate altered structural characteristics.
    1. Shrinkage or swelling of cells occurs, depending on the location.
    2. The nucleus of the cell appears atypical and may be pushed away from the center by an accumulation of lipofuscin (an insoluble, inert compound of lipid, carbohydrate, and protein).
- Senile plaques and neurofibrillary tangles are seen. These changes occur with dementia, but also are seen in individuals who did not exhibit signs and symptoms of dementia.
- The outer cortex of the brain appears yellow-brown because of the lipofuscin deposits.
- Sizable losses occur in the number of nerve fibers (usually axons) outside of the central nervous system, but axons and dendrites continue to form throughout old age.
- The rate of nerve conduction may decrease.
- The blood supply to the brain decreases, and, therefore, there is a decrease in the amount of available oxygen.
- Cerebrovascular resistance increases.
- Simple reflexes may be diminished or absent.
- There are decreases in the metabolic rate and in the metabolism of the catecholamines (needed for nerve transmission).

- Both monoamine oxidase (MAO) and serotonin increase while norepinephrine (precursor of epinephrine) and dopamine decrease

IMPLICATIONS

- The nervous system has a reduced capacity to perform its normal regulatory function in times of stress.
- The elderly individual may have more difficulty maintaining normal body temperature with external changes.
- Decreases in the senses of touch and pain may allow cuts, burns, and infection to go unnoticed and untreated. Heating pads can be especially dangerous.
- Reduced message transmission from the baroreceptors can cause difficulty in blood pressure regulation (*e.g.,* orthostatic hypotension).
- Sleep patterns in the elderly usually change.
    1. Levels 3 and 4 (deep sleep) become less prominent, and brief arousals become more frequent.
    2. Total sleep time is only *slightly* reduced.
    3. Sedatives may improve the situation briefly, but then may become ineffective while producing unwanted side-effects.
    4. Explain that the arousals are normal and brief and that they do not usually impair the effectiveness of the total sleep period.
- Declines in intelligence are variable and are significantly related to the person's past life-style and educational and cultural background.
- In the healthy individual, declines in performance are frequently caused by physical changes rather than intellectual impairment. Reactions are slower and the elderly individual needs more time to perform such tasks as bathing, dressing, and eating. However, the formation of activity habit patterns (engrams) continues, and repeated performance of an activity enables the elderly individual to adapt his or her performance to changing abilities. Performance may be altered, but it is still satisfactory and satisfying.
- Short-term memory loss may occur.
- Confusion and disorientation are *not* part of the normal aging process. However, elderly persons newly admitted to the hospital may experience periods of confusion, especially at night. A new environment, sensory changes, fear, and medication effects are contributing factors. Sedation and restraints compound the problem. A night light and frequent explanations and reassurance are much more effective. It may be possible for a family member or friend to stay with the elderly person until he or she adjusts to the new environment.
- The concurrent increase in MAO and decrease in norepinephrine may contribute to the high incidence of depression seen in the elderly population.

BIBLIOGRAPHY • Neurologic System

BOOKS

Brunner L, Suddarth D: The Lippincott Manual of Nursing Practice, 3rd ed, pp 701–751. Philadelphia, JB Lippincott, 1982

Carini E, Owens A: Neurological and Neurosurgical Nursing, 7th ed. St. Louis, CV Mosby, 1978

Chin T: Encephalitis, In Wehrle P, Top, F (eds): Communicable and Infectious Diseases, 9th ed. St Louis, CV Mosby, 1981

Chusid, J. Guillain-Barre Syndrome and Myasthenia. In Krupp M, Chatton M (eds): Current Medical Diagnosis and Treatment. Los Altos, CA, Lange Medical Publications, 1983

Davis J, Mason C: Neurologic Critical Care. New York, Van Nostrand Co, 1979

Donovan W, Bedbrook G: Comprehensive Management of Spinal Cord Injury. CIBA Clinical Symposia 32(2):2, 1982

Friedman W: Head Injuries. Ciba Clinical Symposia, 35(4):2, 1983

Flynn I, Schwetz K, Williams D: Muscular Dystrophy: Comprehensive Nursing Care. Nurs Clin North Am 14(1), 1979

Gall G B: The Nervous System. In Gall G B Handbook of Clinical Nursing. New York, McGraw Hill, 1979

Greenlee J: Encephalitis. In Stein J (ed): Internal Medicine. Boston, Little, Brown, 1983

Haynes R, Azimi P, Sherard E: Infectious encephalitis. In Youmans G, Paterson P, Sommers H (eds): The Biologic and Clinical Basis of Infectious Diseases. New York, Harper & Row, 1982

Kinney M, Schenk E: Problems of the Nervous System. In Phipps WJ, Long B, Woods N (eds): Surgical Nursing: Concepts and Clinical Practice, 2nd ed. St. louis, CV Mosby, 1979

Mace N, Rabins P: The 36-hour Day. Baltimore, The Johns Hopkins University Press, 1981

Mandell G, Douglas R, Bennett J: Principals and Practice of Infectious Diseases, pp 769–775. New York, John Wiley, 1979

Merritt HH: A Textbook of Neurology, 6th ed. Philadelphia, Lea & Febiger, 1979

Reisberg B: Brain Failure. New York, The Free Press, 1981

Taylor J, Ballenger S: Neurological Dysfunctions and Nursing Intervention. New York, McGraw Hill, 1980

Yoshikawa T: Meningitis and encephalitis. In Yoshikawa T, Chow A, Guze L (eds): Infectious Diseases: Diagnosis and Management. Boston, Houghton Mifflin, 1980

MSN

CONFERENCES

- Spinal Injury. Sponsored by the Maryland Institute of the Emergency Medical System, March 22, 1983.
- Recent advances in the Diagnosis and Treatment of Multiple Sclerosis. Dale McFarlin, M.D., Chief, Neuroimmunology Branch, National Institute of Neurological Diseases, NIH April 29, 1983

- Neurological Assessment. Sponsored by the Clinico-Patho-Physiology Associates, August 24, 1982. Wash D.C.

Normal Aging Changes in the Neurologic System

BOOKS

Finch C, Hayflick L (eds): Handbook of the Biology of Aging. New York, Van Nostrand Reinhold, 1977

Reff M, Schneider E: Biological markers of Aging. U.S. Department of Health and Human Services, 1982 (NIH Publication No. 82-2221)

Rockstein M, Sussman N: Biology of Aging. Belmont, Wadsworth Publishing, 1979

JOURNALS

Barnes, R., Raskin, M., Scott, M., and Murphy, C. Problems of families caring for Alzheimer patients: Use of a support group. J Am Geriatr Soc 29(2):80–85, 1981

Glenner G: Alzheimer's disease (senile dementia): A research update and critique with recommendations. Geriatr Soc 30(1):59–62, 1982

Gwyther L, Matteson M: Care for the caregivers. Gerontol Nurs 9(2):92–95, 1983

LaPorte H: Reversible causes of dementia: A nursing challenge. Gerontol Nurs 8(2):74–80, 1982

Mackey A: OBS and nursing care. Gerontol Nurs 9(2):75–85, 1983

Palmer M: Alzheimer's disease and critical care. Gerontol Nurs 9(2):86–90, 1983

Wells C: Chronic brain disease: An update on alcoholism, Parkinson's disease, and dementia. Hosp Comm Psychiatry 33(2):111–126, 1982

RESPIRATORY SYSTEM

CANCER OF THE LUNG

DESCRIPTION

Lung cancer is classified according to the type of cancer cell identified by microscopic examination of biopsy material. The four most common types are squamous cell, oat cell, adenocarcinoma, and large-cell cancers. The bronchus is the most common site of lung cancer. Frequently the cancer metastasizes to the liver, bone, brain, and adrenal glands. The lung is also a common site of metastases from other areas of the body.

Common Diagnostic Tests

- X-rays and tomograms of the chest usually are done. (A tomogram provides a 3-dimensional picture of lung tissue)
- Bronchoscopy with bronchial brushing for microscopic study may be ordered (see NR, Endoscopic procedures).
- For sputum cytologic studies, an early morning specimen should be obtained as soon after awakening as possible; multiple specimens usually are needed.
- Alkaline phosphatase, when elevated, is an indicator of liver and bone metastases.
- Bone, liver, brain, and CT scans can be used to detect signs of metastases (see NR, Scans).
- Mediastinoscopy is used to evaluate mediastinal lymph nodes for metastases (see NR, Endoscopic procedures).

Observations

- A productive and increasingly persistent cough
- Increasing fatigue
- Anorexia (loss of appetite)
- Sudden weight loss
- Dyspnea, hoarseness, and chronic chest pains

Treatment

- Surgery is the first choice of treatment in the early stages of squamous cell, adenocarcinoma and large cell cancers. It is not usually attempted in oat cell because this type is frequently widespread at the time of diagnosis.
  1. Lobectomy is performed if the cancer is confined to a segment or lobe.
  2. Pneumonectomy is performed if the cancer involves more than one lobe.
  3. Over half of the patients presenting with x-ray evidence of lung cancer are inoperable. A lung cancer has to be 2 cm distal to the origin of the bronchus (carina) in order to be able to suture the bronchus following lobectomy (pneumonectomy). Also, when there is metastases to the mediastinal nodes, surgery usually is not done.
- See MSN, Pulmonary surgery, for additional information.
- Radiation
  1. Radiation may be useful for symptomatic relief of chest wall metastases or pain resulting from bone metastases, or for reduction of the tumor mass. Radiation to the chest may cause inflammation of the mucosa of the trachea and bronchial tree.

Radiation pneumonitis is a complication that may occur several weeks after the radiation treatment. Patients develop a cough, increased sputum, and fever.

- Chemotherapy can be useful in treating widespread oat cell lung cancer with resulting shrinkage of the tumor.

Nursing Considerations

- See MSN, Pulmonary surgery.
- See Oncology Nursing Considerations.

CHRONIC OBSTRUCTIVE PULMONARY DISEASE

Description

Chronic obstructive pulmonary disease (COPD) may result from the following conditions:

1. *Chronic bronchitis* is a constant inflammation of the bronchi that produces large amounts of heavy mucous secretions. Permanent dilatation of one or many bronchi is called bronchiectasis.
2. *Asthma* is a spasm of the bronchi that causes the airways to narrow. It may result from an allergy, infection, or emotional upset and is the leading cause of chronic illness in children. The lungs are unable to empty out used air, and thus cannot completely fill with new air. Status asthmaticus refers to an asthmatic episode that lasts for hours to days and is resistant to therapy.
3. *Emphysema* occurs when the elasticity of the lungs diminishes and they are no longer able to effectively perform their principal function of exchanging oxygen for carbon dioxide. Ultimately, they are destroyed by inflammation and infection. Emphysema often is associated with chronic bronchitis.

Common Diagnostic Tests

- Chest x-ray
- Arterial blood gases (ABGs) (See LAB.)
- Pulmonary function tests
- Lung scan with flow studies (See NR, Scans.)

Observations

- Check the nature of the respirations to see if they are shallow, rapid, and labored. Note whether the patient's shoulders, neck, or abdominal muscles are used in breathing, especially during exhalation.

- Check the color of the skin. A very pink skin color indicates oxygen retention. Cyanosis indicates an oxygenation failure.
- A PaO_2 below 50 mmHg and a $PaCO_2$ greater than 50 mmHg, or both, at sea level usually are considered as respiratory failure.
- Jugular vein distention (JVD), a sign of right-sided heart failure, often is associated with respiratory distress.
- Cerebral anoxia is demonstrated by restlessness and confusion.
- Clubbing of the fingers is common in some types of long-standing pulmonary, disease, *e.g.,* pulmonary fibrosis.
- A cough is usually present.
- Listen for chest sounds.
- Check for symptoms of upper respiratory infection (URI).

Treatment

- Inhalation therapy with the introduction of bronchodilator drugs, by aerosal: e.g. isoproterenol hydrochloride (Isuprel.) Inhalation: e.g. Melaproteronol (Alupent) may be started (see PH).
- Water by mouth, a nebulizer, or a vaporizer to aid in liquifying mucous secretions may be ordered.
- Chest physical therapy and postural drainage are recommended.
- Medications, *e.g.,* steroids (prednisone), bronchodilators
- (aminophyllin), and antibiotics, may be ordered (See PH).
- Endotracheal suctioning may be necessary to remove any accumulation of bronchial secretions.
- Oxygen administration is a treatment that must be monitored carefully through blood-gas analyses. Individuals with chronic lung disease are often limited to 1 liter or less of oxygen per minute. They *must* not be given more. Never give more than 2 liters (per minute) to *any* patient without a physician's order (see NR, Oxygen administration).

Nursing Considerations

- The normal stimulus to increase the depth of breathing is an increase in the carbon dioxide (CO_2) level in the blood. Patients with severe COPD become habituated to a high CO_2 level, and their resultant lack of stimulus to breathe produces an insufficient oxygen (O_2) level or hypoxia. A secondary stimulus then takes over, which is triggered by the hypoxia. If this hypoxia is relieved by administering high concentrations of O_2 to the patient, then the secondary stimulus does not function, and the patient may breathe too slowly or even cease to breathe. This results in a further build-up of CO_2, which may rapidly lead to coma, or CO_2 narcosis. Thus, either too little or too much oxygen will be harmful, and the flow rate must be monitored carefully.

- At the beginning of each shift, check patients receiving oxygen for correct liter flow. The oxygen also must pass through humidification. Be sure that the water bottle is kept full. Extension tubing should enable the patient to move about the room without taking the oxygen mask on and off.
- Sedatives, tranquilizers, hypnotics, and narcotics should be avoided since they suppress the respiratory drive and the cough reflex, and thus may be fatal.
- Instruct patients in the use of hand nebulizers; teach them to blow out as much air as possible, placing the nebulizer in the mouth, inhaling slowly, and then exhaling through pursed lips. Caution about the overuse of nebulizers, which may decrease their effectiveness and may aggravate arrhythmias, which are very common with COPD.
- Damaged lungs display a high degree of infection; normal lungs are seldom infected. Antibiotics generally should not be started until a sputum specimen for culture is obtained, and then a specific antibiotic is selected. It is best to collect a sputum specimen shortly after the patient awakens and coughs it up. It also can be obtained during a respiratory therapy treatment, when the patient may find it easier to produce sputum. Also, it may be collected while suctioning in a special tube attached for this purpose. Document the volume, consistency, color, and odor of sputum collected during each shift. Do not allow sputum to collect at the bedside for longer than 24 hours.
- There is a need to reduce the work of breathing for these patients. Teach abdominal breathing to those with emphysema by placing one of their hands on their chest and one on the abdomen. In abdominal breathing, the abdomen moves while the chest remains immobile.
- Breathing through pursed lips prolongs the time it takes to exhale. This enables the patient to perform the actions that require the greatest exertion, *e.g.,* sitting up in bed and moving to a chair, while exhaling.
- Milk and milk products thicken mucous secretions and should be avoided.
- The most common cause of a severe increase in symptoms of asthma is an upper respiratory infection. Hospitalization usually occurs if the $PaCO_2$ level is elevated and there is need for IV hydration and medication.

PNEUMONIA

Description

In pneumonia, the alveoli (small chambers) of the lung become inflamed and fill with an exudate. As this process continues, the lung tissue becomes consolidated, and inspired air is unable to contact blood for gas exchange. Pneumonias generally are referred to by their causative agents: *e.g.*, pneumococcal, gram-negative, staphylococcal, and viral. Pneumococcal pneumonias usually follow upper respiratory infections (URI). Staphylococcal and gram-negative pneumonias frequently are complications of other diseases in weak and debilitated patients. Viral pneumonias occur suddenly without any preexisting condition. Pneumonia also may result from aspiration of a liquid or solid, or circulatory congestion in the lungs (hypostatic pneumonia).

Common Diagnostic Tests

- Chest x-ray
- Sputum culture
- Nasopharyngeal cultures
- Blood culture
- Arterial blood gases

Observations

- Rapid and shallow respirations
- A high temperature that may be accompanied by chills
- Chest pain which, if severe, may indicate pleurisy
- Coughing, which may produce thick or greenish-yellow colored sputum

Treatment

- Antibiotics specific for organisms involved
- Antitussives, expectorants, and antipyretics
- Analgesics
- Isolation, depending on causative agent (See NR, Isolation.)
- Oxygen, if indicated, and humidification of room (See NR, Oxygen therapy.)
- Increased fluid, PO or IV

Nursing Considerations

- The causative agent needs to be identified before antibiotics are started. Thus, it is of the utmost importance that blood and sputum cultures are obtained as soon as possible.
- Use common sense in the choice of roommate for the patient if isolation is not required. It is preferable to have these patients in a private room.

- Patients who, for any reason, require suctioning of the upper respiratory tract, are especially susceptible to pneumonia. Always use strict sterile technique while suctioning (see NR, Nasopharyngeal suctioning).
- Be alert to the possibility of reactions to antibiotics, and check for fungal infestation after several days of antibiotics. This appears in the mouth or vagina as patches on the mucosa.
- Increased fluid intake will help loosen thick airway secretions.
- Bath blankets placed under and above the patients help absorb moisture from these often very diaphoretic patients.
- Even though it is often painful for these patients to turn and cough, insist that this be done. Mucous plugs can easily form and block airways, resulting in atelectasis (lung collapse).

PNEUMOTHORAX

Description

Pneumothorax is a condition in which air enters the pleural space. It may occur as the result of a leak in the lung (spontaneous pneumothorax) or from air entering through an opening in the chest wall. When air is admitted into the pleural space, it tends to collapse the lung or prevent its full expansion. A tension pneumothorax occurs if the air becomes trapped within the pleural space, causing pressure within the space to exceed atmospheric pressure. A mediastinal shift may then result, with the heart and other organs within the mediastinum shifting toward the opposite side of the chest. This disturbs the normal function of the heart and of the healthy lung.

Common Diagnostic Test

- Chest x-ray with inspiratory and expiratory films

Observations

- A sudden, sharp chest pain with a lack of chest movement on one side may occur, frequently after severe coughing. This is followed by anxiety, dyspnea, tachycardia, and, possibly, a fall in blood pressure.
- Tension pneumothorax and mediastinal shifts are *extreme emergencies* because shock and cardiac failure may occur within minutes.

Treatment

- Thoracentesis (See NR, Thoracentesis.)
- Chest tubes (See NR, Chest tube drainage.)

- Oxygen (See NR, Oxygen administration.)
- Analgesics
- Surgical correction of a leak within the lung

Nursing Considerations

- Because the patient is usually extremely apprehensive, stay with the patient as much as possible.
- Patients are usually most comfortable with the head of the bed elevated.
- Chest tubes cause pain, and the pain often continues for several days after their removal. Pain relief is imperative.
- Pneumothorax may be a complication of chronic obstructive pulmonary disease (see MSN, Chronic obstructive pulmonary disease).
- Pneumothorax is not often seen in pediatric patients, but it does occur, especially in premature infants.

PULMONARY EMBOLISM

Description

Pulmonary embolism generally is the result of a thrombus that originates in the venous system (most often in the deep veins of the legs or pelvis) or in the heart. Part of the thrombus breaks off and becomes an embolus. An embolus, called a fat embolus, also may occur after a long bone fracture. The embolus moves into the pulmonary circulation and blocks one or more arteries, thus becoming a pulmonary embolism. An infarction with necrosis of lung tissue results because of curtailed blood supply. If sufficient arterial blood supply to the lungs is obstructed by an embolism, sudden death results.

Common Diagnostic Tests

- Pulmonary arteriogram
- Lung scan (See NR, Scans.)
- Chest x-ray
- Arterial blood gases (See LAB.)
- PT and PTT measurements (See LAB.)

Observations

- The intensity of the symptoms is indicative of the severity of the obstruction.
- Common symptoms are dyspnea; sudden chest pain, with in-

creased pain on inspiration; diaphoresis; tachycardia; weakness; cough (perhaps hemoptysis); and mildly elevated temperature.

- A positive Homans' sign (pain in the calf of leg when foot is dorsiflexed) may be the first indication of deep vein thrombosis.
- Large emboli usually occur in veins above the knee.
- Low PaO_2 levels are found on blood-gas analysis.

Treatment

- *Immediate treatment is necessary.*
- Introduce an IV line for vein access (see NR, IV therapy).
- Oxygen may be administered (see NR, Oxygen therapy).
- Analgesics may be ordered (see PH).
- Anticoagulants, *e.g.,* heparin and warfarin (Coumadin) are ordered (see PH).

Nursing Considerations

- Prevention should be the first consideration. Hospitalized patients must be assessed daily for any indication of deep vein thrombosis.
- Pain, inflammation of the lower calf or thigh, or a positive Homans' sign should be reported immediately to the physician.
- Elastic stockings should be used and should fit well, extending to just below the knee. They can be removed twice a day for 5 minutes to 10 minutes.
- These patients usually are on anticoagulants for many days. Be aware of any unusual bleeding. Daily PT and PTT measurements are done. Be sure the physician is notified of daily results.
- The use of cough pillow (a very firm surface) pressed against the chest helps relieve some of the chest pain that occurs with coughing or other chest movement.

PULMONARY SURGERY

Description

Pulmonary surgery includes exploratory thoracotomy and resection of all or part of a lung. A resection most frequently is performed for removal of cancer, but it also may be necessary following a lung abscess or bronchiectasis.

The following are types of pulmonary surgery. A pneumonectomy is the removal of a lung. A lobectomy is the removal of a lobe. A segmented resection is the removal of one of the lung segments.

And, a wedge resection is the removal of a small amount of lung tissue.

Common Diagnostic Tests

- Chest x-ray, which includes tomography to check for any lesions
- Sputum for cytologic examination
- Pulmonary function tests and blood-gas studies (See LAB).
- Bronchoscopy with biopsy (See NR, Endoscopic procedures.)

Nursing Considerations

Preoperative

- Encourage smokers to stop smoking at least two weeks before surgery to help decrease mucus production and increase oxygen saturation of lungs.
- Patients may routinely go to an intensive care unit (ICU) after chest surgery. If this is the case, arrange for an ICU nurse to visit the patient and explain ICU procedures and equipment. Assess how receptive a patient is before scheduling the visit or conference.
- Patients and family members should be told about oxygen equipment, possible use of a ventilator, nasogastric tubes, IV lines, chest tubes, and the frequency of nursing checks of vital signs.
- Demonstrations of turning, coughing, and deep breathing, along with range of motion (ROM) and arm exercises (see NR, Range of motion exercises), should be done several times. Have the patient return the demonstration. Explain that coughing and deep breathing are most effective in a sitting position. Sputum will probably be bloody at first. During the first 24 hours after surgery, there will be little rest because of the necessity of maintaining circulatory and respiratory efficiency.
- Patients should be aware that, although pain is to be expected, narcotics will be given to minimize severe discomfort.

Postoperative

- In any postoperative patient, respiratory change is an important indicator of physical status. Restlessness, disorientation, or change in the level of consciousness (LOC) can indicate respiratory distress.
- Congestive heart failure and pulmonary edema are possible complications of a pneumonectomy.
- Hemorrhage may first become evident by a drop in blood pressure, tachycardia, and a large amount of blood in pleural drainage. Mark with a pencil the drainage on the bandage at the beginning of each shift. Increases will be obvious.

- Chest tubes must be milked each hour. When two tubes are in place, the anterior tube removes air and the posterior tube removes serosanguineous fluid. Chest tubes usually are not used after a pneumonectomy (see NR, Chest tube drainage).
- Oxygen therapy after pulmonary surgery is critical because of the possibility of inadequate alveolar perfusion and increased oxygen demand (see NR, Oxygen administration).
- Suctioning is important in order to maintain an open airway if the patient is unable to expectorate mucus (see NR, Nasopharyngeal suctioning).
- A central venous pressure (CVP) line may be used following pulmonary surgery to monitor cardiac performance and establish infusion rates (see NR, Central venous pressure). However, pulmonary artery catheters (Swan-Ganz catheters) have replaced CVP lines in many hospitals, and this procedure usually is done in ICUs.
- Hourly measurement of chest drainage is done for the first 24 hours.
- Positioning orders should be written specifically. A patient should not lie on the unoperated side following a pneumonectomy because of the necessity of maximum expansion of the remaining lung.
- Turning, coughing, and deep breathing must be done every hour for the first 24 hours. Then, the period may be extended to every two hours or four hours. Note the color of the sputum, which can be an early indication of infection, if, e.g., it changes from bloody to nonclear mucus.
- When the patient is told to cough and deep breathe, the nurse should splint the chest by placing one hand on the front incision line and the other on the back incision line.
- Passive (with support) exercises involving the arm and shoulder on the affected side should begin as soon as the patient regains consciousness. These are done every four hours. They should be changed gradually to active (independent) exercises. Encourage use of the arm on the affected side by placing the bedside table on that side.
- Pain is usually severe and continues for the first 24 hours to 48 hours, and may continue after the chest tubes are removed. Medicate the patient to keep him or her comfortable and cooperative when required movements are to be performed. Check the quality of respirations before and after the administration of narcotics.
- Check the dressing and surrounding tissue every hour for the first 24 hours, and then as indicated. Subcutaneous emphysema first becomes apparent as edematous tissue that "crackles"when touched.

PULMONARY TUBERCULOSIS

Description

Tubercle bacilli most commonly gain access to the lung, and an inflammatory reaction occurs, producing a tubercle (nodule). If the body's resistance is high, calcification occurs, and the disease is arrested at this stage. If the disease progresses, purulent material forms within the tubercle, which eventually breaks down, a cavity forms, and the disease spreads into adjacent tissues.

Common Diagnostic Tests

- A tuberculin intradermal test (PPD intermediate) is considered positive if, in 48 hours, an indurated (swollen) area 10 mm or larger appears at the site of test.
- A chest x-ray is necessary
- Sputum culture: collect early in the morning. It often takes 4 weeks to 8 weeks to produce a positive growth of acid-fast bacilli (AFB) (see LAB).

Observations

- Fatigue, weight loss, elevated temperature (late in the day), chronic cough, and hemoptysis are possible. These symptoms usually only occur when the disease is well advanced.

Treatment

- Modern treatment consists predominantly of drug therapy, in contrast to extended sanatorium care.
- The principal drugs that are include ethambutol (Miambutol), isoniazid (INH), and Rifampin (see PH).

Nursing Considerations

- Today, most patients with tuberculosis are treated as out-patients by their physicians. Those seen in hospitals have advanced disease or are diagnosed while hospitalized for other reasons.
- Respiratory isolation is ordered until the patient's AFB smears are negative, usually after 1 week to 2 weeks of therapy. This could be longer in some cases.
- If there is a productive cough, teach the patient to cover his or her mouth, to place used tissue in a disposable bag, and to wash hands afterwards.

- Be prepared to give the patient information about the medication and review it with him or her. Emphasize the necessity for taking medication daily, without missing any days.
- It is important that adequate rest and a good diet be maintained. Ask the dietitian to talk to the patient.
- The patient's family needs as much education as the patient. Be sure the family members understand the treatment and have been tested for tuberculosis themselves.

NORMAL AGING CHANGES IN THE RESPIRATORY SYSTEM

- A significant degree of kyphosis (exaggerated curvature of the spine) occurs in approximately 70% of the elderly.
- There is a gradual increase in the anterior-posterior diameter of the chest resulting from vertebral and rib calcification.
- The chest wall stiffens and becomes harder.
- Respiratory muscles (diaphragm and intercostals) are weakened.
- An increase in size of the alveoli occurs, and alveolar ducts become dilated.
- There is a loss of capillaries surrounding the alveoli, with resulting decreased diffusing capacity.
- Epithelial (cellular covering) atrophy occurs in the bronchi and bronchioles; ciliary action is diminished.
- Total lung volume (TLV) does not change, but forced vital capacity is decreased and residual volume is increased.
- PaO_2 (partial pressure of oxygen) decreases with age, but $PaCO_2$ (partial pressure of carbon dioxide) remains the same.

IMPLICATIONS

- Despite age-related changes, the ability to maintain oxygenation is *not* seriously impaired if the person is healthy and moderately active. However, an elderly individual's functional reserve ability decreases with anxiety, disease, and severe exercise.
- Because of anatomic changes, it may be more difficult to distinguish breath sounds. Auscultate laterally as well as on the back.
- The elderly person may have difficulty taking deep breaths and may have a weak cough; coughing and deep breathing are extremely important for the older ill person.
- Diminished ciliary activity causes difficulty in mobilizing secretions.
- Pulmonary blood flow normally favors the capillaries of the lower lungs, but the airways of the elderly are open predominantly in the upper lung areas, and contribute to a decreased PaO_2. This

"mismatching" will be worse when the elderly individual is supine and taking shallow breaths.

- Respiratory acidosis may present as severe agitation in the elderly person.
- Improper use of sedation can depress the respiratory centers and lead to respiratory arrest.
- Continuous bedrest is extremely hazardous to the elderly patient.

BIBLIOGRAPHY • Respiratory System

BOOKS

Baum G, Wolinski E: Textbook of Pulmonary Diseases, 3rd ed. Boston, Little Brown, 1983

Blodgett D: Manual of Respiratory Care Procedures. Philadelphia, JB Lippincott, 1980

Craig R (ed): Symposium on Respiratory Care. Nurs Clin North Am 16(2) 1981

Fisher D, Marsh J: (eds): Cancer Therapy. Boston, GK Hall, 1982

Glauser F (ed): Signs and Symptoms in Pulmonary Medicine. Philadelphia, JB Lippincott, 1983

Grenville-Mathers R: The Respiratory System, 2nd ed. Edinburgh, Churchill-Livingston, 1983

Netter F: The CIBA collection of Medical Illustrations, Vol 7, Respiratory System. CIBA Pharmaceutical Co, 1980

Traver G (ed): Respiratory Nursing: The Science and the Art. New York, John Wiley, 1982

Wade J: Comprehensive Respiratory Care, 3rd ed. St. Louis, CV Mosby, 1982

Youmans G: Tuberculosis. Philadelphia, WB Saunders, 1979

JOURNALS

Bakow E (ed): Acute respiratory care update. Crit Care Quarterly 6(2): 1983.

Brodoff A, (ed): When your patient's asthma is mild; When asthma causes "moderate" trouble. Consultant 15(19):115, 1981

Brodoff A (ed): When your patient's asthma is severe. Consultant 15(20):59, 1981

Callahan M: COPD: A special post-op challenge. RN 47(5):44, 1984

Chin R, Pesce R: Practical aspects in management of respiratory failure in chronic obstructive pulmonary disease. Crit Care Quarterly 6(2):1, 1983

Coleman D: TB: The disease that's not dead yet. RN 47(9):48 1984

Kaufman J, Woody J: For patients with COPD: Better living through teaching. Nursing '80(10):57, 1980

Kiblawi S, Jay S: Management of status asthmaticus. Resp Ther 11(2):48, 1981

Knepil J: The control of breathing. Nurs Mirror 156 (19):44, 1983

Krzysko A, Erdel S, Greiner M, Lawrance A: Guidelines for nursing care of patients with altered ventilation. Oncol Nurs Forum 10(2):113, 1983.

Matthay R: Management of acute respiratory failure: Conference summary. Resp Care 28(5):672, 1983

Penney M: Pneumonia. Am J Nurs 81(3):517, 1981

Raffin T, Roberts P: The prevention and treatment of status asthmaticus. Hosp Pract 71 (80A–Z–6), 1982

Snider G: Under the umbrella of COPD. Emerg Med 14(21):100, 1982

Smith M: Respiratory emergencies. Nurs Mirror 154 (11 Clinical Forum) 3, II–X 1982

Strieder D: Cystic fibrosis in adults. Resp Ther 11(4):71, 1981.

Turner-Warwick M: Some clinical problems in airway obstruction. Chest 82(1):35, 1982

Weber-Jones J, Bryant M: Over-the-counter bronchodilators. Nursing '80 10:34, 1980

Wenger N: Pulmonary embolism: Recognition and management. Consultant 20(6):85, 1980

Williams M: Severe asthma. Consultant 20(3):294, 1980

5
Obstetrics (OB)

PREGNANCY AND ANTENATAL CARE

Description

Human pregnancy lasts approximately for nine calendar months or for 266 days from conception. Some variation is common. For purposes of description, the nine calendar months frequently are divided into three trimesters, *i.e.,* the first, second, and third.

Perinatal care refers to care of the health needs of a woman through the entire pregnancy and three months of the postpartum period.

Gestation refers to the period of intrauterine fetal development from conception to birth. *Abortion* describes loss of pregnancy, whether spontaneous or induced, before the point of viability of the fetus. *Gravida* describes the number of times a woman has been pregnant. *Primigravida* indicates that a woman is pregnant for the first time; *multigravida* means that a woman has been pregnant more than once. *Para* indicates past pregnancies that continued to the point of viability of the fetus, regardless of whether the fetus was delivered alive or dead. *Nullipara* indicates that a woman has not carried a fetus to the point of viability; *multipara* means that she has had two or more pregnancies that continued to that point. Gravida and para refer to the pregnancy and not the fetus.

Common Diagnostic Tests

- Urinalysis: Screening for protein and glucose is done at every prenatal visit. Urine culture may be ordered if there is suspicion of infection.
- Blood tests
  1. Complete blood count
  2. Blood typing, Rh typing, and antibody screening
  3. Rubella titer and antibody screen
  4. Serologic tests for syphilis: VDRL is used most commonly for screening, but may produce biologic false-positive results. Positive results are tested further by the FTA-ABS absorption test, in which there is a higher degree of accuracy.
  5. Screen for sickle cell anemia for black patients
- Culture for gonorrhea
- Papanicolaou (Pap) smear
- Tests for pregnancy

1. Immunodiagnostic tests provide results with increasing accuracy after the 40th day following the first day of the last menstrual period (LMP). Examples include the hemagglutination inhibition test (Pregnosticon R) and agglutination inhibition test (Gravindex) on urine; and the radioreceptor assay (RRA), and beta HCG (human chorionic gonadotropin) by radioimmunoassay (RIA) on serum.
2. Pregnancy tests for home use are now available in over-the-counter kits.
3. Hormonal tests include the Aschheim-Zondek, Friedman's test, frog tests, and Kuppman or rat hypermic tests, which rarely are used now.

- Additional tests may be tailored to the client's special needs.
- Tests that assess the well-being of the fetus are described in a separate section (see Assessing Fetal Status).

Screening for the High-Risk Pregnancy

The pregnancy is considered to be high risk when the health or life of the mother or fetus is endangered. Prematurity is the greatest single factor in infant mortality or morbidity. Screening for risk factors continues throughout pregnancy. Common ones include the following:

- Personal
  1. Age of the patient—younger than 16 years or over 35 years
  2. Parity over four, especially when the woman is over 35 years
  3. Delayed or absent prenatal care
  4. Poor nutritional status
  5. Economic deprivation
  6. Heavy cigarette smoking, alcohol or drug abuse
  7. Exposure to disease or any substance that could damage the developing fetus
  8. Previous cesarean section or uterine surgery
  9. History of problems in past pregnancies, either with the woman or with the fetus/baby, including repeated spontaneous abortions, bleeding, still births, or preterm births
  10. Family history of genetic disorders
- Coexisting problems
  1. Diabetes
  2. Hypertension
  3. Cardiac disorders
  4. Thyroid problems
  5. Uterine fibroids
  6. Sickle cell anemia

7. Anemia
8. Infections, particularly rubella, toxoplasmosis, and sexually transmitted diseases

- Present pregnancy
  1. Preterm labor
  2. Bleeding, especially in the third trimester
  3. Preeclampsia, eclampsia
  4. Abnormal presentations
  5. Multiple pregnancy
  6. Hydramnios (excessive amniotic fluid)
  7. Intrauterine growth retardation (IUGR)

Observations

History includes screening for risk factors (see above).

- General factors, *e.g.,* age, marital status, family support systems, socioeconomic status, planned or unplanned pregnancy, educational needs regarding pregnancy
- Previous medical history
- Previous pregnancies, including dates, number, length of labor, birth weight of infant(s), problems encountered with the pregnancies or infants
- Present pregnancy, symptoms of pregnancy, weight at the onset of pregnancy
- Estimated date of confinement (EDC), calculated using Nägele's rule: Count back three months from the first day of the LMP and add seven days. Dating the pregnancy is important for the assessment of fetal growth. Ultrasound and measurement of fundal height are other methods of assessing gestational age.

Physical assessment includes the following:

- General appearance of physical and emotional health
- Vital signs
- Weight
  1. Measuring a baseline weight is essential during the first prenatal visit. A weight gain of 11 kg to 13 kg (24–28 lb) during the entire pregnancy is considered normal for most women, but it may not be restricted to that. Allowances are made for initial underweight or overweight patients. Weight loss, or a sudden, rapid weight gain, requires evaluation.
- Mouth, eyes, ears, nose, and throat, including palpation of the thyroid
- Heart and lungs
- Skin

1. Changes in the pigmentation of the skin are common, *e.g.*, linea nigra (pigmented skin on the midline of the abdomen) and facial chloasma or "mask of pregnancy" (darkened skin over the forehead and around the eyes that appears late in pregnancy, but almost always fades after delivery). Striae gravidarum, or stretch marks, may appear on the abdomen, buttocks, and breasts.

- Breasts and nipples
  1. Normal breast changes include enlargement, tenderness, and tingling sensations, especially during the first and third trimesters. Nodular tissue may be present. Veins become increasingly visible. Striae may appear.
  2. Increase in size and pigmentation of the nipples, darkening of the areolas (the pigmented area around the nipples), and the appearance of Montgomery tubercles (sebaceous glands of the areola that become enlarged during pregnancy) are common. Colostrum, a thin liquid precursor to milk, may be expressed from the nipples after the twelfth week.
- Abdomen

  Gradual enlargement of the abdomen is seen, with the fundus of the uterus being palpable near the end of the tenth to twelfth week.
  1. Fundal height—uterine size
     a. From approximately the 20th to the 36th week, the height of the uterine fundus is an indicator of gestational age in a normal singleton pregnancy. The distance between the notch of the symphysis pubis and the tip of the uterine fundus is measured with a flexible tape measure that is calibrated in centimeters.
     b. During this period, fundal height increases approximately 1 cm/week, and usually correlates roughly with gestational age in weeks; *e.g.*, a fundal height of 24 cm would indicate a gestational age of 24 weeks.
     c. A plus or minus of 4 cm in fundal height when compared with gestational age is considered abnormal and may indicate intrauterine growth retardation (IUGR), a multiple pregnancy, hydramnios, or inaccurate dates. While obesity and uterine fibroids may cause confusion, an abnormal fundal height is an indication for further study. Ultrasound provides a more accurate estimate of gestational age.
  2. Fetal heartbeats (normally 120–160 beats/min) may be heard with Doptone (portable ultrasound) at 10 weeks to 12 weeks, and with a fetoscope at 20 weeks. It is best heard over the area where the fetal back lies.
  3. Uterine souffle (a soft blowing sound caused by blood pulsating through the placenta) may be heard when auscultating

over the uterus. It beats at the rate and rhythm of the maternal pulse.

4. Funic souffle (a sharp, whistling sound caused by blood rushing through the fetal umbilical arteries) is sometimes heard. It beats at the rate of the fetal heart.
5. Fetal movement may be felt by the mother between 16 weeks and 20 weeks (quickening), and by an examiner after 20 weeks.
6. Ballottement describes the rebound of the fetal part when the abdomen of the mother is tapped lightly by an examiner.

- Pelvic examination
  1. Changes in the pelvic organs usually include the following: Chadwick's, Goodell's, Hegar's, and Ladin's signs
  2. Ovaries (size, shape, and position)
  3. Pelvimetry measures the dimensions of the bony pelvis, the angles and planes through which the fetus must pass for vaginal delivery. Ultrasound or an x-ray provides exact measurements, but measurements also can be estimated through vaginal examination.
     a. Most critical pelvic measurements estimate the size of the pelvic inlet, pelvic cavity, and pelvic outlet.
     b. When doing a vaginal examination, the examiner must know the length and width of his fingers by having actually measured them.
- Evidence of varicose veins of the lower extremities, the anorectal area (hemorrhoids), vagina, and vulva

Nursing Considerations

Prenatal visits should be made every month during the first 28 weeks of gestation, every 2 weeks from the 29th week until the 36th week, and on a weekly basis thereafter. More frequent visits may be required. These visits provide opportunities for assessment of fetal and maternal well-being, early treatment of problems, health education, and the development of a supportive relationship between the patient and health-care provider.

Health teaching regarding hygiene during pregnancy should include the following:

- Adequate rest: This may mean more than normal amounts especially during the first and third trimesters when fatigue is common. A break in the day for a short rest period is helpful.
- Nutrition: Adequate maternal nutrition is one key to delivering a normal-birth-weight baby. Diet during pregnancy should adequately meet the needs of both the mother and developing fetus. It should be balanced and meet the recommended daily dietary allowances (RDA) for pregnant women. Calories, protein, vita-

mins, and minerals should be increased. (Iron, and often vitamin, dietary supplements frequently are prescribed.)

1. Weight gain during pregnancy should take into account the woman's prepregnant weight and nutritional status.
2. For most women, a weight gain of from 11 kg to 13 kg (24–28 lb) over pregravid weight is recommended, but not mandated.
3. Weight loss or failure to gain, or a sudden weight gain should be investigated.
4. A diet history in which the patient writes down everything she eats for a specified time period (*e.g.*, 1–3 days) may provide data on which to base nutritional counseling.
5. For more information, consult the dietitian affiliated with your agency or hospital. Nutritional information is available from many sources, including the American College of Obstetricians and Gynecologists, the Public Health Service, and the March of Dimes-Birth Defects Foundation. If for financial reasons the patient is unable to meet her nutritional needs, refer her to an appropriate public assistance agency.

- Exercise in normal amounts: Walking outdoors is an especially appropriate form of exercise. The patient should check with her clinician regarding participation in strenuous sports.
- Clothing should be clean, comfortable, and nonrestricting.
  1. Maternity girdles are not necessary but may be helpful in providing support for a pendulous abdomen. Cotton undergarments are recommended. Tight leg bands or elastic garters may restrict circulation and should not be worn.
  2. Comfortable, well-fitting shoes with low to moderate heels provide stability and do not aggravate back discomfort by accentuating curvature of the back.
- Bathing
  1. Showering has the advantage of ease and safety when getting in and out. It also is recommended for women who are subject to urinary tract infections.
  2. Tub bathing is allowable, except in the presence of ruptured membranes or vaginal bleeding. Side rails, a rubber bath mat, and warm, but not hot, water increase safety.
- A dental check up early in pregnancy—proper dental hygiene: Bleeding gums are common. Patients should brush teeth gently with a soft brush, and use dental floss or a Water Pic regularly. Major dental work, including x-rays, requires consultation between dentist and physician or midwife.
- The patient should avoid cigarette smoking during pregnancy. Smoking is believed to be associated with low-birth-weight babies.
- Alcohol consumption, even in minimal to moderate amounts, may be harmful to the fetus.

- Many drugs, when taken during the first trimester of pregnancy, have a damaging effect on the fetus. Teratogenic effects are most likely to occur during the time between fertilization and the end of the first trimester when organogenesis (the development of body organs from embryonic tissues) is taking place. Any medications taken during pregnancy should be taken under the direct supervision of the clinician (see Table 5-1). A drug history should be a part of the initial prenatal visit.
- Immunizations made with attenuated live viruses, *e.g.*, mumps and rubella, are contraindicated during pregnancy because of possible teratogenic effects on the developing embryo. Immunizations for poliomyelitis, influenza, smallpox, yellow fever, cholera, and hepatitis-A are given only in special circumstances.
- Breasts should be supported with a clean, comfortable, well-fitting, cotton brassiere with wide, non-elastic straps. All breast tissue should fit comfortably into the cup. The bra should adjust to accommodate enlarging breasts. Lack of support causes tissue to sag.

  Crusts caused by colostrum secreted from the nipples should be softened with an ointment such as lanolin cream or vitamin E oil, and then removed with warm water. Soap, because of its drying effect, should not be used on the nipples.

  Using care not to injure them, the patient can toughen her nipples in preparation for breast feeding by

  1. Using a rough towel to dry nipples after bathing
  2. Nipple-rolling, accomplished by grasping the nipple between the thumb and the forefinger and gently rolling it several times a day
  3. Oral stimulation by the woman's sex partner throughout pregnancy, if pleasurable to both

  Inverted nipples can be identified by gently pinching the areola at the base of the nipple with a forefinger and thumb. An inverted nipple retreats. If it comes out even a little, preparation, as described above, may make nursing possible. Some breast shields specially made to correct inverted nipples may correct the problem if worn during pregnancy.

- Vaginal irrigations (douches) should be done only with permission of the clinician.
- Perineal-tightening or Kegel's exercises should be encouraged in an effort to maintain good support for the pelvic organs. The patient is instructed to tighten the muscles of her vagina by stopping and starting the flow while urinating.
- Sexual activity

  Sexual intercourse is only restricted if membranes have ruptured, bleeding exists, or there are other factors that might lead to premature delivery.

OB

(*Text continues on page 467*)

TABLE 5-1 EFFECTS OF MATERNAL DRUG INGESTION ON THE NEONATE

1. *Teratogenesis*
   Alcohol*
   Anticonvulsants
   Cancer chemotherapeutic agents
   Corticosteroids
   Diazepam (Valium)
   Dicoumarol
   Hallucinogenic agents
   Lead
   Lithium
   Mercury
   Estrogens
   ? Ovulatory agents
   Progestagens
   ? Psychotropic agents
   Quinine
   Radiation
   Radioisotopes
   Stilbestrol (DES)
   Tetracyclnies

   Barbiturates
   Bromides
   Cholinesterase inhibitors
   Diazepam
   Hexamethonium
   Indomethacin
   Lithium
   Magnesium sulfate
   Narcotics
   Oxytocin
   Oxytocin + diuretic + IV fluids
   Paraldehyde
   Phenothiazines
   Pyridoxine
   Reserpine
   Salicylates*

6. *Convulsions*
   Local anesthetic agents
   Magnesium sulfate

   Glutethimide
   Hydroxyzine HCl
   Meprobamate
   Narcotics
   Pentazocine
   Trifluoperazine

9. *Effects on Metabolism*
   (a) Hypoglycemia
       Alcohol (IV and oral)
       Chlorpropamide
       Insulin
       Tolbutamide
       Propranolol
   (b) Hyperglycemia
       Diazoxide
   (c) Electrolyte imbalance
       Corticosteroids
       Diuretics + hypotonic IV fluids + oxytocin

Thalidomide
Warfarin

2. *Carcinogenesis*
? Cancer chemotherapeutic agents
Radiation
Radioactive drugs
Stilbestrol

3. *Effects on Somatic Growth*
Alcohol*
Anticonvulsants
Drugs of abuse

4. *Effects on Birth Weight*
Alcohol*
Cigarette smoking
Corticosteroids
Drugs of abuse
Ovulatory agents

5. *Effects on Immediate Adaptation to Extrauterine Life*
Aminophylline
Anesthetic agents

Oxytocin + diuretic + IV fluids
Pilocarpine
Pyridoxine

7. *Fetal Death*
Chloral hydrate*
Chlorpropamide
Dicoumarol
Ergot
Lead
Salicylates*

8. *Withdrawal Symptoms*
Alcohol*
Amitriptyline
Amphetamines
Anticonvulsant agents
Barbiturates
Chlordiazepoxide
Chlorpromazine
Dextropropoxyphene
Diazepam
Diphenhydramine
Drugs of abuse
? Ethchlorvynol

(d) Thyroid function
Iodine
Lithium
Radioactive drugs
Radiopaque dyes
Thioureas

10. *Hematologic Changes*
(a) Hemorrhage, anemia, platelets
Alcohol
Barbiturates
Dicoumarol
Diuretics
Local anesthetic agents†
Menaphthone (menadione) sodium bisulfite
Nitrofurantoin
Phenytoin
Promethazine
Quinine
Salicylates
Sulfonamides
Thioureas

(*continued*)

TABLE 5-1 EFFECTS OF MATERNAL DRUG INGESTION ON THE NEONATE

(b) Jaundice
- Menaphthone (menadione) sodium bisulfite
- Oxytocin
- Sulfonamides (long and short acting)

11. *Sexual Reproduction*
- Cigarette smoking
- ? Cancer chemotherapeutic agents
- ? Stilbestrol

12. *Effects on Mental Ability*
- Alcohol
- Anticonvulsants
- Carbon monoxide
- Dicumarol
- Mercury
- Radiation
- Radioisotopes
- Thioureas

13. *Renal failure*
- Acetaminophen (Tylenol)

* Excessive doses
† Methemoglobinemia
(From Stern L, Hill R: Drugs and pregnancy. Drugs 17(3):183,1979)

(continued from page 463)

Because of the discomforts of early and late pregnancy, sexual desire and response may vary from normal. The second trimester is probably the optimum time during pregnancy for sexual activity. The woman may experience more sexual satisfaction than prior to pregnancy because of increased vascular congestion of the pelvis.

Alternative positions, *e.g.*, female superior, rear entry, or side-lying, may have to be used as the woman's abdomen grows. Sexual needs may be nurtured by cuddling, kissing, and being held by one's sexual partner. Mutual masturbation may be a pleasurable alternative to sexual intercourse, as long as both partners feel comfortable with it.

Orgasmic changes may occur in the last trimester. The woman may experience a contraction lasting up to one minute instead of usual rhythmic orgasmic contractions. These contractions do not cause premature labor in the majority of pregnant women.

Expectant couples need to be aware of changing sexual desires during pregnancy, the need for sharing these feelings, and finding satisfying adaptations to them.

- Patients should know that any deviation from normal (*e.g.*, diabetes mellitus, heart disease, hypo- or hyperthyroidism, and any kind of infection) should be called to the attention of the obstetrician so that the condition can be treated and monitored.
- "Lightening" occurs near the end of pregnancy, usually 2 weeks to 3 weeks before term in a primigravida and just before or during labor in a multigravida. The fetus "drops" to a lower position in the abdomen. The patient will find breathing easier. She will feel more out of balance as lordosis increases. Urinary frequency increases because of pressure on the bladder.
- Every patient should know the danger signs of pregnancy and recognize the importance of reporting them immediately.

Danger Signals of Pregnancy

The appearance of any of these symptoms should be reported to the physician immediately.

Vaginal bleeding

Abdominal pain

Sudden chills or fever

Headaches

Dizziness, blurred or double vision, spots before the eyes

Edema of the face, hands, or feet

Sudden weight gain

Persistent vomiting

Unusual vaginal discharge, itching, or burning

Frequency, pain on urination

- The patient should also know the signs of approaching labor—bloody show (mucous plug often tinged with blood), rupture of the membranes (slow or sudden gush of fluid from vagina), and the establishment of regular, frequent, strong contractions.

COMMON DISCOMFORTS OF PREGNANCY AND MEASURES THAT MAY HELP

(Discomforts are listed alphabetically)

- Backache
    1. Pelvic tilt exercises help relieve the exaggerated lumbosacral curvature of the back during pregnancy. They may be done while lying supine, standing, or on hands and knees. Yoga exercises also may be helpful.
    2. Proper body mechanics, including good posture, are important.
    3. Low-heeled shoes can help prevent backaches.
    4. For sleep, the side-lying (Sims') position with a pillow between the knees and a firm support mattress are recommended.
    5. A maternity girdle can be worn to provide external support for the pendulous abdomen.
- Constipation
    1. Increase fluid intake to up to 8 glasses of water a day.
    2. Increase roughage and fiber in the diet (*e.g.*, bran, fruits, celery, potato skins, and whole-grain breads).
    3. Prunes and prune juice are effective natural laxatives.
    4. Follow a daily exercise program.
    5. Improve bowel habits.
        a. Establish a regular, uninterrupted time of the day for having a bowel movement.
        b. Don't ignore the sensation of the urge to defecate.
    6. When natural methods fail, mild laxatives, stool softeners, or suppositories occasionally may be needed.
    7. Sometimes oral iron supplements are constipating. One that contains a stool softener may help.
- Dependent edema
    1. Avoid prolonged standing or sitting with legs dependent.
    2. Avoid tight garters and sitting with crossed legs.
    3. Elevate legs when sitting or lying. Do it several times a day for at least 15 minutes at a time.
    4. When sitting for extended periods of time, get up and walk around at intervals.
    5. When standing, shift weight from one foot to the other, and flex the feet frequently to exercise the calf muscles and propel venous blood upward.

6. Lying on the left side enhances renal blood flow and venous return.
7. Be aware that edema associated with eclampsia and pre-eclampsia tends to be generalized—including the face, hands, and abdomen.

- Dyspnea or shortness of breath, most common in the last trimester, is relieved in the primigravida patient when lightening occurs.
  1. Good posture and having the upper part of the body elevated relieves the pressure of the uterus on the diaphragm.
- Heartburn
  1. Small frequent meals are recommended.
  2. Avoid spicy, fatty, or highly acid foods.
  3. Avoid constrictive clothing around the waist.
  4. Sleep with the head elevated.
  5. Specific antacids such as aluminum hydroxide (Amphojel), magnesium trisilicate (Gelusil), and magnesium hydroxide (Maalox) may be recommended. Soda bicarbonate (baking soda), Tums, Rolaids, and Alka-Seltzer should be avoided because of their high sodium contents.
- Hemorrhoids (varicosities of the anal area) (See MSN, Gastrointestinal system, anorectal conditions.)
  1. Avoid constipation (see above).
  2. Chilled witch hazel soaks (Tucks) can be used.
  3. Avoid long periods of standing and sitting.
  4. Elevate hips, as well as lower extremities, several times a day and at night.
  5. Topical ointments, anesthetic agents, and warm soaks may be helpful.
  6. After each bowel movement, using a lubricant, gently reinsert internal hemorrhoids.
  7. Sitz baths are recommended.
- Leg cramps
  1. With the patient lying down, straighten the leg and dorsiflex the foot.
  2. Dietary modifications may be recommended on the assumption that cramps are caused by an imbalance in the calcium/phosphorus ratio. Emphasis is usually on increasing calcium intake and decreasing phosphorus intake.
  3. Daily exercise to improve circulation is important.
- Morning sickness

  Nausea, with or without vomiting, may occur when the stomach is empty at any time during the day or night. Most commonly, it is a symptom during the early months of pregnancy, and is relieved by the fourth month. If severe and unrelieved after that time, it may indicate hyperemesis gravidarum or hydatidiform mole.

1. Dietary modifications include the following:
   a. Eat three or four dry crackers before sitting up in bed in the morning.
   b. Eat six small meals a day, including a low-fat bedtime snack.
   c. Avoid greasy, fatty, and spicy foods, or any foods that are known to precipitate the problem.
   d. Take adequate amounts of vitamin B complex daily. Vitamin B_6 (pyridoxine hydrochloride) is particularly recommended.
2. Rising from bed slowly minimizes orthostatic hypotension.
3. Rushing in the morning should be avoided.

- Urinary frequency
  1. During the first and third trimesters, the pregnant uterus presses directly on the mother's bladder and causes symptoms of urinary frequency and urgency.
  2. The pregnant woman should limit fluids after dinner, to reduce nocturia.
  3. Symptoms should be evaluated to rule out urinary tract infection (see MSN, Urinary tract infections).
- Vaginal discharge

  Increased vaginal discharge (leukorrhea) is normal during pregnancy. Excessive foul-smelling discharge, itching, or burning may indicate infection and should be evaluated.
  1. Showering or bathing can help.
  2. Cotton underpants should be changed several times daily.
  3. No constricting clothing, *e.g.*, tight jeans, should be worn.
  4. Cornstarch may help maintain a dry perineum.
- Varicosities (See MSN, Cardiovascular system, varicose veins.)
  1. See notes under dependent edema above.
  2. Support stockings, including those made-to-measure on prescription, should be put on before getting out of bed in the morning.
  3. Elevating the foot of the bed on shock blocks may be indicated in severe cases.
  4. Varicosities of the vulva (as well as hemorrhoids) may be helped by elevating the hips on two pillows while elevating the legs, several times of the day.
  5. A sanitary napkin held in place by a belt will support vulvar varicosities. It should be changed frequently.
  6. Be alert for signs and symptoms of complicating thrombophlebitis or phlebothrombosis (see MSN, Cardiovascular system, thrombophlebitis).

COMPLICATIONS OF PREGNANCY

BLEEDING DISORDERS

Vaginal bleeding during pregnancy is a danger signal that must be evaluated. (See Table 5-2 for differential diagnosis.) In all cases, the immediate danger is hypovolemic shock that leads to renal damage and disseminated intravascular coagulation (DIC). The ultimate danger is fetal or maternal death.

Nursing Considerations

Elements of care of the pregnant patient who is bleeding include the following:

- A history of the pregnancy, including onset, duration, and severity of bleeding and any relevant medical history, should be obtained. A more complete medical history can be taken when bleeding is under control.
- Constant monitoring of vital signs is necessary.
- Observe for signs of shock—pallor, clammy skin, perspiration, dyspnea, or restlessness.
- Record the estimated blood loss. (To estimate it pour 30 ml of water on a pad to see how 30 ml of fluid looks.) Count the number of pads used and the estimated amount of blood on each one. Expelled tissue or clots should be saved.
- Monitor fetal and labor status, including the presence or degree of abdominal pain.
- Intravenous fluids will be started. Use a large-bore needle (*e.g.*, #18) so that blood may be started when available (see NR, Intravenous therapy).
- Organize laboratory work for type and cross-match, coagulation studies, hematocrit and hemoglobin, and other blood work as indicated.
- Oxygen therapy may be initiated (see NR, Oxygen therapy).
- Monitor urinary output hourly. A Foley catheter and measurement of specific gravity may be ordered.
- Prepare the patient for examinations and procedures.
- Emotional support for the patient and her support person, including an examination of what is happening, is essential.

OB

HYDRAMNIOS (POLYHYDRAMNIOS)

Description

Hydramnios (polyhydramnios) is a condition in which there is an excessive amount of amniotic fluid. Although the cause is unknown, the condition is frequently associated with fetal anomalies, espe-

(*Text continues on page 478*)

TABLE 5-2 BLEEDING DURING PREGNANCY—DIFFERENTIAL DIAGNOSIS

Description	Causes	Observations	Treatment
Abortion (Spontaneous) Termination of the pregnancy prior to viability of the fetus. It usually occurs early in pregnancy—before the 16th week. *Spontaneous*—implies natural causes (non-induced) *Threatened*—pregnancy in doubt, but may continue *Inevitable*—no chance for salvage of the pregnancy *Complete*—all products of conception expelled. *Incomplete*—partial expulsion of products of conception *Missed*—uterus retains products of conception for 2 or more months after the death of the fetus	Fetal defects Maternal factors, *e.g.*, diabetes, trauma, dietary deficiencies, incompetent cervix Unknown	History of pink discharge for several days, or a scant brownish discharge for several weeks Vaginal bleeding Uterine cramping Backache Products of pregnancy usually expelled Signs and symptoms of pregnancy disappear Pregnancy tests, questionable or negative	When abortion threatens: 1. Bed rest 2. Abstinence from sexual intercourse 3. Sedation Treatment for hemorrhage (See Nursing considerations for the care of a patient who is bleeding during pregnancy.) Dilatation and curettage (D & C) or dilatation and evacuation (D & E) may be required to remove all products of conception in cases of incomplete abortion. Analgesics and oxytocin may be ordered. An Rh-negative mother with a negative indirect Coombs' test

Habitual—spontaneous loss of three or more consecutive pregnancies

should receive $Rh_o(D)$ immune human globulin (Rh_oGAM) within 72 hours.

Most physicians urge women to go through two to three menstrual cycles before attempting to become pregnant again.

For the woman with habitual abortions:

1. Thorough examinations of both husband and wife are necessary.
2. If an incompetent cervix is found, surgical reinforcement of it may be recommended (Shirodkar-Barter procedure). Sutures may be removed after about 14 to 16 weeks; or they may be left in place and the patient delivered by cesarean section.

See OB, Abortion—induced.

(*continued*)

TABLE 5-2 BLEEDING DURING PREGNANCY—DIFFERENTIAL DIAGNOSIS

Description	Causes	Observations	Treatment
Hydatidiform Mole 1. A developmental anomaly of the placenta, in which chorionic villi degenerate into a mass of fluid-filled, grapelike vesicles 2. Although the mole is benign, the incidence of choriocarcinoma following it is high. 3. It is seen early in pregnancy in 1 out of 2,000 pregnancies. It is more common in multipara patients over 40 years old, and is seen more often in Asia than in the United States.	Unknown	Brownish, bloody vaginal discharge with appearance of grapelike vesicles Hyperemesis during the first trimester Fundal height in advance of gestational age Elevated HCG levels after 100 days past LMP Absence of fetal heart tones or fetal movement Sonography reveals no fetal skeleton Elevated blood pressure	Suction curettage of the uterus with complete evacuation of the mole Sharp curettage performed 1–2 weeks later Hysterectomy, if patient wants no more children Intensive medical follow-up because of incidence of choriocarcinoma following this condition Prevention of pregnancy for at least 1 year Frequent evaluation of HCG titers Treatment for hemorrhage, if it occurs. (See Nursing Considerations.)

Placenta Previa (See Fig. 5-1) 1. The placenta is abnormally implanted in the lower segment of the uterus, either partially or completely covering the cervical os; or it is low-lying so that the placental edge is very close to, but does not cover, the os. 2. It is seen late in pregnancy in 1 out of 200 pregnancies. 3. It is more common in multipara patients, especially those with a history of previous placenta previa or low cervical cesarean section.	Unknown	Painless, bright red vaginal bleeding during the third trimester In the first episode, bleeding is usually scanty, with more profuse bleeding during each subsequent episode. Evidence of placenta previa by ultrasound only can be diagnosed accurately after 28 weeks.	When and how (whether vaginally or by cesarean section) to deliver the baby are dependent upon its maturity (see OB, Assessing fetal status), and the amount of bleeding. Vaginal examination may cause overt bleeding, so it is avoided unless absolutely necessary. When a vaginal examination must be done to determine the extent of the placenta previa, a double set-up should be provided so that either cesarean or vaginal delivery can be accomplished on an emergency basis. Treatment for hemorrhage if it occurs. See Nursing Considerations.

(*continued*)

TABLE 5-2 BLEEDING DURING PREGNANCY—DIFFERENTIAL DIAGNOSIS

Description	Causes	Observations	Treatment
Ectopic Pregnancy			
Abnormal implantation of fertilized ovum outside the uterine cavity, *e.g.*, in the fallopian tubes, ovary, or abdominal cavity Seen early in pregnancy in 1 out of 200 pregnancies; 98% of these are tubal implantations	Factors that affect tubal contractibility, ciliary action, or patency, or sperm mobility, *e.g.*, salpingitis, pelvic inflammatory disease	Symptoms usually appear after tubal rupture. They include sudden, severe, unilateral pain in the lower abdomen; and shock—elevated pulse rate, falling blood pressure. Other symptoms include abnormal menstrual periods; symptoms of pregnancy, *e.g.*, nausea, breast discomfort; vaginal bleeding, frequently with passage of tissue. Pregnancy tests may be negative. Laparoscopy, culdoscopy, or laparotomy may confirm the diagnosis.	Surgical removal of affected organs, with an effort made to leave a normal fallopian tube, ovary, and the uterus for potential future childbearing Treatment for hemorrhage if it occurs. (See Nursing Considerations.)

Placental Separation or abruptio Placentae (See Fig. 5-2) 1. Separation of the placenta from the uterine wall occurs. 2. It is seen late in pregnancy in 1 out of 150–200 pregnancies. 3. It is more common in women with parity over 5, who are over 30 years old.	The cause is unknown, but common predisposing factors include multiple pregnancy, a short umbilical cord, sudden decompression of the uterus on rupture of the membranes (especially in hydramnios), hypertensive disorders, trauma, and precipitous labor.	Bleeding may or may not be apparent, depending upon where the separation is. Symptoms of shock appear—falling blood pressure, rapid pulse, pallor, and dyspnea. Sudden, severe uterine pain with rigidity and tenderness are common. Excessive fetal movement, indicating fetal anoxia, occurs. Loss of fetal heart tone may indicate fetal death.	Treatment is dependent upon the severity of the separation; the fetus may be delivered vaginally or by cesarean section. Supportive treatment includes blood transfusions, clotting mechanism evaluation, and, frequently, infusion of fibrinogen to decrease the risk of DIC. Treatment for hemorrhage if it occurs. (See Nursing Considerations.)

(*continued from page 471*)

cially those involving the central nervous system, such as spina bifida and anencephaly. It also is associated with diabetes mellitus, hypertensive disorders, Rh sensitization, and multiple gestation. Premature labor, malpresentations, cord prolapse, abruptio placentae, and postpartum hemorrhage are common complications. Diagnosis is confirmed by ultrasound.

Observations

- Maternal symptoms of shortness of breath, edema, and, in severe cases, pain
- A grossly distended abdomen
- A fundal height that is large for gestational age (LGA)
- Difficulty in palpating fetal parts
- Difficulty in hearing fetal heart beats

Treatment

- Removal of excess fluid may be required. Pressure must be relieved slowly, usually by amniocentesis.

Nursing Considerations

- Carefully monitor maternal and fetal conditions.

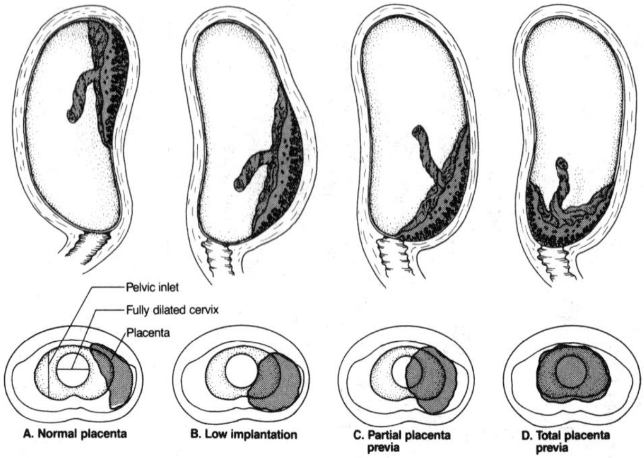

Fig. 5-1. *Placenta previa. (A) Normal placenta. (B) Low implantation. (C) Partial placenta previa. (D) Total placenta previa. (Redrawn from Benson RC: Handbook of Obstetrics and Gynecology, 6th ed. Los Altos, CA, Lange Medical Publications, 1977)*

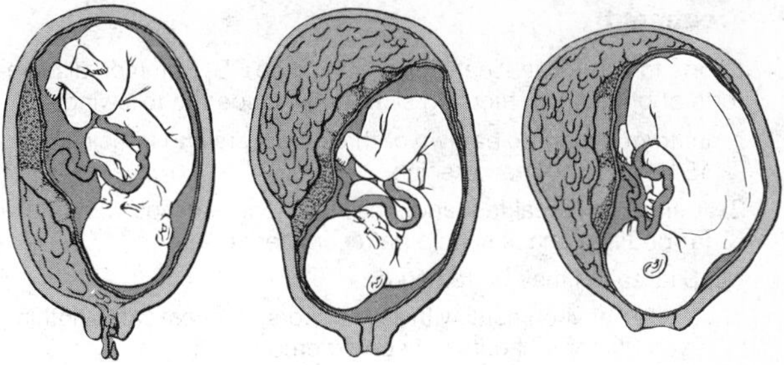

Fig. 5-2. Abruptio placentae at various separation sites.

HYPEREMESIS GRAVIDARUM

Description

Hyperemesis gravidarum describes pernicious, uncontrolled vomiting during pregnancy that leads to weight loss, electrolyte imbalances, ketosis, and nutritional and vitamin deficiencies. Ultimately, if the condition is not controlled, severe metabolic damage leading to death may ensue. Although the etiology is unknown, it seems to be related to elevated gonadotropin production. Psychological factors are believed to contribute to the condition. Other causes of vomiting must be ruled out, *e.g.*, infectious diseases, intestinal obstruction, or hydatidiform mole.

Common Diagnostic Tests

- In urinalysis, the urinary specific gravity is elevated.
- Electrolyte screen is usually ordered.
- Complete blood count may show anemia and hypothrombinemia.

Observations

- Nausea and vomiting that persist unrelated to meals
- Inability to control nausea
- Signs of dehydration, weight loss, electrolyte imbalances (particularly acidosis), ketosis with acetonuria, jaundice, and hemorrhage caused by vitamin C and B-complex deficiencies, bleeding from hypothrombinemia

Treatment

- Efforts to control nausea and vomiting (see OB, Common discomforts of pregnancy, morning sickness) include the following:
  1. Instruct patient to eat two or three crackers and remain in bed 15 minutes after awakening.
  2. A small dry breakfast and small frequent feedings with a low-fat bedtime snack should be recommended.
- Hospitalization may be required.
  1. A quiet environment with few visitors, bedrest, and nothing given PO for 48 hours may be ordered.
  2. Parenteral fluids to correct dehydration, electrolyte imbalances, vitamin deficiencies, and anemia may be given as needed. (Vitamins B_1 and B_6, nicotinamide, and calcium pentothenate may be ordered and given slowly IV.)
- Psychiatric evaluation and treatment may be ordered.

Nursing Considerations

- Efforts to control nausea and vomiting should be made (see OB, Common discomforts of pregnancy, morning sickness).
- Provide a quiet, nonstressful environment.
- Monitor parenteral fluids and laboratory tests.
- As the patient's condition improves, six small dry feedings followed by clear liquids in one hour may be resumed, on the physician's orders.
- Work with the dietitian to meet the patient's nutritional needs.
- Evaluate the patient's mental and emotional status.
- Provide physical and emotional support for the patient.

INTRAUTERINE GROWTH RETARDATION

Description

Intrauterine retarded growth (IURG), which describes the condition of the fetus that does not grow at a rate consistent with its gestational age, may be associated with maternal hypertension (including preeclampsia), chronic third trimester bleeding, vascular or renal disease, diabetes, multiple gestation, viral disease, poor nutrition, drug abuse, high altitude, or fetal infection or anomaly.

IURG is indicated by a fetal growth pattern two or more weeks smaller than normal for its gestational age. When born, an infant is considered growth retarded or small for gestational age (SGA) if his or her birth weight is below the 10th percentile for the gestational age.

Perinatal and neonatal asphyxia, meconium aspiration, and metabolic disturbances are some of the common problems seen in SGA infants.

Common Diagnostic Tests

- Measurement of fundal height (See OB, Pregnancy and antenatal care.)
- Serial ultrasound (See NR, Ultrasound.)
- Serial plasma and urinary estriol determinations (See OB, Fetal assessment.)
- Nonstress testing—may be done weekly. (See OB, Fetal assessment.)
- Amniotic fluid studies to rule out abnormalities and assess lung maturity (See OB, Fetal assessment.)

Observations

- Accurate estimation of gestational age is important. Check dates (see OB, Pregnancy and antenatal care).
- Decreased fetal movements often are associated with chronic fetal distress. Ask the patient to record the number of fetal movements in 30-minute time periods monitored 3 times/day. (Fewer than 10 movements in 12 hours indicate a need for stress testing. See OB, Assessing fetal status.)
- Absent fetal movements may indicate fetal death. (The fetus may be stimulated to move by palpation of the abdomen.)

Treatment

- A high-protein diet (up to 100 g protein/day) should be ordered.
- Bedrest, with the patient lying on the left side as much as possible, is recommended.
- The patient should avoid cigarette smoking.
- Avoid diuretic treatment, when possible.
- Treat maternal complications of pregnancy that may be causing IURG.
- Time the delivery for maximum safety for infant. Have a neonatologist present in the delivery room.

Nursing Considerations

- Emphasize good nutrition, and educate the patient as to what to include in a high-protein diet.
- Encourage bedrest, and help patient plan for it.

- Monitor the patient on a weekly basis for weight gain and fundal height.
- Educate the patient regarding her condition and testing that will be required. Provide emotional support.

PREECLAMPSIA–ECLAMPSIA

Description

Preeclampsia–eclampsia is the major progressive hypertensive disruption of pregnancy usually seen during the third trimester and in the first hours following delivery. Although the exact cause is unknown, peripheral arteriolar vasoconstriction and vasospasm lead to changes in maternal organ functions. The kidneys, the central nervous system, and the liver may be affected. Decreased uterine blood flow may endanger the fetus. Preeclampsia denotes the nonconvulsive disorder, and eclampsia indicates its progressive outcome when convulsions occur. It also is known as toxemia of pregnancy.

Common predisposing factors include age (younger than 20 or older than 35 years); parity (more common in primiparas); coexisting diabetes, renal disease, hydatidiform mole, hydramnios; multiple pregnancy; socioeconomic factors (including inadequate access to prenatal care or good nutrition); and psychological status.

Common Diagnostic Tests

- Urinalysis shows proteinuria (1+ or greater in a clean catch specimen).
- Elevation of hematocrit implies hemoconcentration, and usually is taken serially.
- Clotting studies show fibrinogen depletion.
- Serum uric acid is increasingly elevated. (Note that thiazide diuretics can cause increased uric acid levels.)
- In eclampsia, greatly reduced blood CO_2 combining power and content, and increases in serum nonprotein nitrogen and blood urea nitrogen (BUN) also are seen. Serum electrolytes and serum protein are determined prn. Type and cross-match should be done (see LAB).
- Assessment of fetal status, including serial estriols, nonstress testing, is important (see OB, Assessing fetal status).
- The "roll over" test, if positive in the third trimester, is an indicator of preeclampsia in 90% of patients; if it is positive earlier, it usually is an indicator of diabetes or another pathologic condition. The patient is asked to lie on her left side. Blood pressure is taken until two stable readings are obtained. The patient then turns on her back. The blood pressure is taken immediately and again in

5 minutes. In a positive test, the diastolic reading usually will be 10 to 15 mm Hg higher when the patient is in the supine position than when she is on her side.

Observations

- Blood pressure elevation (either persistent or a sudden increase) when compared with the baseline (Increases of 30 mm Hg systolic or 15 mm Hg diastolic are considered significant, although any change should be noted.)
- Proteinuria
- Sudden excessive weight gain greater than 2 lb/week (1 kg/week)
- Edema of the face, hands, abdomen, or sacral area
- Signs of cerebral or neurologic involvement: frontal headache; dizziness; hyperreflexia; visual disturbances (*e.g.,* scintillating scotomas, blurring or double vision) caused by retinal edema, hemorrhage, and detachment; irritability; convulsions
- Epigastric pain, nausea, liver tenderness, and enlargement thought to be due to congestion and thrombosis of the periportal system (Epigastric pain often occurs just before convulsions.)
- Bleeding gums, easy bruising, oozing from IV sites (signs of fibrinogen depletion)

Treatment

- Prompt vigorous treatment is essential.
- Many patients with preeclampsia can be managed at home with bedrest, a quiet environment, and a high-protein, high-carbohydrate, low-fat diet. Careful monitoring includes accurate recording of intake and output, frequent blood pressure checks, and daily urine protein determinations.
- If improvement is not seen in 48 hours with this regimen, hospitalization will be considered.
- Early termination of the pregnancy, either by induction of labor or cesarean section, may be recommended. It will be based on assessment of both maternal and fetal status.
- When the patient is hospitalized, elements of care include the following:
  1. A stimuli-reduced environment: all visitors may be prohibited.
  2. Bedrest in a side-lying position is believed to increase the blood flow to the kidneys and the placenta.
  3. A diet high in protein, low in fat, and high in carbohydrates is recommended. (Most authorities favor salt restriction.)

4. Sedatives, diuretics, and antihypertensive drugs may be indicated.
5. Oxygen therapy may be indicated (see NR, Oxygen therapy).
6. Intravenous therapy may be required. Typed and cross-matched whole blood must be available (see NR, Intravenous therapy).
7. Magnesium sulfate may be ordered for the prevention and control of convulsions (see PH).
8. The baby will be delivered as soon as it is safely possible.

Nursing Considerations

- Maintain a quiet, stimuli-reduced environment, *e.g.*, a darkened room. Do not disturb patient with unnecessary procedures.
- Monitor vital signs, q 4 h., or up to q 15 min if the patient's condition indicates it. Leave blood pressure cuff in place to minimize disturbing the patient.
- Assess fluid retention with daily weight measurements, observations about location, and degree of edema.
- Intake and output must be recorded accurately.
- A Foley catheter with a urine meter for hourly urinary output measurement may be inserted if indicated.
- Monitor biceps, patellar, and ankle reflexes frequently to assess for increased irritability (hyperreflexia), or for diminished reflexes, which is a sign of toxicity, if magnesium sulfate is being administered.
- Monitor fetal status (see separate section).
- Maintain seizure precautions. Have at the bedside a tray containing a rolled wash cloth or a padded tongue blade; emergency drugs (*e.g.*, magnesium sulfate, calcium gluconate—the specific antidote for magnesium sulfate), syringes, and needles; emergency equipment (*e.g.*, suction, oxygen); and padded side rails (see PH, Endocrine system; NR, oxygen therapy; NR, nasopharyngeal or oropharyngeal suctioning).
- When the patient is receiving magnesium sulfate
  1. Serum magnesium levels should be monitored. Adverse reactions appear when levels are greater than 10 mg/dl.
  2. Check for signs of toxicity, including flushing, muscle flaccidity, and depressed reflexes that lead to respiratory and cardiac arrest.
  3. Do not give magnesium sulfate if knee jerk is absent, urinary output is less than 100 ml in the past 4 hours, or respirations are less than 16 per min.
  4. Have calcium gluconate available.

- Observe for signs of placental separation, which is more common in women with severe preeclampsia. Signs include vaginal bleeding (although it is not always seen), uterine tenderness, sustained abdominal pain, and changes in fetal activity and heart rate (see OB, Bleeding disorders).

PRETERM LABOR

Description

A preterm or premature labor is one that occurs between the 20th and 37th weeks of gestation, often producing a viable fetus. The patient is carefully managed in an attempt to postpone delivery until the fetus is more ready for extrauterine life. Prematurity is still the leading cause of infant death.

While the cause of premature labor is unknown, there are many associated factors. These include other complications of pregnancy discussed in this section, genetic factors, previous premature births, closely spaced pregnancies, abdominal surgery during pregnancy, a blow to the abdomen, uterine anomalies (including incompetent cervix), and maternal or fetal infections.

Common Diagnostic Tests

- Tests to assess fetal status (See OB, Assessing fetal status.)
- Fetal and maternal monitoring
- Routine laboratory work and tests specific for complicating factors

Observations

- Uterine contractions occurring for 1 hour in a regular pattern, with or without pain (Progressive changes in the cervix during observation period include cervical dilation or effacement.)
- Menstrual-like cramps, with a sensation of pelvic pressure
- Low backache
- Change in vaginal discharge
- A sudden gush or slow leak of fluid from the vagina, signaling rupture of the membranes

Treatment

- Arresting premature labor is the goal in most cases. Elements of treatment include the following:
  1. Bedrest
  2. Hydration, with intravenous fluids, if necessary (See NR, Intravenous therapy.)

3. Treatment of underlying problems
4. Glucocorticoids, to hasten fetal lung maturity, may be ordered.
5. Drugs to arrest premature labor, *e.g.*, ritodrine hydrochloride, isoxsuprine (Vasodilan), and terbutaline sulfate (Brethine) (See PH.)

- Premature rupture of the membranes, active labor with cervical dilation of 4 cm or more, presence of severe preeclampsia–eclampsia, and serious fetal complications (*e.g.*, isoimmunization, or evidence of cross anomalies) are indications to allow labor to continue.

Nursing Considerations

- Monitor conditions of the patient and the fetus carefully by observation and the use of fetal and maternal monitors. Keep accurate records.
- Vaginal examinations are avoided when possible.
- If delivery seems imminent, have a neonatologist in the delivery room. Alert the nursery staff.
- Provide emotional support for the patient and her family, preparing them gently for the possibility of premature birth.

Rh SENSITIZATION

Description

Rh sensitization most commonly occurs when an Rh-negative woman delivers an Rh-positive fetus. Fetal red blood cells (RBCs) invade the maternal circulation and stimulate production of maternal Rh antibodies. If left untreated, maternal Rh antibodies pass through the placenta in subsequent pregnancies and attack fetal RBCs, causing a severe hemolytic disease known as *erythroblastosis fetalis.* Rh sensitization also can occur following accidental transfusion of Rh-negative patients with Rh-positive blood.

This condition rarely is seen today because of routine screening that identifies Rh-negative patients (with subsequent testing for the father's blood type and Rh factor), and immunization with Rh_o(D) immune globulin (see below).

Common Laboratory Tests

- Blood typing, including Rh factor
- Coombs' test

1. Indirect Coombs' test measures the amount of antibodies present in maternal serum. Rh_o(D) immune globulin (*e.g.* RhoGAM, Gamulin) should be administered only if the results of the Coombs' test are negative.

2. Direct Coombs' test should be done on cord blood collected at time of delivery.

- Amniotic fluid studies, for bilirubin

Treatment

- Prevent sensitization by immunizing every Rh-negative woman who is carrying a Rh-positive fetus with $Rh_o(D)$ immune globulin within 72 hours after delivery, amniocentesis, or abortion or termination of ectopic pregnancy. Following a transfusion in which Rh-positive blood has been given accidentally to an Rh-negative woman, $Rh_o(D)$ immune globulin must be given within 3 hours. It is given IM.
- $Rh_o(D)$ immune globulin administration should be repeated in each subsequent situation where sensitization could occur. It may be given prophylactically to the Rh-negative patient between the 28th and 32nd weeks of gestation.
- *Caution:* $Rh_o(D)$ immune globulin is given only to the mother, and not to the infant.
- Intrauterine transfusions of Rh-negative blood cells into the amniotic sac may be indicated.
- Early delivery, for the well-being of the infant, may be indicated.
- After delivery, complete transfusions may be given to the infant through the umbilical vein.

Nursing Considerations

- $Rh_o(D)$ immune globulin is cross-matched in the laboratory. Verify its lot number and cross-match form with those on the vial. Return the empty vial and identification form to the lab with the time of injection noted.
- Jaundiced infants may require phototherapy (exposure to "bilirubin lights").

COEXISTING MEDICAL CONDITIONS COMPLICATING PREGNANCY

ANEMIA

Description

A significant reduction of hemoglobin, the volume of packed red cells (hematocrit), or the number of erythrocytes (RBCs) will cause anemia, a decrease in the oxygen-carrying capacity of the blood. There are a number of underlying causes that must be diagnosed and treated appropriately.

During pregnancy, there is a normal dilution of hemoglobin

caused by an expanded plasma volume that peaks and then stabilizes during the second trimester of pregnancy. In addition to this physiologic anemia of pregnancy, inadequate nutrition, and increased iron requirements associated with pregnancy, plus other causes (*e.g.,* repeated infections and chronic blood loss, before conception), make anemia one of the most common problems of pregnancy.

Common Diagnostic Tests

- Complete blood count
- Serum iron
- Total iron-binding capacity
- Hemoglobin electrophoresis for diagnosis of sickle cell (See MSN, Cardiovascular, Sickle cell anemia.)
- Glucose-6-phosphate dehydrogenase (G6PH)

Treatment

- On the basis of the precise diagnosis

Nursing Considerations

- Encourage the patient to eat an iron-rich diet—one high in such foods as liver, kidneys, beef, egg yolks, dried fruits, and green leafy vegetables. Give relevant advice if supplemental iron or folic acid has been ordered.
- The enzyme G6PH is deficient in 15% of black women. In this condition, destruction of RBCs is caused by certain foods and drugs. The clinician should provide the patient with G6PH deficiency with a list of specific foods and drugs to be avoided. She should carry it with her at all times.

DIABETES MELLITUS

Description

Keeping the diabetic patient's condition under control is made more difficult by the normal changes in metabolism during pregnancy. Insulin requirements fluctuate during pregnancy and in the early postpartum period. Even when diabetes is managed carefully, the pregnant diabetic patient and her baby are at risk.

Gestational diabetes is caused by the metabolic changes during pregnancy. Diabetes becomes apparent during pregnancy and usually disappears after delivery.

In addition to the common problems associated with diabetes control, the incidence of obstetric complications such as hydramnios, hyperemesis gravidarum, preeclampsia–eclampsia, infections (particularly urinary tract infections), and prematurity is increased. Infants, while usually large for gestational age (LGA), also usually are immature. They frequently suffer from respiratory distress syndrome secondary to hyaline membrane disease; congenital anomalies; metabolic disturbances including ketoacidosis, hypoglycemia, hypocalcemia, and hyperbilirubinemia; and birth injuries. Fetal and neonatal death rates are still high.

Careful management by an interdisciplinary health team is required (see MSN, Endocrine system, Diabetes mellitus). White's classification of diabetes in pregnancy is widely used in planning this management.

Common Diagnostic Tests

- Urinalysis for glucose and ketone (See LAB.)
- Fasting blood sugar (FBS) and 2-hour postprandial blood sugar (See LAB).
- Glucose tolerance tests
- Tests that assess placental functioning as well as fetal status
  1. Ultrasound (See NR, Ultrasound.)
  2. Plasma and urinary estriols (See OB, Assessing fetal status.)
  3. Lecithin/sphingomyelin ratios (See OB, Assessing fetal status.)
  4. Nonstress testing (See OB, Assessing fetal status.)
- Examination of the eyes: Diabetic retinopathy seems to progress during pregnancy, and may regress following delivery.

Observations

- See MSN, Endocrine system, Diabetes mellitus.

Treatment

- Frequent antenatal check-ups (*e.g.,* biweekly until the 28th week of gestation, and weekly thereafter) aimed at careful monitoring of maternal and fetal status, and control of the diabetes through adjustments in insulin dosage and diet are required (see MSN, Endocrine system, Diabetes mellitus).
- It is recommended that oral hypoglycemia agents not be used during pregnancy and lactation.
- Hospitalization may be required.
- Early delivery, usually before the 37th week, is recommended with most diabetic patients.
- Diet and insulin dosage are adjusted carefully during labor, delivery, and the postpartum period.
- Cesarean section is common.

Nursing Considerations

- Education is a must. The patient must understand diabetes and the self-care required, especially during pregnancy. Emphasize how important it is for her to keep appointments with her health-care providers.
- Special instructions should be given for the collection of specimens for specific tests.
- During late pregnancy and lactation, Tes-Tape, Diastix, or Chemstrip can be used for urine testing because they test for glucose specifically. (Benedict's and Clinitest are not reliable for this.)
- Psychological support is vital.
- See MSN, Endocrine system, Diabetes mellitus.

HEART DISEASE AND PREGNANCY

Description

About half of the cases of heart disease diagnosed during pregnancy have been undiagnosed previously. Mitral stenosis of either congenital origin or caused by rheumatic heart disease (RHD) accounts for the majority of cases. Congenital cardiac anomalies such as atrial septal defect, patent ductus arteriosus, ventricular septal defect, pulmonary stenosis, and coarctation of the aorta account for most of the remaining cases.

Normal cardiovascular changes during pregnancy put additional strain on the heart. Cardiac output may be increased by 30% to 40% throughout pregnancy. It may precipitate cardiac decompensation leading to congestive heart failure (CHF) in patients with preexisting cardiac disease. Early diagnosis and subsequent management, usually as a joint effort of the cardiologist and obstetrician, can do much to avoid this complication that endangers the well-being of both the mother and the fetus (see MSN, Cardiovascular, Congestive heart failure).

Common Diagnostic Tests

- Chest x-ray showing cardiac enlargement
- Arterial blood gases (ABGs) (See LAB.)
- Careful monitoring of both maternal and fetal conditions. (See OB, Assessing fetal status, Fetal and maternal monitoring.)

Observations

- Progressive symptoms indicate CHF. They include coughs (with or without hemoptysis), shortness of breath (progressive with exertion), rales at the base of the lungs, progressive generalized edema, heart murmurs, and arrhythmias.

Treatment

- Frequent prenatal evaluations: Depending upon the severity of symptoms, visits may be required as often as two times a week. Hospitalization may be required.
- A diet low in sodium and calories and high in protein, iron, and vitamins is usually prescribed.
- Adequate rest and decreased physical activity are recommended.
- Emotional support for patient and family is important.
- Efforts should be directed to prevent any kind of infection. Prompt treatment is necessary if an infection occurs.
- Drug therapy will be ordered, as indicated.
  1. Digitalis preparations, antiarrhythmic medications, and diuretics may be ordered.
  2. Antibiotics may be given prophylactically against bacterial endocarditis at the time of delivery and immediately postpartum.
  3. Heparin is usually ordered if anticoagulant therapy is needed (see PH).
  4. Analgesics are usually ordered for relief of pain during delivery.
- The patient and her support person should attend childbirth classes to learn relaxation techniques.
- Oxygen therapy may be indicated (see NR, Oxygen therapy).
- Regional block or local anesthesia and low forceps delivery are done frequently in these patients to reduce the stress of the second stage of labor.
- Intensive maternal and fetal monitoring during labor is necessary. The immediate postpartum period is most critical.

Nursing Considerations

- See MSN, Cardiovascular system, Congestive heart failure.
- Continuous monitoring of maternal and fetal status, including assessment for CHF, is essential.
- Emotional support, as well as practical guidance on ways to reduce physical and emotional stress, is helpful.
- Advise the patient to seek immediate medical attention at the first appearance of symptoms of upper respiratory or urinary tract infections (see MSN, Urinary system, Urinary tract infections).
- During labor, in addition to the above, remember the following points:
  1. The patient should be in a semi-Fowler or side-lying position with head and shoulders elevated.
  2. Assist with breathing and relaxation techniques.

3. *Caution:* Use of scopolamine hydrobromide is avoided because of side-effects, *e.g.*, tachycardia or agitation.

- Observe for signs of CHF and shock during the critical immediate postpartum period.
- *Caution:* Ergot preparations should be avoided because they may elevate blood pressure.

INFECTIONS

Maternal infections during pregnancy increase the risk for both the mother and fetus. In many cases, damage to the fetus may be devastating, even though the mother's symptoms are minimal. Prompt, effective evaluation and treatment are essential. In some cases, the risk of congenital anomalies in the fetus is so high that therapeutic abortion may be an option.

The acronym TORCH represents a group of infections with particularly severe effects on the fetus. These are toxoplasmosis (TO), rubella (R), cytomegalovirus (C) and herpes virus type 2 (H), and are so identified to assist health-team members to recognize the risk factors associated with them.

Toxoplasmosis is a protozoal infection that usually is transmitted through the feces of cats. Pregnant women should be counselled to avoid handling a cat's litter box.

Sexually transmitted diseases (STD) present special problems during pregnancy. Gonorrhea and syphilis must be reported and treated. Herpes virus type 2 or cytomegalovirus (or a history of infection) dictate special management. Repeated cultures for herpes are taken during the third trimester; delivery is by cesarean section if the cultures are positive. Infections of *Candida albicans, Trichomonas vaginalis,* and *Gardnerella vaginalis* are frequently more persistent during pregnancy (see MSN, Sexually transmitted diseases).

Infections of the Urinary Tract During Pregnancy

Hormonal changes plus alterations of the anatomy caused by the enlarging uterus increase the risk of acquiring urinary tract infection (UTI) during pregnancy. Ascending UTIs cause pyelonephritis. While it is a comparatively rare complication, it is a major cause of hospitalization during pregnancy. The onset of premature labor is triggered by UTI often enough so that any patient in premature labor should be evaluated with UTI in mind.

The patient should be aware of the symptoms of UTI and of the importance of reporting them promptly to her physician should they appear (see MSN, Genitourinary system, Urinary tract infection).

ASSESSING FETAL STATUS

AMNIOCENTESIS

In amniocentesis, amniotic fluid is withdrawn through a needle inserted into the amniotic sac through the abdomen (usually suprapubically).

Ultrasound is used to locate the fetus, the placenta, and the pocket of amniotic fluid.

- The patient's bladder should be empty.
- Fetal heart rate (FHR) and the patient's vital signs should be taken before the procedure and monitored for 30 minutes to 40 minutes following it.
- The procedure should be done near a delivery room in case emergency delivery should be required.
- An informed consent slip must be signed by the patient. Complications caused by inadvertent puncturing of the placenta, cord, fetus, or maternal bladder are rare, but they do occur.
- Lightheadedness, nausea, and diaphoresis may be experienced by the patient during the procedure because of the pressure of the gravid uterus on her abdominal vessels when she is lying on her back.
- Watch for signs of fetal distress, maternal hemorrhage, preterm labor, and infection. Following the procedure instruct the patient to report any of the following:
    1. Either excessive fetal activity or lack of it
    2. Vaginal discharge, either bloody or clear drainage
    3. Uterine contractions or abdominal pain
    4. Chills or fever

Examination of Amniotic Fluid

- Amniotic fluid tests for the lung maturity of the fetus include:
    1. *Shake test (Foam Stability Test)*
    2. *Lecithin/spingomyelin ratio (L/S ratio):* Lecithin and spingomyelin are two components of surfactant whose concentrations in amniotic fluid vary as pregnancy progresses. When fetal maturity is attained, the amount of lecithin is at least two times greater than that of sphingomyelin, achieving a 2:1 ratio.
- Creatinine levels in the amniotic fluid usually are indicators of fetal kidney maturity. Levels greater than 2 mg/100 ml usually correlate with a GA of 36 weeks to 37 weeks.
- Lipid (fetal fat) cells greater than 10% usually correlate with a GA of 35 weeks.

- Optical density measures the amount of pigment bilirubin present in amniotic fluid, an indicator of the severity of hemolytic disease in the fetus of a Rh-sensitized mother.
- Tests for specific genetic or congenital disorders may be done.
- Increases in alpha fetoprotein (AFP) may indicate threatened abortion, or possible open neural tube defect in the fetus, *e.g.*, anencephaly or spina bifida.
- Meconium staining (a green tint) of amniotic fluid indicates probable fetal distress.

AMNIOSCOPY

- An amnioscope, introduced through the cervix, is inserted into the amniotic sac to look for meconium staining of the amniotic fluid.

ESTRIOL DETERMINATIONS

Estriol is a breakdown product of estrogen that circulates in the maternal blood and is excreted in her urine. Estriol levels in both the blood and the urine increase as a normal pregnancy progresses. Its increasing presence reflects the well-being of the maternal-placental-fetal unit.

Tests must be done serially and must show a continuous rise in estriol levels. A sudden drop (if the test has been done accurately) indicates a serious problem with the fetus.

- Serial plasma estriol studies are accurate and easy.
- Serial urinary estriol studies require 24-hour urine collection. Some labs require that the specimen be refrigerated.
    1. The most common cause of error is incorrect collection of the urine. The specimen is invalid if any urine is missing.
- A serial study may require specimens to be collected every other day.

FETAL MOVEMENTS

- The first fetal movements felt by the mother (quickening) usually are sensed at about 16 weeks to 19 weeks. This event is one of the indicators of GA.
- As pregnancy progresses, fetal movements usually are felt by the mother several times an hour.
- Any marked decrease or cessation of fetal activity should be called to the immediate attention of the clinician.
- In high-risk pregnancies, the mother may be asked to count and record the number of fetal movements while she is lying on her left side. It is done for one-hour periods, morning, noon, and night.

FETAL SCALP BLOOD SAMPLES (FSB)

- This test is done during labor after the membranes have ruptured and dilatation is sufficient for a portion of the scalp to be exposed with a speculum.
- A small blood sample is taken from the head of the fetus and tested for its pH. This test has a high degree of accuracy in predicting fetal outcome.
  1. A pH above 7.25 is always a positive sign. A pH below 7.2 is always an indicator that the fetus is acidotic and in serious trouble.
  2. An amnioscope is inserted, and a stilette stabs the fetal scalp briskly. Blood is collected in a capillary tube. The specimen must go directly to the laboratory. The lab must be notified that the specimen is coming.

FETAL TRANSCUTANEOUS PO_2 AND PCO_2 (FETAL $TCPO_2$ AND $TCPCO_2$)

- New, promising, noninvasive transcutaneous (TC) PO_2 and PCO_2 fetal monitors yield information on fetal oxygenation. Although they are still in development, it is believed that they will be helpful in predicting fetal distress more accurately.
  1. An electrode is glued to the fetal scalp for measurement of O_2 tension on the skin surface. Oxygen diffuses through the skin, particularly if the skin has been rubbed or heated. These $TCPO_2$ and $TCPCO_2$ values usually correlate well with conventional blood-gas values.

NONSTRESS TESTING (NST)

- The fetal heart rate (FHR) is monitored over a period of 40 minutes under normal (non-labor) conditions, as an initial screening for fetal jeopardy (see OB, Fetal and maternal monitoring). The mother marks the strip (with a button) when she feels fetal movement. A "reactive" test shows FHR acceleration with every fetal movement and is considered a sign of general fetal well-being. If fetal movements come less often than four in 20 minutes, efforts are made to stimulate the fetus by palpating the fundus and shaking the fetus; making sounds near the abdomen with a clap or whistle; or shining a flashlight on the abdomen.
- A "non-reactive" test indicates possible fetal danger, and is an indication for further testing. Nipple rolling (rolling one nipple between the thumb and forefinger for 10 minutes, then the other nipple, and then both) after 34 weeks GA frequently stimulates fetal movement.

OXYTOCIN CHALLENGE TEST (OCT) OR CONTRACTION STRESS TEST (CST)

- The OCT evaluates the respiratory reserve of the uterine-placental-fetal unit by indicating the response of the FHR to stress of uterine contractions.
- The patient is asked to void.
- External fetal and maternal monitoring devices are attached to the patient's abdomen (see OB, Fetal and maternal monitoring).
- Baseline measurements are taken during the first 15 minutes, including blood pressure, fetal activity, variations of FHR with fetal movement, and spontaneous contractions.
- Efforts are made to stimulate spontaneous uterine contractions.
- If contractions are insufficient, an IV infusion is started with oxytocin delivered piggy back at a rate ordered by the physician or by the protocol of the hospital. A constant infusion pump is used to provide utmost accuracy in the delivery of the medication. After three good quality contractions lasting 40 seconds to 60 seconds occur in ten minutes, the oxytocin is discontinued.
- Occasionally, the patient may go on into real labor.
- OCTs generally are begun with patients at risk only after the 32nd to 34th week of gestation.
- When late decelerations recur repeatedly, they usually are associated with fetal compromise. Their presence indicates a positive OCT. The test may be repeated in 24 hours for validation (see OB, Fetal and maternal monitoring).
- OCTs are contraindicated in patients who are at high risk for premature labor, or in those with placenta previa or previous uterine surgery.

ULTRASOUND

- See also NR, Ultrasound
- Except for amniocentesis when the placenta is being localized, the patient's bladder should be full during sonography.
- Ultrasound is used widely in obstetrics today to:
  1. Estimate gestational age
  2. Identify intrauterine growth retardation (IUGR)
  3. Identify multiple fetuses
  4. Detect fetal anomalies, placental maturity or abnormalities, hydramnios, oligohydramnios (volume of amniotic fluid less normal)
  5. Identify the appropriate place for tap in amniocentesis
  6. Determine fetal position and presentation
  7. Make fetal surgery possible
  8. Identify the sex of the fetus

FETAL AND MATERNAL MONITORING

Description

The fetal heart rate (FHR) is an indicator of fetal well-being. It responds to changes in the placenta where fetal oxygen and carbon dioxide are exchanged, and to changes in the autonomic nervous system of the fetus. It can be monitored intermittently with a fetoscope or continuously with electronic devices. Electronic monitoring is an adjunct to, but not a replacement for, careful observation.

Equipment

- *Intermittent fetal monitoring* is done with a fetoscope between contractions. Auscultation for FHR should be done immediately after a contraction for 30 seconds every 15 minutes during the second stage of labor.
  1. Use the Leopold maneuvers (see Fig. 5-5) to determine fetal position for auscultation of the fetal heart. If there is no time to complete the maneuvers, try the midline between the pubis and umbilicus. This is frequently the best place to listen when the presentation is cephalic.
- *Electronic fetal monitoring* records both baseline FHR and "periodic FHR," (the FHR during contractions). Two tracings are recorded on graph paper simultaneously. The top tracing records the time and frequency of FHR; the bottom one, intensity, frequency, and duration of uterine contractions. Monitoring can be done externally or internally.
  1. In external monitoring systems (EMS) or indirect continuous monitoring, an ultrasound transducer is placed on the mother's abdomen to monitor the FHR. Uterine contractions are monitored by a simple pressure gauge (a tocodynamometer) also anchored to her abdomen. Maternal position and bowel sounds, and fetal movement interfere with accurate tracings and require adjustments in the placement of the ultrasound transducer.
  2. Internal monitoring systems (IMS) or direct continuous monitoring are more accurate. After the membranes have ruptured, a cardiac electrode is attached to the presenting part, and a water-filled catheter is inserted directly through the dilated cervix into the uterine cavity behind the presenting part to measure the intensity of uterine contractions. With IMS, the patient must stay in bed. Some reports of fetal scalp abscesses and postpartum uterine infections have been associated with IMS.
- *Telemetry* appears to be safe. It allows the patient to be out of bed, walking, and still have the FHR and intrauterine pressure continuously monitored. It is especially useful during nonstress testing.

Nursing Considerations

- Establishing a baseline FHR, (that between or in the absence of contractions) is important. Normally it will range between 120 to 160 beats/min, with short-term variability of 6 to 10 beats/min. Look for and report tachycardia, bradycardia, and decreased variability. (See Table 5-3, Monitoring FHR, Baseline changes in FHR.)
- To ascertain periodic FHR changes, cover the monitor strip on either side of the contraction (on the left side from where it begins and on the right from where it ends) to see if deceleration extends beyond the contraction. (See Table 5-3 and Fig. 5-3.)
- The tonus or pressure within the uterus between contractions is normally between 10 to 12 mmHg. If the uterus is not relaxing, there will be interference with the fetal blood supply; frequently, oxytocin is the problem.
  1. Notify the physician.
  2. In most institutions, the nurse can stop oxytocin without an order; this would be an indication to do so.
- Monitor strips are a legal record. They, as well as the patient's chart, should have all interventions marked on them at the time the procedure is done, *e.g.,* vaginal examination, administration of all medications (with dosage and route), turning of the patient, administration of oxygen, the patient's vital signs, and the time when the physician was called because of suspicious tracings.
  1. Since the monitor strips go with the chart, be sure each strip is marked in consecutive order.

LABOR

Description

Labor is divided into four stages, but the progress is on a continuum. The first stage begins with true labor contractions and ends with the complete dilatation of the cervix. When the cervix is almost effaced (thinned) and dilatation (opening) progresses 3 cm. it is described as "early labor" or "the latent phase." In the "active phase," contractions become stronger and more frequent, and dilation progresses to approximately 8 cm. The short but intense "transition" stage begins at the 8-cm dilation and ends with full dilatation (10 cm). Contractions are frequent and strong. The second stage of labor begins with complete dilatation and ends with the birth of the baby. The third stage begins with delivery of the baby and ends with delivery of the placenta. The fourth stage begins after delivery of the placenta and continues until the postpartum condition of the patient becomes stable, a period of usually one hour, but sometimes lasting up to four hours.

The "mechanisms of labor" are related primarily to the move-

(*Text continues on page 504*)

TABLE 5-3 MONITORING FETAL HEART RATE

Condition	Causes	Nursing Considerations
Baseline Changes in Fetal Heart Rate (FHR) that Occur in the Absence of or Between Contractions		
Tachycardia (FHR above 160 beats/min)	Maternal causes: fever (the most common cause), dehydration, anxiety, and hyperthyroidism	Check the patient's temperature. Check the patient's intake and output to be sure she is hydrated adequately. Check urine's specific gravity (see LAB). Concentrated urine may indicate dehydration. Assess the patient's emotional state. Help her to relax.
	Certain drugs, *e.g.*, ritodrine hydrochloride, isoxsuprine hydrochloride, atropine, scopolamine, increase FHR.	Check the patient's medication record.
	Fetal causes: hypoxia cardiac arrhythmias, and infection	Position the patient on her left side to improve placental perfusion. Notify the physician.
Bradycardia (FHR below 110 beats/min)	Fetal hypoxia (a sign of fetal distress) is the most common cause.	Discontinue IV oxytocin, if applicable. (See PH.) Prepare to give oxygen through a face mask, if ordered (see NR, Oxygen therapy). Position patient on her left side to improve placental perfusion. Notify the physician.

(continued)

TABLE 5-3 MONITORING FETAL HEART RATE

Condition	Causes	Nursing Considerations
	The cervix is fully dilated, the patient is pushing and ready to deliver—the FHR suddenly drops	Check the patient's perineum. Delivery may be imminent.
	Maternal hypothermia and fetal heart block	Check the patient's temperature.
	Certain drugs, including some agents used as paracervical and epidural blocks	Check the patient's chart and monitor strips to see when analgesics and anesthesia have been given. Prepare for possible procedures. 1. Vaginal examination 2. Fetal scalp blood sample (FSBS): A pH value at or below 7.2 is a serious danger sign (see assessing fetal status). 3. Cesarean section
Variability—normal (6–10 beats/min)	Short-term variability or irregularity indicates a responsive, healthy, fetal nervous system.	
Decreased variability (less than 6 beats/min)	Fetal hypoxia	This requires immediate evaluation. Position the patient on her left side to increase placental perfusion. Prepare to give oxygen through a face mask (see NR, Oxygen therapy).

		Observe for late decelerations, an ominous danger sign (see Fig. 5-3), especially when combined with decreased variability.
		Try to rule out other causes of decreased variability.
	Fetal sleep cycle—usually lasts 20 min	With hands on the head and rump, stimulate the fetus by moving him gently. Sounds and light shown on the maternal abdomen also may arouse the fetus. Variability should return.
	Analgesia and anesthesia also depress variability.	Check the patient's chart for times of administration of analgesics and anesthesia. They also should be recorded on the monitor strip.
		Notify the physician if variability does not return promptly.
		Prepare for oxygen therapy, FSBS, and cesarean section, if condition does not improve.

Periodic FHR Changes that Occur with Contractions

Early decelerations occur with uterine contractions. Onset and recovery of FHR mirror contractions. FHR may drop to 100–140 beats/min.	Fetal head compression during labor, especially late transition and second stage	These are not considered a sign of fetal distress. Check the perineum. Early decelerations are common just before delivery of the head.

(*continued*)

TABLE 5-3 MONITORING FETAL HEART RATE

Condition	Causes	Nursing Considerations
Late decelerations—their onset occurs after the uterine contraction. An ominous FHR pattern that is insidious because the FHR range usually is within normal limits.	Fetal hypoxia resulting from insufficient oxygen and carbon dioxide exchange through the placenta—uteroplacental insufficiency (UPI)	Discontinue IV oxytocin, if applicable. Position the patient on her left side to improve placental perfusion. Prepare for possible procedures: 1. Oxygen through face mask (See NR, Oxygen therapy.) 2. FSBS (See Assessing fetal status.) A pH of 7.2 is the critical level for FSBS. 3. Cesarean section
Variable decelerations occurring at irregular times during uterine contracting	Compression on the umbilical cord	Change the patient's position.
Sudden or severe decelerations	Prolapsed cord	Perform a vaginal examination. If you feel something soft and pulsating (like moving worms), call for help, and keep the presenting part away from the cord until help arrives.

		If side-to-side changes in position do not help, or if the cord is prolapsed, have the patient assume the knee-chest position (see OB, Complications of labor, prolapsed cord).
More pronounced variable decelerations just before delivery of fetal head	Cord around the neck	Prepare for possible procedures: 1. Vaginal examination 2. Oxygen therapy through face mask (See NR, Oxygen therapy.) 3. FSBS (See Assessing fetal status.) 4. Emergency delivery, either vaginally or by cesarean section
Accelerations during labor—usually considered normal	Not much is known	If accelerations precede decelerations, it is considered a dangerous sign.

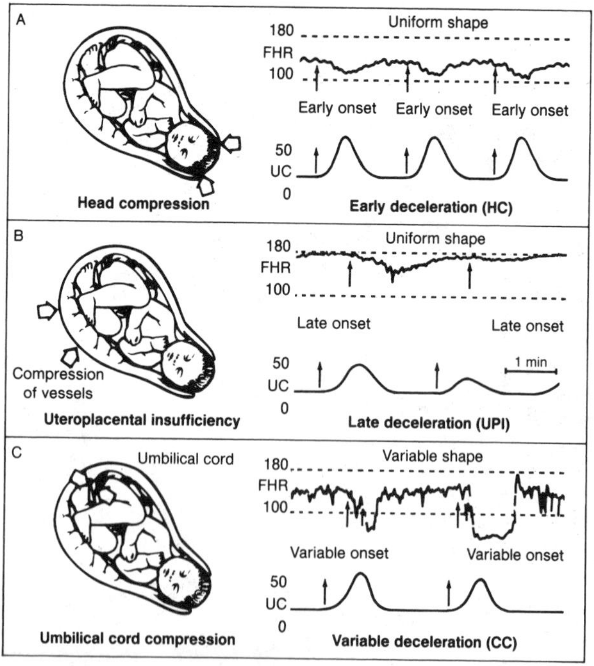

Fig. 5-3. *(A) Early decelerations may be caused by head compression during labor. They are uniform in shape and occur early during the contraction. This is a clinically innocuous sign. (B) Late decelerations occur during the late stage of the contraction. Their shape is uniform, and they are associated with uteroplacental insufficiency. This is an ominous sign. (C) Variable decelerations have no relationship to the contraction curve. "Variable" is used to describe form rather than time of decelerations. This pattern is probably caused by umbilical cord compression. (Hon EH: An Atlas of Fetal Heart Patterns. New Haven, Conn, Harty Press, 1968)*

(continued from page 498)

ments of the fetus during the second stage of labor (Fig. 5-4). *Engagement* describes the entrance of the fetal presenting part into the superior pelvic strait and the beginning of the descent through the pelvic canal. *Descent* is the movement of the presenting part toward the pelvic outlet. *Station* of the presenting part is described in centimeters above (minus) and below (plus) the level of the ischial spines (zero). *Flexion* refers to the fetal head's being tucked against his chest. *Internal rotation* brings the anterior-posterior (AP) diameter of the fetal head into alignment with the AP diameter of the mother's pelvis. Unless the baby is very small, internal rotation is essential for vaginal delivery. *Extension* occurs when the suboccipital

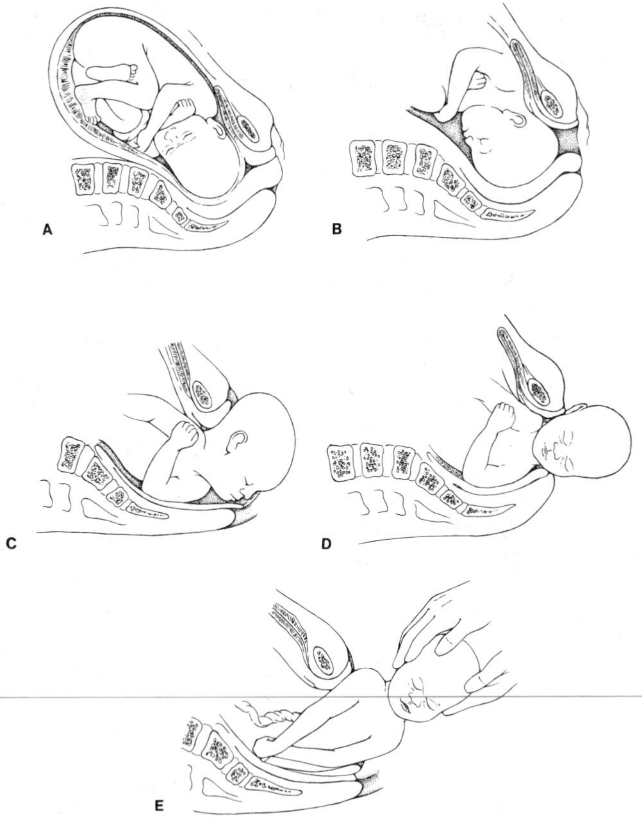

Fig. 5-4. *Vertex presentation. (A) Engagement. (B) Internal rotation. (C) Extension. (D) External rotation. (E) Expulsion.*

region (nucha) of the fetal head pivots under the mother's symphysis pubis. *Crowning* occurs when the fetal head is encircled by the vaginal orifice. *Restitution* and *external rotation* describe the untwisting of the neck after the head is delivered so that the head realigns with the shoulders. The anterior shoulder comes under the symphysis pubis and emerges first, followed by the posterior shoulder and the remainder of the body.

False labor describes contractions (usually occurring near term) that never become regular or effective. They do not continue. These Braxton Hicks contractions do assist in ripening the cervix for effacement.

Common Diagnostic Tests

- Urinalysis
- Complete blood count and blood typing
- Fetal and maternal monitoring
- Other diagnostic tests as indicated

Observations

Probable signs of approaching labor include:

- Regular uterine contractions become closer together and increase in intensity.
- The painful contractions are felt in both the back and the abdomen.
- Rupture of the membranes occurs, and may be a slow leak or a sudden gush of fluid.
- "Bloody show"—blood-tinged mucus appears in the perineum.
- The presenting part descends.
- Contractions do not stop with moderate sedation.
- Effacement of the cervix occurs.
- Dilatation of the cervix is the only true sign.

Guide for Evaluating the Patient's Labor Status and Progress*

On admission, obtain a history by asking questions that will provide the following information.

1. Age, parity of patient, estimated date of confinement (EDC), weight gain
2. Course, problems, complications of *this* pregnancy
3. Course, problems, complications with *previous* pregnancies, labors, deliveries, babies, or postpartum periods
4. Size of largest and smallest babies
5. Events prior to admission
   a. Time of onset of regular contractions, and observed changes
   b. Occurrence of vaginal bleeding
   c. Signs and time of rupture of membranes
   d. Occurrence of show; changes in amount and character
   e. When fetal movement was last felt

*Adapted from a presentation by Susan M. Ludington, PhD, CNM, at a Regional Perinatology Conference, Georgetown University, Washington, DC, April 1983.

Observe the patient's appearance and behavior during and between contractions. (Note changes over a period of time.)

- Positioning of the body
  1. Are the legs together or apart?
  2. Is there vaginal quivering, labia separation, or mucous show?
  3. Asymmetric sit position usually indicates that the baby is at 0 station.
- Facial expression and verbal behavior. Be prepared for great differences in the way individuals and people from different cultures respond to pain and stress.
  1. What does the patient say about how she is feeling?
  2. When cervix dilatation is about 7 cm, she may say something like, "I can't take it any more."
  3. During the transition period just before the dilatation reaches 10 cm, moaning and groaning are common.
  4. A primal scream is not unusual.
- Physical activity
  1. Is activity random or rhythmic? Note the frequency of movement.
  2. Rhythmic activity is typical of the active phase.
  3. Clawing and holding on tight are typical behaviors of the patient whose dilatation is near complete.
- Abdominal examination
  1. Using the Leopold maneuvers (Fig. 5-5), determine
     a. Lie (the relationship between the long axis of the fetus and that of the mother): Is it longitudinal or transverse? Transverse lie will have an oval contour.
     b. Presentation (what fetal part lies over the pelvic inlet), *i.e.*, cephalic (the head), breech (the buttocks), or the shoulder
     c. Position (relationship of presenting part to maternal pelvis)
     d. Descent of the presenting part (whether engagement has taken place). In a cephalic presentation, if the head is engaged, it will not be movable in the pelvis.
  2. Height of fundus in relation to EDC (See OB, Pregnancy and antenatal care, Physical assessment.)
  3. Character of abdominal wall
     a. Tone: If there is poor wall support, the patient may be unable to push well. She may be more prone to postpartum hemorrhage.
     b. Scars: Patients who had cesarean sections before 1975 are rarely able to subsequently deliver vaginally.
     c. Striae: They are associated with an overdistended abdomen and poor tone, which predisposes to postpartum hem-

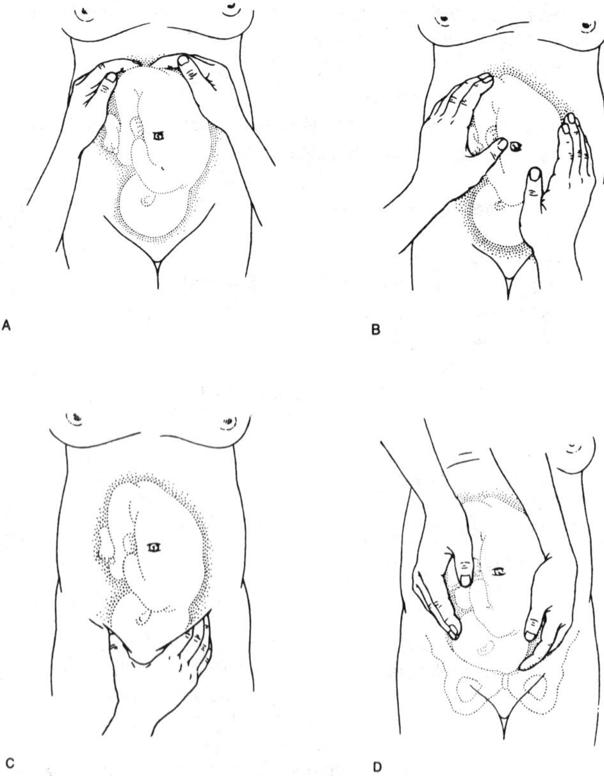

Fig. 5-5. *Leopold maneuvers, or palpation of fetal position. (A) Palpate upper abdomen to determine contents of fundus. (B) Locate fetal back in relation to right and left sides. (C) Locate presenting part at inlet and check for engagement by evaluating mobility. (D) Palpate just above the inguinal ligament on either side to determine the relationship of the presenting part to the pelvis.*

orrhage. Overdistention may be caused by fetus LGA, multiple gestation, severe anemia, a constitutionally large fetus, maternal diabetes mellitus, hydramnios (the abdomen ripples when tapped).

4. Fetal heart rate: fetal activity (See OB, Fetal and maternal monitoring.)
5. Evidence of bladder distention

- Vaginal examination always requires sterile technique procedures in accordance with your agency's policy. It determines

1. Lie, presentation, position, and station (Fig. 5-6.)
2. Attitude (the degree of flexion or extension of the fetal head as it presents)
3. Status of the membranes: intact or ruptured
4. Conditions of the cervix: Compare during and between contractions
   a. Consistency, effacement (thinning), dilatation, and location
5. Presence of edema of the fetal scalp or molding of the head.
6. Station of presenting part: Compare with and between contractions.
7. Adequacy of pelvis for passage of fetus

- Respirations
  1. What is the rate? Is the patient holding her breath? Is there a catch in her breath?
  2. Grunting, especially between contractions, is common when the baby is low (at +1 or +2 station), and when legs are apart.
- Ability to respond to support, comfort measures, and coaching
  1. At 9- to 10-cm dilatation, the patient can only respond to short, one- or two-word commands.
- Contractions: Note changes over a time period.
  1. Frequency, duration, and quality; time from the beginning of one contraction to the beginning of another
  2. Patient's reactions to the contractions
  3. Effect on the contractions by changes in position, ambulation, enema, medication, paracervical block, and so forth
- Patient's perception of pain
  1. While variable, the intensity of the pain of uterine contractions progresses between the first and second stages of labor. In transition, it may be described as "coming apart at the seams." By the third stage, it may be described as "bursting."
  2. Suprapubic pain may be described as "cramping," "tightening," and "aching"; low back pain, as "aching" and "tightening."
  3. Pain in the upper abdomen frequently indicates a breech presentation.
  4. If uterine tenderness is generalized, and the pain is continuous and out of proportion to the intensity of contractions, consider placental separation (see OB, Complications of pregnancy, Bleeding during pregnancy, Differential diagnosis, Table 5-2).
- Perineum
  1. Watch for bulging of the perineum.
  2. Check the show for changes in character and amount. It usually is tinged with blood.

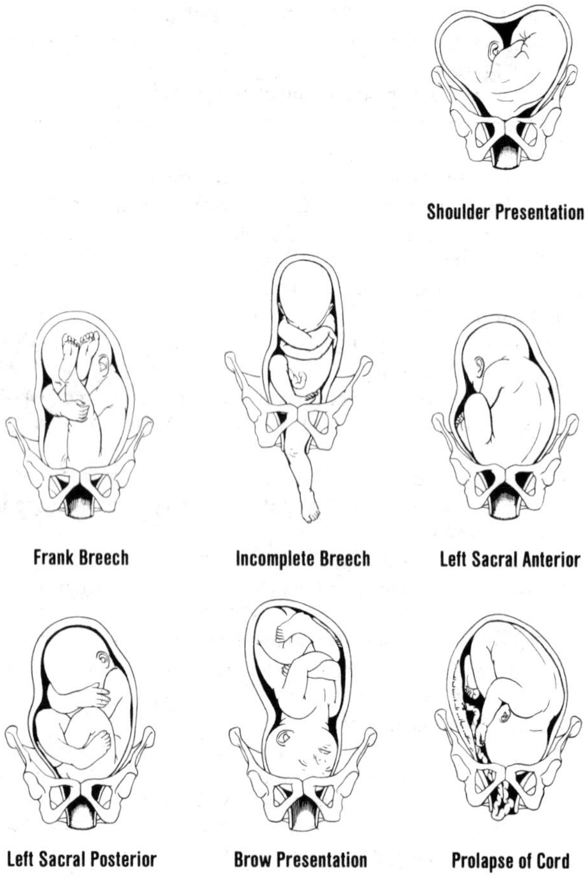

Fig. 5-6. *Categories of presentation. (Mechanism of Normal Labor [Clinical Education Aid No. 13], Ross Laboratories, Columbus, Ohio)*

3. Look for evidence of ruptured membranes. Note the color and character of amniotic fluid.

   a. Amniotic fluid has a characteristic odor.

   b. Watch for meconium staining of the fluid. It may appear to be green to black. It is a sign of fetal distress that requires immediate notification of the physician.

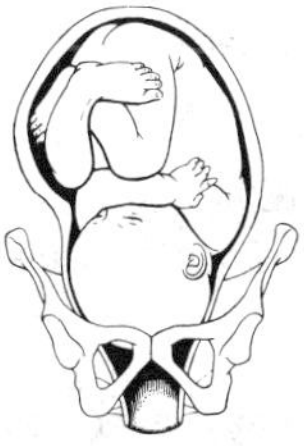
Left Occipital Posterior

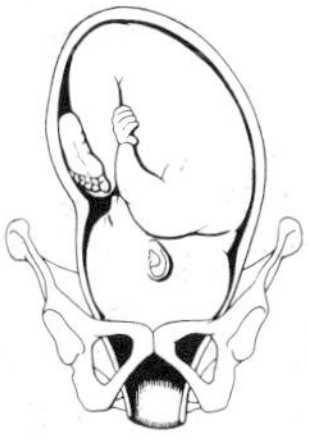
Left Occipital Transverse

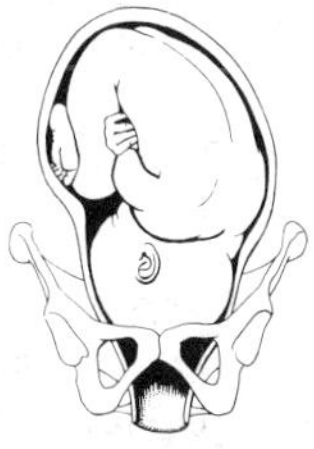
Left Occipital Anterior

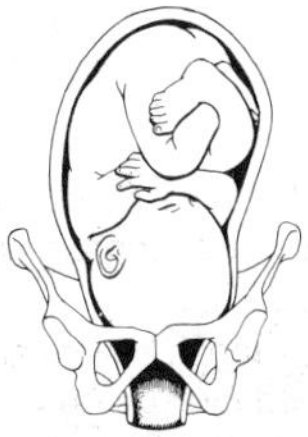
Right Occipital Posterior

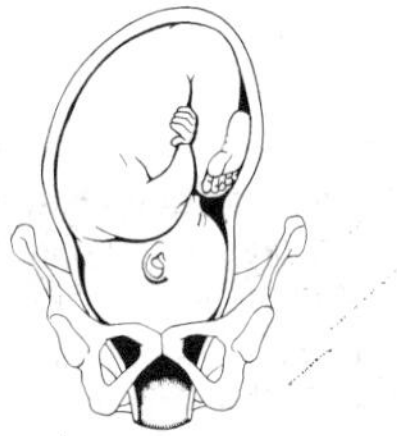
Right Occipital Transverse

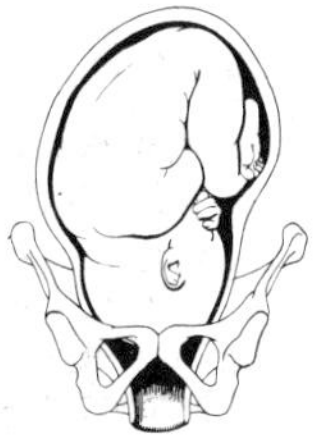
Right Occipital Anterior

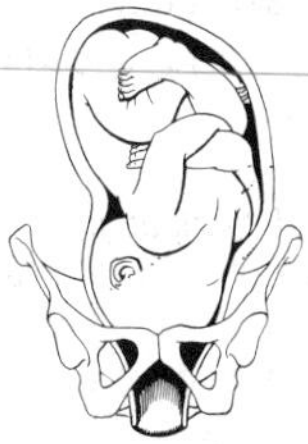
Left Mentum Anterior

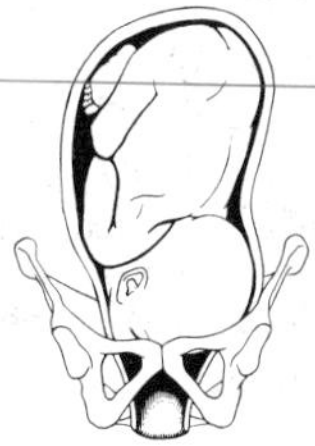
Right Mentum Posterior

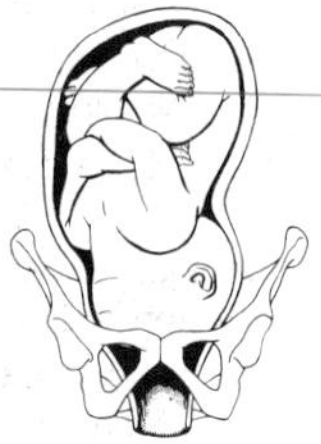
Right Mentum Anterior

Fig. 5-6. *(continued)*

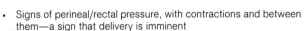

- Signs of perineal/rectal pressure, with contractions and between them—a sign that delivery is imminent
  1. Vaginal quivering
  2. Opening of the vaginal canal—caput visible
  3. Bulging of the perineum, with a shiny appearance
  4. Passage of flatus or fecal matter (caused by the baby's chin pressing on the rectum)

5. Changes in the anus—puffiness, open, rectal mucosa exposed or everted

- Frank bleeding during labor
    1. Placenta previa (see OB,. Antenatal care, Bleeding disorders): This constitutes an emergency and may require immediate delivery.
        a. No vaginal examinations should be done.
        b. Provide a double set-up in the delivery room, one for a possible cesarean section.
    2. Differential diagnoses for frank bleeding include placenta abruptio, lacerations of the cervix or vagina, and bleeding varices.

Treatment

- An enema may be ordered, on admission.
    1. The traditional belief has been that an empty bowel facilitates the descent of the presenting part, reduces fecal contamination, and stimulates uterine activity.
    2. One recent study raises doubt as to whether these beliefs are justified. It suggests that enemas be reserved for women who have not had a bowel movement in the past 24 hours, or for those found to have fecal matter in the rectum on initial pelvic examination.
- Partial shaving of the pubic area occasionally is ordered.
- Support and coaching throughout labor and delivery is important (see Nursing Considerations).
- Relief of pain is usually necessary
    1. In addition to education, coaching, and comfort measures, analgesia and anesthesia, and other methods of pain relief are often ordered (see OB, Pain Management).
- Vaginal delivery is normal (see OB, Normal birth process and delivery technique).
- An episiotomy may be done.
- Deviations from normal labor and delivery must be treated (see OB, Intrapartal deviations).

Nursing Considerations

- Upon the patient's admission, her answers to questions regarding her history will help you plan her nursing care.
    1. If the baby is premature, a pediatrician will be needed at the delivery. An episiotomy may be indicated to make delivery less stressful for the baby.

2. Multipara patients normally deliver more quickly than primipara women.
3. Problems during the pregnancy are usually conditions that require special attention during labor. Remember that bleeding constitutes an emergency.
4. The size of previously delivered babies gives an indication as to how the pelvis has been tested.
5. If the patient has not felt fetal movement in the last 10 hours, listen for the fetal heart beat. If it is not heard, notify the physician immediately.

- Follow your hospital's admission policy and the patient's physican's orders for admission procedures. (See previous sections on assessment, and on fetal and maternal monitoring.)
- Vital signs should be taken upon admission and at least every four hours. Blood pressure should be measured every hour, and up to q 15 min after epidural anesthesia or in cases of toxemia. Temperature may be taken as often as q 2 hours if membranes have been ruptured over 5 hours.
- Explain procedures and what is happening (including the progress of labor) to the patient.
- Encourage the baby's father to participate and provide appropriate support for the patient.
- Assuming that it is permitted by the physician, keep the patient upright and walking as long as possible if membranes are intact.
- A warm tub bath or shower during labor prior to the rupture of the membranes is a comfort measure.
- Vaginal examinations usually are done only when the information to be obtained is critical to some sort of intervention, *e.g.*, an epidural block or a move to the delivery room.
    1. The patient's bladder should be emptied before a vaginal examination.
- Remind the patient to void frequently. A full bladder is uncomfortable and may impede fetal descent.
- If she has had prenatal education, she should be encouraged to follow what she's been taught. Breathing techniques vary.
- During early labor, the following are recommended:
    1. Breathing techniques should be started when the clinician advises it.
    2. Distraction and relaxation are most important during this stage.
- During active labor, it is important to do the following:
    1. Have the patient focus on an immobile object, keep her limbs relaxed, stroke her abdomen, and have her begin breathing techniques.

2. If the patient has had no prenatal education, instruct her to say, "Hut, hut, hut, who." Emphasis on the "T" sound prevents hyperventilation.
3. Coach her to rest between contractions.
4. Remind her to urinate frequently.
5. Offer mouthwash and a cool washcloth.

- During the transition stage, remember the following:
  1. Do not leave the patient alone.
  2. Give only short, one- or two-word commands.
  3. Encourage a pant-blow breathing pattern.
     a. Have her blow out forcefully when the early urge to push comes at the end of transition.
     b. Breathe with her when she loses the rhythm.
  4. The patient should avoid pushing until she has the permission of her clinician.
  5. Reassure her that she will soon be able to push and that it will bring some relief, and that the baby is almost here.
  6. Offer encouragement, comfort measures, a wet washcloth, mouthwash, and ice chips.
  7. There may be pressure at the base of the spine; back rubs may relieve the backache.
- From full dilatation to birth of the baby, these measures are important:
  1. The patient should be ready to move into the birthing or the delivery room, if she is not already there.
  2. Coach her with each contraction with these directions:
     a. Take two deep cleansing breaths; then with the third breath, hold it and bear down. At the same time, try to relax the perineum. Push to the end of the contraction.
     b. Keep elbows out and head forward.
     c. In the delivery room, hands go on the handgrips.
     d. Think in the direction you are pushing—down and out.
     e. Be ready to blow when the doctor tells you to "stop pushing" as the baby's head is being delivered.
     f. Rest between contractions.
  3. Give her praise and encouragement.
  4. Wipe her face with a cool, wet cloth.

PAIN MANAGEMENT DURING LABOR AND DELIVERY

Description

Many individual and cultural differences influence a woman's perception of pain during labor and delivery. Ideal pain relief does not adversely affect the fetus or the progress of labor. Systemic analgesics and anesthesia cross the placental barrier and affect not only the mother, but the fetus. The problem for the physician is to prescribe the minimum amount of medication that will cover the pain (see Fig. 5-7 and Table 5-4).

Most authorities agree that a woman's preparation for childbirth and the support provided by a trained loved one and that of a knowledgeable sympathetic nurse are vital factors in pain reduction.

Nurse midwives have been in the forefront in promoting noninvasive methods of pain relief. Breathing techniques, support, and coaching through the labor and delivery process help reduce the amount of analgesia or anesthesia required (see Labor and delivery, and Normal birth process).

NORMAL BIRTH PROCESS, DELIVERY TECHNIQUE, AND THE FOURTH STAGE OF LABOR

In most cases, birth will be attended by a physician or a certified nurse midwife. In an emergency, a less-qualified person may be

(*Text continues on page 522*)

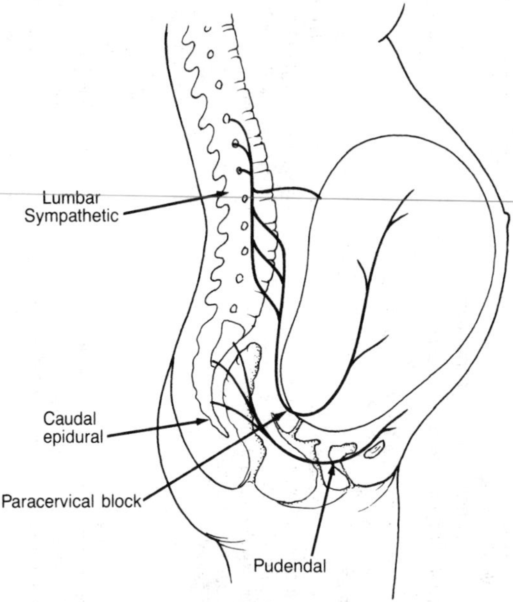

Fig. 5-7. *Pain pathways during labor and appropriate techniques of nerve block. (After Bonica JJ: Principle and Practice of Obstetric Analgesia and Anesthesia. Philadelphia, FA Davis, 1967)*

TABLE 5-4 ANALGESIA AND ANESTHESIA DURING LABOR AND DELIVERY

Description	Observations	Nursing Considerations
Systemic Analgesia Analgesics, tranquilizers, and sedatives		See PH
Regional Analgesia/Anesthesia (see Fig. 5-7) A local anesthetic agent is injected into a specific site to block nerves supplying a specific area.		An IV line always should be in place before administration of anesthetic agents. Adverse reactions can occur.
Some commonly used agents are bupivacaine (Marcaine), procaine (Novocain), dibucaine (Nupercaine), lidocaine (Xylocaine), tetracaine (Pontocaine), and mepivacaine (Carbocaine)	Adverse maternal reactions to these agents may include palpitations, vertigo, tinnitus, slurred speech, metallic taste, apprehension, confusion, headache, nausea and vomiting, hypotension, muscle twitching, convulsions, and loss of consciousness.	
The most common causes of adverse reactions are excessive dose and accidental intravascular injection of the drug.	Signs of respiratory distress, *e.g.*, dyspnea, apnea, anxiety, discomfort, may occur. Miosis (constriction of the pupils) may occur before breathing difficulties appear.	*Caution:* With either epidural or spinal anesthesia, the risk of the anesthetic agent rising in the spinal cord high enough to affect nerves involving respiration requires

	Maternal hypotension can cause fetal bradycardia/distress from resultant hypoxia.	that emergency equipment and drugs necessary for respiratory resuscitation be available.
1. *Paracervical block* a. A local anesthetic is injected into both lateral fornices of the vagina when the patient is in active labor and the cervix is dilated between 4 and 9 cm.	Fetal bradycardia lasting up to 10 minutes occurs rather frequently. Because of this side-effect, this method of anesthesia usually is limited to use in normal labor with an uncompromised fetus. Adverse effects of anesthetic agents are possible (see above).	Monitor FHR carefully. If it slows, position the patient on her left side; increase fluid intake (see OB, Fetal and maternal monitoring).
2. *Epidural or peridural block* a. An anesthetic is injected into the epidural space between L2–3 or L3–4 when dilatation is approximately 5 cm. It may be done by single injection or continuously through a plastic catheter. It is widely used for either vaginal or cesarean delivery. b. One disadvantage of its use is that the patient may be unable to bear down efficiently, thus making forceps delivery common.	Maternal hypotension is possible. Adverse effects of local anesthetics may occur (see above). Watch for signs of respiratory distress (see above).	Have an IV line in place (see NR, IV therapy). Establish baseline vital signs. Monitor them carefully. Check blood pressure, pulse, and respirations q 2 min for the first 15 min after injection of anesthetic, and q 15 min thereafter.

(*continued*)

TABLE 5-4 ANALGESIA AND ANESTHESIA DURING LABOR AND DELIVERY

Description	Observations	Nursing Considerations
		Position the patient according to the preference of the physician for administration of the block.
		Immediately thereafter, position the patient on her left side for 15 min. Then she may move *ad lib.*
		If signs of maternal hypotension are present, administration of oxygen (see NR, Oxygen therapy) and an increase in the IV flow rate usually will be ordered. Turn the patient on to her left side.
	FHR decelerations, resulting from maternal hypotension may occur.	Monitor FHR carefully (see OB, Fetal and maternal monitoring).
	Bladder distention may be present.	Remind the patient to void frequently.

3. *Spinal anesthesia (subarachnoid or saddle block)*

a. The anesthetic is injected into the spinal fluid in the subarachnoid space to provide anesthesia for cesarean section and for vaginal deliveries, including those using forceps.

b. When properly administered, it has a low failure rate. But maternal hypotension (with resulting fetal hypoxia), maternal postspinal headaches, and problems in maintenance of uterine tone are real disadvantages.

Maternal hypotension is a common side-effect, with resultant fetal bradycardia/distress.

Adverse reactions to anesthetic agents may occur (see above).

Establish baseline vital signs.

Have an IV line in place (see NR, IV therapy).

Position the patient sitting with her head down, and the lower back arched while the physician administers the anesthetic.

The patient may have to remain sitting for a few minutes so that the anesthetic can descend to the desired level.

Take blood pressure readings every minute for the first five minutes following the spinal block, and q 5 min for 30 min after the BP becomes stable. Monitor FHR carefully (see OB, Fetal and maternal monitoring).

(*continued*)

TABLE 5-4 ANALGESIA AND ANESTHESIA DURING LABOR AND DELIVERY

Description	Observations	Nursing Considerations
c. The anesthetic may be administered by single injection or continuously.		The IV infusion rate may be increased if the BP falls or if there are signs of respiratory compromise.
	Watch for signs of respiratory distress (see above).	In respiratory compromise, support for ventilation and cardiac resuscitation may be needed.
	A spinal headache may occur.	Maintain the patient flat in bed for 8–12 hours postpartum.
	A distended bladder may result.	Encourage voiding. Force fluids.
4. *Caudal block*	Side-effects, similar to those seen in epidural block, may occur.	See the considerations for the epidural block.
a. The anesthetic agent is introduced into the peridural space at the lower end of the sacrum.		
b. Although it was once a popular form of anesthesia, it is less widely used today.		
c. The patient is less able to push, and a forceps delivery is common.		

5. *Pudendal block*		
a. The pudendal nerve is anesthetized and provides relief from perineal pain.		Explain to the patient that the entire perineum, the vulva, and the clitoris will be anesthesized.
b. It is used immediately before a spontaneous or low forceps delivery, in uncomplicated breech delivery, and in repair of episiotomy and significant laceration.	Reduction or elimination of the urge to bear down during the second stage of labor may occur.	With appropriate coaching, the patient usually can bear down.
6. *Local anesthesia (perineal infiltration)*		Explain that a local anesthesia only affects the area injected.
a. An anesthetic is injected into the intracutaneous, subcutaneous, and intramuscular layers of the perineum.		
b. It may be used at the time of delivery, especially for repair of simple lacerations or episiotomy.		
7. *General anesthesia*	Watch for changes in vital signs.	Monitor maternal vital signs and FHR.
a. It may be indicated when there is a need for rapid induction of anesthesia, especially in emergency situations.	Check for changes in FHR (see OB, Fetal and maternal monitoring).	Provide the pulmonary care given postoperatively following general anesthesia. Include turning, coughing, and deep breathing (see MSN, Postoperative care).
b. The presence of hypovolemia is another indication to choose general anesthesia over regional blocks.	Look for return of consciousness during recovery.	Postion patient on her side so that aspiration cannot occur if the patient should vomit.

(*continued from page 515*)
called upon to assist with a delivery until help arrives. In most cases, delivery is a normal process. Most babies are delivered with a cephalic presentation in a left occiput anterior (LOA) or right occiput anterior (ROA) position. The following guidelines are usually applicable.

- When delivery seems imminent, the patient is prepared in the delivery or birthing room by positioning her and draping her with sterile linens. The perineum is cleansed with an antiseptic solution. (In an emergency delivery, try to use as clean a technique as possible. Attempt to avoid fecal contamination of the birth canal and baby.)
- As the head crowns, the attendant applies firm, gentle, steady pressure to it in the direction of the perineum, using the flat of his or her hand with fingers and thumb close together. This maneuver maintains flexion and controls the speed of advancement of the head. There should never be an attempt to hold or push it back, but delivery of the head must be controlled, and it must not be allowed to pop out.
- The patient is instructed not to push after the delivery of the head. The attendant then wipes the baby's face with gauze sponges and suctions the mouth and nares.
- While gently supporting the head during restitution and external rotation (Fig. 5-8), the attendant will palpate around the neck for the umbilical cord, pulling gently to slacken it if necessary. If it is too tight and does not slip easily over the head, two clamps are applied close together and gripped firmly. The cord is cut between the clamps, and then unwrapped.
- The mother is asked to bear down for the delivery of the shoulders with the attendant using the technique shown in Figure 5-9.
- The baby's head is lowered to promote drainage of secretions, and more suctioning is done, if indicated.
- Some clinicians place the baby on the mother's abdomen and chest (on a sterile field). The baby should be thoroughly dried and wrapped in a warm blanket (including the head). The baby is safest in the mother's arms if she is alert and able to hold the infant.
- At this point, a pediatrician (if present) or the circulating nurse assumes responsibility for the baby.
- Many obstetricians and nurse midwives urge putting the baby immediately to the mother's breast. Nursing stimulates uterine contractions.
- The cord is clamped in two places and cut between the clamps. Controversy exists as to the appropriate time to clamp and cut the cord. In an emergency, the cord can be left attached until clamps, ties, and scissors can be sterilized.
- The third stage of labor, completed with delivery of the placenta and membranes, may take from 5 minutes to 30 minutes.

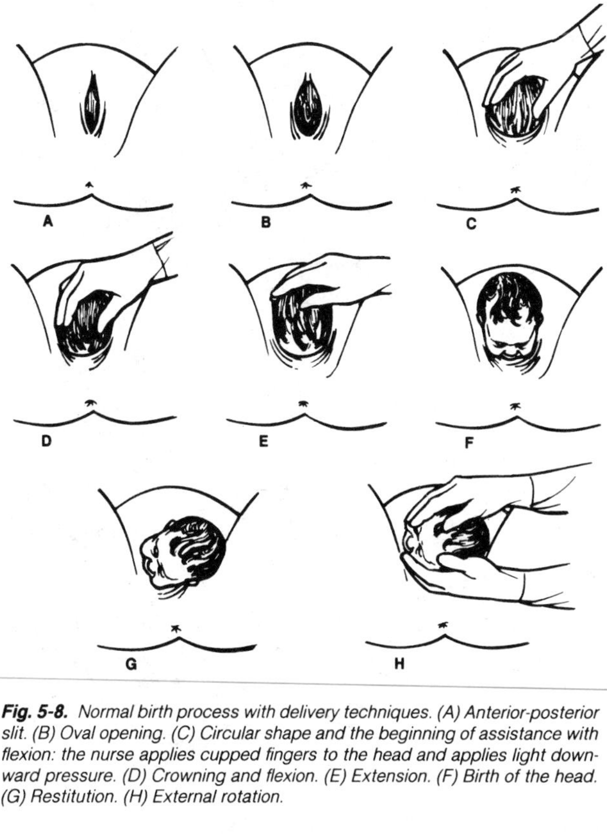

Fig. 5-8. *Normal birth process with delivery techniques. (A) Anterior-posterior slit. (B) Oval opening. (C) Circular shape and the beginning of assistance with flexion: the nurse applies cupped fingers to the head and applies light downward pressure. (D) Crowning and flexion. (E) Extension. (F) Birth of the head. (G) Restitution. (H) External rotation.*

- Signs of placental separation are the following:
  1. Uterine contractions
  2. Uterine fundus rising in the abdomen, becoming globular in shape
  3. Visible lengthening of the external part of the umbilical cord
  4. A variable amount of bleeding
  5. The empty fundus may become freely movable in the abdomen
- To deliver the placenta the following is done:
  1. The patient is asked to gently bear down.
  2. The attendant places the flat of one hand gently but firmly on

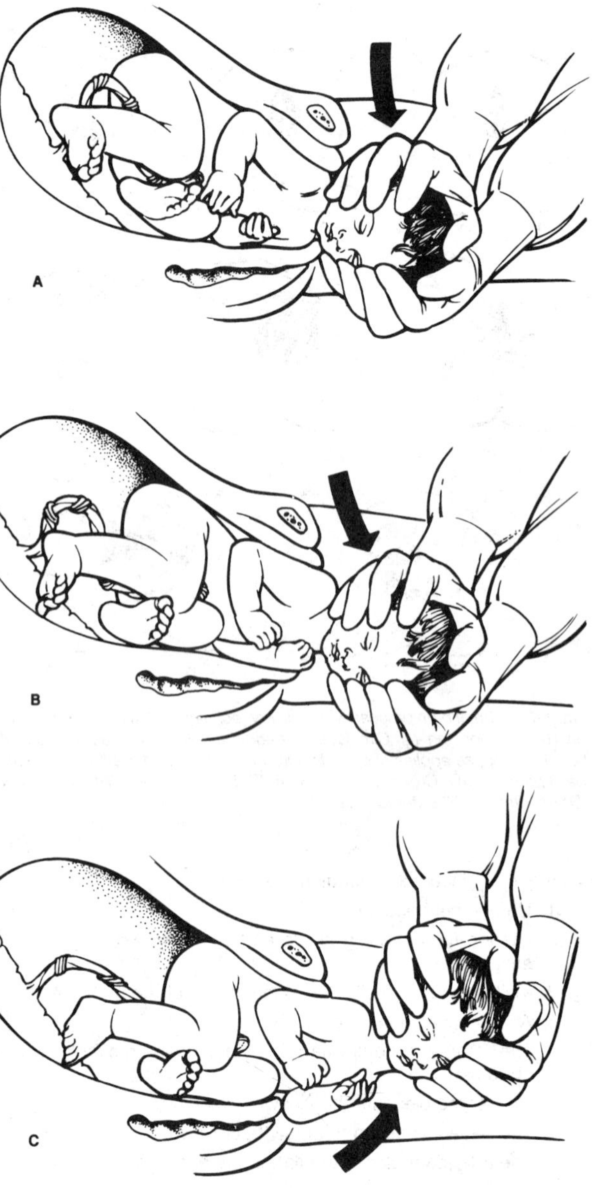

A

B

C

the patient's lower abdomen just above the symphysis pubis (to prevent uterine inversions).

3. With the other hand, he or she holds the umbilical cord near the introitus and pulls gently.
4. After delivery of the placenta and membranes, the fundus is massaged gently.

- Bleeding is carefully monitored and controlled. Gentle massage of the uterine fundus promotes its contraction.
- Oxytocic drugs (those that promote uterine contraction) may or may not be ordered before or after delivery of the placenta. Oxytocin (Pitocin or Syntocinon), ergonovine maleate (Ergotrate), and methylergonovine maleate (Methergine) are used most commonly. *Caution:* Ergonovine maleate and methylergonovine maleate are contraindicated in women who have hypertension or cardiac disease because these drugs increase blood pressure.
- Once bleeding is controlled and the patient's vital signs are stable, the umbilical cord, membranes, and placenta are examined for abnormalities, including possible missing pieces.
  1. The fetal surface (usually delivered first) is smooth and shiny.
  2. The maternal surface is rough, red, and somewhat irregular in appearance. Separate cotyledons fit together exactly to form a continuous margin.
  3. The cord normally has two arteries and one vein.
  4. Membranes are held up to check for completeness. Ragged edges suggest retained fragments.
- The episiotomy (see section on operative deliveries), and cervical and perineal lacerations, if present, are repaired.
- The immediate care of the newborn is described in OB, The normal neonate.

Nursing Considerations

During the fourth stage of labor, the immediate postpartum period, the following should be done.

- Do a quick general physical assessment.
- Blood pressure, pulse, respiration, the condition of the uterine fundus, and the character and amount of vaginal flow (lochia rubra) are checked at least q 15 min during the first hour postpartum and until the patient's condition is stable. Deviations from normal prompt more frequent checking, although one can expect

Fig. 5-9. *Delivery of the shoulders. The pressure direction is indicated by an arrow. (A) Lowering of the baby's head. (B) Delivery of the anterior shoulder. (C) Delivery of the posterior shoulder.*

minor fluctuation in vital signs. Unless elevated, temperature is taken once.

- If the mother has not had an opportunity to hold the baby, allow her to do so before she leaves the delivery room. Positive interaction between parents and baby should be encouraged.
- Wash the patient's perineum and legs.
- In most institutions, a sterile ice pack and/or perineal pad is applied immediately to the perineum. (The ice pack provides comfort and reduces swelling.)
- The patient is taken to the recovery room, given a sponge bath, a fresh gown, and warm blankets. Shivering occurs rather frequently during this period, and may occur during transition.
- Perineal care can be done by the patient.
  1. Instruct the patient to cleanse her perineal area with clean soapy water with at least three strokes—front to back.
  2. A fresh surface of the washcloth or fresh gauze squares should be used for each stroke.
  3. Rinse in the same manner, and pat dry.
  4. A sterile perineal pad is applied, again from front to back.
  5. Hospital protocol varies, but the basic concept is to avoid contamination from the anus to the perineum and vagina.
- Check for firmness of the uterine fundus, which when contracted will usually be at the midline. When it is contracted, bleeding is usually minimal.
  1. A gentle massage usually will cause a boggy uterus to contract.
  2. Avoid a vigorous massage, which can cause relaxation resulting from exhaustion of the muscle.
  3. Nursing causes uterine contraction and furthers involution.
  4. Oxytocic drugs may be ordered.
  5. To express clots, place one hand on the fundus. Cup the other hand under the fundus just above the symphysis pubis. Apply gentle pressure.
- Observe the amount and character of the lochia when the patient is both supine and in lateral position.
  1. A saturated perineal pad holds approximately 100 ml of blood.
  2. The saturation of more than one perineal pad an hour indicates more than normal bleeding.
  3. Watch for pooling of blood under the buttocks.
  4. Check for uterine firmness (see above).
  5. If bleeding continues, notify the physician. Maintain or restart IV therapy with a large-bore needle. Type and cross-match, and have blood available, if needed.
- Check urinary bladder for distention every 15 minutes. (Oxytocin has an antidiuretic effect.)

1. If bladder becomes distended, it is palpated easily. (The uterus moves to the right or left.)
2. Using nursing measures, encourage the patient to void. If she is unable to do so, catheterization may be ordered (see NR, Urinary bladder catheterization and drainage).

- Observe the perineum for the following:
  1. Hematoma (vaginal or perineal), noting increase in size (It may not be visible, but if the patient complains of severe perineal pain, think of hematoma.)
     a. Notify the physician.
     b. Apply an ice pack.
  2. Oozing from or separation of the episiotomy suture line
     a. Notify the physician.
     b. Reapply the ice pack.
     c. Apply gentle, steady pressure to the site with a sterile dressing.
- Administer analgesics, as indicated.
- Observe the patient's emotional reaction to the baby and to the birth process. Immediately after delivery, some women experience euphoria and may laugh and talk. Others may cry. Still others, depending upon the labor experience, may withdraw, wanting to sleep and rest.
- Provide a relaxed, warm, loving atmosphere for the new family unit.
- Document your observations and all interventions.
- The patient is transferred to the postpartum floor after 1 hour or 2 hours and her condition is stable.

INTRAPARTAL DEVIATIONS

Description

Labor and delivery is a normal physiologic process in most cases. When deviations occur, in addition to specific appropriate nursing care, the patient needs extra sympathetic emotional support and accurate information about what is happening. The following are some of the common deviations from normal labor and delivery that are not covered in the section on complications of pregnancy.

CESAREAN SECTION

Description

In *cesarean section* the fetus is delivered through an incision made through the abdomen and the uterus.

Common indications for cesarean section include failure of labor to progress, previous cesarean section or uterine surgery, third trimester bleeding (*e.g.,* placenta previa or abruptio placentae), medical complications (*e.g.,* diabetes), cephalopelvic disproportion, malpresentation, prolapsed cord, breech presentation, and fetal distress.

The classic cesarean section involves a vertical incision through the uterine fundus. It may be used when the fetus is in transverse lie, or when there is an anteriorly implanted placenta. Danger of uterine rupture in subsequent pregnancies is slightly higher than in low-segment cesarean section.

Cesarean section with a low-segment, transverse, or low-cervical incision is currently most popular. In many centers, if there are no other indications for a cesarean section, women who have previously delivered by low-segment incision cesarean are being given an opportunity to deliver vaginally in subsequent pregnancies.

Nursing Considerations

- Provide educational and emotional support for the patient and her support person(s).
- Monitor the fetal and maternal well-being preoperatively and intraoperatively.
- If the cesarean section is elective, the patient should have preoperative care consistent with preparation for any abdominal surgery (see MSN, Preoperative care).
- Postpartum care includes that of normal delivery and routine postoperative care (see MSN, Postoperative care, and OB, Postpartum). In addition
  1. Provide an opportunity for the patient to see her baby as soon as possible, and to hold him or her as soon as she is alert enough to do it safely.
  2. Palpate the fundus (to be sure it is remaining firm) by putting hands to the side of the incision. Direct pressure on the incision is painful.
  3. Observe for bleeding by checking the perineal pad, the dressing on the incision, and by feeling underneath the patient where blood can pool, at least q 15 min for the first hour, and prn thereafter.
  4. If the patient has had epidural or spinal anesthesia, check the level of return of sensation and movement in the lower extremities q 30 min until it has returned fully. Remind the patient who has had spinal anesthesia to stay flat in bed for 6 hours to 12 hours to prevent headaches caused by leakage of spinal fluid.
  5. Monitor fluid intake and output.
     a. An indwelling catheter usually will be in place until intravenous fluids have been discontinued.
     b. Check for bladder distention after the catheter is removed. Record the amounts of first two voidings.

c. Watch for blood-tinged urine, a possible sign of bladder trauma.

6. Provide analgesic medication as needed. If the mother is nursing, advise the pediatrician of the medication(s) she is taking.

EPISIOTOMY

Description

An episiotomy is a surgical incision of the perineum that is done when the presenting part is crowning. It provides a larger perineal outlet. The goal is to prevent possible perineal laceration or less trauma to the fetal head. Routine use of episiotomies is becoming increasingly controversial.

Mediolateral episiotomy begins at the midline and extends at a 45-degree angle in a mediolateral direction to the right or left (see Fig. 5-10). The cut goes through the perineal muscles. It is less commonly done now, the only advantage to it being that there is little or no risk of extension involving the rectum.

A *median or midline episiotomy* cuts down the midline through the perineal body. It provides better approximation, and heals more

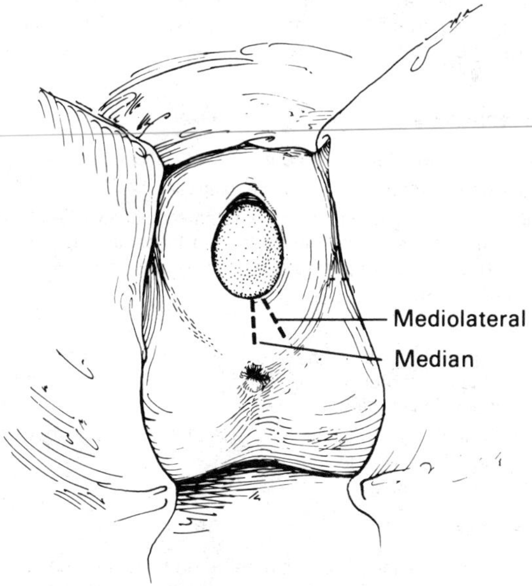

Fig. 5-10. *Types of episiotomies.*

easily and with less discomfort. Dyspareunia is a less common sequela.

Nursing Considerations

- See care of episiotomy and perineal lacerations under Postpartum care.

HYPOTONIC UTERINE CONTRACTIONS

Descriptions

Hypotonic uterine contractions, occurring in the active phase of labor, are contractions that are so inefficient and infrequent that there is failure of the cervix to dilate, or the fetus to descend. (Hypertonic uterine contractions are rare, but usually begin during the latent phase.)

While the cause may be undiagnosed, hypotonic contractions may occur in cases of cephalopelvic disproportion, fetal malposition or malpresentation, multiple gestation, polyhydramnios, and when analgesia or regional anesthesia have been given too early or in excessive amounts.

Unless corrected, a prolonged labor may lead to maternal exhaustion, postpartum hemorrhage, and ascending infection that may affect both mother and baby.

Observations

- Frequency and intensity of contractions
- Evaluation of labor status, cervical dilatation
- Changes in FHR (see Fetal and maternal monitoring): Fetal tachycardia may be seen late in prolonged labor as a result of increased maternal temperature caused by infection.
- Maternal exhaustion, if labor is prolonged
- After delivery look for
    a. Changes in vital signs, *e.g.,* elevated pulse rate and dropping blood pressure could indicate hemorrhage or fever, an indication of infection
    b. Softening (or relaxation) of the uterine fundus that could allow hemorrhage

Treatment

- Stimulation of labor by oxytocin delivered by IV infusion or amniotomy may be tried (if not contraindicated) (see Induction or augmentation of labor).

- IV fluids may be given to maintain maternal hydration.
- Cesarean section may be required.

Nursing Considerations

- Maintain IV therapy.
- Encourage ambulation (if allowed by physician), and position changes that reduce exhaustion.
- Provide emotional support and information as different interventions are planned.
- If cesarean section becomes necessary, provide normal pre- and postoperative care (see MSN, Preoperative and postoperative care).
- After delivery the following are necessary.
  1. Palpate the uterus to be sure it remains contracted.
  2. A gentle massage will usually stimulate contraction.
  3. Overmassage can cause it to relax completely.
  4. Observe the infant carefully for signs of sepsis. Alert the nursery staff to that possibility.

INDUCTION OR AUGMENTATION OF LABOR

Description

Induction of labor means the establishment of effective labor using artificial means. *Augmentation* or *stimulation* of labor indicates that artificial means are used to stimulate effective uterine contractions after labor already has been established.

Amniotomy, or the artificial rupture of the membranes, is the most common and, in most cases, an effective method of inducing labor, if the cervix is ready and the fetal head is dipping into the pelvis. After labor has been established and cervical dilatation is progressing, amniotomy stimulates labor. Amniotomy, when combined with oxytocin, shortens labor. (A prolapsed cord is a possible complication of amniotomy, particularly if the fetus is high in the pelvis or the fluid is released too suddenly.)

The use of prostaglandins to ripen the cervix for favorable induction, as well as to actually induce labor, is under study. Oxytocin (Pitocin) is commonly used to induce or augment labor (see PH). It must be administered accurately, and the effects monitored very carefully. Written hospital policies and procedures should be available to any team member responsible for its use.

Indications for induction with oxytocin include medical complications of pregnancy that can no longer be managed safely, *e.g.,* preeclampsia or eclampsia, Rh incompatibility, postmaturity, or evidence of fetal compromise or demise.

Risks include prematurity of the infant, uterine rupture, amniotic fluid embolism, and fetal hypoxia. Contraindications include previous uterine surgery, transverse lie, fetopelvic disproportion, placenta previa, significant fetal distress, uncertain fetal maturity (unless other complications outweigh risk of prematurity), breech presentation, and multiple gestation.

Observations

- Abnormal changes in FHR may occur. Electronic monitoring is standard in most centers (see OB, Fetal and maternal monitoring).
- Frequency and character of uterine contractions must be monitored.
- The resting pressure during the relaxation period between uterine contractions (tonus), can be determined when direct continuous monitoring is used. It should not exceed 10 to 12 mmHg. An elevated resting tonus over an extended period of time can compromise the fetus, lead to placental separation, uterine tetany, and uterine rupture (see OB, Fetal and maternal monitoring).
- A prolapsed cord, especially after amniotomy, is possible. Palpate for it during vaginal examinations.
- Progress of labor, as evidenced by cervical dilatation, should be monitored.
- Tetanic contractions, lasting over 90 seconds, may occur and are an indication to discontinue oxytocin.

Treatment

- Oxytocin is administered intravenously by continuous drip. The solution in which it is mixed, its dilution, and the rate of flow are prescribed by the physician or hospital policy.
- The dosage delivered may be increased gradually or maintained at the same level, depending upon the course of labor and the physician's preference.
- Two-bottle set-ups with an electronic infusion pump are strongly recommended to ensure accuracy. One bottle contains the oxytocin in the prescribed dilution; the second, an IV fluid that can run to keep the vein open if oxytocin is discontinued (see NR, IV therapy).

Nursing Considerations

- The procedure should be explained to the patient and her support person. They should be advised of the reasons for doing it, as well as possible complications, including the possibility of failed induction and of fetal distress that could lead to cesarean section.

- A signed informed consent is required.
- Continuous monitoring of uterine contractions and internal or external fetal monitoring is indicated (see Fetal and maternal monitoring).
- The physician or a knowledgeable nurse should remain with the patient continuously while oxytocin is infusing.
- The attending physician must be immediately available at all times.
- If electronic monitoring is not available, auscultation of the FHR during and after every contraction is required.
- If signs of fetal distress occur, *e.g.,* bradycardia (<120 beats/min) or tachycardia (>160/min), discontinue the oxytocin, and keep the line open by letting the other IV fluid infuse slowly. Turn the patient on her left side to maximize circulation to the fetus. Nasal oxygen may be given (see NR, Oxygen therapy). Notify the physician immediately.
- Discontinue oxytocin if contractions last more than 90 seconds. Notify the physician.
- Any increase of oxytocin dosage is prescribed by the physician.
- Monitor and record fluid intake and output. Oxytocin may have an antidiuretic effect.

INSTRUMENTAL DELIVERY

Description

Vaginal deliveries assisted by the use of *forceps* or *vacuum extractor* are considered instrumental. Such deliveries are relatively infrequent today, because cesarean section is considered safer for both the fetus and mother in most cases.

In a *low or outlet forceps delivery,* the fetal head has reached the perineal floor and is visible during contractions. *Midforceps delivery* denotes that the fetal head is higher than the level of the ischial spines. Midforceps deliveries also involve rotations of the fetal head.

Forceps may be used to expedite delivery in cases of fetal distress, maternal exhaustion, or lack of progress in the second stage of labor, when there is inability to push effectively (which is rather common when regional anesthesia is used), and in medical conditions where a shortened second stage is advisable (such as heart disease or hypertension). Outlet forceps may be used to protect the fetal head, especially when the fetus is premature. Piper forceps are used to allow controlled delivery of the aftercoming head in breech delivery. Complete cervical dilatation, ruptured membranes, and knowledge of fetal position and presentation are essential before forceps are used.

The vacuum extractor (widely used in Europe instead of midforceps delivery) includes a suction cup that is attached to the fetal head to which gradual negative pressure and traction are applied by means of a pump. The extractor's use in this country is controversial.

Nursing Considerations

- Provide an explanation of the procedure and support for the patient.
- Provide the physician with the type of forceps requested.
- Encourage the mother to maintain her breathing techniques and to refrain from pushing.
- Continuously monitor the FHR.
  1. Early deceleration due to head compression is not uncommon (see Fetal and maternal monitoring).
- Pediatric assistance and adequate resuscitation equipment should be available when a midforceps delivery is anticipated.

Observations

- Postpartum
  1. Check for the integrity of the perineal repair, the amount of postpartum bleeding, and evidence of hematoma.
  2. Signs of postpartum hemorrhage occasionally are seen after midforceps delivery when the second stage of labor has been prolonged.
  3. Signs of urethral trauma include pain on urination, excessive delay in first voiding, and hematuria.
  4. Perineal discomfort sometimes is increased as a result of trauma.
- In the neonate
  1. Check for facial bruising, lacerations, cephalohematomas, facial nerve paralysis, and cerebral trauma.
  2. Assure the parents that most of the common injuries will disappear.

LACERATION REPAIR

Description

A perineal laceration or tear may occur when there is no episiotomy, not enough room, or not enough control in the delivery of the presenting part. Repair is similar to repair of an episiotomy. Lacerations are classified as follows.

- A *first-degree laceration* is a tear that begins at the fourchette and involves the perineal skin and the vaginal mucosa.
- A *second-degree laceration* involves all of the above and extends to the muscles and fascia of the perineal body.

- A *third-degree laceration,* in addition to all of the above, extends to the anal sphincter.
- In a *fourth-degree laceration,* the lumen of the rectum is exposed.

Nursing Considerations

- See care of episiotomy and perineal lacerations under Postpartum care.

PROLAPSED CORD

Description

Prolapse of the cord occurs when the umbilical cord comes down with or ahead of the presenting part. It occurs when the presenting part does not fit firmly against the cervix, in situations such as breech presentations of all types, transverse lie, contracted inlet, prematurity, multiple gestation, hydramnios, and an extra long cord.

Prolapse constitutes an obstetric emergency requiring action that prevents the presenting part from obstructing the fetal circulation by compressing the cord. Unless vaginal delivery is imminent, cesarean section usually is performed immediately.

Observations

- Immediately after rupture of the membranes look for the following:
  1. Presence of the cord in the vaginal introitus
  2. Sensation of a pulsating cord of rope while doing a vaginal examination
- FHR irregularity, variable decelerations (See Fetal and maternal monitoring and Fig. 5-3).

Treatment and Nursing Considerations

Caution: This is a life-threatening situation; the fetus can die in 2.5 minutes if cord compression is unrelieved.

- Exert upward pressure on the presenting part manually through the vagina, pushing the part away from the cord and out of the pelvis—continue until relieved of this responsibility.
- Call for help! Others will do the following.
- Position the patient in steep Trendelenburg or a knee-chest position; elevate the hips.
- Keep the cord moist with a sterile towel moistened with sterile normal saline.
- Observe the FHR on a fetal monitor. A change of maternal position to side-lying may help.

- Oxygen therapy may be instituted to increase oxygenation of the fetus (see NR, Oxygen therapy).
- Start an IV with a large-bore needle. Send blood for typing and cross-matching.
- Obtain consent for imminent cesarean section.
- The urinary bladder may be filled (500–700 ml) with normal saline. Ritodrine hydrochloride by IV infusion may be started in an effort to reduce contractions.
- Alert the staff that cesarean section is an immediate probability.
- Be sure that the patient and her support person(s) understand what is happening and the seriousness of the situation.

POSTPARTUM CARE

Description

The *puerperium* or postpartum period is described as that time between the birth of the baby and the return of the mother to a near prepregnant state physiologically and psychologically. It usually takes approximately six weeks.

The focus of nursing care is on the assessment of the patient, identification and correction of deviations from the normal anticipated changes, relief of common discomforts, and teaching and support for the mother that will ensure her good health and ease the happy integration of the baby into the family. For more information, particularly regarding complications of the puerperium, see the references listed in the bibliography at the end of this section.

Common Diagnostic Tests

- On the second postpartum day
  1. Hemoglobin should drop no more than 2 g below the value on admission.
  2. Hematocrit should drop less than 3 ml/100 ml below the value at admission.
  3. Urine, glycosuria, or acetonuria may be present in the first three days. Red blood cells may be present in uncatheterized specimens. No bacteria should be present. Specific gravity should be 1.020.
     a. Presence of bacteria, white blood cells, and a specific gravity greater than 1.020 indicate a urinary tract infection.
- Blood
  1. Type and cross-match in case of hemorrhage.
  2. Coombs' tests—indirect on maternal serum and direct on cord blood—determine the need for Rh_o(D) immune globulin (RhoGam, Gamulin) administration to the mother and treat-

ment of isoimmune hemolytic disease (if present) in the neonate. If required, Rh_0(D) immune globulin must be administered to the mother within 72 hours of delivery.

Observations and Nursing Considerations

- Some important elements in post partum physical assessment include: breasts, uterus, bladder, bowels, lochia, episiotomy (BUBBLE).
- See Table 5-5 for more details.

THE NORMAL NEONATE

Description

The first 4 weeks of life constitute the neonatal period. The newborn's first 24 hours are a critical period of transition from intrauterine to extrauterine life, with specific changes taking place in the circulatory and respiratory systems.

Physical and psychosocial assessment, rough assessment of gestational age, identification of deviations from normal, nursing management of the infant in the delivery room, nursery, and postpartum units, and anticipatory parent education are essentials of neonatal nursing. Space and scope limit this presentation to the highlights of the care of the normal newborn. More information is essential for nurses actually working in the delivery room and nursery. Some references of greater depth are listed in the Bibliography at the end of this section.

Common Screening Tests

- Coombs' test, blood typing, and serologic examination may be done on cord blood. A second tube of cord blood may be saved for use in case further testing is required.
- Metabolic screening is necessary.
  1. Phenylketonuria (PKU): PKU is an inherited genetic defect that results in the body's inability to metabolize the essential amino acid phenylalanine. Accumulation of phenylalanine and its derivatives seems to prevent normal development of the brain and central nervous system, causing mental retardation and a variety of clinical manifestations if their levels are not lowered. Screening for PKU is mandatory in many states.
     a. The Guthrie test on blood from a heel stick is done after the infant has been receiving milk for at least 3, preferably 4, days. A second test is run 2 weeks to 6 weeks later, after milk feedings have been well established.
     b. A Phenistix urine test, done at 2 weeks to 6 weeks, may be used at some centers.

(Text continues on page 549)

TABLE 5-5 POSTPARTUM CARE

Observations	Nursing Considerations
History	
Gravida, para, time of delivery, course of labor and delivery (including complications, if any), type of anesthesia/analgesia and when administered, presence of an episiotomy or repaired lacerations, whether the mother intends to breast feed or bottle feed the baby, presence of support people, condition of the infant, general level of knowledge or experience about parenting	
Vital Signs	
Pulse, respirations and blood pressure (BP). (There is a normal drop in pulse rate for approximately the first two weeks postpartum.)	1. Watch for variations that might indicate hemorrhage, *e.g.*, elevated pulse and respirations, and falling BP. 2. Orthostatic hypotension may occur the first time the patient gets up. Caution her to do it slowly and with assistance. 3. BP may be elevated in the immediate postpartum period in the preeclamptic patient, and should be measured hourly.
Elevated temperature may indicate infection. Try to identify the site (see below).	Force fluids and administer antibiotics as ordered. Bedrest may be ordered.

Uterine Involution

The uterus should remain firm, well contracted, and at the midline, with the height of the fundus decreasing about one finger breadth each day.

1. The uterine fundus should be massaged gently q 2 hr for the first 8 hr after delivery and q 8 hr thereafter. Under many circumstances, this may be done by the patient, if she has been well taught. (Do not overmassage, which can cause uterine muscle exhaustion.)
2. Encourage the patient to lie in the prone position.
3. Early ambulation usually is encouraged.
4. Breast-feeding hastens involution. The patient may find that "afterpains" accompany or follow the baby's nursing. Emphasize that this is temporary and healthy. Analgesics may be ordered.
5. Administer oxytocic drugs, as ordered.

Lochia (the discharge from the uterus during the puerperium)

1. The lochia rubra is dark red in color, and is similar to a menstrual flow. It lasts about three days, and normally saturates around six peri-pads per day.
2. A slow continuous ooze of blood when the fundus is firm may indicate cervical or perineal lacerations.

Caution: A continuous flow of bright red blood or large clots are abnormal and signal postpartum hemorrhage. They may be caused by uterine atony, retained placental fragments, or clots. Check the uterine fundus for firmness.

1. If clots are reported by the patient but not seen by you, ask the patient to save her pads and to call you before flushing the toilet. When compared with a menstrual flow, bleeding may seem heavy.

(continued)

TABLE 5-5 POSTPARTUM CARE

Observations	Nursing Considerations
	2. If heavy bleeding is reported, ask the patient how long she wore the pad. Replace it and check soon thereafter. 3. Monitor vital signs and confirm that the uterus is contracted. 4. Notify the physician if bleeding continues. Usual protocol includes the following: a. Start an IV infusion with a large-bore needle. b. Have blood typed and cross-matched, and available for possible transfusion. c. Give oxytocic drugs, as ordered. d. Prepare the patient for a return to surgery, if the situation does not improve.
3. Lochia serosa is a pinkish discharge during the fourth to tenth days. The odor is inoffensive. 4. Foul-smelling lochia may indicate infection. 5. Lochia alba is a whitish discharge that appears roughly from the tenth day to 2 weeks after the delivery. 6. Lochia of women who have undergone cesarean section may be very light the first 24 hours.	

Assessment	Intervention
Perineum (Assess q 8 hr) Check for the integrity of the episiotomy or laceration repair for redness, edema, ecchymosis, discharge, and approximation (REEDA). 1. Discomfort is most marked on days 2–3. 2. Hematoma formation causes marked discomfort.	1. Apply a cold pack during the first 24 hours. 2. Thereafter, apply heat with Sitz baths or perineal light. 3. An analgesic spray, such as Dermoplast, may be used. 4. Teach hand washing before and after perineal care. Apply the pad from front to back. Cleanse from front to back, and blot until dry. 5. Encourage tightening exercises (Kegel) to increase tone of perineal muscles. Have the patient stop and start the flow during urination, to help her identify the correct muscles. These exercises should be done at least 10 times several times a day, starting on day 1.
Hemorrhoids See MSN, Anorectal conditions.	1. Provide Sitz baths, witch hazel pads, local analgesics, and stool softeners (as ordered). 2. Teach the patient to avoid constipation by including roughage in her diet, forcing fluids, and establishing regular bowel habits.

(*continued*)

TABLE 5-5 POSTPARTUM CARE

Observations	Nursing Considerations
Breasts (Assess Daily) Tenderness, redness, warmth, firmness, and presence of colostrum changing to milk are common. 1. Engorgement (fullness, tenderness, and prominent venous pattern) usually occurs on the second or third day.	
a. Milk production increases in breast-feeding mothers.	1.a. To relieve discomfort in breast-feeding mothers a. Increase frequency of feedings. b. Apply warm compresses. c. Breasts should be alternated for nursing. d. A support brassiere should be worn. e. Nipple care should be done (see below). f. Encourage rest and relaxation.
b. Engorgement subsides in bottle-feeding mothers, usually between four and seven days.	1.b. For mothers who are bottle-feeding a. Administer medication to suppress lactation, *e.g,* analgesics, prn, as ordered. b. A support brassiere should be worn. c. Apply cold compresses. d. Avoid any stimulation of the nipple and any expression of milk. e. Fluids may be restricted for 24 hr to 48 hr after engorgement.

2. A hard, warm, reddened, and tender area, usually in the upper outer quadrant of the breast, may indicate a blocked milk duct.

3. Fissures, cracks, soreness, and erectibility of the nipples of the breast-feeding mother may occur.

2. Meticulous hand-washing is a must.
   a. Rotate the position of the nursing baby's gums so that a different sinus is compressed each time.
   b. Be sure the breast is emptied completely, using manual or mechanical expression, if necessary.
   c. As the infant nurses, gently stroke from the point farthest away on caked area down toward the nipple.
   d. With these measures, a true mastitis usually can be avoided.

3. Teach measures to prevent or relieve discomfort.
   a. Keep nipples clean and free from build-up of secretions. Avoid harsh soaps and alcohol.
   b. Lanolin-based creams or vitamin E keep nipples supple.
   c. Exposure to air toughens nipples.
   d. Be sure the baby's mouth grasps entire areola.
   e. Show the mother how to break the suction before taking the baby from her breast by inserting her finger into the baby's mouth.

(*continued*)

TABLE 5-5 POSTPARTUM CARE

Observations	Nursing Considerations
Signs of Thrombophlebitis	
Pain, tenderness, local warmth and redness, cordlike sensation, and positive Homan's sign (in which pain is felt in the calf on dorsiflexion of the foot when the leg is extended) may be present.	1. In order to prevent thrombophlebitis, early ambulation usually is encouraged; support hose may be ordered. 2. See MSN, Thrombophlebitis, varicose veins, for treatment and nursing considerations. 3. *Caution:* Estrogens are to be avoided in the patient with predisposition to thrombophlebitis.
Urinary Tract	
Inability to void in first hours postpartum may occur.	Monitor fluid intake and output during first 24 hours. Note the first voiding. Diuresis is common immediately postpartum.
Check for evidence of bladder distention by palpation, or the displacement of the uterus to the right.	Provide privacy, warm water over the perineum, sound of running water, and assistance to the toilet (if allowed). Catheterization should be a last resort.
Incomplete emptying of the bladder (urinary retention) is possible.	Encourage ambulation as soon as permitted.
Frequency, urgency, pain on urination, nocturia, and fever are signs of urinary tract infection (UTI).	When these symptoms appear 1. Force fluids. 2. Clean-catch or catheterized specimen for microscopic examination, culture for sensitivity, may be ordered. 3. Administer antibiotics, as ordered. Breast-feeding may have to be curtailed. 4. See MSN, Genitourinary system for more on UTI.

Bowels Constipation is not uncommon, and is caused by decreased tone, and reduced fluid intake and bowel emptying during labor and delivery.	1. Encourage ambulation as soon as permissible. 2. Encourage the intake of fluids and foods containing roughage. 3. Administer stool softener or enemas, if ordered. 4. Urge development of regular bowel habits.
Pain Some causes include the following: Afterpains are caused by contraction of the uterus, and are especially common during breast-feeding.	Administer analgesics as ordered. If the mother's breast-feeding, the pediatrician should be questioned as to when analgesics may be given.
Episiotomy, hemorrhoids, breast engorgement, and sore nipples cause pain.	See above.
In cases of cesarean section, discomfort compounds that of normal postpartum course and lower abdominal surgery.	Normal postoperative care is required, and should include early ambulation (as ordered), position changes, analgesics, and all of the above (see MSN, Postoperative care).
Psychological Adjustment Watch for evidence of bonding (parent–child attachment) in which the parent seeks eye contact with the infant, exhibits interest in the baby, and responds to his or her behavior, *e.g.*, crying, smiling, or cooing.	Provide a relaxed environment for parents to become acquainted with their baby. 1. Provide information about the care of an infant as opportunities present themselves. Particularly support and help with breast-feeding.

(*continued*)

TABLE 5-5 POSTPARTUM CARE

Observations	Nursing Considerations
Mood swings and some negative feelings may occur.	"Postpartum blues" seem to be part of the normal let-down following delivery. If it is prolonged, the physician should be notified. Intervention may be required.
Excessive fatigue, marked depression or preoccupation with her physical status, evidence of low self-esteem, lack of support systems, or family problems may be clues to future problems.	Provide for rest and graduated activity, relief of pain, and ventilation of feelings. Referral for follow-up to an appropriate professional, *e.g.*, public health nurse or a psychiatrist, may be required.
Postpartum psychosis with a break from reality does sometimes occur.	
Opportunities to Counsel Concerning Rest, Graduated Activity, and Exercise	
	Help the patient organize her time so that periods of rest alternate with gradually increasing activity.
	Emphasize the importance of adequate rest not only for her postpartum recovery, but for her baby and her family.
	Encourage simple exercises (Fig. 5-11) that begin in the hospital and can be repeated several times a day for 5-minute intervals. Include Kegel perineum-tightening exercises, which are best explained as the sensation felt in stopping and starting a stream of urine.

Opportunities to Counsel Concerning Nutrition

A well-balanced diet including all of the basic food groups will provide most of the recommended nutrients for lactation, with enough increases in proteins, calories, minerals, and vitamins to meet the recommended daily dietary allowances.

Need for Contraceptive Information

The patient should understand that ovulation may resume before menstruation and that a nursing mother may become pregnant.

A final choice of contraceptive is made at the time of the 4- to 6-week examination.

Spermicidal foam and condoms frequently are recommended for the period before a final choice is made.

While many clinicians urge patients not to resume intercourse until after the 4- to 6-week postpartum examination, some now say that there is no reason to prohibit it once lochia has ceased and the perineum has healed. But the patient must understand that she can become pregnant during this period if not protected by a contraceptive during sexual intercourse. She must also understand that some contraceptives are not appropriate during this period before the body has returned to its prepregnant state.

Sterilization by tubal ligation may be done during the postpartum period. It should be done on the basis of a well-thought-out decision to have no more children. The patient and her spouse should consider it a permanent procedure (although infrequently it can be reversed). Vasectomy is another option.

Adequate counseling, a waiting period between the decision and the procedure, and a signed consent form are required.

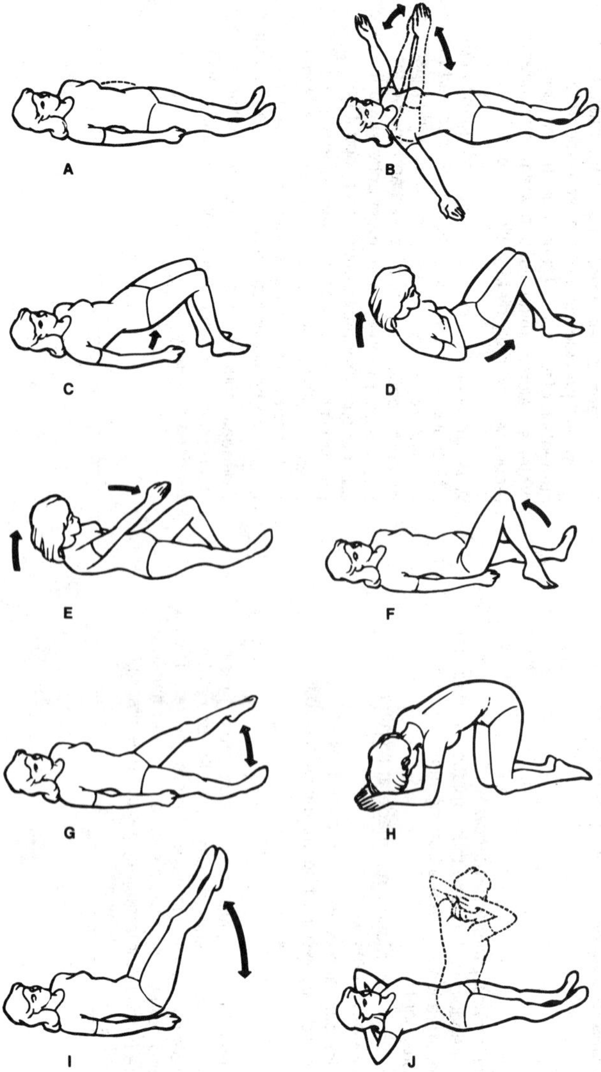

Fig. 5-11. *Postpartum exercises. (A) Day 1: Breathe deeply, expanding the abdomen. Slowly exhale and draw in the abdominal muscles. (B) Day 2: Assume a supine position with legs slightly parted. Place arms at right angles to torso and slowly raise them, keeping the elbows stiff. Gradually return to original position and repeat. (C) Day 3: Assume a supine position with arms at the side. Draw knees up slightly and arch back. (D) Day 4: With knees and hips*

(continued from page 537)

c. Other tests may be used for confirmation and diet monitoring.

2. Serum thyroxine (T4)

- Dextrostix is used to determine blood glucose level in infants of diabetic mothers. Blood from a heel stick is tested with a Dextrostix reagent stick. (See the Dextrostix bottle for instructions.) If the color change indicates a glucose level below 45 mg/dl, a prompt second test is required. For confirmation of hypoglycemia, a test for blood glucose on a serum sample is necessary.

Observations

- Heart rate, respiratory effort, muscle tone, reflex irritability, and color are evaluated and scored according to the Apgar Scoring System (See Table 5-6), at 1 minute and at 5 minutes after birth in an effort to identify an immediate need for resuscitation.
- Respiratory distress is evaluated using the Silverman and Anderson criteria (Fig. 5-12).
- General condition, need for resuscitation, number of cord vessels, and gross abnormalities are the focus of delivery room assessment.
- More complete assessment provides a data base, identifies risk factors, estimates gestational age, and establishes needs for teaching and anticipatory guidance for the parents.

1. History includes family, past medical, prenatal, labor and delivery, and immediate post-delivery information.
2. An assessment for gestational age should be done within 24 hours after birth (Fig. 5-13).

a. The physical assessment can be done soon after delivery; the neurologic assessment, 24 hours after birth, when the infant's neurologic status has stabilized.

b. The assessment of gestational age has become an important key in identifying the high-risk infant. Weight is related

flexed, lift head and pelvis upward and contract buttocks. (E) Day 5: With legs straight, raise head and left knee slightly. Reach for, but do not touch, knee with right hand. Repeat with other leg and hand. (F) Day 6: On back, flex one knee and thigh toward abdomen. Lower foot toward buttocks, then straighten and lower the leg. (G) Day 7: In supine position, with toes pointed and knees straight, raise one leg and then the other as high as possible, using abdominal muscles to slowly lower. (H) Day 8: On elbows and knees, keep elbows and lower legs together. Hump back upward (cat position), contracting buttocks and drawing in abdomen. Relax and breathe deeply. (I) Day 9: Same as for day 7, but lift both legs at once. (J) Day 10: In supine position, with hands clasped behind head, sit up and lie back slowly. (Feet may be hooked under furniture, at first.)

TABLE 5-6 THE APGAR SCORING CHART

Sign	0	1	2
Heart rate	Absent	Slow (less than 100)	Over 100
Respiratory effort	Absent	Slow, irregular	Good, crying
Muscle tone	Flaccid	Some flexion of extremities	Active motion
Reflex irritability	No response	Weak cry or grimace	Vigorous cry
Color	Blue, pale	Body pink, extremities blue	Completely pink

to gestational age by plotting both on a standardized graph (Fig. 5-14).

c. The infant whose weight is appropriate for gestational age is assumed to have grown at a normal rate no matter when he or she was born—preterm, term, or postterm. The *small-for-gestational age* (SGA) infant is presumed to have had a slow intrauterine growth rate or weight loss. The *large-for-gestational-age* (LGA) infant presumably grew more rapidly than normal prenatally. Gestational age is more closely related to maturity than is birth weight.

3. See Table 5-7 for reminders concerning physical assessment of full-term infants. (Look to references of greater depth for more information on neonatal assessment. Some of them are listed in the Bibliography.)
4. The baby's status of alertness should be noted.
5. Any sign of distress in the newborn should be called to the physician's attention immediately (see common signs of distress in the newborn).
6. Hints for doing a good physical assessment include the following:
   a. Find a quiet environment and a comfortable position.
   b. Undress the baby, but keep him or her warm.
   c. Concentrate, using a systematic approach.
   d. Move from general to specific, from external to internal.
   e. Be opportunistic, auscultating the baby's chest when the baby is quiet. A finger in the mouth may help.

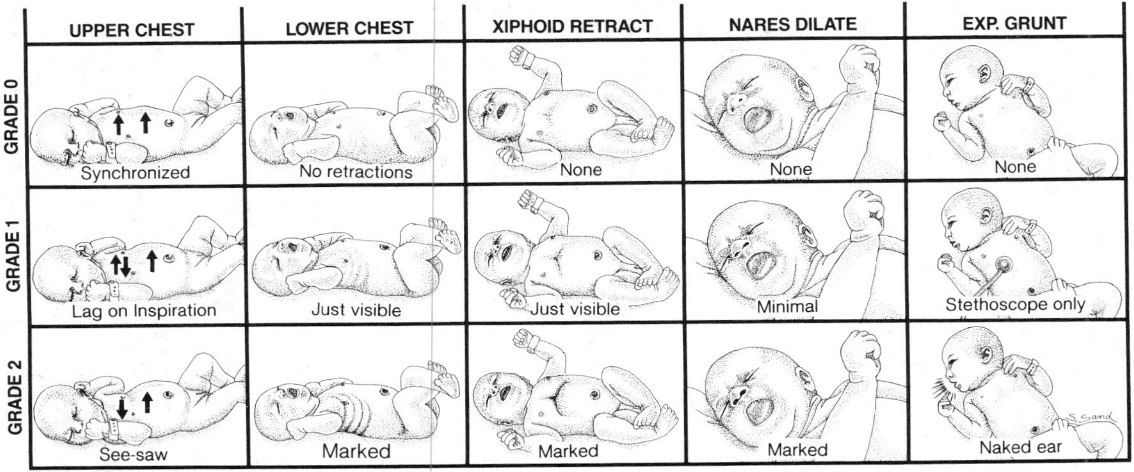
UPPER CHEST
LOWER CHEST
XIPHOID RETRACT
NARES DILATE
EXP. GRUNT
GRADE 0
GRADE 1
GRADE 2
Synchronized
No retractions
None
None
None
Lag on Inspiration
Just visible
Just visible
Minimal
Stethoscope only
See-saw
Marked
Marked
Marked
Naked ear
S. Sand

Fig. 5-12 *Criteria for evaluating respiratory distress.*

Symbols: X - 1st Exam O - 2nd Exam

NEUROMUSCULAR MATURITY

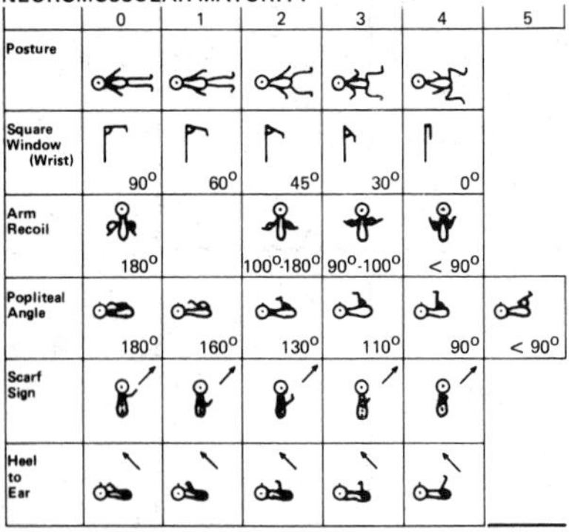

	0	1	2	3	4	5
Posture						
Square Window (Wrist)	90°	60°	45°	30°	0°	
Arm Recoil	180°		100°-180°	90°-100°	< 90°	
Popliteal Angle	180°	160°	130°	110°	90°	< 90°
Scarf Sign						
Heel to Ear						

Gestation by Dates ________ wks

Birth Date ______ Hour ______ am pm

APGAR ______ 1 min ______ 5 min

MATURITY RATING

Score	Wks
5	26
10	28
15	30
20	32
25	34
30	36
35	38
40	40
45	42
50	44

PHYSICAL MATURITY

	0	1	2	3	4	5
SKIN	gelatinous red, trans-parent	smooth pink, visible veins	superficial peeling &/or rash, few veins	cracking pale area, rare veins	parchment, deep cracking, no vessels	leathery, cracked, wrinkled
LANUGO	none	abundant	thinning	bald areas	mostly bald	
PLANTAR CREASES	no crease	faint red marks	anterior transverse crease only	creases ant. 2/3	creases cover entire sole	
BREAST	barely percept.	flat areola, no bud	stippled areola, 1–2 mm bud	raised areola, 3–4 mm bud	full areola, 5–10 mm bud	
EAR	pinna flat, stays folded	sl. curved pinna, soft with slow recoil	well-curv. pinna, soft but ready recoil	formed & firm with instant recoil	thick cartilage, ear stiff	
GENITALS Male	scrotum empty, no rugae		testes descend-ing, few rugae	testes down, good rugae	testes pendulous, deep rugae	
GENITALS Female	prominent clitoris & labia minora		majora & minora equally prominent	majora large, minora small	clitoris & minora completely covered	

SCORING SECTION

	1st Exam=X	2nd Exam=O
Estimating Gest Age by Maturity Rating	____ Weeks	____ Weeks
Time of Exam	Date ____ Hour ____ am pm	Date ____ Hour ____ am pm
Age at Exam	____ Hours	____ Hours
Signature of Examiner	____ M.D.	____ M.D.

Fig. 5-13 *Estimation of gestational age by maturity rating. (Courtesy of Mead Johnson Company, Evansville, Indiana)*

f. Use a good stethoscope that fits your ears well. It should have a diaphragm and a bell small enough for an infant.

7. A number of tools are available for the assessment of developmental, behavioral, temperamental, and environmental factors that affect the baby, including tools to assess parental–neonatal perceptions, and mother–infant and father–infant interaction. One of those is Reiser's Mother-Infant Screening Tool (MIST) (see Table 5-8). Others are listed in the Bibliography.

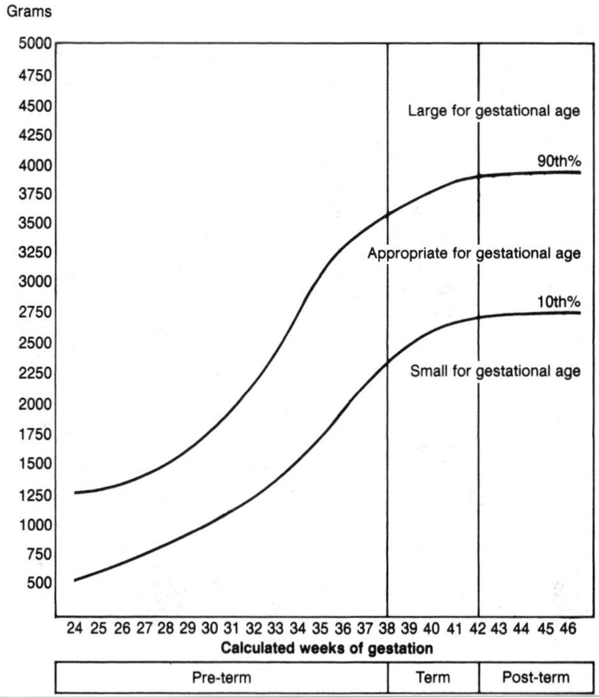

Fig. 5-14 *Classification of newborn infants by birth weight and gestational age. (Brenner WE, Edelman DA, Hendricks CH: A standard of fetal growth for the United States of America. Am J Obstet Gynecol 126:555–564, 1976)*

Common Signs of Distress in the Newborn

- Changes in behavior; lethargy, irritability, "not looking right"
- Respiratory difficulties, including increased rate (greater than 60/min), any retractions, nasal flaring, grunting, apnea greater than 20 sec (see Fig. 5-12).
- Rapid, slow, or irregular pulse (normal heart rate is between 120–160/min)
- Cyanosis—generalized or persistent circumoral
- Excessive mucus
- Abdominal distention, tenseness, mass, scaphoid abdomen (concave), ecchymosis

(*Text continues on page 564*)

TABLE 5-7 THE NEWBORN PHYSICAL EXAMINATION

Physical Examination	Findings in Normal Full-Term Infants	Common Abnormalities
General Appearance		
Color	Pink, acrocyanosis	Generalized cyanosis, pallor, jaundice, "tomato red"
Position	Flexion of extremities	Flaccidity with extension of extremities
Activity	Spontaneous movement	Decreased or absent spontaneous movement
Cry	Vigorous and sustained after stimulation	Weak, high pitched, hoarseness aphonia
Facial appearance		Unusual familial facies
		Syndromes: Down's, Potter's, Cornelia de Lange's, and so forth
		Facial nerve paralysis
		Cretinism
Measurements		
Weight	See gestational age chart. (Fig. 5-14)	Small for gestational age: large for gestational age
Length	Average: 49.4 cm (19.5 in) with a range between 45.8 cm–52.3 cm (18–20.5 in)	Long: Marfan's syndrome
		Short: dwarf (achondroplasia), osteogenesis imperfecta, and so forth
Head circumference	Average: 33–35 cm (13–14 in)	Large: hydrocephalus
	Head 1–2 cm greater than chest in full-term infant	Small: microcephaly

Skin		
Color	Pink, acrocyanosis	Generalized cyanosis, mottling, jaundice, petechiae, and ecchymosis
Pigmentation	Mongolian spot	Meconium stained
Vernix	Vernix caseosa, lanugo	Absence of vernix caseosa or lanugo
Lesions	Milia, erythema toxicum, occasional petechiae	Multiple petechiae
	Telangiectasia	Multiple hemangiomas
	Mild peeling	Massive peeling: postmaturity and congenital ichthyosis
Head		
Shape	Molded (secondary to compression in labor)	Cephalohematoma, hydrocephalus, oxycephaly, brachycephaly, microcephaly
	Caput succedaneum	
Fontanels	Soft, flat; open anterior and posterior fontanel	Bulging (caused by increased intracranial pressure)
		Small: cranial synostosis or microcephaly
		Large: hypothyroidism
	Occasionally third fontanel	Third: mongolism
Eyes		
Conjunctiva	Clear	Conjunctivitis: chemical, bacterial, or viral
	Occasionally subconjunctival hemorrhage	

(*continued*)

TABLE 5-7 THE NEWBORN PHYSICAL EXAMINATION

Physical Examination	Findings in Normal Full-Term Infants	Common Abnormalities
Cornea	Clear	Corneal opacity syndromes: rubella, Hurler's, Lowe's congenital idiopathic hypoparathyroidism
Eyelids	Lid edema (especially with brow or face presentation)	Edema: congestive heart failure
		Coloboma
		Ectropion: lamellar ichthyosis
		Entropion: Horner's syndrome with or without brachial palsy
Ears		
Shape		Preauricular skin tag, sinus Large, small, or malformed ear (rule out renal anomalies)
Place		Low-set ears (rule out renal anomalies and/or trisomies)
Consistency of ear lobe	Stiff cartilage	Cartilage abnormalities
Nose		
Patency	Bilateral patency of nares	Choanal atresia (bilateral or unilateral) or "stuffy nose"
Discharge	No discharge	Mucosanguineous discharge of syphilis
Mouth		
Lips		Harelip
Palate	Epstein's pearls	Cleft or high-arched palate
Tongue	Geographic tongue	Large: Syndromes: Beckwith's, cretinism, mongolism (very small jaw)
		Glossoptosis with micrognathia: Pierre Robin syndrome

Teeth	None	Natal teeth, ranula
Mucous membrane	Epithelial pearls (inclusion cysts)	Thrush
		Epulis
Saliva	Moist mucous membranes	Excessive saliva; esophageal atresia, tracheo-esophageal fistula
Neck		
Shape	Short (head seems to sit on neck)	Web: Turner's syndrome
		Excessive tissue back of neck: mongolism, Turner's syndrome
Masses	No palpable mass	Cystic hygroma, goiter, brachial cysts, hematomas, ectopic thyroid
		Torticollis
Thorax		
Shape	Symmetric	Asymmetric: pigeon breast, funnel chest, pneumothorax, atelectasis
Breast	>7 mm palpable breast tissue	Mastitis
	Engorgement with or without "witches milk"	Supernumerary nipples
Lungs		
Breath sounds	Presence of breath sound bilaterally	Unilateral absence of breath sounds; pneumothorax or atelectasis
		Peristaltic sounds; diaphragmatic hernia
Grunting	Grunting normal during the first hour of life	After first hour of life, grunting abnormal

(*continued*)

TABLE 5-7 THE NEWBORN PHYSICAL EXAMINATION

Physical Examination	Findings in Normal Full-Term Infants	Common Abnormalities
Rales	Rales normal during the first hour of life	After first hour of life, rales abnormal
Respiratory rate	60/minute for first hour of life, 35–40/minute thereafter	After first hour of life, above 60/minute
Retractions (intercostal, substernal, suprasternal)	Retractions normal during the first hour of life	After the first hour of life, retractions indicate ventilatory insufficiency
Heart		
PMI	Fifth intercostal space on midclavicular line	Shifted to the right, left, or displaced downward; dextrocardia, pneumothorax, atelectasis
Rate	After 15 minutes of age, 100–175/minute; can drop to 70/minute during sleep	Tachycardia; cardiac, respiratory metabolic, infectious, or hematologic disease
		Bradycardia; hypoxia, intracranial disorder, heart block
Murmurs	Grade I–II/VI systolic murmur in the first 24 hours of life	After 24 hours of life, systolic or diastolic murmurs
Abdomen	Flat, not distended	Distended; intestinal obstruction sepsis, prune-belly syndrome
		Scaphoid abdomen; diaphragmatic hernia
Liver	Palpable about 2 cm below the right costal margin	Enlarged: congestive heart failure, sepsis, hepatitis, rubella, glycogen-storage disease, and so forth
		Palpable on the left side in situs inversus

Spleen	Tip palpable in 25% of normal infants	Enlarged: sepsis, rubella, cytomegalic inclusion disease, and so forth
Kidney	Easily palpable bilaterally	Enlarged: renal vein thrombosis, polycystic kidney
Anus	Patent	Imperforate anus with or without fistula
Umbilicus		
Vessels	Two arteries and one vein	Single umbilical artery; gastrointestinal, genitourinary, CNS, cardiovascular system anomalies
Color	Translucent	Green, yellow, meconium stained resulting from fetal distress
Genitalia		
Male: Testes	Descended into scrotum or palpable in canal	Testes in abdomen (may descend spontaneously later)
Urethral opening	At center of shaft	Hypospadias: opening on ventral surface of penis Epispadias: opening on dosal surface of penis
Swelling	Noncommunicating hydrocele	Communicating hydrocele, trauma secondary to breech presentation
Female: Hymen	Hymenal tag	Hydrometrocolpos behind a bulging imperforated hymen
Clitoris	Large clitoris in premature infant	Large clitoris: Adrenogenital syndrome, maternal drug ingestion, hermaphroditism
Discharge	Mucoid vaginal discharge or bleeding caused by maternal hormone withdrawal	

(*continued*)

TABLE 5-7 THE NEWBORN PHYSICAL EXAMINATION

Physical Examination	Findings in Normal Full-Term Infants	Common Abnormalities
Extremities		
Position and movement	Full range of joint motion	Passive motor limitation
	Position abnormalities passively corrected are normal	Lower extremities: talipes equinovarus, calcaneovalgus anomalies, or spinal cord injury
		Upper extremities: brachial plexus injury, clavicular or humerus fracture
Hip	Full abduction of flexed hip	Congenital subluxation or dislocation of hip: Ortolani's sign
Neurologic examinations		
Reflexes	Moro's, sucking, rooting, grasping, walking, pupil, supraciliary tap	Absence of appropriate reflexes
Movement	Spontaneous movement	Flaccidity, rigidity, convulsions

(From Harper K, Yoon J: Handbook of Neonatology. Chicago, Year Book Medical Publishers, 1974)

TABLE 5-8 MOTHER–INFANT SCREENING TOOL (MIST)

A	B	C	D
Tactile			
Mother			
Holds infant close to her body	Holds infant on forearm	Holds infant away from body	Doesn't hold infant
Infant			
Curls up close to mother	Keeps some distance	Moves away when touched	Stiffens-up when held
Mother			
Comfortable touching infant, strokes head or face	Looks comfortable, pats infant's back	Tentative when touching infant	Avoids touching infant
Infant			
At ease; turns toward mother's touch	Looks at ease	Looks tense	Cries when touched
Visual			
Mother			
Establishes eye contact	Looks at infant's face	Does not look at infant's face	Does not look at infant
Infant			
Establishes eye contact	Looks at mother's face	Does not look at mother's face	Does not look at mother

(*continued*)

TABLE 5-8 MOTHER–INFANT SCREENING TOOL (MIST)

A	B	C	D
Mother			
Smiles and makes faces in play	Smiles	No special facial expressions	Looks unhappy
Infant			
Laughs or big smile	Smiles	No special facial expression	Looks unhappy
Auditory			
Mother			
Talks to infant in soothing or playful way	Talks to infant in calm way	Talks but just gives directions	Doesn't talk to infant
Infant			
Infant makes happy sounds, coos and goos	Makes ah-ah sounds	Cries	Doesn't talk
Mother			
Understands meaning of infant's cries	Differentiates most of infant's cries	Seldom differentiates infant's cries	Never differentiates infant's cries
Infant			
Exhibits different cries	Usually exhibits different cries	Seldom exhibits different cries	Never exhibits different cries

Feeding			
Mother			
Shows signs of pleasure during feeding—smiles, rocks, sings	Looks content during feeding	Acts unsure during feeding—stops and starts	Agitated or irritable
Infant			
Shows pleasure in being fed—smiles, coos	Looks content during feeding	Restless during feeding	Agitated—cries during feeding
Mother			
Looks pleased after feeding	Looks satisfied after feeding	Looks uneasy after feeding	Looks agitated after feeding
Infant			
Looks happy after feeding	Looks satisfied after feeding	Looks restless after feeding	Looks agitated after feeding
Total	MOTHER		
SCORE	INFANT		
DATE			

How to score MIST: B describes a middle range of mother–infant interactions. A mother or infant with two or more checks in C or D warrants reevaluation. A mother or infant with four or more checks in C or D warrants reevaluation and nursing intervention, *e.g.*, counseling and teaching. Reevaluation and possible intervention are warranted if there is an inconsistency in either the mother's or the infant's results.
(Reiser SL: A tool to facilitate mother–infant attachment. JOGN Nurs 10(4): 294, July/Aug 1981.)

(*continued from page 553*)

- No meconium stool in 48 hours
- Delayed voiding past 24 hours; or dribbling or interrupted urinary stream
- Vomiting
- Jaundice appearing before 24 hours to 48 hours, or persisting beyond 7 days
- Seizures, tremors
- Cord bleeding, odor, exudate, or erythema
- Signs of dehydration—weight loss, small amounts of concentrated urine, dry mucous membranes
- Temperature instability
- Petechiae
- Bulging fontanel
- Poor feeding

Nursing Considerations

Immediate Care of the Newborn in the Delivery Room

- Apgar scoring is done at 1 minute and at 5 minutes after birth to evaluate the infant's physical condition and need for immediate resuscitation (see Table 5-6).
- The preservation of warmth is of the utmost importance.
  1. Place the baby under radiant heat as you dry him or her. (Because the heat warms the baby's outer surface, no garments or blanket is needed.)
     Caution: The setting for the radiant warmer should be 36.5°C. Care must be taken not to overheat the baby.
  2. Dry the baby's head and keep it covered to prevent cooling by evaporation from a large surface.
  3. Wrap the baby in a dry warm blanket, either separately or with the mother. The infant can be put on the mother's chest and in her arms if she is alert.
- Place baby in a modified Trendelenburg position on the left side to promote gravity drainage of mucus.
- Gently suction with a bulb syringe prn. Avoid deep oropharyngeal suctioning.
- Hospital protocol may call for the administration of oxygen if pallor or cyanosis is present.
- Stimulate prn by gently rubbing the back or soles of the feet.
- Immediate care of the cord includes:
  1. Examination of the cut end of the cord for the presence of two arteries and one vein (the larger of the blood vessels).
  2. Apply the cord clamp approximately 0.5 to 1 inch from the abdomen, taking care not to include skin. Use aseptic technique.

- Instillation of 1 to 2 drops of 1% silver nitrate solution or ophthalmic antibiotic (either in single-dose containers) into the lower conjunctival sac of each eye is required prophylaxis against gonorrheal ophthalmia neonatorum.
  1. This may be done in the delivery room or upon admission to the nursery.
- Prophylactic IM injection of 0.5 mg to 1.0 mg of vitamin K_1 (phytonadione) is given within 1 hour of birth to prevent hemorrhage.
- Identification of the baby is done in the delivery room.
  1. Bands or bracelets applied to the mother's wrist and two applied to the infant should contain identical identifying information, including sex of the baby and the family name. In some institutions, the date and time of birth and the clinician's name also will be included. *Caution:* Bracelets applied to newborn should be snug enough so they won't fall off after the infant's normal, postdelivery weight loss.
  2. Some institutions include footprinting of the baby and fingerprinting of the mother. Vernix must be wiped off the baby's foot in order to get a good print.
- A brief physical assessment for general condition, gross abnormalities, and a quick determination of gestational age, is done by the delivery room nurse, with indepth physical and neurologic assessment reserved for the nursery (see Table 5-7 and Fig. 5-13.)
- Promotion of attachment or bonding is important.
  1. As soon as possible, provide an opportunity for the mother and father to hold and examine the baby.
  2. Encourage eye contact by placing the infant in the parent's arms.
  3. Breast-feeding may be started while the mother is still on the delivery table. It stimulates bonding, milk production, and uterine involution.
  4. Direct skin contact between the baby and mother is encouraged as long as the baby is kept warm.
  5. When showing the baby to the parents, try to point out something attractive about him, *e.g.,* "Doesn't he have a cute little nose?"

Post Delivery Room Care of the Newborn

- The care of the neonate in the hospital is on a continuum, from delivery through discharge.
- The nurse continues skilled observation, assessment, and care; intervention when indicated; teaching and guidance of the parents, whether the infant is transferred to the nursery, to rooming-in, or is cared for at home, as is usual after home births or delivery at birthing centers.

- Retention of warmth is essential. Axillary temperature should stabilize around 36.6° C (97.8° F) within 24 hr. The baby's temperature is taken q 4 h during the first 24 hr, and bid thereafter. If the temperature drops, return the infant to the warmer, and take it q 1 h until it becomes stable. *Caution:* If a radiant warmer is being used, be sure the probe is touching the baby's skin at all times. Monitor the temperature of any warmer.
  1. Axillary temperature should be taken for at least 3 minutes. Apical pulse and respirations should be counted for a full 60 seconds.
- Protect infant from infection. Detailed recommendations are given in control of infections in obstetric and nursery areas, in Guidelines for Perinatal Care, by the American Academy of Pediatrics/The American College of Obstetricians and Gynecologists, 1983. Based on these guidelines hospital protocols* usually include the following:
  1. Handwashing
     a. An initial 2-minute scrub of hands and arms with an antimicrobial agent is required before entering the nursery, before providing care for neonates highly susceptible to infection, before performing invasive procedures, and after the care of infected neonates.
     b. A 15-second soap and water wash should be done between neonates.
  2. Dress code
     a. Scrub suits or dresses, and caps and gowns for special procedures, should be worn.
  3. Maternal infections
     a. The febrile postpartum patient without a specific diagnosed site of infection usually is allowed to handle and feed her baby, if she feels like it; she should wash her hands thoroughly and wear a clean hospital cover gown to prevent the baby's contact with contaminated items.
     b. For an upper respiratory infection, the mother's handwashing and use of a surgical mask are recommended.
     c. Breast-feeding is usually possible, even if the mother is taking antibiotics.
  4. Infected neonates
     a. Protocol varies with the type and severity of the infection.
     b. High-risk neonates with infections usually are cared for in a special setting (admission/observation area, or intensive care nursery).
- Weigh the baby on admission to the nursery, and thereafter daily, usually before the bath. The scale is covered to prevent cross-

*Check for protocols specific to your hospital.

infection and heat loss, and is balanced before each baby is weighed.

1. Infants normally lose between 5% to 10% of their birth weight during the first five days, but generally regain it in about 2 weeks. (At 6 months, the baby's birth weight usually is doubled, and it is tripled by the first birthday.)

- Measurements of length, head, and chest circumference are taken.
- Stools and voiding are recorded each time, the first time being especially important.
  1. Meconium stools, the first, are sticky, black, and odorless, and should be passed within 24 hr to 48 hr.
  2. Transitional stools go from greenish-brown to brownish-yellow to bright yellow in color.
  3. Bottle-fed infants have stools that are more solid, usually one or two a day.
  4. Stools of breast-fed infants are loose and more frequent.
- Feeding
  1. Assess the infant's sucking, gagging, and swallowing reflexes.
  2. If the mother is breast-feeding, put the baby to the breast during the first hour, if possible.
     a. Generally, the infant should be offered the breast q 3 hr.
     b. Supplementary water and glucose water are controversial and should be cleared with the physician and mother.
     c. The pediatrician should be made aware of any medication prescribed for the mother.
  3. If the baby is to be bottle-fed, offer sterile water or 5% glucose water according to your hospital's protocol—usually about 4 hr to 6 hr after birth.
  4. Try to keep the feeding schedule moderately flexible.
  5. The physician may order vitamin or iron supplements.
  6. After feeding, the infant should be positioned on the right side to prevent aspiration. A rolled blanket may be put at the baby's back.
- Bathing
  1. The first bath may be given after the baby's temperature is stabilized.
  2. The bathing area should be free from drafts, the water temperature about 37°C to 38°C (98°F–100°F), or comfortable to your wrist or elbow.
  3. The entire body should be washed with water and a mild soap. The head should be shampooed gently to prevent cradle cap (thick, flaky patches on the scalp). Avoid oils and lotions.
  4. When bathing, start with the cleanest areas first. Using a clean cotton ball for each eye, wipe from the inner canthus out.

5. Use a clean washcloth to wash the nose and ears, and do not use cotton swabs.
6. Do not submerge the baby in water until the cord has dropped off—usually at about 1 week to 2 weeks. If the base of the cord remains moist, rubbing alcohol may be applied at the base to hasten drying. Fasten the diaper below the cord.
7. Wipe the genitalia clean with cotton balls or a wash cloth. To cleanse the penis, gently retract the foreskin only as far as it will go without resistance.

- In *circumcision,* the prepuce (or foreskin) of the penis is separated from the glans, and a portion is removed surgically. The value of the procedure is somewhat controversial at present. Whether or not it is done, is now largely a matter of family preference. Options should be discussed with the parents.
- When circumcision is chosen, nursing responsibilities include the following:
  1. Confirmation that consent form has been signed
  2. Assembly of equipment needed according to the physician's preference
  3. Positioning the infant on a restraining board
  4. Keeping the wound clean and watching for bleeding, following the procedure
     a. Bleeding usually can be controlled with gentle pressure. If it continues, notify the physician immediately.
     b. Advice varies, but usually the circumcised area is covered with a sterile gauze pad and a little sterile petroleum jelly to keep the dressing or diaper from adhering to the incision. The circumcised area may be gently washed and patted dry. The dressing is changed when diapers are changed. Diapers should be loosely secured.
     c. A whitish yellow exudate forms around the glans. It is normal and will disappear. It should not be forcibly removed.
- Accident prevention is another focus of parent teaching. Accidents are the leading cause of death in infants and young children, with suffocation, falls, burns, and automobile accidents high on the list.
  1. Start by urging that the infant ride in an approved car seat with appropriate restraints, when going home from the hospital.

BIBLIOGRAPHY • Obstetrics

BOOKS

Brunner L, Suddarth D: The Lippincott Manual of Nursing Practice, 3rd ed., Philadelphia, JB Lippincott, 1982

Buckley K, Kulb N: Handbook of Maternal-Newborn Nursing. New York, John Wiley & Sons, 1983

Christman B, Nemchik R, O'Connor M, et al: Managing Diabetics Properly. Horsham, Intermed Communications, 1978
Krupp M, Chatton M: Current Medical Diagnosis and Treatment 1983. Los Altos, Lange Medical Publications, 1983
Olds S, London M, Ladewig P, et al: Obstetric Nursing. Menlo Park, Addison-Wesley, 1980
Pritchard J, MacDonald P: William Obstetrics, 16th ed. New York, Appleton-Century-Crofts, 1980

JOURNALS

Atkinson L: Prenatal nipple conditioning for breast feeding. Nurs Res 28(5):267, 1979
Aumann G, Blake G: Ritodrine hydrochloride in the control of premature labor—implications for use. JOGN Nurs 11(2):75, 1982
Brown S: The devastating effects of congenital rubella. Matern Child Nurs J 4(3):171, 1979
Carr K, Walton V: Early postpartum discharge. JOGN Nurs 11(1):29, 1982
Chesley L: Severe rheumatic cardiac disease and pregnancy. Am J Obstet Gynecol 136(5):552, 1980
Cohn S: Sexuality in pregnancy: a review of the literature. Nurs Clin North Am 17(1):91, 1982
Curet L, Olson R: Oxytocin challenge tests and urinary estriols in the management of high risk pregnancies. Obstet Gynecol 55:296, 1980
Gabbe S: Diabetes mellitus in pregnancy: Have all the problems been solved? Am J Med 70(3):613, 1981
Gilstrap L, Cunningham F, Whalley P: Acute pyelonephritis in pregnancy: an anterospective study. Obstet Gynecol 57(4):409, 1981
Hayes B: Inconsistencies among nurses in breast feeding knowledge and counseling JOGN Nurs 16(6):430, 1981
Jones M: Hypertensive disorders of pregnancy. JOGN Nurs 8(2):92, 1979
Katz M, Creasy R, Herron M: Evaluation of a preterm birth prevention program: preliminary report. Obstet Gynecol 59(4):452, 1982
Katz Z, Lancet M, Borenstein R: Management of labor with umbilical cord prolapse. Am J Obstet Gynecol 142(2):239, 1982
MacLaughlin S, Taubernheim A: Epidural anesthesia for obstetric patients. JOGN Nurs 10(1):9, 1981
Martin B, Reeb R: Oral health during pregnancy: A neglected nursing area. MCN 7(6):391, 1982
Peck T: Electric monitoring evidence of fetal distress in high-risk pregnancies. J Reprod Med 24(3):103, 1980
Pirong G: An in-house program of continuing education for perinatal nurses. JOGN Nurs 11(11):109, 1982
Rang M: Bibliography for nutrition in pregnancy. JOGN Nurs 9(1):5, 1980
Rayburn W, Green J, Donalson, M: Nonstress testing and perinatal outcome. J Reprod Med 80(24):191, 1980

Snyder D: The high-risk mother viewed in relation to a holistic model of the child-bearing experience. JOGN Nurs 8(3):164, 1979

Sugue D, Blake S, Macdonald D: Pregnancy complicated by maternal heart disease at the National Maternity Hospital, Dublin, Ireland 1969–1978. Am J Obstet Gynecol 139(1):1, 1981

Timm M: Prenatal education evaluation. Nurs Res 28(6):338, 1979

White P: Pregnancy and diabetes: Medical aspects. Med Clin North Am 49(4):1015, 1965

TEACHING MODULES

March of Dimes Birth Defects Foundation

Herron M, Dulock H: Preterm labor a staff development program in perinatal nursing care. Series 2, Prenatal Care, Module 5

Derby V, Williams J: Antepartal predictors of fetal and neonatal risk: a staff development program in perinatal nursing care. Series 2, Prenatal Care, Module 6

Wheeler L, Duxbury M: Fetal assessment, a staff development program in perinatal nursing care. Series 2, Prenatal Care, Module 3

Fetal and Maternal Monitoring

BOOKS

Brunner L, Suddarth D: The Lippincott Manual of Nursing Practice, 3rd ed. Philadelphia, JB Lippincott, 1982

Buckley K, Kulb N: Handbook of Maternal-Newborn Nursing. New York, John Wiley & Sons, 1983

Olds S, London M, Ladewig P, et al: Obstetric Nursing. Menlo Park, Addison-Wesley, 1980

JOURNALS

Applegate J, Haverkamp A, Orleans M, et al: Electronic fetal monitoring: Implications for obstetric nursing. Nurs Res 28(6):369, 1979

Cranley M: Antepartal fetal assessment. Am J Nurs 78(12):2098, 1978

Haukkamoa M, Purhonen M, Teramo K: The monitoring of labor by telemetry. J Perinat Med 10(1):17, 1982

Katz M, Shan N, Meizner I: Is end-stage deceleration of the fetal heart ominous? Br J Obstet Gynecol 89(3):186, 1982

Calvert J, Newcombe R, Hibband B: An assessment of radiotelemetry in the monitoring of labor. Br J Obstet Gynecol 89(4):285, 1982

Peck T: Electronic monitoring evidence of fetal distress in high-risk pregnancies. J Reprod Med 24(3):103, 1980

The Neonate

BOOKS

American Academy of Pediatrics/The American College of Obstetricians and Gynecologists: Guidelines for Perinatal Care. Evanston, The American Academy of Pediatrics, 1983

Buckley K, Kulb N: Handbook of Maternal-Newborn Nursing. New York, John Wiley & Sons, 1983
Chow M, Durand B, Feldman M, et al: Handbook of Pediatric Primary Care. New York, John Wiley & Sons, 1979
Kempe C, Silver H, O'Brien D: Current Pediatric Diagnosis and Treatment 1976, 5th ed. Los Altos, Lange Medical Publications, 1982
Ludington-Hoe S: Summation report: Essential tools and techniques of infant stimulation. Washington, DC, ISEA Publication, 1980
Olds S, London M, Ladewig P, et al: Obstetric Nursing. Menlo Park, Addison-Wesley, 1980
Powel M: Assessment and Management of Developmental Changes in Children, 2nd ed. St Louis, CV Mosby, 1981
Whaley L, Wong D: Nursing Care of Infants and Children. St Louis, CV Mosby, 1981

JOURNALS

Apgar V: A proposal for a new method of evaluation of the newborn infant. Anesth Analg 32(4):260, 1953
Battaglia F, Lubchenco L: Classification of newborn infants by birthweight and gestational age. J Pediatr 71(2):160, 1967
Brodish M: Perinatal assessment. JOGN Nurs 10(1):43, 1981
Frankenburg W, Dodds J: The Denver Developmental Screening Test. J Pediatr 71(2):181, 1967
Gibbons M: Why circumcise? Pediatr Nurs 5(4):9, 1979
Moss J: Swaddling then there and now: Historical, anthropological, and current practices. MCN 8(3):137, 1979
Poole C: Neonatal circumcision. JOGN Nurs 8(4):207, 1979
Sullivan R, Foster J, Schneiner R: Determining a newborn's gestational age. MCN 8(1):38, 1979
Vanderzanden E: Anticipatory guidance for the first two months of life. J Nurse Midwifery 24(5):28, 1979

TOOLS FOR NEONATAL ASSESSMENT

Brazelton T: Neonatal behavioral assessment scale. Clinics in Developmental Medicine No. 50. Philadelphia, JB Lippincott, 1973
Caldwell B: Home observation for measurement of the environment 1970. In Erickson M: Assessment and Management of the Developmental Changes in Children. St Louis, CV Mosby, 1976
Chow M, Durand B, Feldman M, et al: Neonatal perception inventory I and II, Handbook of Pediatric Primary Care. New York, John Wiley & Sons, 1979
Cropley C: Assessment of mothering behaviors. In Johnson S: High Risk Parenting. Philadelphia, JB Lippincott, 1979
Murphy C: Assessment of fathering behaviors. In Johnson S: High Risk Parenting. Philadelphia, JB Lippincott, 1979

6
Pediatrics (PED)

BLOOD PRESSURE, PEDIATRIC

Pediatric Blood Pressure Tables

A blood pressure measurement should be part of the physical examination of all children over the age of 3 years. There may be wide variations in the blood pressure of children and adolescents; therefore, a single elevation is not reliable. However, those with diastolic blood pressure levels consistently above the 90th percentile on three or more occasions, taken at one- to two-week intervals, require further diagnostic investigation. (see charts on pages 574, 575)

CHILD ABUSE AND NEGLECT

Description

Child abuse encompasses sexual, emotional, and physical maltreatment; child neglect is characterized by lack of concern for physical and educational well-being. Sexual abuse is not only physical molestation, but also the use of children in pornographic pictures or movies. Legally, "child" usually refers to a person up to the age of 18 years. However, most cases of abuse or neglect start at the infant or young child stage. The maltreatment of children is receiving increasing attention. It has become obvious that child abuse and neglect produce acute and chronic medical problems, as well as increase the risk of juvenile delinquency, psychiatric problems, sexual dysfunction, and, later, poor parenting attitudes.

Observations

- See Table 6-1.

Nursing Considerations

- There are typical situations that predispose an individual to child abuse. These include a handicapped or premature infant; a child born of a teenager or of an unwanted pregnancy; lack of maternal–child bonding; a stressed family; parental alcoholism; parents who have been abused as children; and a parent with a personality unable to cope with normal family living.
- A normal bonding pattern between a parent and child is important for healthy growth and development. Lack of proper bonding

often is evidenced by an impersonal attitude of the parent, including no eye contact with the infant and little verbal support or friendly physical contact.

- Any child under 24 months of age with an unkempt appearance merits further investigation. An assessment of parent attitude should be done and should include observations of any aggressive, hostile, critical, or over demanding manner of the parent toward the child. Unusual behavior of a parent such as euphoria or depression calls for immediate referral.
- An implausible story of injury should lead to detailed questioning regarding the accident. This should include the following: Who was the care giver? How did the accident take place? What did the child do after the accident? And, what immediate care was given? A delay in seeking medical care is suggestive of abuse. Careful documentation of the injury is necessary, especially in cases where separation of child and family may be necessary.
- All 50 states require nurses and other designated professionals to report suspected cases of child abuse. Most states provide civil and criminal penalties when this is not done. Those who report in good faith are immune from liability. Nurses should learn the reporting process in their community.
- It is extremely important to be nonjudgmental in dealing with those involved in child abuse and neglect. The reaction from the family or care giver is often hostile. The protection of the child is the immediate objective; the rehabilitation of the family is the long-term objective.

CLEFT LIP AND CLEFT PALATE

Description

A cleft lip and a cleft palate, which may occur together or separately, are developmental defects of the face and mouth. A cleft lip may be unilateral or bilateral. It can vary from a simple notching of the lip to a defect that extends from the lip edge through the floor of the nostril. A cleft palate may involve either the hard or soft palate, or both. When the cleft is in the hard palate, there is a direct opening between the mouth and the nose.

Observations

- A cleft lip is an obvious deformity of the lip that may extend up into the floor of the nostril.
- If an infant is unable to suck, has swallowing problems, or if liquids taken in through the mouth appear in the nose, an examination for a cleft palate is necessary.

(*Text continues on page 579*)

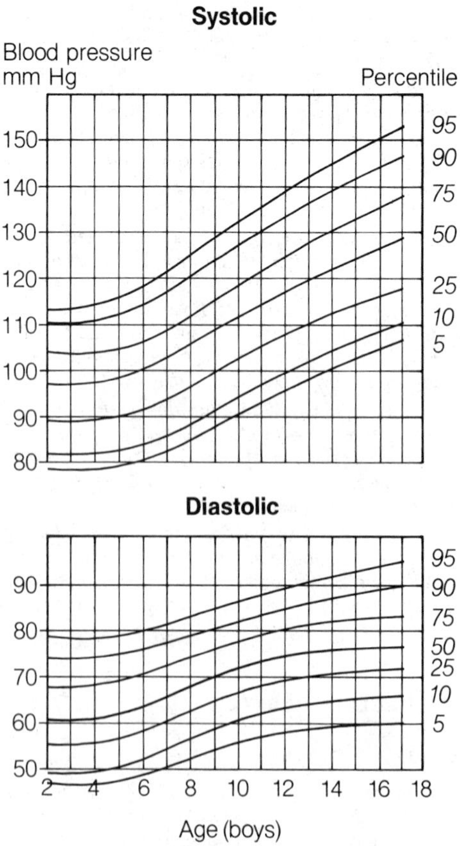

Percentiles of blood pressure measurement in boys (right arm, seated). (The National Heart, Lung, and Blood Institute's Task Force on Blood Pressure Control in Children: Report of the Task Force on Blood Pressure Control in Children. Pediatrics *(Suppl)59(5):797–820, May 1977)*

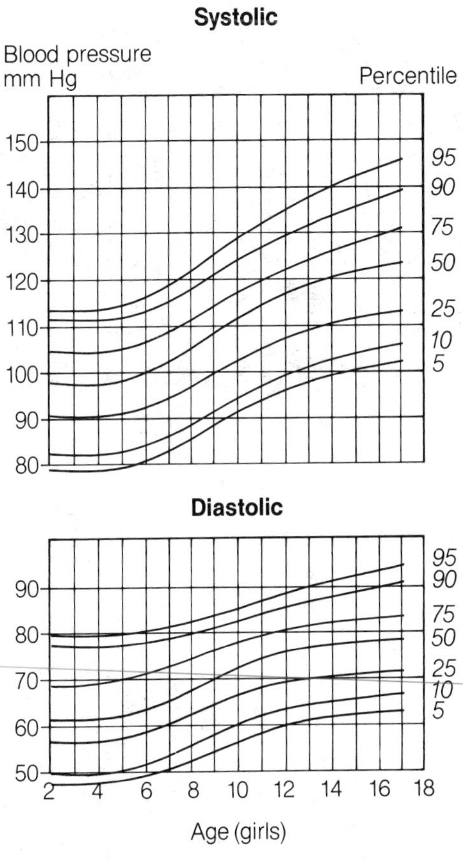

Percentiles of blood pressure measurement in girls (right arm, seated). (The National Heart, Lung, and Blood Institute's Task Force on Blood Pressure Control in Children: Report of the Task Force on Blood Pressure Control in Children. Pediatrics *(Suppl)59(5):797–820, May 1977)*

TABLE 6-1 PHYSICAL AND BEHAVIORAL INDICATORS OF CHILD ABUSE AND NEGLECT

Physical Indicators	Behavioral Indicators
Physical Abuse Unexplained bruises and welts On face, lips, mouth On torso, back, buttocks, thighs In various stages of healing Clustered, forming regular patterns Reflecting shape of article used to inflict (electric cord, belt buckle) On several different surface areas Regularly appear after absence, weekend, or vacation Unexplained burns Cigar and cigarette burns, especially on soles, palms, back, or buttocks Immersion burns (sock-like, glove-like, doughnut-shaped on buttocks or genitalia) Patterned like electric burner, iron, and so forth Rope burns on arms, legs, neck, or torso Infected burns, indicating delay in seeking treatment Unexplained fractures/dislocations To skull, nose, facial structure In various stages of healing Multiple or spiral fractures Unexplained lacerations or abrasions To mouth, lips, gums, eyes	Feels deserving of punishment Wary of adult contacts Apprehensive when other children cry Behavioral extremes Aggressiveness Withdrawal Frightened of parents Afraid to go home Reports injury by parents Vacant or frozen stare Lies very still while surveying surroundings Will not cry when approached by examiner Responds to questions in monosyllables Inappropriate or precocious maturity Manipulative behavior to get attention Capable of only superficial relationships Indiscriminately seeks affection Poor self-concept

To external genitalia	
In various stages of healing	
Bald patches on the scalp	
Physical Neglect	
Underweight, poor growth pattern, failure to thrive	Begging, stealing food
Consistent hunger, poor hygiene, inappropriate dress	Extended stays at school (early arrival and late departure)
Consistent lack of supervision, especially in dangerous activities or for long periods	Rare attendance at school
Wasting of subcutaneous tissue	Constant fatigue, listlessness, or falling asleep in class
Unattended physical problems or medical needs	Inappropriate seeking of affection
Abandonment	Assuming adult responsibilities and concerns
Abdominal distention	Alcohol or drug abuse
Bald patches on the scalp	Delinquency (*e.g.,* thefts)
	States there is no caretaker
Sexual Abuse	
Difficulty in walking or sitting	Unwilling to change for gym or participate in physical education class
Torn, stained, or bloody underclothing	Withdrawal, fantasy, or infantile behavior
Pain, swelling, or itching in genital area	Bizarre, sophisticated, or unusual sexual behavior or knowledge
Pain on urination	Poor peer relationships
Bruises, bleeding or lacerations in external genitalia, vaginal or anal areas	Delinquent or run away
Vaginal/penile discharge	

(*continued*)

TABLE 6-1 PHYSICAL AND BEHAVIORAL INDICATORS OF CHILD ABUSE AND NEGLECT

Physical Indicators	Behavioral Indicators
Venereal disease, especially in pre-teens	Reports sexual assault by caretaker
Poor sphincter tone	Change in performance in school
Pregnancy	
Emotional maltreatment	
Speech disorders	Habit disorders (sucking, biting, rocking, and so forth)
Lags in physical development	Conduct/learning disorders (antisocial, destructive, and so forth)
Failure-to-thrive	Neurotic traits (sleep disorders, inhibition of play, unusual fearfulness)
Hyperactive/disruptive behavior	Psychoneurotic reactions (hysteria, obsession, compulsion, phobias, hypochondria)
	Behavior extremes Complaint, passive Aggressive, demanding
	Overly adaptive behavior Inappropriately adult Inappropriately infant
	Developmental lags (mental, emotional)
	Attempted suicide

(From DHEW Publication No. (OHDS) 79-30202)

(continued from page 573)

Treatment

- *Cleft lip:* Surgical repair may be done when the infant is a few days old or within the first few weeks of life. When both cleft lip and cleft palate are present, the lip is repaired first.
- *Cleft palate:* Surgical repair ideally is done when the child is between 12 and 18 months of age, after some normal growth of mouth structure but before speech habits are affected. In cases where repair is delayed, a special denture plate may be used to cover the cleft, thereby enabling more normal speech.

Preoperative Care

- Breast-feeding may be difficult because clefts inhibit the infant's ability to suck. It is best attempted when the breast is firm and full of milk. Hold the nipple in the baby's mouth and the baby in an upright position. Direct the flow of milk to the side of the infant's mouth.
- Starting a newborn feeding from a small cup is possible, or a long soft nipple with large holes may be used. The nipple should extend back into the mouth so that liquid can be dropped slowly on to the base of the tongue and then swallowed. When long nipples are unsatisfactory, a bulb syringe or a medicine dropper with a soft rubber extension is useful. The feeding device should not be inserted through the cleft in the lip, but rather through the normal part of the lip.
- These infants tend to swallow large amounts of air with feedings, and thus requiring frequent burping.
- A feeding takes a long time, and choking and gagging may occur. These possibilities, and the facial deformity, can alter parents' reactions to the child. Thus, when they are learning to feed and care for the infant, they need all the help and emotional support possible.
- Start the feeding method that will be used after surgery *before* surgery.
- Introduce arm restraints for increasing periods of time *before* surgery.
- A myringotomy may be performed before surgery, especially in the case of children with cleft palates. They often have a history of frequent ear infections because of malfunctioning eustachian tubes.

Postoperative Care

- The operative site must be protected. Therefore, arm restraints are an *immediate* need. The patient's arms and hands must be secured so that they cannot touch the face. Remove the restraints as often as possible, and, while holding the infant or child, exercise the limbs, and check for reddened areas.

- Try to anticipate needs so that crying, possibly resulting in damage to the suture lines, can be avoided.
- Explain to the parents what you are doing and the reason why as you care for their child. They must be prepared for at-home care.

Cleft Lip Repairs

- Following the repair, watch for respiratory difficulties. The head of the crib should be kept slightly elevated; an oxygen tent or croupette will be in use.
- Cleft lip repairs often are protected with a metal device to prevent tension on the suture line. A body restraint can be used to prevent lying on the abdomen, which is contraindicated for several weeks, to prevent damage to the suture line.
- The feeding method is the surgeon's choice, but is best started before the surgery. Sucking may be avoided until after the lip has healed.
- Daily weight measurements are important to ensure that the child is receiving adequate nourishment.
- The suture line on the lip must be kept clean to prevent crusts from forming, which could lead to infection and scarring. Half-strength hydrogen peroxide, dabbed on the area with an applicator, then rinsed with sterile saline, and patted dry, often is used after each feeding. This may also be followed with an application of an antibiotic ointment.
- If a palate repair remains to be done after the cleft lip repair, formula may flow from the nose after feeding. The lip closure allows for more effective suction, permitting the formula to enter the nose. Also, an open palate makes the ear more susceptible to infection. Parents need to know the signs and symptoms of this problem.

Cleft Palate Repairs

- The child must be weaned from the bottle before a cleft palate repair is done.
- Parents need a good preoperative explanation of their child's care following surgery, and should be included in the care as much as possible. The child will probably be in an intensive care unit during the immediate postoperative period. The parents should see the unit and be shown the equipment that will be in use.
- Hemorrhage and respiratory distress are two complications that may occur very suddenly.
- Some oozing of bloody mucus from the mouth or nose is normal. Any suctioning must be gentle and must avoid the suture line.
- Position the child as ordered, but *never* on his or her back.
- An IV line will be maintained until liquid can be taken from a paper

or styrofoam cup. No object (straws, nipples, or spoons) should enter the mouth until the suture line is healed. China cups should not be used.

- When pureed food is fed, the child must be fed by the parent or nurse using the side of the spoon. The child's mouth must be rinsed with water following meals.
- Observe for restlessness or other signs of discomfort, and administer medication as needed.
- These children will be discharged with elbow restraints in place. They will be necessary for about three weeks postoperatively, or until the suture line is healed.
- Parents should be aware of the possibility of ear infections, and also that consultation, over a long period of time, will be needed with a speech therapist; dentist; ear, nose, and throat specialist; as well as with the plastic surgeon.

COMMUNICABLE DISEASES AND IMMUNIZATION SCHEDULES

- See Tables 6-2 and 6-3.

CONGENITAL HEART DISEASE

Description

Congenital heart disease (CHD) most often occurs because structural defects in the heart and major vessels result in an alteration in the normal circulation. It also may result if patterns of circulation normal for the developing fetus persist. With many types of CHD, the disease manifests itself by an increase in cardiac workload and a decrease in cardiac output. This may be accompanied by increased pulmonary resistance and shunting, leading to decreased oxygen saturation of the arterial blood. The symptoms depend on the type and severity of the defect which are classed as cyanotic or acyanotic lesions. CHD may be immediately evident in the infant, or may not be detected until later in childhood when the defective heart is unable to satisfy the need for oxygenated blood.

Common Diagnostic Tests

- ECG; echocardiography (See NR.)
- Chest x-ray
- Cardiac catheterization/angiocardiography
- Complete blood count; an increased hemoglobin and hematocrit may occur to compensate for a reduced level of oxygen in the blood; some types of CHD have a normal oxygen saturation of the blood.
- Arterial blood gases (See LAB)

(*Text continues on page 589*)

TABLE 6-2 COMMUNICABLE DISEASES OF CHILDHOOD

	Chicken Pox	Diphtheria	Measles	Mumps	Poliomyelitis
Cause	A virus present in secretions from the nose, throat, and mouth of infected people	Diphtheria bacillus present in secretions from nose and throat of infected people and carriers	A virus present in secretions from the nose and throat of infected people	A virus present in saliva of infected people	Three strains of polio virus have been identified and are present in discharges from the nose, throat, and bowels of infected people.
How Spread	Contact with infected people or articles used by them; very contagious	Contact with infected people and carriers or articles used by them	Contact with infected people or articles used by them; very contagious	Contact with infected people or articles used by them	Primarily, contact with infected people
Incubation Period (from Date of Exposure to First Signs)	13–17 days; sometimes 3 weeks	2–5 days; sometimes longer	About 10–12 days	12–26 (commonly 18) days	Usually 7–12 days

Period of Communicability (Time When Disease is Contagious)	From 5 days before, to 6 days after the first appearance of skin blisters	From about 2 to 4 weeks after the onset of disease	From 4 days before until about 5 days after the rash appears	From about 6 days before symptoms to 9 days after; principally at about the time swelling starts	Apparently greatest in late incubation and first few days of illness
Most Susceptible Ages	Under 15 years	Under 15 years	Common at any age during childhood	Children and young people	Most common in children 1 to 16 years
Seasons of Prevalence	Winter	Fall, winter, and spring	Mainly spring; also fall and winter	Winter and spring	Summer and early fall (June through September)
Prevention	No prevention	Vaccination with diphtheria toxoid (in triple vaccine for babies)	Measles vaccine	Mumps vaccine	Polio vaccine

(*continued*)

TABLE 6-2 COMMUNICABLE DISEASES OF CHILDHOOD

	Chicken Pox	Diphtheria	Measles	Mumps	Poliomyelitis
Control	Exclusion from school for 1 week after eruption appears; avoid contact with susceptibles. Immune globulin may lessen severity. (Cut child's fingernails.) Immunity usually follows after one attack.	Booster doses; antitoxin and antibiotics used in treatment and for protection after exposure. One attack does not necessarily give immunity.	Isolation until 7 days after appearance of a rash. Immune globulin between 3 and 6 days after exposure can lighten attack. Antibiotics can be given for complications. Immunity is usual after one attack.	Isolation for 9 days from onset of swelling. Immunity is usual after one attack, but second attacks can occur.	Booster doses; isolation for about one week from onset. Immunity to infecting strain of virus is usual after one attack.

	Rheumatic Fever	Rubella	Smallpox	Streptococcal Infection	Tetanus	Whooping Cough
Cause	Direct cause is unknown. Precipitated by a streptococcal infection.	A virus present in secretions from the nose and mouth of infected people	A virus present in skin pocks and discharges from the mouth, nose, and throat of infected people; rare in US	Streptococci of several strains cause scarlet fever and strep sore throats; present in secretions from the mouth, nose, and ears of infected people	Tetanus bacillus present in a wound so infected	Pertussis bacillus present in secretions from the mouth and nose of infected people
How Spread	Unknown, but the preceding strep infection is contagious.	Contact with infected people or articies used by them, very contagious	Contact with infected people or articles used by them	Contact with infected people; rarely from contaminated articles	Through soil, contact with horses, street dust, or articles contaminated with the bacillus	Contact with infected people and articles used by them

(*continued*)

TABLE 6-2 COMMUNICABLE DISEASES OF CHILDHOOD

	Rheumatic Fever	**Rubella**	**Smallpox**	**Streptococcal Infection**	**Tetanus**	**Whooping Cough**
Incubation Period (from Date of Exposure to First Signs)	Symptoms appear about 2 to 3 weeks after a strep infection.	14–21 (usually 18) days	From 8–17 (usually 12) days	1–3 days	4 days to 3 weeks; sometimes longer; the average is about 10 days.	From 7–10 days
Period of Communicability (Time When Disease Is Contagious)	Not communicable, but the preceding strep infection is communicable.	From 7 days before to 5 days after onset of the rash	From 2–3 days before rash, until disappearance of all pock crusts	Greatest during acute illness (about 10 days)	Not communicable from person to person	From onset of first symptoms to about third week of the disease
Most Susceptible Ages	All ages; most common from 6 to 12 years	Young children, but also common in young adults	All ages	All ages	All ages	Under 7 years
Seasons of Prevalence	Mainly winter and spring	Winter and spring	Usually winter, but anytime	Late winter and spring	All seasons, but more common in warm weather	Late winter and early spring

Prevention	No prevention, except proper treatment of strep infections. (See Streptococcal infections.)	Rubella (German measles) vaccine	Vaccination (*no longer* given routinely in the US)	No prevention; antibiotic treatment for those who have had rheumatic fever	Immunization with tetanus toxoid (in triple vaccine for babies)	Immunization with whooping cough vaccine (in triple vaccine for babies)
Control	Use of antibiotics; one attack does not give immunity.	Isolation, when necessary, for 5 days after onset; immunity is usual after one attack.	Vaccinia immune globulin may prevent or modify smallpox if given within 24 hours after exposure. Isolation is necessary until all pock crusts are gone. Immunity is usual after one attack.	Isolation for about 1 day after the start of treatment with antibiotics—used for about 10 days; one attack does not necessarily give immunity.	A booster dose of tetanus toxoid for protection is given on day of injury. Antitoxin is used in treatment and for temporary protection for child not immunized. One attack does not give immunity.	Booster doses; special antibiotics may help to lighten attack for a child not immunized. Isolation from susceptible infants for about 3 weeks from onset or until cough stops is necessary. Immunity is usual after one attack.

(Based on The Control of Communicable Diseases, American Public Health Association, 1975, and Report of Committee on Control of Infectious Diseases, American Academy of Pediatrics, 1974)

TABLE 6-3 IMMUNIZATION SCHEDULES

	Diphtheria Pertussis Tetanus	Polio	Measles	Rubella	Mumps
If Your Child Is Two Months Old. . .					
Age					
2 mo	+	+			
4 mo	+	+			
6 mo	+	+ (optional)			
15 mo			+	+	+
18 mo	+	+			
4–6 yrs	+	+			

If Your Child Is One Through Five Years of Age. . .*

First Visit	Diphtheria, pertussis, tetanus (DPT) Polio
1 mo after first visit	Measles, rubella, mumps†
2 mo after first visit	Diphtheria, pertussis, tetanus (DPT) polio
4 mo after first visit	Diphtheria, pertussis, tetanus (DPT) Polio (optional)
10–16 mo after first visit	Diphtheria, pertussis, tetanus (DPT) Polio

If Your Child Is Six Years of Age or Older. . .*

First Visit	Tetanus–diphtheria (Td) Polio
1 mo after first visit	Measles, rubella, mumps
2 mo after first visit	Tetanus–diphtheria (Td) Polio
8–14 mo after first visit	Tetanus–diphtheria (Td) Polio
Age 14–16 years	Tetanus–diphtheria (Td), repeat every 10 years

Notes: Measles, rubella, and mumps vaccines can be given in a combined form, at about 15 months of age, with a single injection. Children should receive a sixth tetanus-diphtheria injection (booster) at age 14–16 years.

*Your doctor may recommend schedules that differ somewhat from those that appear here. Generally, though, the first schedule in this table shows the immunizations that children one through five years of age will get on their first visit to the doctor, and on each visit thereafter. The second schedule is recommended for children six years of age and older.

†Not routinely given before 15 months of age.

Names				
Birth dates				
DPT	First			
	Second			
	Third			
	Fourth			
	Boosters			
Polio	First			
	Second			
	Third			
	Booster			
	Booster			
Measles Rubella Mumps				

Immunization record. (U.S. Department of Health, Education, and Welfare, Public Health Service, Centers for Disease Control no. [os]77-50058)

(continued from page 581)

Observations

- Learn the cause and physical manifestations of each individual case of CHD. Base the observations and nursing care, as well as the teaching of other health care givers, especially the parents, on this knowledge.
- Tachypnea at rest in an infant (respiration rate of 60/min or more) can be an early sign of heart failure. Also, dyspnea and cyanosis at rest, or while crying or feeding, may occur.
- Respirations should be counted for a full minute by observing the chest and abdominal movements of an infant. Observe the chest motion for asymmetry, unusual pulsations of the chest wall, or intercostal or substernal retractions with breathing
- Heart murmurs and tachycardia (heart rate of 160 beats/min or more in infants) frequently occur.
- Cyanosis is best observed in the mucous membranes of the mouth in newborns, and later around the mouth, in the lips, or in the nailbeds. Within a few months, clubbing of the fingers may develop.

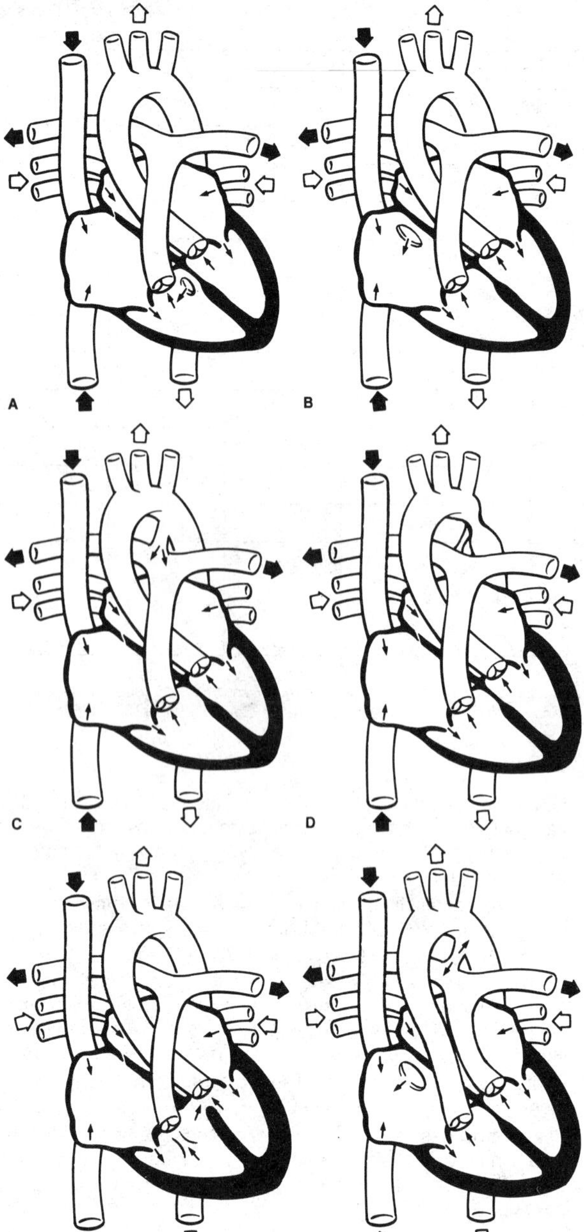
A
B
C
D
E
F

- Anorexia in the infant and growing child may result from fatigue associated with the eating process. An infant may be unable to suck for more than a few moments before falling asleep, and will then awaken shortly after from hunger. Ascites or pulmonary congestion seen in congestive heart failure may also be responsible for anorexia. Weight loss and retarded growth result from few calories being available for growth.
- A side-lying, knee-chest position is often assumed by an infant with CHD. Older children rest frequently during any activity, and characteristically assume a squatting position. These positions restrict the return of blood from the extremities, thus decreasing the work load of the right side of the heart.

Treatment

- Surgical procedures may be used to repair or alleviate symptoms, depending on the child's age and anatomy of the cardiac defect.
- Small defects may close or the child may adapt to limitations of activity.
- See MSN, Congestive heart failure.

Nursing Considerations

- Generalized cyanosis in a newborn, which is unrelieved with oxygen administration and persists for three or more hours after birth, may indicate a serious cardiac defect and needs to be investigated.
- Infants and young children with pulmonary vascular engorgement or CHD are very susceptible to chest colds. With infants, this can rapidly result in pneumonia, which precipitates congestive heart failure.
- Prophylactic antibiotics are given to children with congenital heart defects before any surgery, including tooth extraction. This is done because of the danger of systemic *Streptococcus* infection, resulting in infective endocarditis.
- Small, slow, and frequent feedings are necessary. A nipple with a large hole is helpful for infant feedings. Burp after each one-half ounce; there is increased air swallowing with these infants.
- Dehydration can exacerbate polycythemia. The resulting viscosity of the blood adds to the workload of the heart, increasing the risk of thrombosis and cerebrovascular accidents.
- Hypoxic (lack of oxygen) episodes, also called "Tet" spells are characterized by a sudden increase in dyspnea and cyanosis

PED

←

Congenital heart defects. A. Ventricular septal defect. B. Atrial septal defect. C. Patent ductus arteriosus. D. Coarctation of the aorta. E. Tetralogy of Fallot. F. Complete transposition of great vessels. (From Clinical Education Aid, No. 7, Ross Laboratories, Columbus, Ohio, 1970.)

leading to unresponsiveness, and need *immediate attention.* Place the patient in a knee-chest position and administer oxygen. If left untreated, this can lead to seizures caused by decreased oxygen to the brain.

- Discharge planning should start with the hospital admission. The effect on the family, their ability for appropriate care and observation as well as their understanding of the growth and development of an infant or child with CHD determines the teaching.

CONGENITAL HIP DISLOCATION

Description

Congenital dislocation of the hip (CDH) is the displacement of the head of the femur outside of the socket (acetabulum). In most cases of CDH the acetabulum is shallow. CDH usually occurs just before birth or immediately following delivery; most frequently seen in females, it is also more common in breech deliveries. The dislocation is described as complete or incomplete; incomplete is also called subluxation or a dislocatable hip. In most cases of CDH, there is a shallow acetabulum. CDH should be diagnosed at birth. The longer the problem exists, the more difficult it is to correct.

Common Diagnostic Tests

- At birth, the Ortolani and Barlow tests are commonly used to diagnose the unstable hip joint.
    1. In the Ortolani test, the infant is placed on his or her back, and the hips are flexed one at a time to 90 degrees, and gently abducted. Simultaneously, your index finger should apply gentle pressure over the greater trochanter. If the head of the femur is dislocated, a "clunk" will be felt or heard as it falls into place.
    2. In the Barlow test, the infant is placed on his or her back, and the hip and knee are flexed to 90 degrees, and abducted gently downward. An unstable hip will be felt as the femoral head easily slips out of the acetabulum.
- An arthrogram may be performed when treatment with splints or braces has been ineffective. It is done under anesthesia, and a contrast material is injected into the hip joint for x-ray visualization.

Observations

- Watch for signs of an unstable hip joint when changing an infant's diapers.
- Infants having a dislocated hip for more than two weeks will have, on the affected side, a shortened thigh with excess folds of skin and a significant loss of hip abduction.

- When the child reaches the weight-bearing stage, the physical signs become very obvious. The child walks with a limp and, when standing on the leg of the dislocated hip with the other leg lifted off the floor, the pelvis tilts downward on the normal side. This is called a "Trendelenburg sign."

Treatment

- A hip may be held in a position of abduction, using several diapers or a pillow sling (Frejka Pillow sling) to achieve this effect. If this does not produce the desired hip placement, a harness (commonly the Parlik harness) or splint is applied. Whatever is used must be left on continuously so that the head of the femur is kept in the acetabulum. This is less difficult when a brace or harness is used, since these do not have to be removed for routine care.
- When the hip is not easily reducible, traction is applied to stretch the leg muscles and line up the femoral head for placement into the acetabulum. This traction is maintained for two to three weeks. A general anesthetic is given when the attempt is made to reduce the hip. A plaster cast (hip spica cast) is applied when the proper positioning is obtained. This cast is usually kept on for 8 weeks to 12 weeks, and may need to be changed two to three times to allow for normal growth.
- An open reduction of the hip is necessary if a closed reduction does not correct the condition.

Nursing Considerations

- Force must never be used to reduce a hip.
- Maintaining extreme abduction of the hip can result in necrosis of the femoral head, which results when the blood supply is cut off. This causes irreversible damage.
- Parents should be thoroughly familiar with cast care before they take the child home.
- There must be a major effort to keep the cast clean and dry in the perineal area. Keeping the shoulders propped up lessens the problem of urine running back down under the cast.

CONGESTIVE HEART FAILURE IN THE CHILD

Description

Congestive heart failure (CHF) develops when the heart is unable to pump an adequate supply of blood, causing circulatory congestion. In children, CHF most often occurs in infancy as the result of congenital heart disease, and is often precipitated by a general or respiratory infection. Heart failure can be left-sided failure (LSF) or right-sided failure (RSF), and can range from mild to life-threatening.

LSF results in lung congestion which can lead to pulmonary edema. RSF has systemic effects resulting in generalized edema and liver congestion. In infants, RSF and LSF usually occur at the same time.

Common Diagnostic Tests

- Chest x-ray
- Electrocardiogram; echocardiogram
- Arterial blood gases (See LAB.)

Observations

- Tachycardia (heart rate at or above 160 beats/min in infants) can occur.
- Tachypnea (respirations at or above 60 breath/min in infants) often with nasal flaring, grunting, and intercostal and subcostal retractions may be present.
- Cyanosis along with dyspnea, orthopnea, wheezing, and rales is possible.
- Pulmonary edema is rare in infants, but may occur in the older child. It may first be evident by increased coughing.
- An enlarged and tender liver is an early sign of CHF in infants and children.
- Generalized edema results from water retention, and usually is first noted as an unexplained weight gain. Periorbital edema also may be noted in infants.
- Infants in CHF are often listless, fall asleep after a small amount of feeding, sweat excessively, and fail to thrive.
- Dyspnea on exertion, chronic fatigue, and delayed growth are evident in the older child.

Treatment

- Correction of underlying pathology should be done, if possible.
- Oxygen therapy can be started (see NR, Oxygen therapy).
- Medications include diuretics (*e.g.*, furosemide), digitalis preparation, and potassium supplements (see PH).
- Rest is necessary to decrease cardiac demand. Sedation (*e.g.*, morphine sulfate) may be necessary.
- Diet and fluid restrictions may be required. Often, avoiding added salt or salty foods is sufficient. Any fluid restriction must be monitored carefully to avoid dehydration.

Nursing Considerations

- Assess the child's condition, including the lungs, at the beginning of the shift and as often as indicated. Vital signs should be taken in a resting state, and significant changes reported immediately.

Pulse and respiration should be counted for a full minute; respirations can be counted by observing chest or abdominal movements in an infant.

- Encourage parents to stay with the child as much as possible to help alleviate anxiety and prevent crying. Also, for teaching purposes, parents should be included in the care.
- Weigh children daily on the same scale, after voiding, and before breakfast. Diuretics should be given early in the day to prevent night-time voiding. Infants are often weighed every 8 hours. Be sure to use the same scale and the same amount of clothing. Diapers can be weighed dry and later when wet to determine urine output. An increase in weight of 1 g is counted as 1 ml of urine output. Catheterization may occasionally be indicated to monitor output.
- An accurate intake and output measurement at least every 8 hours is essential. A decrease in urinary output (less than 1 ml/kg/hr) is indicative of uncompensated failure.
- It is extremely important that a shift above or below the normal serum potassium level be reported to the physician at any hour of the day or night. Severe cardiac arrhythmias may develop from potassium imbalance.
- Measure abdominal girth daily using a tape measure at the level of the umbilicus, marking where the tape is placed with a magic marker.
- The use of an upright infant seat can help relieve dyspnea in an infant.
- The stress of crying may worsen dyspnea; therefore, infants should be fed before they cry for a feeding. Small, frequent feedings with a large hole nipple or gavage feeding may be necessary if sucking requires too much energy. A more concentrated formula may be given to decrease the volume. Nasogastric or gastrostomy tube feedings may be necessary.
- Chilling should be avoided, but there should be no restrictive clothing around the chest or abdomen. Diapers are pinned loosely.
- Discharge planning is critical. Parents should participate in the hospital care to prepare for home care.

CROUP (LARYNGOTRACHEOBRONCHITIS)

Description

Croup is a description of symptoms arising from an acute inflammation of the larynx, trachea, and bronchus. This usually is caused by a common virus infection. It is most often seen in children under the age of 3 years, because their airway is small and the edematous and inflamed tissue causes some airway obstruction. However, adults also can have croup.

Observations

- Harsh barking cough and hoarseness
- Noisy labored breathing with "crowing" sound (stridor) during inspiration
- Complaints of a sore throat

Treatment

- Moist warm air and increased hydration can help liquify secretions.
- Administer oxygen to alleviate hypoxia.
- A tracheostomy, or endo- or nasotracheal tube may be necessary in severe cases of airway obstruction.

Nursing Considerations

- These patients usually are cared for at home. A hot shower producing a steamy bathroom will often provide relief of symptoms.
- If breathing becomes increasingly labored, if cyanosis is apparent, or if the temperature is very high, hospitalization is indicated.
- Children need constant observation during the period of acute respiratory distress. Be aware of the possibility of complete airway obstruction in these patients. Try to keep children from crying in order to minimize breathing difficulty.

CRYPTORCHIDISM (UNDESCENDED TESTICLE)

Description

Failure of one or both testes to descend into the scrotal sac is called *cryptorchidism.* The testes may remain in the abdomen or the inguinal canal arrested in descent (which usually occurs during the seventh to ninth month of gestation). This condition is seen most commonly in premature infants, and in these infants especially, the testes may descend spontaneously during the first year.

It is important to get the testes into a scrotal position by the time the child is 5 years old. Testes left in the abdomen are subjected to a higher degree of body heat, and are likely to be damaged, resulting in sterility. Testis cancer is more frequent in undescended testes.

Treatment

- Hormonal therapy with human chorionic gonadotropin for testes below the external inguinal ring may be prescribed.
- Orchiopexy (surgically bringing the testes down into the scrotum) may be necessary, if hormonal therapy fails. While the rubber

band technique described below may be used, it is more common now to create a scrotal pouch that secures the testis in the scrotum.

Nursing Considerations

- Following orchiopexy, the testis may be secured in position in the scrotum for about 5 days to 7 days by attaching one end of a rubber band to a retraction suture in the scrotum. The other end is secured with adhesive tape to the inner thigh.
  1. The tension on the rubber band must be preserved to prevent the testis from reascending.
- Prevent infection of the operative site by keeping it clean.
- Administer antibiotics, as ordered.

CYSTIC FIBROSIS

Description

Cystic fibrosis is a hereditary disease found primarily in Caucasians. The signs and symptoms arise from the malfunction of exocrine glands (glands that secrete through ducts). An abnormal amount of thick mucus is produced, which obstructs the normal flow from the exocrine gland ducts. The major signs and symptoms arise from the effects of this blockage on the gastrointestinal and pulmonary systems, although the function of almost any organ can be affected. Also found in this disease is abnormally high secretion of sodium and chloride by the sweat glands.

Cystic fibrosis is the most common of the life-threatening genetic diseases in children. If it is found in one member of a family, diagnostic studies should be done on all siblings. It can be diagnosed in infancy and the survival is dependent on the severity of system involvement. Many patients die at an early age, generally from advanced lung disease, but those with a milder form of the disease survive through adulthood with appropriate treatment. The median survival time is now 20 years of age.

Common Diagnostic Tests

- Sweat analysis for sodium and chloride should be done. A level of these electrolytes greater than 60 mEq/l (normal, 20–30 mEq/l), induced by pilocarpine iontophoresis, is indicative of cystic fibrosis. In adults, normal levels may be as high as 60 to 80 mEq/l; however, the test is much less reliable in adults.
- Pancreatic function tests will show a pancreatic enzyme deficiency with cystic fibrosis.

- Stool analysis will indicate pancreatic enzyme deficiency and a high fat content in this disease.

Observations

- Intestinal obstruction resulting from a meconium ileus is strongly suggestive of cystic fibrosis in infants; chronic fecal impactions may occur in older children and adults. A prolapsed rectum or intussusception may follow if the condition is left untreated.
- Respiratory symptoms are the most prevalent and usually begin as chronic wheezing and a dry cough in an infant. As the disease progresses, secretions of thick and tenacious mucus plug the airways of the pulmonary system and lead to recurrent infection, tissue damage, and eventual deterioration of respiratory function. Chronic sinusitis, bronchitis, and recurrent pneumonia are common; atelectasis can result if total airway obstruction occurs.
- The development of a barrel chest and clubbing of the fingers is symptomatic of progressive obstructive lung disease leading to cor pulmonale. Respiratory acidosis occurs if there is a significantly decreased ability to exhale carbon dioxide.
- Symptoms of maldigestion appear because the pancreatic ducts become plugged with mucus, thus preventing the digestive enzymes from entering the small intestine. Failure to thrive, with delayed growth despite a voracious appetite, are common in cystic fibrosis; also, foul, oily, and bulky stools occur frequently. Deficiency of the fat-soluble vitamins A, D, E, and K is usually present.
- Heat exhaustion is a danger in periods of excessive sweating. In hot weather, infants have a particularly high risk of symptoms associated with a severe salt loss.
- Cirrhosis of the liver may develop in adolescence or in adulthood as a result of biliary obstruction.

Treatment

- The frequency of postural drainage and breathing exercises is based on individual need; this can vary from twice to several times a day. (See NR Postural Drainage)
- Mucolytic agents (to thin secretions), aerosal therapy with bronchodilators, and antibiotics are given to prevent or treat respiratory infections.
- Missing pancreatic enzymes are replaced with a supplement; *e.g.,* in infants, the supplement is mixed with a small amount of applesauce, not liquid formula. A cystic fibrosis diet is high in protein and calories, and water-soluble vitamins are given. When there is excessive sodium and chloride loss through abnormal

sweating in periods of hot weather or fever, an increased salt intake may be advised.

Nursing Considerations

- Large amounts of sodium and chloride excreted in the sweat can cause an infant to taste salty when kissed.
- Any infant with chronic wheezing should have a sweat test.
- Be aware of changes in sputum color and the frequency and amount of coughing as early indications of a respiratory infection.
- A respiratory infection that does not respond to oral antibiotics is the most frequent reason for hospitalization of these patients.
- Daily weight measurements are very important to monitor nutrition as well as to check for fluid retention.
- Measles and pertussis immunizations and annual flu vaccine should be given, because these diseases cause a severe increase in the symptoms of cystic fibrosis.
- Families as well as the patients need intensive instruction about the nature of this disease, and on the procedures necessary to sustain life.
- There are more than 100 cystic fibrosis care centers in the United States. Patients and families should be referred to these centers for outpatient care and support. Information may be obtained from the Cystic Fibrosis Foundation, 6000 Executive Boulevard, Suite 309, Rockville, Maryland 20852.

DEHYDRATION

Description

Dehydration results when fluid output is greater than fluid intake. In infants and young children, the metabolic rate is more than twice that of adults. The ratio of skin surface to body weight in children is also considerably higher. These factors result in a much greater percentage of body fluid being exchanged daily in infants and young children as contrasted to adults. In an infant, as much as one-half of the extracellular fluid is exchanged daily. Thus, fluid imbalance can quickly become life threatening, and fluid therapy needs careful attention and accurate calculation, especially in infants. When dehydration occurs, electrolyte balance also tends to change. Recovery is not complete until electrolyte balance is restored, along with lost intra- and extracellular water.

Common Diagnostic Tests

- BUN, serum creatinine, and serum protein usuallly will be elevated in dehydration.

- Serum electrolyte tests establish the electrolyte status of the body.
- Arterial blood gases are indicators of the metabolic balance of the patient.
- A complete blood count will show an increase in red blood cell count, hematocrit, and hemoglobin concentration if vascular fluid volume deficit is present.
- Complete urinalysis will help determine the status of kidney function.
- Stool and blood cultures are done if an infectious agent is suspected as the cause of illness.
- An ECG is run to detect if the heart has been affected by electrolyte imbalances; alteration in plasma potassium concentration is the principal concern.

Observations

- A sick-appearing and irritable infant or child with recent vomiting or diarrhea, and whose appetite and level of activity are decreased, requires immediate attention.
- A decrease in the amount and frequency of urinary output; also an increase in urine concentration.
- The amount of weight loss in an infant or small child during an illness is roughly equivalent to the percentage of fluid loss. A 10% or more weight loss in an infant or young child, or a 5% or more in older children, requires immediate treatment. Progressive circulatory failure leading to shock results from the loss of plasma volume.
- When weight loss is unknown, the degree of dehydration can be quickly estimated by the severity of signs and symptoms associated with poor peripheral circulation. These symptoms are low blood pressure; a weak, rapid pulse; gray, mottled skin with cool extremities; poor skin turgor (tested by quickly releasing a pinch of skin on the abdomen and observing if it remains elevated for several seconds); dry mucous membranes with longitudinal lines on the tongue; and, in infants, the anterior fontanel and eyeballs are depressed.
- Seizures, rather than circulatory symptoms, may occur when high serum sodium levels accompany dehydration.

Treatment

- Restoration of fluid volume with the prescribed type and amount of fluid to prevent shock, restoration of renal function, and correction of mild to severe metabolic acidosis are necessary. Since the immediate need is the treatment of dehydration, the correction of the underlying pathology may be delayed.

- Mild dehydration is treated with oral fluids, often containing electrolytes, which are given as prescribed. It is very important to observe and report the response to the feedings. Continued anorexia or vomiting and diarrhea require immediate attention.
- Intravenous therapy is used in severe dehydration, or when oral feeding is not possible.
- The reintroduction of a regular diet is determined by the physical condition. Early resumption of milk feedings may exacerbate diarrhea. However, breast-feeding generally is not interrupted unless the diarrhea is intractable.

Nursing Considerations

- Change in body weight is the most useful physical indicator in treating dehydration. Weighing is done frequently during the initial stage of treatment. Be sure to use the same scale and the same amount of clothing or equipment, *e.g.,* armboards and dressings, each time.
- *Absolutely accurate* intake and output measurements of *all* sources of fluid, including sweat, drainage from a wound or nasogastric tube, and IV fluid, is essential.
- Urine volume should be checked frequently, along with the urine specific gravity (sp gr) and pH. The urine output of an infant averages 17 to 25 ml/hr, and that of an older child, 20 to 40 ml/hr. The sp gr of the urine will increase in dehydration because the kidney, in an attempt to conserve salt and water, will produce only a small amount of concentrated urine. The pH of the urine will indicate the acidity or alkalinity of the urine.
- Check vital signs as often as every 15 minutes to 30 minutes during the critical phases of treatment.
- All stools must be checked for blood, and their volume and characteristics described.
- Diarrhea causes a loss of water and electrolytes as does vomiting; however, vomiting also prevents the intake of water and salts. Observe and note any cramping or vomiting when oral feeding is resumed.
- Potassium losses in diarrheal stools are great and, if diarrhea persists more than 24 hours, can be significant. Potassium is given if the urinary output is within normal limits.
- Nurses are in the unique position of being able to observe and evaluate conditions that may lead to dehydration, such as disorders of the skin (perspiration, burns), gastrointestinal tract (vomiting, diarrhea, suctioning), renal system (diabetes mellitus, diabetes insipidus), lungs (hyperventilation), and vascular system (hemorrhage).
- Parents need support and explanations of why oral fluid and food may need to be withheld from their often hungry and thirsty in-

fant. Careful instruction as to feeding and care at home needs to begin early.

EMOTIONAL PROBLEMS OF THE HOSPITALIZED CHILD

Description

To the child, hospitalization means separation from parents, siblings, and familiar surroundings. Illness and hospitalization of an infant can affect normal emotional as well as physical growth and development. The bonding process, which is the natural path to devotion and orderly behavior in the parent–child relationship, tends to be disrupted in hospitalized infants. Young children tend to perceive any separation as abandonment or punishment. A child between the ages of six months and four years has a limited ability to cope with strange and anxiety-producing situations. Children in this age group are very susceptible to adverse reactions to hospitalization. In older children, the loss of independence and control over activities, often accompanied by pain or discomfort, can trigger regressive or antisocial behavior, including harmful changes in the parent–child relationship. A significant number of hospitalized children suffer some form of psychological upset, which continues after discharge.

The active evidence of affection by the parents during the hospitalization of a child significantly lessens the impact of separation. Communications between parents and nurses should attempt to alleviate the anxiety of the parents, support the parent–child relationship, provide the nurse with valuable insight into the child's response to the stress of illness and hospitalization, and plan for care that is responsive both to the needs of the child and the parents.

Observations

- The child between 6 months and 1 year of age tends to react strongly to separation from parents. Inconsolable crying may be followed in hours or days by quiet, withdrawn behavior, and later by a detachment from human contact. Parents may react to their child's detachment with anger or a deep sense of guilt.
- Older children, although they may have been prepared for the separation, often are disturbed by having their routine altered. Regressive behavior, anorexia, or withdrawal from human contact can occur. These children are frequently very fearful of anesthesia.
- Behavior, at any age, that does not fit the normal for the stage of development, or which is significantly different from that reported by the parent as pre-hospital behavior, is indicative of emotional stress.

- The reaction of the family to the illness of a child is important. Parents often have feelings of guilt, anxiety, fear, and grief which limits their parenting ability.

Nursing Considerations

- Eighty percent of all hospitalization of children under 5 years of age occurs on an emergency basis. Twenty-four-hour visiting for parents, as well as rooming-in accommodations, should be provided. The need for a parent or other family member to stay with this child is critical. Parental presence during stressful events lessens the stress and anxiety of the child.
- An assessment of the emotional state, level of concern, and level of understanding of the child's illness by the parents is necessary while planning their participation in the child's care. Anxiety and stress are transmitted easily to the child; parents may need as much help as their child during hospitalization.
- The parents and the child must have an honest and comprehensible explanation of what is happening and what to expect. Also, emotional support before, during, and after medical and surgical procedures is imperative.
- Children under 6 years of age fear separation from parents; school-age children fear body damage and have difficulty understanding why pain is associated with getting well; older children tend to be concerned with possible alterations in their appearance.
- When a parent or family member cannot stay, continuity of care with a primary nurse providing consistent, nurturing care is the best alternative. Initially, a detailed admission history should provide information as to home routines, names for routine activities (especially natural functions), fears, favorite toys, and the health history. Frequent communication with the family is necessary to update this and to keep the family informed. It is important that parents not perceive their roles as parents being usurped by the hospital staff.
- Siblings, school friends, and others important to the child should be encouraged to visit the child who is hospitalized.
- Opportunities for play must be provided; it is necessary for normal development. Play helps the child be self expressive and is a way of coping with problems. In the structured environment of a hospital, play allows choice as well as control of activities which is very necessary for the child's feelings of self esteem. The play area must provide an escape from tests and procedures.
- When possible, hospitalization of children should be avoided, using out-patient services providing home-care support. If this cannot be done, discharge planning should be started on admission to help minimize the hospital stay.

- If hospitalization is necessary and an admission is scheduled, an orientation visit should be planned for the child and the parents. Information as well as a tour should be included. Parents also should receive special help in preparing their child for hospitalization.
- Sources of Information: Association for the Care of Children's Health, 3615 Wisconsin Avenue, NW, Washington, DC 20016.

EPIGLOTTITIS

Description

When the tissue of the epiglottis and surrounding area becomes swollen and inflamed, it is called epiglottitis. This usually is caused by a bacterial infection. It is a *true emergency.* Swallowing is difficult and loss of airway is imminent especially in children. It is most common in children of 1 year to 5 years of age, but it also is seen in adults.

Common Diagnostic Tests

- Visualization is the most direct method, but this carries a risk of laryngospasm if the epiglottis is touched. A tracheostomy set *MUST* be on hand for emergency use.
- Lateral neck x-ray can be done to show a swollen epiglottis. Often, there is no time to do this because of rapid airway closure.

Observations

- Children are usually restless and apprehensive, and will have symptoms of a sudden, very sore throat, painful swallowing, drooling, high temperature, dyspnea, tachycardia, and tachypnea. The child often will be sitting up with mouth open and chin forward, trying to keep the airway open.
- In adults, there is usually a longer period (1–2 days) in the development of the symptoms indicated above, which also may include a muffled voice.

Treatment

- Use of oxygen with humidification is helpful; a mist tent often is used for children.
- IV antibiotics are started immediately after direct laryngoscopy and intubation.
- Tracheostomy or endotracheal intubation is necessary in children because of the severe airway obstruction caused by this disease.

Nursing Considerations

- Anyone with these symptoms needs help *immediately.* Don't try to look down the throat because the mere touch of a tongue depressor on the epiglottis can cause laryngospasm and the airway will close.
- In children, suspected epiglottitis is diagnosed or ruled out in the operating room under direct vision. At that time, throat and blood cultures are taken *after* intubation.
- These patients need constant observation, and are cared for in intensive care units.

GLOMERULONEPHRITIS

Description

In *acute glomerulonephritis* there is a diffuse, inflammatory process in the glomeruli, usually precipitated by an antigen–antibody reaction to exogenous (*e.g.,* bacterial—particularly streptococcal, viral, chemical, and drugs) or endogenous (*e.g.,* circulating mature DNA, tumor antigens, thyroglobulin) causes.

The disease most often is seen in children or young adult males; 80% recover within about 2 weeks, but a few go into latent or chronic glomerulonephritis.

The disease is considered chronic when symptoms extend beyond a year, although this may develop without the patient having exhibited symptoms of the acute phase. *Chronic glomerulonephritis* is characterized by periods of exacerbations and remissions with progressive decline in renal function.

Common Diagnostic Tests

- The antibody titer against the causal organism usually is elevated in acute glomerulonephritis.
- Urinalysis usually shows the presence of protein red blood cells (RBCs) and RBC hyaline and granular casts (see LAB).
- BUN and serum creatinine levels are elevated in acute glomerulonephritis, and in chronic glomerulonephritis renal function is impaired markedly (see LAB).
- Complete blood count and hemoglobin and hematocrit may show the presence of anemia (see LAB).
- Kidney function tests may show decreased renal ability to concentrate urine (see MSN, Kidneys, Common diagnostic tests).
- Renal biopsy for differential diagnosis in chronic disease may be done (see NR, Renal biopsy).

Observations

In Acute Glomerulonephritis

- Usually, there is a history of sudden onset of symptoms occurring about 10 days to 12 days following a streptococcal infection (*e.g.*, strep throat, scarlet fever, impetigo), exposure to hydrocarbons, or evidence of systemic lupus erythematosus (SLE).
- Urine is scanty and may appear red, brown, or smoky.
- Hypertension may be present. (The course of the disease may be followed by monitoring the blood pressure.)
- Edema may be mild and generalized. Retinal edema causes decreased visual acuity.
- Headaches, malaise, nausea and vomiting, and low-grade fever may occur.

In Chronic Glomerulonephritis

- Hypertension
- Edema
- Easy fatigue, weakness, and lassitude (signs of anemia)
- Visual disturbances caused by retinopathy
- Nocturia: evidence of kidneys' decreased concentrating ability
- Symptoms of complications or progression of renal impairment: uremia, cardiac failure, and convulsions

Treatment

- Bedrest is usually ordered until urinary symptoms have subsided
- Penicillin and other broad-spectrum antibiotics may be prescribed.
- Antihypertensive medications may be ordered.
- A diet high in carbohydrates and low in sodium is usually prescribed. Protein is usually restricted in acute disease, but amounts may be liberalized in chronic disease, as long as patient maintains a normal BUN level.
- Fluid may be restricted if edema is present in acute disease. Liberal fluid intake is desirable in chronic glomerulonephritis.
- Renal failure is treated, if present (see MSN, Renal failure).
- In the chronic disease, the female patient usually is advised that pregnancy should be avoided.

Nursing Considerations

- Monitor blood pressure carefully.
- Monitor intake and output carefully. Note the color of the urine.

- Daily weight measurements should be taken in the same clothing, before breakfast each day.
- Try to prevent infections, especially upper respiratory infections.
- Elevate the head of the bed to minimize facial edema.
- Provide good skin care. This is especially important for the edematous patient.
- Provide general, supportive care similar to that given for renal failure, if indicated.
- Assess for complications, such as renal failure, congestive heart failure, hypertensive encephalopathy (drowsiness, confusion, severe headache, nausea, blurred vision, with progression from stupor and coma).
- In cases of chronic glomerulonephritis, educate the patient and family as to the importance of following the prescribed regimen. Emotional support is required for dealing with long-term illness. Arrangements for home care may need to be arranged.

GROWTH AND DEVELOPMENT CHARTS

- See charts on following pages.

HYDROCEPHALUS

Description

Hydrocephalus describes an abnormal accumulation of cerebrospinal fluid (CSF), usually with increased pressure, within the cranial cavity. It may be caused by an excess secretion of CSF, but more commonly is caused by an obstruction to the flow within the ventricles of the brain or a decrease in the normal absorption of CSF. It may be a developmental defect recognizable at birth, sometimes caused by an intrauterine infection, or it may occur later as the result of a brain tumor, infection, or trauma. Hydrocephalus often is the result of an obstruction caused by adhesions secondary to inflammation of brain tissue. As the volume of CSF increases, the ventricles enlarge and compress on the adjacent brain tissue. This eventually results in brain atrophy. In older adults there is a syndrome called normal pressure hydrocephalus in which the ventricles become very large, the CSF pressure usually remains normal, and brain atrophy occurs. The cause is unknown, but this often follows a head injury, meningitis, or encephalitis.

Common Diagnostic Tests

- Measure head circumference of infant to see if it is larger than the normal range.
- A neurologic examination will identify signs of increasing intracranial pressure (IICP), as well as neurologic impairment.
- Skull x-rays will show separating suture lines of the skull.

**GIRLS: BIRTH TO 36 MONTHS
PHYSICAL GROWTH
NCHS PERCENTILES***

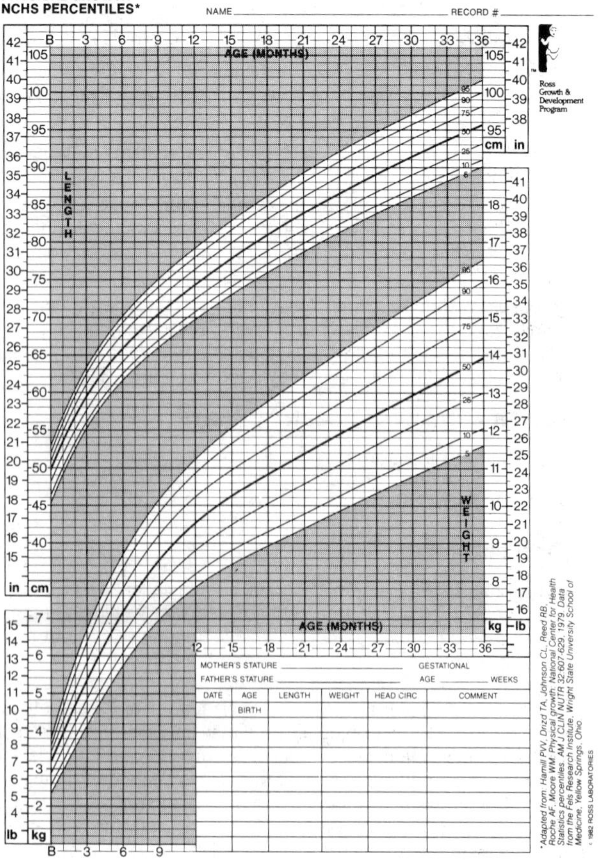

- A computed tomography (CT) scan will demonstrate ventricular dilatation (see NR, Scans).

Observations

- An enlarged head with bulging fontanels and dilated scalp veins usually is seen in infants with hydrocephalus. These infants are often irritable and have a high-pitched cry.

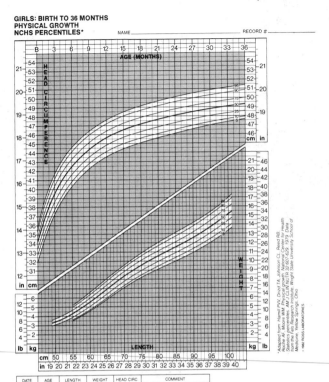

GIRLS: BIRTH TO 36 MONTHS
PHYSICAL GROWTH
NCHS PERCENTILES*

NAME ______________________ RECORD # __________

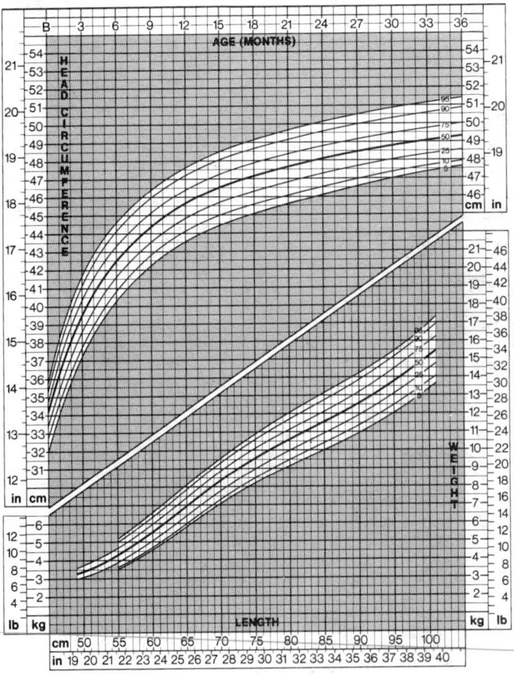

*Adapted from: Hamill PVV, Drizd TA, Johnson CL, Reed RB, Roche AF, Moore WM: Physical growth: National Center for Health Statistics percentiles. AM J CLIN NUTR 32:607-629, 1979. Data from the Fels Research Institute, Wright State University School of Medicine, Yellow Springs, Ohio

DATE	AGE	LENGTH	WEIGHT	HEAD CIRC.	COMMENT

- Increasing head circumference of a growing infant or child that is beyond the normal range of head growth is often an indication of hydrocephalus.
- Early symptoms that may be indicative of IICP are headache that is relieved by emesis or by sitting in an upright position or by standing, lethargy in an infant, and drowsiness and confusion in an older child or adult.

BOYS: BIRTH TO 36 MONTHS
PHYSICAL GROWTH
NCHS PERCENTILES*

NAME ______________________ RECORD # ____________

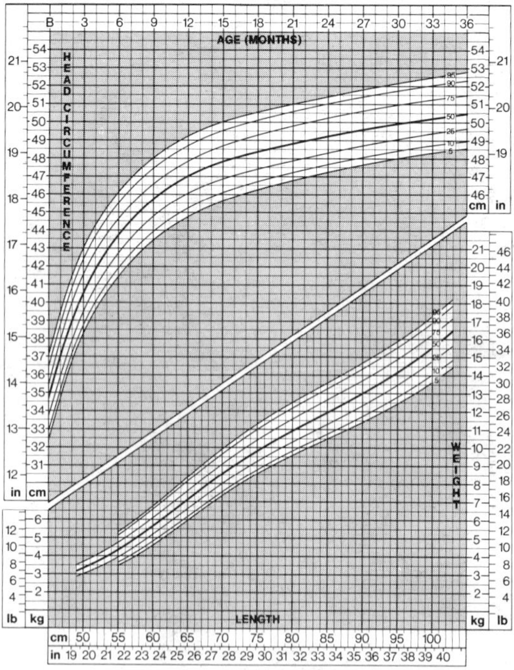

*Adapted from: Hamill PVV, Drizd TA, Johnson CL, Reed RB, Roche AF, Moore WM: Physical growth: National Center for Health Statistics percentiles. AM J CLIN NUTR 32:607-629, 1979. Data from the Fels Research Institute, Wright State University School of Medicine, Yellow Springs, Ohio

DATE	AGE	LENGTH	WEIGHT	HEAD CIRC	COMMENT

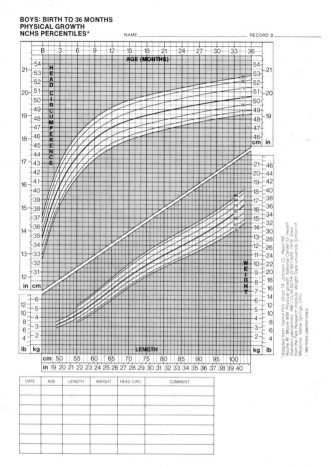

- In normal pressure hydrocephalus, dementia, gait changes, and incontinence represent the characteristic triad of symptoms.

Treatment

- Surgical correction of the defect may be possible, or a tumor may be removed.
- The insertion of a catheter in a ventricle is used as a permanent shunt to drain off the CSF into another area for absorption. A ventriculoatrial or ventriculoperitoneal shunt may be done.

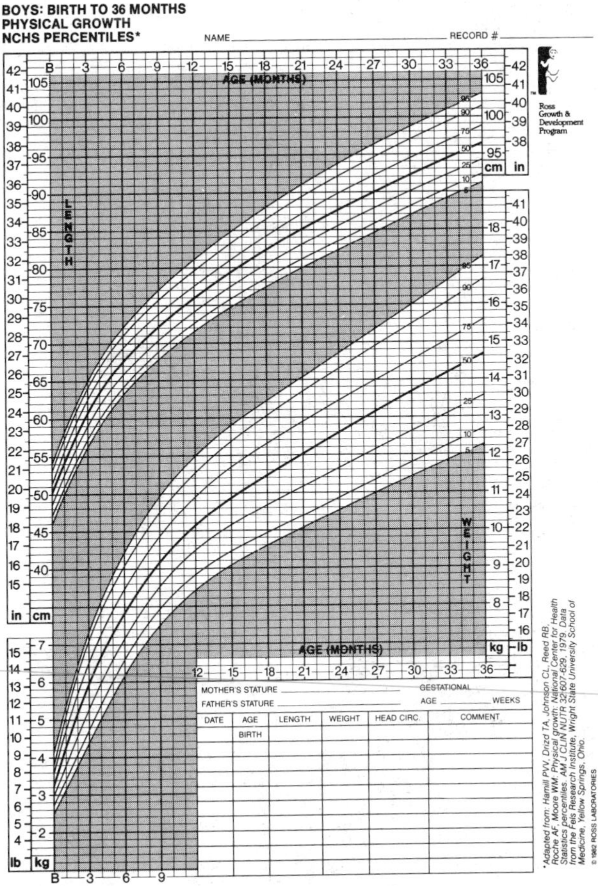

- The type of catheter used will have a valve designed to open when the pressure within the ventricle reaches a predetermined pressure. The valve also prevents a reflux of blood into the catheter when it drains into the jugular vein.

Nursing Considerations

- Infants need to be fed with small and frequent feedings. Poor sucking ability or vomiting after feeding are often the first signs of IICP in an infant.

GIRLS: 2 TO 18 YEARS
PHYSICAL GROWTH
NCHS PERCENTILES*

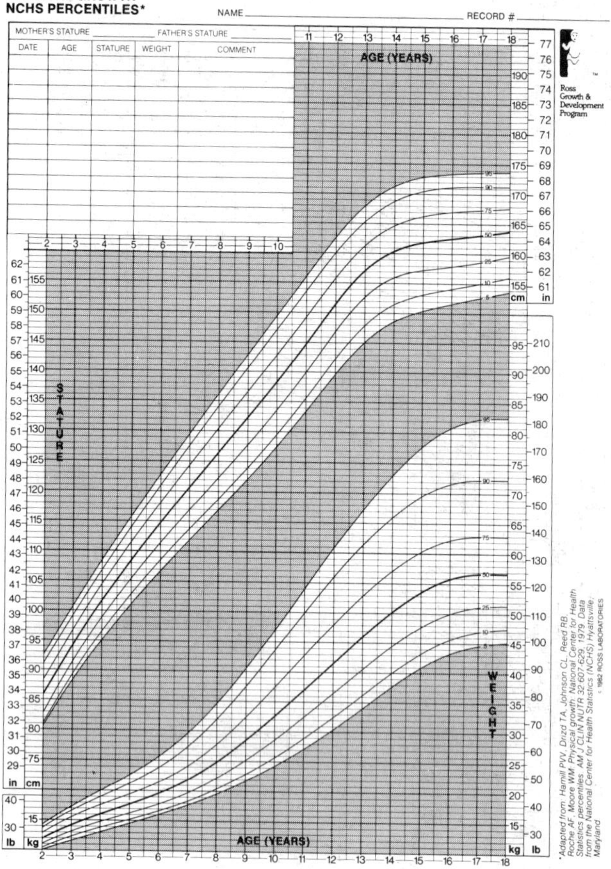

- Mark with an indelible marker the proper placement of the tape on the head for the daily measurement.
- The size and weight of the enlarged head restricts the infant's ability to move. Position changes are necessary at least every two hours.
- In mild hydrocephalus, a neurologic disability may not be noted until later in life.

GIRLS: PREPUBESCENT PHYSICAL GROWTH NCHS PERCENTILES*

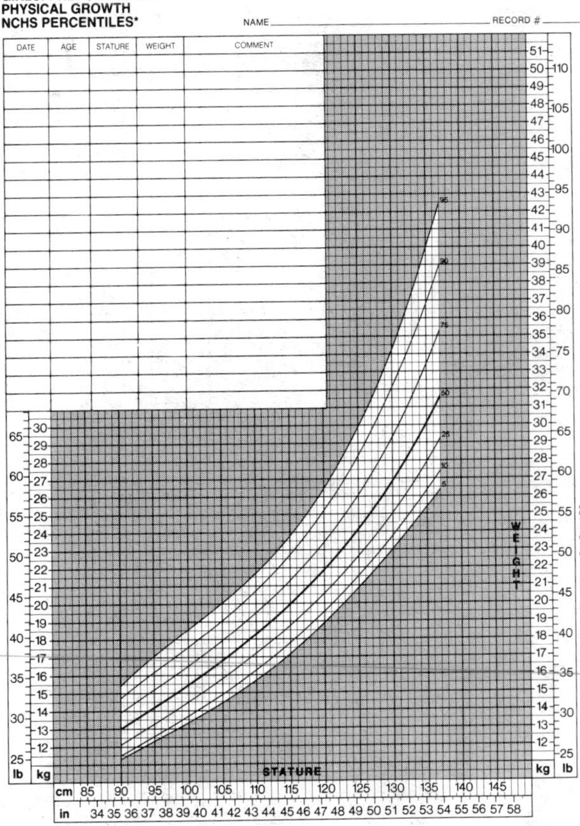

*Adapted from: Hamill PVV, Drizd TA, Johnson CL, Reed RB, Roche AF, Moore WM: Physical growth: National Center for Health Statistics percentiles. AM J CLIN NUTR 32:607-629, 1979. Data from the National Center for Health Statistics (NCHS) Hyattsville, Maryland

Post-Shunt Insertion Care

- Specific orders should be written as to the side the patient is to lie on and the elevation of the head of the bed.
- Complications following a craniotomy are bleeding, signs of infection, or leakage of CSF. Also, be aware of signs of IICP (see MSN, IICP).

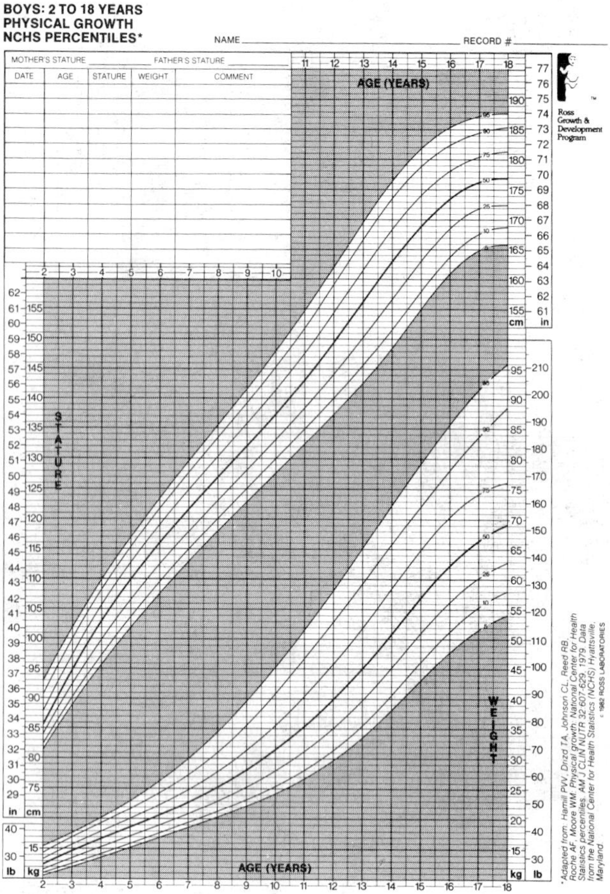

- Shunt insertion sites should be checked for inflammation or tenderness, which are signs of a local infection.
- Shunts may have mechanical failure. When there is an order to "pump a shunt," locate the valve; it usually is above or behind the right ear and feels like a soft spot between two firm spots. Press and release this soft spot; the emptying and filling of the valve should be felt in a properly working valve.
- A shunt catheter may have to be replaced as the child grows. It is rarely removed unless infection or a malfunction occurs.

BOYS: PREPUBESCENT PHYSICAL GROWTH NCHS PERCENTILES*

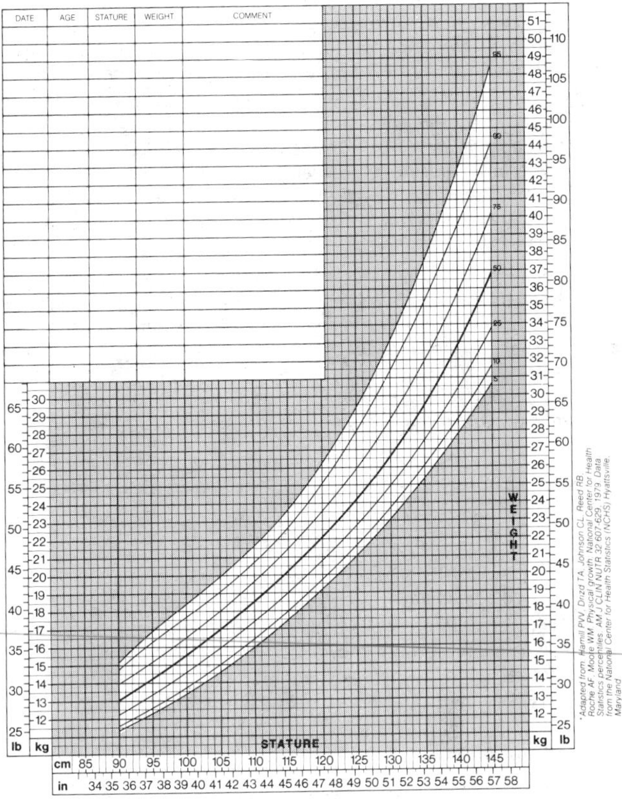

PED

NEPHROTIC SYNDROME

Description

Nephrotic syndrome describes a complex of symptoms in which there is a massive loss of urinary protein as a result of increased glomerular permeability. It may occur during the course of several different kidney diseases.

Nephrotic syndrome has been classified as the following:

- *Congenital nephrotic syndrome* has symptoms that appear early, usually within the first months of life. The disease does not respond to usual treatment. Death usually occurs within the first year or two of the infant's life.

- *Idiopathic nephrotic syndrome* occurs in approximately 80% of nephrotic children. The cause of the condition is unknown, but prednisone seems to hasten remission. The condition may relapse many times.
- *Secondary nephrotic syndrome* usually occurs as a result of glomerulonephritis (see PED, Glomerulonephritis). These are antigen-antibody reactions sometimes caused by systemic diseases, such as systemic lupus erythematosus. Causative antigens may come from drugs, or rarely from venoms or stings, but are usually from unknown sources.

The course of the nephrotic syndrome is that of the underlying disease: acute glomerulonephritis may go away after a few weeks, idiopathic nephrotic syndrome may remit and relapse again and again, and chronic glomerulonephritis may proceed to permanent renal failure.

Common Diagnostic Tests

- Urinalysis reveals marked proteinuria. (Most nephrologists use the standard of more than 3.5 g of protein in a 24-hour urine collection.)
  1. Red blood cells and casts may be present.
- Blood chemistry usually shows
  1. Low serum albumin
  2. High serum triglycerides and cholesterol
     It may show elevated level of serum urea nitrogen (BUN) and creatinine.
- Renal biopsy may be done to make the exact diagnosis.

Observations

Symptoms may begin insidiously.

- Edema is the clinical hallmark.
  1. Periorbital edema (around the eyes), especially upon rising in the morning, frequently occurs.
  2. Generalized edema, especially in dependent parts—the ankles, the scrotum in boys, and the labia in girls—is often seen.
  3. Ascites, if severe, may cause dyspnea (difficult breathing).
  4. Diarrhea, caused by edema of the intestines, may be present.
  5. Paleness of the skin is often seen. If edema is severe, the skin may stretch and weep fluid, making it more susceptible to infection.
- Urine may be frothy (beer-like), and sometimes dark and decreased in volume.
- Irritability, fussiness, lethargy, and fatigability may be seen.

- Orthostatic hypotension caused by hypoalbuminemia may result in dizziness on standing (see NR, Postural hypotension).

Treatment

The goal of treatment is to support the child during the disease.

- Prednisone (or another adrenocorticosteroid) often is ordered (see PH).
- A diet high in protein (to replace urinary protein losses) and low in salt (to minimize further edema formation) is usually ordered.
- Fluid restriction usually is not necessary unless hyponatremia is present.
- Bedrest may be ordered when edema is present.
- Diuretics may be prescribed.
- Intravenous albumin with diuretics may be used for emergency reduction of severe edema or ascites. Results are dramatic, but temporary.
- Cyclophosphamide (Cytoxan) or another alkylating agent may be given for its immunosuppressant action.
- Appropriate antimicrobials are ordered if infections occur. Every effort should be made to prevent skin and systemic infections, to which these patients are susceptible.

Nursing Considerations

- Consider the importance of avoiding infections when assigning a bed or a room to a nephrotic child.
- Assess edema. Measure weight daily at the same time, in the same clothes, on the same scale. Measure girth at the umbilicus daily. Record.
- When edema is present:
    1. Elevate the head of the bed in a semi-Fowler's position to minimize periorbital edema. If present, wipe the eyes with saline wipes.
    2. Provide meticulous skin care.
        a. Provide frequent diaper changes with thorough cleansing. (Expect that older, toilet-trained children may regress.)
        b. Cleanse and powder opposing skin surfaces several times a day. These touching skin surfaces found, for example, in the area of a boy's scrotum, may be separated by soft gauze.
    3. Change the child's position frequently, but maintain good body alignment.
    4. Give injections in the deltoid, and not into edematous thighs or buttocks.
- Measure fluid intake and output accurately, and record.
- Monitor blood pressure and vital signs daily, and prn.

- Encourage the child to eat enough to maintain adequate nutrition. The appetite is frequently poor during the acute phase of the disorder. Provide attractive trays, small servings, with attention to food preferences within the prescribed diet.
- If fluids are restricted (during the acute phase), offer small glasses of water, rather than a few large ones.
  1. A chart showing the amount of fluid allowed during a day may help an older, cooperative child keep track by having him or her color in the amount of fluids as they are taken.
- Collect urine specimens and test for presence of protein, as ordered.
  1. Be sure the child, the parent, and the staff understand the method for collecting timed (24-hour) urine specimens which are ordered periodically.
- Provide suitable diversional activities while the child is on bedrest.
- Encourage increased activity, as allowed, once edema subsides.
- Parents should be taught to detect signs of relapse, and the importance of notifying the physician.
  1. Teach them regarding urine testing, appropriate care, and medication administration. Emphasize the specifics about steroid therapy—the side-effects, and the danger of discontinuing the medication without a physician's supervision.

PYLORIC STENOSIS, HYPERTROPHIC

Description

Hypertrophic pyloric stenosis is the result of a thickening of the pyloric muscle, causing the pyloric canal between the stomach and duodenum to become very narrow. This prevents food from moving out of the stomach into the duodenum. It is the most common cause of gastrointestinal (GI) obstruction in infants, most frequently occurring in full-term male infants.

Common Diagnostic Tests

- It is often possible to palpate an enlarged olive-sized, movable pyloric muscle, located just to the right of the umbilicus. This is felt most easily during a feeding.
- Peristaltic waves moving from left to right across the upper abdomen also may be seen during a feeding.
- An upper GI examination may be done to confirm physical findings.

Observations

- Vomiting tends to occur at about two weeks or three weeks of age; this rapidly progresses from regurgitation to projectile vomiting. Such vomiting usually occurs shortly after feeding. There is no bile in the vomitus because the food cannot progress beyond the stomach.
- The infant is constantly hungry, does not gain weight, is constipated, and begins to show symptoms of dehydration.
- Dehydration is a major complication of this condition (see Dehydration). Watch for sunken eyeballs, a loss of skin turgor, and low potassium, sodium, and chloride serum levels. Metabolic alkalosis may result from the loss of hydrochloric acid in the vomitus.

Treatment

- The correction of electrolyte imbalances must be done before the surgical correction is attempted.
- A Ramstedt pyloromyotomy is the surgical procedure that cuts the muscle fibers of the obstructing pyloric muscle, thereby allowing food to move from the stomach into the duodenum.

Nursing Considerations

Preoperative

- A gastric lavage may be done preoperatively to rid the stomach of its contents.
- IV replacement of fluid and electrolytes is usually necessary.
- Accurate intake and output measurements, daily weights, and urine specific gravity are essential.

Postoperative

- See postoperative care.
- Feeding usually is started four hours to six hours after surgery, with one ounce of glucose water given every two hours. If this is retained, the volume of feeding is increased. Formula is then restarted in about 24 hours, beginning with one ounce, and increasing every two hours to normal feeding.
- Intake and output, daily weights, and the specific gravity of the urine are again very important.

SICKLE CELL ANEMIA

Description

Sickle cell anemia (SCA) is a chronic hemolytic anemia caused by a genetic defect in the hemoglobin molecule. Sickle cells only live 6 days to 12 days, as contrasted to 120 days for normal red blood cells (RBCs). The body cannot produce new cells at the greatly increased rate required to maintain the usual RBC count, and anemia occurs. Normal RBCs are disc shaped and have a cell flexibility that allows them to pass through the tiniest capillaries. RBCs containing sickle hemoglobin assume rigid sickle shapes when they yield oxygen. These abnormal cells are trapped easily in capillaries, where the resulting obstruction of blood flow causes stasis, ischemia, and subsequent infarction of tissue. Dehydration and deoxygenation increase the sickling action of these defective RBCs. Sickle cell vasoocclusive crisis is the result of infarcts, which most commonly occur in the extremities or abdominal organs, but any part of the body may be affected. The pain and fever associated with sickle cell crisis is caused by these infarcts. SCA occurs predominately in dark-skinned people. It results when a sickle cell gene is inherited from both parents. Sickle cell trait occurs when a sickle cell gene is inherited from only one parent. There is a lower percentage of sickle hemoglobin in their blood. Thus, people with sickle cell trait are usually asymptomatic, unless they become severely dehydrated or deoxygenated.

Common Diagnostic Tests

- Hemoglobin electrophoresis detects all major sickle cell variants. It will differentiate between those with the trait and those with the disease.

Observations

- Anemia with accompanying weakness, pallor, and jaundice, which is most frequently apparent in the sclera of the eye may be present. Chronic anemias can lead to cardiomegaly and ultimately congestive heart failure (see MSN, Congestive heart failure).
- An enlarged liver and spleen in infancy and early childhood are common.
- An increased incidence of bacterial infections (*e.g.*, osteomyelitis, pneumococcal pneumonia) and generalized sepsis may be seen. The spleen becomes nonfunctional at an early age because it becomes fibrotic after repeated infarcts. Normally, the spleen filters and destroys infective organisms, especially *Pneumococcus*.
- Recurrent painful and swollen joints mimicking arthritis are present.
- Leg ulcers occur because of vascular insufficiency in the legs. Necroses of the head of the femur, resulting from repeated bone infarctions, may occur in adolescence. The involvement of this weight-bearing bone causes constant discomfort.
- Hematuria may result from kidney damage from an infarction in the kidneys.

- There may be a tendency toward dehydration because of an inability to concentrate urine with resultant high-volume output.
- A stroke may result from thrombosis and resultant ischemia and infarction of brain tissue. This is not uncommon in children; it is seen in 6–12% of these patients (see MSN, Cerebral vascular accident).
- Retarded growth, delayed sexual development, and priapism (constant penile erection) may occur.
- A child with SCA is often thin and small for his age, with disproportionate bone growth of face and skull.
- Sickle cell vaso-occlusive crisis may result, producing mild to severe pain most often in the abdomen, that lasts hours or days along with an elevated temperature. One variation of the vaso-occlusive crisis is called dactylitis or "hand-foot syndrome." It is often the first evidence of SCA, occurring as early as six months of age, but is rarely seen after the age of seven. It is characterized by painful swelling of the hands and feet, often accompanied by a high temperature and an elevated white blood cell count. These symptoms usually subside in about two weeks.
- Sickle cell splenic sequestration crisis is life threatening and is seen before the age of five. There is a sudden pooling of blood in the spleen resulting from the sickling changes in the blood. An enlarged spleen suddenly develops, with the signs and symptoms of shock resulting from a sudden drop in the circulating volume of blood.

Treatment

- There is no known cure for sickle cell anemia. Treatment is directed toward avoiding sickle cell crisis by preventing dehydration, infection, and any activity or stress that depletes oxygen in the tissues.
- The daily fluid intake should be at least two liters.
- Mild sickle cell crisis may be treated at home with analgesics for pain and increased fluids intake.
- During sickle cell vaso-occlusive crisis, pain relief is imperative. This may be accomplished with analgesics given before the pain becomes severe; body positioning with pillows to support and protect extremities; warm baths and warm compresses on affected joints; and the avoidance of unnecessary patient movement.
- Parenteral hydration may be necessary during a crisis. About one and one-half times the daily fluid requirement is given; in children, the volume is based on the total body surface area. Observe for symptoms of fluid overload, *e.g.,* CHF (see MSN, Congestive heart failure) because of the rate and volume of the infusion.

- Transfusions usually are given to decrease the percentage of sickle cell hemoglobin before a surgical procedure or during a pregnancy.
- In the case of splenic sequestration, transfusions are necessary to provide an adequate circulating volume of blood.
- Partial exchange transfusions may be given during a crisis to decrease the percentage of sickle cell hemoglobin.

Nursing Considerations

- SCA most frequently produces its symptoms in early childhood between 6 months and 2 years of age. The crises usually become less severe and less frequent after adolescence, but infection remains a major threat.
- Precipitating factors to a vaso-occlusive crisis are dehydration, infection, and extreme fatigue. Push fluids at the first signs of the slightest temperature elevation.
- Intake and output, with urine specific gravity every eight hours, and daily weights are extremely important to determine the hydration of the patient during a crisis.
- Prompt medical attention is necessary for any symptom of infection. A frequent cause of death in infants and children with this disease is sepsis. A pneumococcal vaccine usually is given at two years of age.
- People with SCA have an increased susceptibility to bacterial meningitis; also, they have an increased incidence of gallstones.
- Persons with sickle cell trait may become symptomatic if they become deoxygenated under such circumstances as prolonged physical exertion, pulmonary disease, or anesthesia.
- There are some milder varieties of SCA that manifest later in life and may primarily produce retinopathy, in contrast to painful crisis.
- Screening for SCA at birth, before surgery, and during pregnancy is important because detection can prevent complications.
- When indicated, genetic counseling is extremely important. The possibility that offspring will have SCA can be determined and its significance explained to prospective parents.
- Although it is still under investigation, amniocentesis is providing a method of prenatal diagnosis.

TONSILLECTOMY AND ADENOIDECTOMY

Description

A tonsillectomy is the removal of lymphoid tissues, called the palatine tonsil, that is located in the pharynx. The most common reasons for performing a tonsillectomy are recurrent inflammations of the tonsil (tonsillitis), peritonsillar abscess, and airway obstruction caused by severe adenotonsillar swelling.

An adenoidectomy is the removal of lymphoid tissue, called the pharyngeal tonsil or adenoid, from the nasopharynx. An enlarged adenoid may cause nasal or eustachian tube obstruction. Serous otitis media causing hearing loss is the principal reason for removal. Also, chronic middle ear infections frequently occur when the eustachian tube is obstructed.

Nursing Considerations

Preoperative

- Surgery is deferred until any acute infection of the tonsils has subsided.
- Explain the procedure to the patient. Mention that the throat will be sore for a few days, and that there will be some blood in the mouth during this time.
- Advise the patient of the need to maintain adequate oral fluid intake postoperatively. Dehydration will make swallowing more difficult and painful.

Postoperative

- Patients should be placed on their side or abdomen, with primary attention toward maintaining the airway.
- Suction equipment should always be at the bedside following a tonsillectomy and/or adenoidectomy (T and A). If suctioning is necessary, avoid traumatizing the throat.
- Hemorrhaging is the most common complication that occurs within the first few postoperative hours. Crying or repeated efforts to clear the throat also can trigger bleeding throughout the week following surgery.
- Any increasing pulse rate, restlessness, pallor, excessive swallowing, or bleeding should be called to the physician's attention.
- Blood will be bright red from fresh bleeding; blood swallowed and then regurgitated has the appearance of coffee grounds.
- Take vital signs as routine in the postoperative period, or as indicated by the patient's condition.
- Liquids may be given by mouth as soon as the patient is alert and not nauseous. It is helpful to give the analgesic ordered about 30 minutes before the first swallowing attempt. Adults often seem to experience more pain than children.
- Complaints of an earache are common. This is the result of referred pain from the pharynx to the ear.

- Saline mouthwashes, *not gargles,* are helpful in clearing the mouth and reducing the odor and bad taste. One teaspoon of salt to a pint of warm water makes a good mouthwash.
- Ice collars may be soothing to the throat.
- A week of restricted activity is suggested after this surgery. Any increase in temperature or new bleeding should be reported to the physician.

WILMS' TUMOR

Description

Wilms' tumor—a malignant mixed tumor of the kidney, also called nephroblastoma, embryoma, or adenomyosarcoma—is the most frequent intraabdominal tumor of childhood. This kidney cancer is seen in early childhood, with the peak incidence at three years. There is evidence of an inherited tendency for this disease. It usually is seen in the presence of congenital defects, *e.g.,* aniridia (the absence of the iris of the eye), hemihypertrophy (hypertrophy of muscles of half of the body or face), and genitourinary anomalies.

Common Diagnostic Tests

- See Cancer of the kidney.

Observations

- Large palpable abdominal mass
- Weight loss, anemia
- Hematuria, a rather rare sign
- Hypertension, frequently present
- Signs of metastases, usually to liver, lungs, bone, or brain

Treatment

- See Cancer of the kidney.
- Wilms' tumor is radiosensitive.

Nursing Considerations

- Caution must be used when handling the infant. Palpation of the abdomen should be avoided. Parents and staff members should be reminded of this by placing a sign stating *"Do not palpate abdomen"* over the bed.
- See MSN, Surgery of the kidneys and ureters, and MSN, Oncology nursing considerations.

BIBLIOGRAPHY • Pediatrics

BOOKS

Avery G: Neonatology, 2nd ed. Philadelphia, JB Lippincott, 1981
Brunner L, Suddarth D: The Lippincott Manual of Nursing Practice, 3rd ed. Philadelphia, JB Lippincott, 1982
Chow M, Durand B, Feldman M, Mills M: Handbook of Pediatric Care. New York, John Wiley & Sons, 1979
DeAngelis C: Pediatric Primary Care, 2nd ed. Boston, Little, Brown, 1979
Farmer T: Intracranial infections, Pediatric Neurology, 3rd ed. New York, Harper & Row, 1983
Farrell J: Illustrated Guide to Orthopedic Nursing, 2nd ed. Philadelphia, JB Lippincott, 1982
Ferguson A: Orthopedic Surgery in Infancy and Childhood. Baltimore, Williams & Wilkins, 1981
Fleisher G, Ludwig S: Textbook of Pediatric Emergency Medicine. Baltimore, Williams & Wilkins, 1983
Given B, Simmons S: Gastroenterology in Clinical Nursing, 4th ed. St Louis, CV Mosby, 1984
Graef J, Cone T: Manual of Pediatric Therapeutics, 2nd ed. Boston, Little, Brown, 1980
Green M, Richmond J: Pediatric Diagnosis, 3rd ed. Philadelphia, WB Saunders, 1980
Hamilton P: Basic Pediatric Nursing, 4th ed. St Louis, CV Mosby, 1982
Hodson M, Norman A, Batten J: Cystic fibrosis. London, Bailliere Tindall, 1983
Hughes J: Synopsis of Pediatrics, 5th ed. St Louis, CV Mosby, 1980
Hughes W, Buescher E: Pediatric Procedures, 2nd ed. Philadelphia, WB Saunders, 1980
Jolly J: The Other Side of Pediatrics. London, Macmillan Press, 1981
Kerkering K, Kendig E: Pediatrics, Respiratory Tract Disease. New York, Harper & Row, 1983
Larson C, Gould M: Orthopedic Nursing, 9th ed. St Louis, CV Mosby, 1978
Latham H, Heckel R, Herbert L, Bennett E: Pediatric Nursing, 3rd ed. St Louis, CV Mosby, 1977
Lerner J, Khan Z: Mosby's Manual of Urologic Nursing. St Louis, CV Mosby, 1982
Lifshitz F (ed): Pediatric Nutrition. New York, Marcel Dekker, 1982
Lloyd-Still J (with contributors): Textbook of Cystic Fibrosis. Boston, John Wright, 1983
McConnell E, Zimmerman M: Care of Patients with Urologic Problems. Philadelphia, JB Lippincott, 1983
Metheny N, Snively W: Nurses Handbook of fluid balance, 4th ed. Philadelphia, JB Lippincott, 1983
Michalck J: Child Abuse, Nursing and Child Protection. Boston, Little, Brown, 1982

Pillitteri A: Child Health Nursing: Care of the Growing Family. 2nd ed. Boston, Little, Brown, 1981
Robinson G, Clarke H: Hospital Care of Children. New York, Oxford Press, 1980
Scipien G, Barnard M, Chard M: Comprehensive Pediatric Nursing, 2nd ed. New York, McGraw-Hill, 1979
Thompson R, Stanford G: Child Life in Hospitals, Theory and Practice. Springfield, Illinois, Charles C Thomas, 1981
Vaughn V, McKay R, Behrman R: Nelson Textbook of Pediatrics, 11th ed. Philadelphia, WB Saunders, 1979
Warner C, Braen G (eds): Management of the Physically and Emotionally Abused. Norwalk, Appleton-Century-Crofts, 1982
Wasserman E, Gromisch D: Survey of Clinical Pediatrics, 7th ed. New York, McGraw-Hill, 1981
Whaley L, Wong D: Nursing Care of Infants and Children, 2nd ed. St Louis, CV Mosby, 1983
Zia M (ed): Pediatrics, 3rd ed. Boston, Little, Brown, 1984

JOURNALS

Bluestone C: Recent advances in the pathogenesis, diagnosis and management of Otitis Media. Pediatr Clin North Am 28(4): 727, 1981
D'Antonio I: Therpeutic use of play in hospitals. Nurs Clin North Am 19(2): 351, 1984
Davis H, Gartner J, Galvia A, Michael R, Mestad P: Acute upper airway obstruction: Croup and epiglottitis. Pediatr Clin North Am 28(4): 859, 1981
Fore C, Holmes S: Sexual abuse of children. Nurs Clin North Am 19(2): 329, 1984
Foster S, Hawkins D: Homecare of the child with a tracheotomy tube. Pediatr Clin North Am 28(4): 855, 1981
Hazinski M: Critical care of the pediatric cardiovascular patient 16 (4): 6 Nurs Clin North Am, Dec 1981
McKittrick C: Child Abuse: Recognition and Reporting by Health Professionals. Nurs Clin North Am 16(1): 103, 1981
Paradise J: Tonsillectomy and Adenoidectomy. Pediatr Clin North Am 28(4): 811, 1981

Child Abuse and Neglect/Emotional Problems of the Hospitalized Child

JOURNALS

Association for the Care of Children's Health: Position Statement on: Critical Care for Children; Care of Children with Chronic Conditions and Developmental Disabilities and Their Families; Care of Infants in Health Care Settings. Position Paper on Ambulatory Care for Children and Their Families; Child Life Position Statement; Statements of Policy for the Care of Children and Families in Health Care Settings.

Feldman K, Brewer D: Child abuse, cardiopulmonary resuscitation and rib fractures. Pediatrics 73(3): 339, Mar 1984

Glen S: Happy families. Nurs Mirror 156(4): 25, Jan 26, 1983

Lamb J, Rodgers D: Assisting the hostile, hospitalized child. MCN 8(5): 336, Sept/Oct 1983

The Nurse's Role in the Prevention and Treatment of Child Abuse and Neglect. U.S. Department of Health and Human Services. Publication No. (OHDS) 79-30202

Perspectives on Child Maltreatment in the Mid '80s. US Department of Health and Human Services. Publication No. (OHDS) 84-303, 38

Porter E: Stress immunization: Techniques to help children cope with hospitalization. Matern Child Nurs J 12(2): 119, Summer 1983

Rosenberg N, Meyers S, Shackleton N: Prediction of child abuse in an ambulatory setting. Pediatrics 70(6): 879, Dec 1982

Swanwick M: Platt in perspective. Nurs Times 79(3): 5, 19, 1983

Cardiovascular

JOURNALS

Abdulla A: The sounds and signs of congenital heart disease. Emerg Med 14(20): 250, Nov 30, 1982

Kneut C: Sickle cell anemia. Iss Compr Pediatr Nurs 4(5–6): 19, Sept–Oct 1980

Modrcin MA, Schott J: An update of congestive heart failure in infants. Iss Compr Pediatr Nurs 3(7): 5, Dec 1979

Morgan B (ed): Symposium on pediatric cardiology. Pediatr Clin North Am Nov 1978

Neal WA, Morgan MF: Care of the critically ill neonate with heart disease. CCQ Crit Care Q 4:47, Jun 1981

Pact B (ed): Symposium on sickle cell. Nurs Clin North Am 18(1): 129, Mar 1983

Report of the Task Force on Blood Pressure Control in Children. Prepared by National Heart, Lung, and Blood Institutes Task Force on Blood Pressure Control in Children, May 1977. Pediatrics 59(5): 19, 1977

Smith K: Congenital heart disease. Recognizing cardiac failure in a neonate. MCN 4(2): 98, Mar/Apr 1979

Strong W: The sick newborn, evaluating cardiorespiratory distress. Emerg Med 15(17): 51, Oct 15, 1983

Dehydration

JOURNALS

Brown K, MacLean W: Nutritional management of acute diarrhea: An appraisal of alternatives. Pediatrics 73(2): 119, Feb 1984

Groshong T: Fluid and electrolyte therapy for infants and young children. Consultant 20(5); 123, May 1980

Ear, Nose and Throat

JOURNALS

Fried E: Acute epiglottitis. Iss Compr Pediatr Nurs 4(5–6): 29, Sept–Dec 1980
Jacobs S: Nursing care of the child with cleft lip and/or palate. Plast Surg Nurs 3(3): 61, Fall 1983
Katz AE: T and A, Recommendations that make sense. Consultant 22(1): 207, Jan 1982
Martin L: A new "gravity-flow" nipple for feeding infants with congenital cleft palate. Pediatrics 72(2): 244, Aug 1983
Maurer JA: The care and feeding of a T and A. Point of View 18(4): 10, Oct 1981
Page H: Croup and epiglottitis. Am Lung Assoc Bull 67(2): 9, Mar 1981
Pashayan H: What else to look for in a child born with a cleft of the lip and/or palate. Cleft Palate J 20(1): 54, Jan 1983
Rayburn R, Gatsh G: Epiglottitis in pediatric patients. AORN 36(1): 59, Jul 1982
Sataloff R, Colton C: Otitis media: A common childhood infection. Am J Nurs 81(8): 1480, Aug 1981
Schneider P: Care of cleft lip and cleft palate patients. Physician Assistant Health Practitioner 6(2):19, Feb 6, 1982
Simmonds S: Cleft lip and cosmetic surgery, A personal account. Nursing (Oxford) 1:1060, Apr 1981
Styer G, Froch K: Feeding infants with cleft lip and/or palate. JOGN Nurs 10:329, Sept/Oct 1981
Teele D, Klein J, Rosner B: Otitis media with effusion during the first three years of life and development of speech and language. Pediatrics 74(2); 282, Aug 1984
Wald E: The middle ear in the early years. Emerg Med 15(18): 94, Oct 30, 1983
Yamaguchi T, Somekawa Y, Ara H, Kataura A: Indications for the use of ventilating tubes for secretory otitis media. Int J Pediatr Otorhinolaryngol 4(1): 29, Mar 1982

Endocrine System

JOURNALS

Gunter-Hunt G, Parker L, Spencer M: Adolescent diabetes clinic: a specialized treatment approach. Diabetes Educ 8(3): 36, Fall 1982

Gastrointestinal System

JOURNALS

Ivenson-Ivenson (ed): Background to congenital hypertrophic pyloric stenosis. Nurs Mirror 150(14): 42, Apr 3, 1980
Kiely E, Deasy J, Harte P, et al: Congenital hypertrophic pyloric stenosis: a review. Ir Med J 74(6): 161, Jun 1981
Markowitz R, Wolfson B, Huff D, et al: Infantile hypertrophic pyloric stenosis congenital or acquired. J Clin Gastroenterol 4(1): 39, Feb 1982
McComas C: Congenital pyloric stenosis. J Nurs Care 13(4): 8, Apr 1980
Wyse M: Pyloric stenosis. Ariz Med 39(2): 96, Feb 1982

Orthopedics

JOURNALS

Hensinger R: Congenital dislocation of the hip. Ciba Clin Symp 31(1): 79, 1979
Hilt N: Musculoskeletal assessment: Screening for congenital dislocation of the hip. Orthop Nurs 1(2): 22, Mar/Apr 1982

Respiratory System

JOURNALS

Cotton E: Respiratory disorders: Treatment in childhood can avert serious adult problems. Consultant 23(4): 78, Apr 1983
Herbst J, Hilman B, Holsclau D, Shuster S: Spotting and sustaining patients with cystic fibrosis. Patient Care 16(4): 16, Feb 28, 1982
Holbreich M, Strunk R: Precipitating factors in childhood asthma. Respir Ther 11(1): 74, Jan/Feb 1981
Huang N, Palmer J: Management of patients with cystic fibrosis, Part 1: Clinical manifestations. Respir Ther 11(1): 49, Jan/Feb 1981
Huang N, Palmer J: Management of patients with cystic fibrosis, Part 2: Principles of treatment. Respir Ther 11(2): 65, Mar/Apr 1981
Huang N, Palmer J: Management of patients with cystic fibrosis, Part 3: Treatment of pulmonary infections and complications. Respir Ther 11(3): 71, May/Jun 1981
Larter N: Cystic fibrosis. Am J Nurs 81(3): 527, Mar 1981
Pearlman D: Bronchial asthma. Am J Dis Child 138(5): 459, May 1984
Richards W, Church J: Self-help for asthmatic children. Respir Ther 12(6): 45, Nov/Dec 1982

Urologic

JOURNALS

Ford B: Nephrotic syndrome. Nurs Times 79(31): 58, Aug 3, 1983

McCrony W: Acute renal failure: A guide to diagnosis during adolescence. Consultant 23(3): 167, Mar 1983

Salcedo J: Focal segmental glomerulosclerosis with idiopathic nephrotic syndrome. J Pediatr 102(2): 325, Feb 1983

Schoeneman M, Spitzer A, Greifer I: Nitrogen mustard therapy in children with frequent relapsing nephrotic syndrome and steroid toxicity. Am J Kid Dis 2(5): 526, Mar 1983

Southby J, Moore J: Nursing diagnosis for a child with end stage renal disease. AANNT J 10(4): 23, Jun 1983

Strauss J: Tips about renal disease in children. Consultant 20: 75, Apr 1980.

7

Pharmacology

MATHEMATICS OF DOSAGE

METRIC SYSTEM

- In the hospital situation three types of metric measurements are of main concern: length, volume, and weight.
- The basic unit for length is a *meter;* for volume, it is a *liter;* and for weight, a *gram.*
- There are larger and smaller units of measurement for each basic unit. They will always contain the name of the basic unit (*e.g.*, milli*liter* refers to volume, and milli*gram* refers to weight). The larger and smaller units are designated by the following prefixes: kilo, milli, and micro.
  1. *Kilo* indicates a quantity larger than the basic unit and multiplies it by 1000 (*e.g.*, 1000 meters = 1 kilometer; 1000 grams = 1 kilogram).
  2. *Milli* indicates a quantity smaller than the basic unit and divides it by 1000 (*e.g.*, 1 liter = 1000 milliliters; 1 gram = 1000 milligrams).
  3. *Micro* indicates a quantity smaller than milli and divides a milli by 1000 (*e.g.*, 1 milligram = 1000 micrograms).
- Abbreviations are commonly used. Official abbreviations (from the National Bureau of Standards) are as follows:
  1. Basic units use the first initial in small letters: meter = m; liter = l; gram = g.
  2. The larger unit uses the following: kilo = k.
  3. Smaller units are the following: centi = c; milli = m; and micro = mc.
  4. Unofficial abbreviations commonly used are: gram = gm, milligram = mgm, and microgram = mcgm.
  5. The following are some official examples: kilogram = kg; milliliter = ml; microgram = mcg.
- To ensure accuracy and avoid misunderstanding when using the metric system, always observe the following:
  1. Use Arabic numbers (*e.g.*, 1, 2, 3).
  2. Place the number in front of the abbreviation (*e.g.*, 2 ml, 4 mg).
  3. Express a part of a whole in decimals (*e.g.*, 0.5 ml).
  4. If a whole number is not present in front of the decimal point,

PH

place a zero there to emphasize the decimal point (*e.g.*, 0.4 ml, 0.2 mg).

5. Omit unnecessary zeros to the right of the decimal point (*e.g.*, 0.4 ml, not 0.40 ml).

- The metric system is a decimal system. To *convert* from larger to smaller or from smaller to larger units of measure, you simply move the decimal point.
  1. The following units of weight commonly used are listed from highest to lowest value: kg, g, mg, mcg.
  2. The units of volume (highest to lowest) are as follows: l, ml or cc [1 ml is considered equivalent to 1 cc [cubic centimeter], and the abbreviations can be used interchangeably].
  3. Each of the above units differs from the next by 1000, so when converting from one "neighbor" to another, you move the decimal point three places.
  4. When converting from a higher to a lower value, move the decimal point three places to the *right* (*e.g.*, 4.1 g = 4100 mg; 0.132 l = 132 ml).
  5. When converting from a lower to higher value, move the decimal point three places to the *left* (*e.g.*, 200 mcg = 0.2 mg; 600 ml = 0.6 l).

APOTHECARY SYSTEM

- In the hospital, two types of apothecary measurement are of main concern: volume and weight.
- The units for volume are ounce, dram, and minim. The unit for weight is a grain.
- The abbreviations and symbols used are as follows: ounce = ℥; dram = ʒ; minim = m; grain = gr.
- To ensure accuracy and avoid misunderstanding when using the apothecary system, always observe the following:
  1. Use Roman numerals (*e.g.*, I, II, III).
  2. The abbreviation or symbol is placed in front of the numeral (*e.g.*, gr v, ʒ ii, ℥ iv).
  3. A part of a whole is expressed in fractions (*e.g.*, gr ¼, gr ½).
  4. $\overline{\text{ss}}$ may be used for ½ (*e.g.*, gr $\overline{\text{ss}}$).

Nursing Considerations

- The following measures and abbreviations are also used: tablespoon = T or tbs; teaspoon = t or tsp; drop = gtt; unit = u.
- A unit is an expression of biologic action rather than weight. Insulin, heparin, and some antibiotics are measured in units.

CONVERSION TABLE: METRIC-APOTHECARY

- At times it will be necessary to convert between the metric and apothecary systems. The *safest* way to do this is to refer to a conversion table (see Table 7-1). The conversions presented are *equivalents.* Therefore, you would find discrepancies if you figured out the same problem mathematically.

CALCULATING DRUG DOSAGE

- The following formula can be used to solve all drug dosage problems. Using a consistent approach helps eliminate errors.

$$\frac{D}{H} \times Q = X$$

where D = the *d*osage you *d*esire to give, the *d*octor's order; H = the dosage you *h*ave on *h*and, what the pharmacy sent; Q = *q*uantity: for solid preparations the drug usually comes in a tablet or capsule, for liquid preparations the drug is usually in milliliters (ml or cc) or ounces; and X = the unknown: what you actually must give to administer the desired dose.

Examples

The doctor's order reads: Lanoxin 0.125 mg, PO.

The label on tablet reads: 0.25 mg per tab.

$$\frac{\text{(D) } 0.125 \text{ mg}}{\text{(H) } 0.25 \text{ mg}} \times \text{(Q) } 1 \text{ tab} = X$$

$X = 1/2$ tab

The doctor's order reads: Keflex 0.5 g, PO.

The label on capsule reads: 250 mg per capsule.

$$\frac{\text{(D) } 0.5 \text{ g}}{\text{(H) } 250 \text{ mg}} \times \text{(Q) } 1 \text{ capsule} = X$$

$X = 2$ capsules

- Change g to mg in the numerator before working the problem. Numerator and denominator must be in the *same* measurement, and it usually is easier to change the larger quantity (*e.g.,* easier to change the grams in the numerator to milligrams).

$$\frac{0.5 \text{ g}}{250 \text{ mg}} \times 1 \text{ cap} = X$$

$$\frac{500 \text{ mg}}{250 \text{ mg}} \times 1 \text{ cap} = 2 \text{ capsules}$$

TABLE 7-1 APOTHECARY DOSES WITH APPROXIMATE METRIC EQUIVALENTS

	Weight				
Volume	**Grains**		**Milligrams**		**Grams**
1 fl oz = 30 ml	30	=	2000	=	2
½ fl oz = 15 ml	15	=	1000	=	1
2½ fl dr = 10 ml	10	=	600	=	0.6
2 drams = 8 ml	7½	=	500	=	0.5
1¼ drams = 5 ml	5	=	300	=	0.3
1 dram = 4 ml	4	=	250	=	0.25
45 minims = 3 ml	3	=	200	=	0.2
30 minims = 2 ml	2½	=	150	=	0.15
15 minims = 1 ml	2	=	120	=	0.12
12 minims = 0.75 ml	1½	=	100	=	0.1
10 minims = 0.6 ml	1	=	60 or 65	=	0.06 or 0.065
8 minims = 0.5 ml	¾	=	50	=	0.05
5 minims = 0.3 ml	½	=	30	=	0.03
4 minims = 0.25 ml	⅜	=	25	=	0.025
3 minims = 0.2 ml	⅓	=	20	=	0.02
1½ minims = 0.1 ml	¼	=	15	=	0.015
1 minim = 0.06 ml	⅙	=	10	=	0.01
¾ minim = 0.05 ml	⅛	=	8	=	0.008
½ minim = 0.03 ml	1/10	=	6	=	0.006
	1/15	=	4	=	0.004
	1/20	=	3	=	0.003
	1/30	=	2	=	0.002
	1/40	=	1.5	=	0.0015
	1/60	=	1	=	0.001
	1/100	=	0.6	=	0.0006
	1/120	=	0.5	=	0.0005
	1/150	=	0.4	=	0.0004
	1/200	=	0.3	=	0.0003
	1/250	=	0.25	=	0.00025
	1/500	=	0.12	=	0.00012
	1/600	=	0.1	=	0.0001
	1/1000	=	0.06	=	0.00006

Note: 1 ml = approx 1 cc; 1 kilogram = 2.2 pounds (lb); 1 liter = 1000 ml.

Household Equivalents

60 drops (gtt) = 1 teaspoonful (t)

3 teaspoonfuls = 1 tablespoonful (T)

The doctor's order reads: Aspirin gr x, PO.

The label on tablet reads: Aspirin 325 mg.

$$\frac{\text{(D) gr x}}{\text{(H) 325 mg}} \times \text{(Q) 1 tab} = X$$

X = 2 tablets

- This problem contains both the apothecary system and the metric system. Use the conversion table to change the gr to mg *before* working the problem. Remember, the two systems are equivalents, not equals. You will find that gr x = 600 mg. When dividing 325 mg into 600 mg, you must round off the answer to two tablets.

The doctor's order reads: Valium 5 mg, IM.

The label on ampul reads: 10 mg per 2 ml.

$$\frac{\text{(D) 5 mg}}{\text{(H) 10 mg}} \times \text{(Q) 2 ml} = X$$

X = 1 ml or cc

- Don't forget that the quantity is 2 ml when calculating the dose.

PEDIATRIC DRUG DOSAGES

- *There are no average dosages for infants and children.* Safe dosages usually are based on the weight or body surface area of the child.
- The determination of body surface area (BSA) requires the use of a nomogram. West devised a nomogram (Fig. 7-1) to estimate BSA from the height and weight of the child.
- Pediatric drug dosages frequently are expressed in mg/kg. The child's weight in pounds is then converted to kilograms (2.2 lb = 1 kg), and the correct dosage can be determined.

Example

How much oral ampicillin should a 30-lb child receive? Patients under 20 kg: 50 to 100 mg/kg/day at 6- to 8-hour intervals.

To change pounds (lb) to kilograms (kg), divide the pounds by 2.2:

$$\frac{\text{30 lb}}{\text{2.2 kg}} = \text{13.6 kg}$$

To determine mg/day, multiply

13.6 kg × 50 mg = 680 mg
13.6 kg × 100 mg = 1360 mg

The child should receive approximately 680 mg to 1360 mg in 24 hr.

Nomogram for Estimating Surface Area of Infants and Young Children

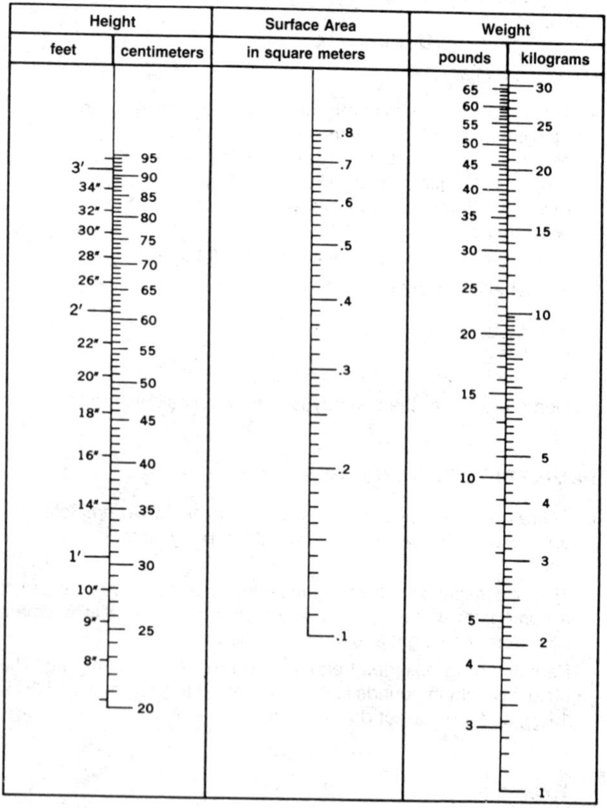

Fig. 7-1. *Nomogram for estimation of surface area. The surface area is indicated where a straight line that connects the height and weight levels intersects the surface area column.*

To determine the 8-hr interval, divide by 3, and to determine the 6-hr interval, divide by 4.

$$\frac{680}{3} = 227 \qquad \frac{1360}{3} = 453 \qquad \frac{680}{4} = 170 \qquad \frac{1360}{4} = 340$$

The child should receive approximately 227 mg to 453 mg every 8 hr, or 170 mg to 340 mg every 6 hr.

- Besides height and weight, factors related to maturation, defects, and disease must be considered when determining drug dosages. Premature infants and newborns have immature enzyme systems in the liver, immaturely functioning kidneys, and lower protein plasma concentrations. They may be unable to metabolize and excrete dosages considered "safe" for their weight or BSA. Any defects or diseases, especially of the liver and kidneys, can alter drug action and safety in children of any age.

CALCULATING INTRAVENOUS FLOW RATES

- Solutions are ordered by the physician in ml per hr, but the nurse regulates flow rates in drops (gtt) per minute.
- The following is the formula needed to convert ml/hr to gtt/min.

$$\text{gtt min (flow rate)} = \text{gtt/ml (calibration of set)} \times \frac{\text{ml/hr}}{60}$$

- The size of the drop varies according to the calibration of the set. Standard or *macrodrip sets* are calibrated at 10 gtt = 1 ml, 15 gtt = 1 ml, or 20 gtt = 1 ml. *Microdrip sets* are calibrated at 60 gtt = 1 ml. This information is found on the package of the IV tubing.

Examples

- Administer an IV at 125 ml/hr, using a set calibrated at 10 gtt/ml.

$$\text{gtt/min} = 10\ \text{gtt/ml} \times \frac{125\ \text{ml/hr}}{60}$$

$$\text{gtt/min} = \frac{125}{6} = 21\ \text{gtt/min}$$

- If tubing calibrated at 10 gtt/min is used consistently, you always will divide the 10 into 60 to get 6. Therefore, you can figure out the flow rate in one step by dividing 6 into the ml/hr.
- Administer an IV at 100 ml/hr, using a microdrip set.

$$\text{gtt/min} = 60\ \text{gtt/ml} \times \frac{100\ \text{ml/hr}}{60}$$

$$\text{gtt/min} = \frac{100}{1} = 100\ \text{gtt/min}$$

- When using microdrip tubing, you always will divide the 60 into 60 to get 1. Therefore, the gtt/min will always *equal* the ml/hr.
- Administer an IV at 3000 ml in 24 hr, using a set calibrated at 15 gtt/ml. First, you must find out how much fluid to give in *one* hour.

$$\frac{3000}{24} = 125\ \text{ml/hr}$$

$$\text{gtt/min} = 15\ \text{gtt/ml} \times \frac{125\ \text{ml/hr}}{60}$$

$$\text{gtt/min} = \frac{125}{4} = 31 \text{ gtt/min}$$

- If the tubing is always calibrated at 15 gtt/ml, you will always divide 15 into 60 to get 4. Therefore, just divide the ml/hr by 4 to get the gtt/min. If you use tubing calibrated at 20 gtt/ml, you simply divide the ml/hr by 3.

DRUG THERAPY

ADMINISTRATION OF MEDICATIONS

Distributing medications is a crucial and often time-consuming responsibility. You *cannot* underestimate the importance of this task. Careless habits or distractions can endanger the safety of your patients.

The following are some facts and safety guidelines to consider. For complete "how to" details, consult a nursing fundamentals textbook.

When administering medications, you aim to achieve either a *local* effect (confined to the site of application) or a *systemic* effect (distributed by the blood and diffused into one or more body tissues), although drugs given for a local effect (*e.g.*, eye drops, skin preparations) can be absorbed by the body and produce systemic effects. To achieve systemic effects, the following routes are used.

- *Oral:* This is the safest, most economical, and most convenient route. There is a slower onset. At times, there are more prolonged but less potent effects than with the parenteral route.
- *Sublingual:* The drug is placed under the patient's tongue and is retained until dissolved and absorbed by way of the venous capillaries. This route prevents drug destruction by the digestive juices and enzymes of the liver.
- *Rectal:* This route is used when the stomach is nonretentive or when the patient is unconscious. The rectum should be free of feces in order to promote optimal absorption.
- *Topical:* Medication applied in a thin, uniform layer to a nonhairy skin surface. Areas commonly used are the chest, abdomen, anterior thigh, and upper arm. Application sites should be rotated to prevent dermal inflammation and sensitization.
- *Parenteral:* This route refers to all forms of drug injection into the body tissues or fluids. Drugs must be sterile and nonirritating. Usually, there is a more rapid onset of action than with the oral route. There are four main categories of parenteral injection.
    1. *Intravenous:* The drug is injected directly into the bloodstream. It is the most rapid acting but least safe. Carefully consider the purpose of the IV when choosing the site and equipment. For

example, emergency situations usually require a large vein and one of the plastic cannulas rather than a butterfly needle. You then are prepared to deliver large volumes of fluid rapidly if this is necessary.

a. *Heparin locks* are a popular means for delivering intermittent IV medications. The butterfly-type needle has a rubber stopper on the end that can receive repeated injections. The vein is kept open by flushing the tubing with a small amount of a dilute heparin preparation after each medication. This allows the patient much greater freedom of movement than the traditional IV setup.

b. *Hickman catheters* are inserted into the external jugular vein by way of a subcutaneous tunnel. Patients receive chemotherapy, TPN, antibiotics, and blood products through this route (see NR, IV therapy).

2. *Intramuscular:* The drug is injected into muscular tissue. Sources differ as to the safe maximum amount to be injected into a single site. Factors to consider are the drug, the site used, and the disease state. An injection of 3 ml is considered safe by most sources. These injections are given at a 90° angle, using a 1-inch to 1½-inch needle with a gauge of 20 to 23 (the larger the gauge, the finer the needle). Sites vary with the age and condition of the patient, as well as the type, purpose, and frequency of the injection (see Figs. 7-2 through 7-6). Sites are chosen to avoid nerves and major blood vessels. The ventrogluteal muscle is often preferable in adults rather than the upper outer quadrant because the injection is further away from the sciatic nerve. When charting the medication, always chart the site given and rotate sites whenever possible.

   a. Some intramuscular injections are given using the Z-track technique (*e.g.*, to administer iron dextran; see Fig. 7-7).
      1. Draw up solution and then change to a fresh needle. Usually a 19- to 20-gauge, 2-inch to 3-inch needle is used.
      2. Draw up 0.5 cc of air into the syringe.
      3. Choose the injection site (*e.g.*, upper outer quadrant of the buttocks) and firmly displace skin, fat, and muscle to one side.
      4. Clean the area, insert the needle, and check for blood return.
      5. Inject the solution slowly, followed by the air in the syringe.
      6. Wait 10 seconds, pull the needle straight out, and release the tissues. Apply direct pressure.

3. *Subcutaneous:* The drug is injected under the layers of the skin. The amount usually ranges from 0.5 to 2 ml in one site. Needle length ranges from ½ to ⅝ inch, with a gauge of 25. Because of the needle length, the injection should be given at a 90° angle. Extremely thin patients may require the 45° angle.

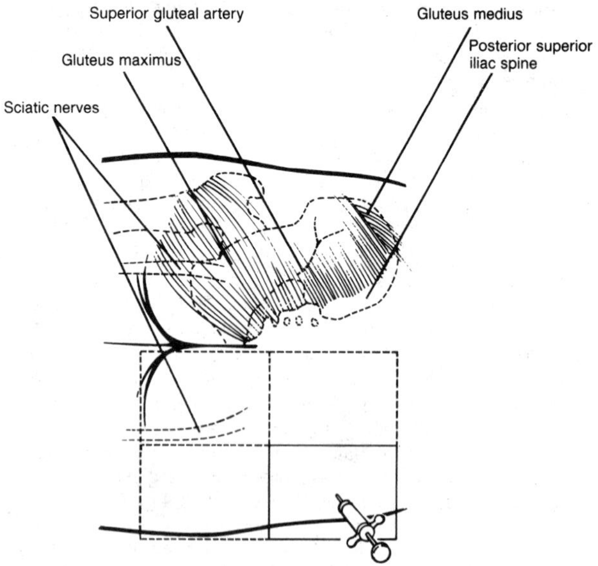

Fig. 7-2. *Dorsogluteal site. Draw an imaginary diagonal line from the greater trochanter of the femur to the posterior superior iliac spine. Inject a site above and outside the diagonal line.*

a. *Hypodermoclysis* is the introduction of large amounts of fluid (500 to 1000 ml) into subcutaneous tissue (*e.g.,* under breasts or upper thighs). It is used for dehydrated patients when IV therapy cannot be done.

4. *Intradermal:* The drug is injected into upper layers of the skin. The amount is small (measured in minims) and absorption is slow. Needle length ranges from ½ to ¾ inch and 26 or 27 gauge. Usually, a 10° to 15° angle is used. This method is used for skin testing for allergic reactions and for administering tuberculosis tests.

Nursing Considerations

- In order to avoid errors, you must concentrate on what you are doing. This means working alone and without interruptions, whenever possible.
- Do not give a medication if you can't read the label; return it to the pharmacy to be relabeled. Many medications are similar in

color and shape. If a patient is being discharged with medications, the pharmacist must relabel them appropriately for home use. Planning ahead for this can avoid delays at discharge time.

- Be sure you have correctly identified your patients. Check their identification bracelets. Some patients (especially if confused) will respond to a name other than their own. Therefore, it is best to ask the patient to tell you his or her name.
- Never chart medications before giving them. Never chart a medication given by another person unless it is clearly stated who administered the drug (*e.g.,* the physician). Chart all medications as soon as possible after giving them, especially prn or STAT drugs. Otherwise, the patient may receive a double dose.
- If a patient has any symptoms of an allergic reaction, report it immediately.

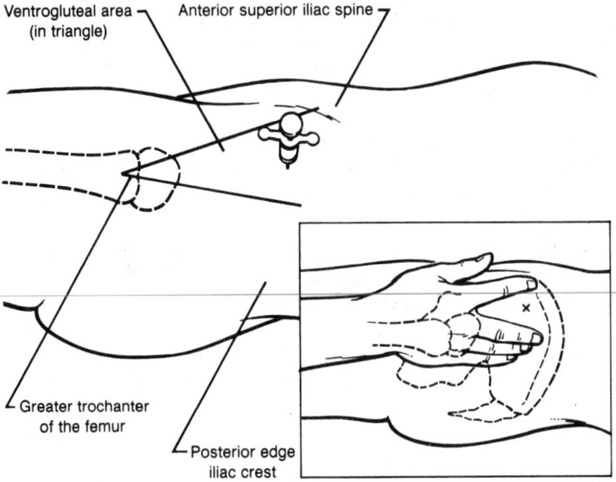

Fig. 7-3. *Ventrogluteal site. Position the patient on his side with his upper knee bent and the leg placed slightly ahead of the bottom leg. This positioning of the legs helps relax the muscle to be injected. Some nurses prefer positioning the patient on his abdomen and having him turn his toes inward, as when injecting the dorsogluteal site. Still others find it convenient to have the patient on his back. Palpate for the greater trochanter at the head of the femur, the anterior superior iliac spine, and the iliac crest. Place your palm on the greater trochanter and your index finger on the anterior superior iliac spine. To locate the proper site, use your right hand when injecting into the patient's left side and your left hand when injecting into the patient's right side. Move your middle finger away from your index finger as far as possible along the iliac crest. Inject the site in the center of the triangle formed by your index and middle fingers.*

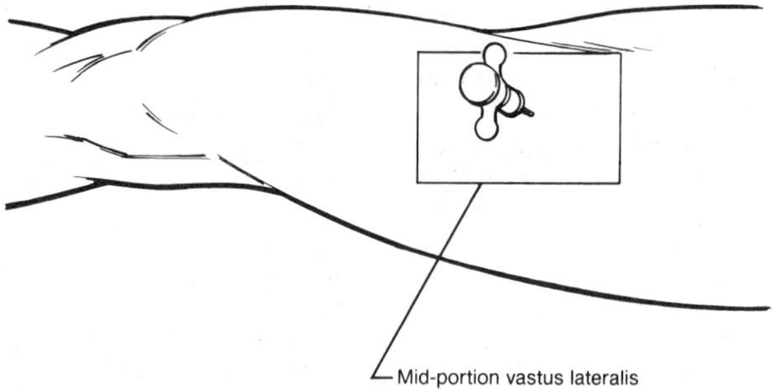

Fig. 7-4. *Vastus-lateralis site. Have the patient lying on his back with the site area well exposed. An injection also can be made in this site satisfactorily when the patient is sitting. Draw these imaginary lines on the thigh: one on the mid-anterior thigh on the front of the leg; one on the mid-lateral thigh on the side; one a hand's breadth below the greater trochanter of the femur; and one a hand's breadth above the knee. Inject a site in the middle of the rectangle you have drawn. The vastus lateralis muscle on the side of the leg is being used more frequently than in the past because it is a thick muscle and there are no large nerves, blood vessels, or joints nearby.*

- If the patient indicates that a drug is different from what he or she has been taking, recheck before giving it. Patients can help you prevent errors too.
- When drugs are omitted intentionally for OR or diagnostic testing, record the omission and the reason on the patient's chart.
- It is very important to maintain therapeutic blood levels of most medications. The physician may want the drug given even if the patient should not eat or drink prior to a diagnostic test. If you have any questions, check with the physician before withholding the drug.
- Report drug errors or omissions immediately, and, for your own protection, fill out an incident report.
- Never give any medication, even a placebo, without a physician's written order. If you are in a position where you must accept phone or verbal orders, be sure the physician signs the order as soon as possible.
- You should have a physician's written order before leaving any medication at a patient's bedside (*e.g.*, nitroglycerin or eye drops).
- When drawing up some medications, double-check your results with another qualified person. When administering such drugs as heparin or insulin, small differences can be crucial to the patient.
- Preparations for internal use should be kept separate from those used externally.

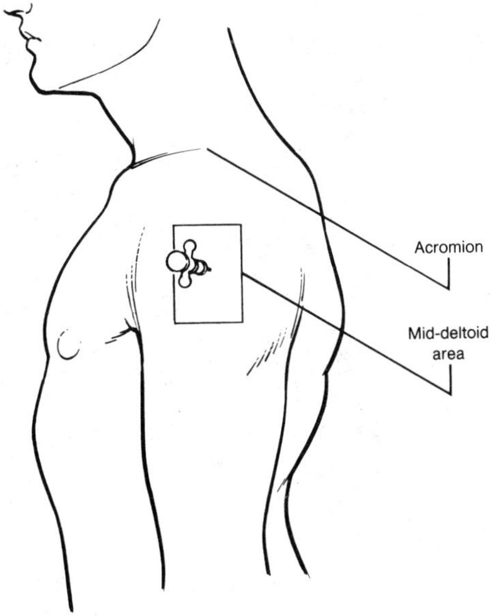

Fig. 7-5. *Deltoid-muscle site. Have the patient lying down, sitting, or standing with the site area well exposed. Draw these imaginary lines: one line along the lower edge of the acromion at the side of the shoulder; one line on the side of the arm opposite the axilla; and two lines parallel to the arm ⅓ and ⅔ around the outer part of the arm. Inject at a site in the center of the rectangle. Bunch the muscle before injecting in order to avoid striking the humerus bone when the patient has a small deltoid muscle. The deltoid muscle is used infrequently because it is a relatively small muscle and only a small amount of solution can be injected comfortably. The muscle should not be used for repeated injections.*

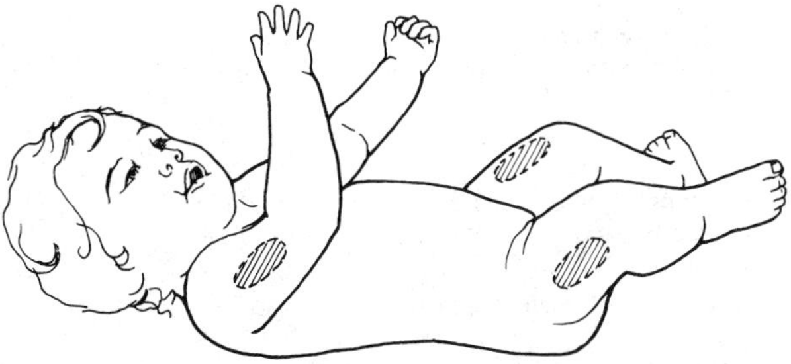

Fig. 7-6. *Injection sites for infants and small children.*

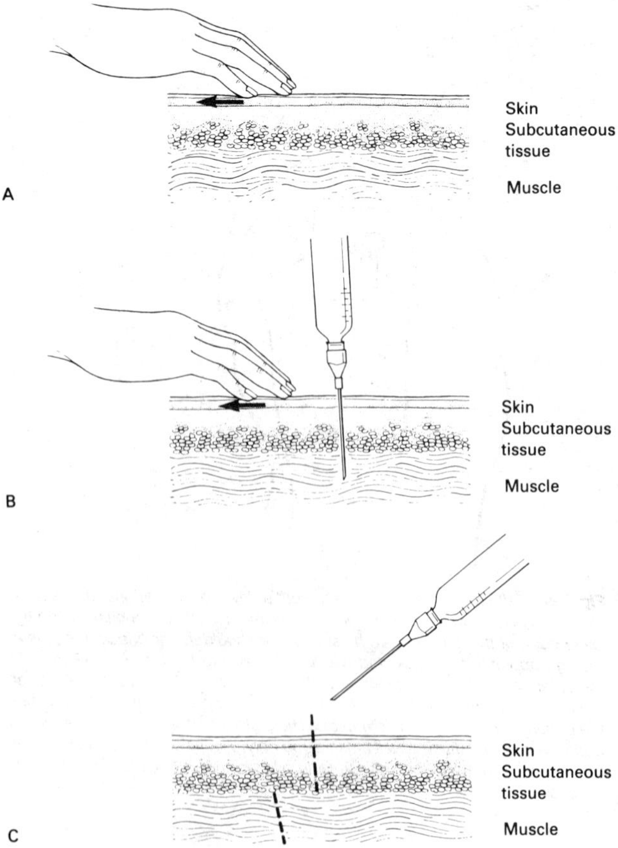

Fig. 7-7. *Z-track technique for injections. Tissue is retracted laterally (A) as needle is inserted (B). After needle is withdrawn (C), tissue returns to normal. The track of needle is thus broken, so medication cannot leak out.*

- Never crush enteric-coated tablets. Your patient may experience gastric irritation, and the effectiveness of the drug may be affected.
- Never divide tablets, suppositories, and so forth, unless they are clearly scored. Return the preparation to the pharmacist and obtain the correct dosage, or have the pharmacist prepare it.
- In order to prevent toxic reactions from some drugs, physicians order measurements of the blood levels of the drug. Timing is

important to ensure accurate results. The blood should be drawn *before* the drug is given, and the nurse is responsible for coordinating drug administration with the laboratory. Examples of drug levels frequently checked are digoxin, gentamicin, heparin, and aminophylline.

- If you feel a medication order is wrong, question it!

PHARMACOKINETICS

Pharmacokinetics refers to the processes by which the body absorbs, distributes, metabolizes, and removes drugs. Also considered are the variables that influence drug action in the body.

- *Absorption:* The drug is transferred from the site of entry to the circulating fluids of the body (*e.g.* blood and lymphatics). Absorption is affected by the following: route of administration (*e.g.,* IV produces immediate absorption), the solubility of the drug and how it is influenced by pH, local conditions at the site of administration (*e.g.,* poor circulation or edema can delay absorption), drug concentration or dosage, and enteric coating.
- *Distribution:* The drug is transferred to its sites of action, metabolism, and excretion. Drugs will diffuse faster to areas of greater blood perfusion (*e.g.,* brain, liver, kidneys). Drugs can combine with plasma proteins and thus remain in the circulating fluids for a longer period of time. Circulatory problems (*e.g.,* atherosclerosis) may slow drug distribution.
- *Biotransformation:* The drug is metabolized, usually in the liver. The drug is converted into products that are generally less active and more easily excreted. The metabolism usually is accomplished by the body's enzyme systems. Factors that depress enzyme function (*e.g.,* hepatic disease or advanced age) will depress metabolism and may allow drugs to accumulate to toxic levels in the body.
- *Excretion:* The drugs, both metabolized and unchanged, leave the body by a variety of routes. Gaseous substances like anesthetics are excreted by way of the lungs. The majority of drugs and drug products are excreted by way of the kidneys.

VARIABLES INFLUENCING DRUG ACTION

- Neonates and elderly patients often have particular problems with drug action because they lack or have diminished enzyme systems.
- The dosage of a drug frequently is calculated on the basis of the ratio of milligrams of the drug to the patient's weight (as expressed in pounds or kilograms).
- Pregnancy is a factor because many drugs easily cross over the placental "barrier" and can cause malformation and other problems in the fetus.

- Sex itself is a variable because body weight, percentage of body fat, and hormonal changes can affect drug action.
- Because of the body's biologic or diurnal rhythms, drugs can be affected by the time of administration. They also may react with food in the stomach.
- Route of administration also may influence drug action.
- Pathologic states, especially of the kidneys and liver, interfere with drug action.
- Genetic differences can produce differences in drug metabolism (usually because of effects on the enzymes).
- A patient's belief in the effectiveness of a drug and the manner in which it is administered can influence drug action.
- Occasionally, a patient's immune system produces antibodies against a drug. Subsequent administration of the drug can produce serious problems for the patient.
- Tolerance, or a decreased physiologic response to repeated administration of a drug, develops in some people.
- Cumulation (drug is excreted more slowly than it is absorbed) can lead to toxic levels of a drug (*e.g.,* digoxin) in the body.
- Interactions between drugs can interfere with the desired effects of a drug. Both prescription and over-the-counter (OTC) medications can cause problems in this manner.

DRUGS AND THE ELDERLY

- The elderly frequently take more medications on a regular basis than other patient populations. This includes both prescription and OTC drugs.
- The elderly are usually at a higher risk for experiencing side-effects because of normal aging changes that can affect drug action. They frequently have one or more acute or chronic illnesses that also can alter drug action. And finally, they are more likely to be taking multiple medications that increase the risk of drug interactions.
- Aging changes can alter sensitivity to drug action. Drug receptor sites may be affected, and the person may experience a decrease in homeostatic mechanisms. However, altered pharmacokinetics appear to cause the main changes in drug action.
- The action of drugs also can be affected by bedrest, dehydration, diet, fever, humidity, malnutrition, stress, and temperature.
- Few references are available that adjust "usual adult dosages" to the particular needs of the elderly population. Standardization would be extremely difficult because two people of the same chronologic age can differ vastly in their biologic age. Medications should be started at lower than "normal" dosages and gradually titrated upward until the desired response is obtained

and adverse effects are controlled or at a minimum. Medication lists should be reviewed frequently by the physician, and all unnecessary drugs should be discontinued.

- It may be very difficult for the elderly individual to keep track of all of his or her medications. Encourage the patient to keep a complete list of all drugs he or she is taking (including OTC preparations) and include the name, dosage, and frequency of administration. Because of specialization and multiple chronic illnesses, an elderly person may have three or four different physicians caring for him or her at the same time. Explain the importance of showing the list to *each* physician.
- When teaching your elderly patients about their medications be aware of the sensory losses that may be present (see EENT, normal aging changes). If you make a list for them to take home, write or print carefully in large script. Taping an example of the medication next to the name may be helpful. Hearing loss may be present. Try to have a quiet environment and sit directly in front of the individual. Discharge from the hospital can be a very stressful event for an elderly person, and teaching done on the morning of discharge may not be retained.
- An elderly person may not consider OTC drugs as medication. When taking a drug history ask specifically about aspirin products, antacids, laxatives, cough and cold remedies, and vitamins.
- OTC medications may be chosen because they are more economical than a visit to the doctor or a prescription medication. They are easily available, which contributes to the belief that they are harmless.
- Particular risks are involved for the elderly individual using OTC preparations. In order to choose a drug, the elderly person must first diagnose his or her own problem. Yet older individuals frequently have atypical reactions to disease and illness. A myocardial infarction can occur without chest pain and confusion may be the presenting symptom of a pneumonia. Both pneumonia and sepsis can exist without a significant rise in temperature. Use of OTC medications can delay the treatment of a serious infection or illness.
- Financial difficulties may interfere with appropriate, safe use of medication. An elderly individual may need assistance in requesting the generic form of his medications. As with all age groups, older persons must be encouraged to discard leftover drugs and not to share these drugs with family members and friends.

ABSORPTION

- Most drugs are absorbed by passive diffusion, which appears to be unchanged by the aging process. The mucosa in the aging intestine may actually be less of a barrier to drugs than that of a younger person.

- Absorption of drugs in the elderly may be delayed or reduced for the following reasons:
  1. Decreased fluid volume and decreased gastric acidity may influence pH and affect the solubility of the drugs.
  2. Decreased peristalsis and gastric emptying could increase local gastric adverse effects.
  3. There may be decreased blood flow to the intestine.
  4. Concurrent administration of other drugs or food may have an effect.

DISTRIBUTION

- The elderly may experience a decrease in plasma proteins to bind with drugs. Both kidney and liver disease may further decrease plasma proteins.
- Increased levels of unbound drugs can enhance drug action and lead to an increase in adverse reactions and toxicity.
- The blood–brain barrier may become more permeable in the elderly, increasing the chance of central nervous system toxicity.
- A decreased cardiac output, increased circulation time, and cardiovascular disease also will alter distribution.
- Multiple drug use may affect distribution by altering the protein binding. Drugs may compete for binding sites, and some drugs may be capable of displacing others. Again, the elderly may be left with increased amounts of free drug and the increased risk of toxicity.

BIOTRANSFORMATION

- Aging changes may depress enzyme function and metabolism in the elderly.
- Decreased blood flow to the liver (*e.g.*, from congestive heart failure) may reduce the rate of metabolism.
- Vitamin deficiency may alter enzyme activity.
- Drugs themselves may either increase or decrease enzyme activity, and again we are concerned with a population that frequently uses multiple drugs.

EXCRETION

- With aging there is a reduction in blood flow to the kidneys and, therefore, a reduction in the glomerular filtration rate. There also may be a reduction in the number of functioning tubules.
- Renal impairment is increased by arteriosclerosis, infections, and hypertension.

DRUGS AND PEDIATRICS

- Drug dosages must be determined carefully and are based on the growth and maturation of the infant or child (see PH, Mathematics of dosage).
- Only a fine line separates therapeutic levels from toxic levels in certain drugs. Besides basing dosages on weight or BSA, the prepared drug should be double-checked by another professional before it is administered. Digoxin, heparin, and insulin are examples of such drugs.
- Consult with parents about the child's capabilities and about the way they administer medication to the child at home.
- Approach the child firmly and positively. Give an explanation appropriate to his level of understanding that includes what you are going to do and what you expect of him.
- When possible, allow choices, but not ones that lead to delaying or refusing the medication. Choice of type of cup or whether the child will hold it are appropriate.
- When administration of the medication involves pain (as an injection), a second person may be helpful and necessary. He or she can provide distraction, security, and assistance in restraining the child.
- A child should be allowed to express his or her feelings and to receive the message that crying is permissible and acceptable. A small reward, such as a colorful sticker, can help the child experience a feeling of achievement from a distasteful situation.
- Most oral medications for children come in liquid form for ease of administration. Suspensions must be mixed thoroughly before administration.
- Honey, jam, syrups, and baby fruits are useful for disguising the taste of disagreeably flavored medications. They should not be mixed in milk, orange juice, or other essential foods.
- The most accurate means of measuring small amounts of oral liquid medication is the syringe (with the needle removed), and the medication can be placed directly in the child's mouth.

ANTIMICROBIALS

Actions

- Antimicrobials exert either *bacteriostatic* or *bactericidal* activity (or a combination of both). Bacteriostatic drugs inhibit the growth of the organism, allowing the person's own defense mechanisms to function. Bactericidal drugs actually kill the organism. Antimicrobials can exert their activity in one of several ways:

1. Synthesis of bacterial cell walls is inhibited.
2. Utilization of substances needed for growth and reproduction is reduced (antimetabolites).
3. The permeability of the cell wall is altered so that essential components may leak out.
4. Protein synthesis is impaired, and genetic information is misread by the cells.

- The action of an antimicrobial is designated as either *narrow spectrum* or *broad spectrum.*
  1. Narrow-spectrum drugs are effective against only a few microorganisms.
  2. Broad-spectrum drugs are effective against a wide variety of microorganisms.
- The action of antimicrobials is complemented by the person's own defense mechanisms (*e.g.,* antibody production and phagocytosis).

Indications

- Antimicrobials are indicated when the problem is caused by a pathogen that will respond to these drugs, especially when the person's own defense mechanisms are depleted. Few drugs are effective against common viral diseases (*e.g.,* colds), and treatment with antimicrobials usually is not indicated in these cases.
- At times, antimicrobials are indicated to prevent infection (*e.g.,* recurrences of rheumatic fever or bacterial endocarditis). Because of the wide variety of antimicrobials available, proper drug selection is crucial. The pathogen causing the infection must be identified. Specimens for culture must be obtained carefully (see LAB, Cultures).
- Certain drugs are known to be effective against certain pathogens. Otherwise, sensitivity testing is done to determine the sensitivity of the infecting pathogen to different antimicrobial agents (see LAB, Cultures).

Adverse Effects, Contraindications

- *Allergic reactions:* These can affect the skin, organs, blood, and bone marrow. These reactions range from simple skin rashes to anaphylactic shock.
- *Lack of selective toxicity* (the antimicrobials will exert their bacteriostatic and bactericidal activities on normal cells as well as on the pathogens): the kidneys, liver, nervous tissue, bone marrow, or gastrointestinal tract are frequently affected.

- *Superinfections:* The patient's own protective bacteria may be eliminated by the antimicrobials, allowing pathogens to grow where they normally would be restrained. The superinfection can be much more dangerous to the patient than the original problem.

Dosage and Administration

- It is extremely important that the antimicrobials be administered in high enough doses and for the proper duration. Otherwise, the infection may recur as a chronic problem, and resistance to the antimicrobial may develop. Although the patient may feel better, he or she must be counseled to finish the entire prescription.
- Resistance also may be delayed or prevented by using two or more antimicrobials at the same time.
- Always check to determine whether or not the antimicrobial should be given with food.

Nursing Considerations

- Be alert for any changes in your patient's condition or behavior in order to identify any allergic reactions or toxic effects that may be occurring. Further administration of the drug could greatly intensify the reaction. Withhold the medication and notify the physician *immediately* if you suspect a reaction.
- Because allergic reactions are relatively common with antimicrobials, obtaining a complete drug history is crucial.
- Some antimicrobials, especially the liquid preparations for children, contain additives for coloring and flavoring. The additives, rather than the medication itself, may cause adverse effects (*e.g.*, CNS stimulation).
- Cultures must be obtained *before* the antimicrobial therapy is begun for accurate results. If therapy cannot be delayed until culture results are returned, a broad-spectrum antimicrobial is used.

AMINOGLYCOSIDES

Actions

- These drugs are both bacteriostatic and bactericidal.
- They cause a misreading of genetic information, thereby altering protein synthesis in the bacteria.

Indications

- These are used mainly to treat severe infections caused by gram-negative bacteria (*e.g.*, bacteremia, meningitis, peritonitis, urinary infections).

- These drugs usually are not indicated to treat gram-positive infections (although they are effective) because less toxic antimicrobials are available.

Adverse Effects, Contraindications

- Ototoxicity—damage to the eighth cranial nerve—may occur and cause permanent deafness and ataxia. Damage is most likely when the medication is given parenterally, but also can occur with oral and topical preparations.
- Nephrotoxicity, or damage to the kidneys, may result. Again, damage is most likely to occur with the parenteral forms given in long-term therapy.
- If the patient has received a neuromuscular-blocking drug (*e.g.*, during surgery), skeletal muscle paralysis can occur.
- Resistance to these drugs develops easily, especially when administered topically.

Dosage, Administration, and Nursing Considerations

- See Table 7-2
- Baseline testing of renal function and eighth cranial nerve function should be done before starting therapy.
- Question patients about ringing in the ears, vertigo, dizziness, and persistent, severe headache. Patients on long-term therapy should have periodic hearing tests.
- Perform laboratory determinations of renal function. Creatinine clearance rates are a good indication of the kidneys' ability to eliminate the drugs (see LAB).
- Do not administer aminoglycosides with other drugs that are nephrotoxic (*e.g.*, polymixins, potent diuretics) or ototoxic (furosemide, edecrin).
- See PH, Antimicrobials, Nursing Considerations.

ANTIFUNGALS

AMPHOTERICIN B (FUNGIZONE)

Actions

- This is a systemic antifungal agent.
- This antimicrobial is both fungistatic and fungicidal.

Indications

- It is used parenterally to treat serious systemic fungal infections (*e.g.*, histoplasmosis or blastomycosis).

- It may be used topically on the skin, nails, and mucous membranes of the mouth to treat infections caused by candidal species.

Adverse Effects and Contraindications

- Intravenous administration frequently causes chills, fever, vomiting, and headache. Rapid IV administration can produce cardiac arrest.
- Kidney and liver toxicity and anemia may occur.
- Severe hypotension and electrolyte imbalances can result.
- Allergic reactions from topical application are infrequent.
- Ototoxicity and blurred vision are possible.

Dosage and Administration

- *Adult and Pediatric:* Initially, 0.25 mg/kg/day, IV, may be given. Increase gradually to 1 mg/kg/day, IV, up to a maximum of 1.5 mg/kg/day.
- Topical: Use 3% cream, lotion, or ointment, and rub well to affected area, bid to qid.

Nursing Considerations

- Intravenous solutions should be used as soon as possible after preparation and should be protected from light.
- Alkalinization of the urine will promote excretion of the drug and thereby help prevent toxic reactions.
- The patient's blood count and kidney and liver function should be monitored closely during therapy (see LAB).
- Concurrent administration of antipyretics, antihistamines, and antiemetics may decrease adverse reactions.
- Amphotericin should not be mixed with other drugs.
- Observe IV site closely for signs of irritation and extravasation.
- Duration of therapy may extend from 6 weeks to 10 weeks up to as long as 9 months to 11 months.

GRISEOFULVIN MICROSIZE (FULVICIN-U/F, GRISACTIN) AND GRISEOFULVIN ULTRAMICROSIZE (FULVICIN P/G, GRIS-PEG)

Actions

- This is a fungistatic drug that binds with keratin and is deposited in diseased hair, nails, and epidermis. New growth of the fungi is prevented.

(*Text continues on page 659*)

TABLE 7-2 AMINOGLYCOSIDES

Drug	Dosage and Administration	Nursing Considerations
Amikacin sulfate (Amikin)	*Adults and Pediatric:* 5 mg/kg every 8 hr, or 7.5 mg/kg every 12 hr, IM or IV; duration of therapy: 7 to 10 days; maximum dosage: 15 mg/kg/day *Neonates:* Initially 10 mg/kg, then 7.5 mg/kg every 12 hr IV infusion administered over a 30- to 60-minute period (infants over a 1- to 2-hr period)	This has broadest range of antimicrobial activity of the aminoglycosides. It is used primarily to treat serious nosocomial gram-negative infections resistant to tobramycin and gentamicin.
Gentamicin sulfate (Garamycin)	*Adults:* 3 to 5 mg/kg/day in three equal doses every 8 hr, IM or IV *Pediatric:* 6 to 7.5 mg/kg/day in three equal doses every 8 hr, IM or IV *Infants and Neonates:* 7.5 mg/kg/day in three equal doses every 8 hr, IM or IV *Premature or less than 1 week:* 5mg/kg/day in two equal doses every 12 hr, IM or IV *Topical:* 0.1% cream or ointment three or four times daily *Ophthalmic solution:* 0.3%, 1 or 2 gtt in affected eye every 4 hr	This is used most frequently to treat serious urinary tract infections, meningitis, and septicemia. Because of the synergistic activity that occurs, gentamicin is combined with ampicillin to treat endocarditis, and with carbenicillin to destroy the *Pseudomonas* bacteria. Gentamicin may be used topically to treat both skin and eye infections. Frequently, gentamicin blood levels are drawn to determine the effectiveness and toxicity of the drug. Blood should

	Ophthalmic ointment: 0.3%, small amount in lower conjunctival sac, two or three times daily	be drawn 0.5 to 1 hr *before* the next dose is administered. Frequency of administration may be reduced to every 12, 18, 24, 36, or 48 hr if kidney function is compromised. Duration of therapy is usually 7 to 10 days.
Kanamycin (Kantrex)	*Adults* 1. Preoperative intestinal preparation: 1 g every 4 hr orally for four doses, then every 6 hr for 36 to 72 hr 2. Intestinal infections: 3 to 4 g/day in divided doses for 5 to 7 days 3. Hepatic coma: 8 to 12 g/day in divided doses 4. *IM:* 15 mg/kg/day in two to four equally divided and spaced doses (maximum 1.5 g) 5. *IV:* maximum 15 mg/kg/day in two to three equal doses *Pediatric* 1. Intestinal infections: 50 mg/kg/day in four to six equally divided doses 2. *IM* and *IV:* same as adult	The parenteral form is used mainly in *short-term* therapy in severe systemic infections (*e.g.,* septicemia, gram-negative urinary infections, some pneumonias). The oral form is used to control infections in the gastrointestinal tract and to destroy normal intestinal flora prior to surgery and in the management of hepatic coma. Ototoxicity from parenteral administration can occur as early as day 5 of therapy. Do not administer with other ototoxic drugs (*e.g.,* potent diuretics).

(continued)

TABLE 7-2 AMINOGLYCOSIDES

Drug	Dosage and Administration	Nursing Considerations
Neomycin sulfate (Myciguent)	*Adults* 1. Preoperative intestinal preparation: 1 g every hour orally, four times, then 1 g every 4 hr for the rest of the 24 hr 2. Hepatic coma: 4 to 12 g/day, orally, in four divided doses for 5 or 6 days 3. Diarrhea: 50 mg/kg/day, orally, in four divided doses for 2 or 3 days 4. Topical: 5 mg/g, ointment or cream *Pediatric* 1. Preoperative intestinal preparation: 10.3 mg/kg, orally, every 4 hr for 3 days 2. Hepatic coma: 437.5 mg to 1.225 g/M^2 every 6 hr for 5 or 6 days 3. Diarrhea: 8.75 mg/kg every 6 hr for 2 or 3 days	This drug *seldom* is used systemically because of its toxicity. It is used orally to suppress the normal bacterial flora of the bowel in hepatic coma and prior to abdominal surgery. It also may be used to treat some types of infectious diarrhea. Topically, it is used to prevent and treat skin infections and, in solution, to irrigate urinary bladders of patients with indwelling catheters. Nausea, vomiting, and diarrhea occur frequently with oral administration. A reversible malabsorption syndrome is a rare occurrence. Overgrowths of bacteria and fungi may cause superinfections. Do not give to patients with large ulcers or intestinal obstruction because of the danger of systemic absorption. Neomycin easily reaches toxic levels in patients with impaired kidney function. Topical administration can lead to hypersensitivity reactions (*e.g.*, skin rashes).

Paromomycin sulfate (Humatin)	*Adults* 1. Intestinal amebiasis: 25 to 35 mg/kg/day, orally, divided in three doses for 5 to 10 days 2. Hepatic coma: 4 g/day, orally, in divided doses for 5 or 6 days *Pediatric:* intestinal amebiasis, same as for adults	The drug is used orally to suppress the normal bacterial flora of the bowel in hepatic coma and prior to abdominal surgery. It also is used to treat acute and chronic intestinal amebiasis and tapeworm.
Streptomycin sulfate	*Adults* 1. Tuberculosis: Up to 1 g/day, IM, used with other drugs. When sputum is negative, it may be stopped or reduced to 1 g, 2 or 3 times/week 2. Other diseases: 1 to 4 g/day, IM, in divided doses every 6 to 12 hr *Pediatric:* 20 to 40 mg/kg/day, IM, in divided doses	It is used mainly with other antitubercular drugs in the treatment of tuberculosis, especially for patients with large lung cavities or for extrapulmonary tuberculosis. It may be combined with other antimicrobials to treat urinary tract infections, nocardiosis, and tularemia. Vertigo is the most frequent side-effect. Optic and peripheral nerves occasionally are affected. Allergic reactions (*e.g.,* skin eruptions) occur in both patients receiving the drug and persons administering it. Blood dyscrasias can develop. Patients with compromised kidney function are susceptible to kidney damage.

(continued)

TABLE 7-2 AMINOGLYCOSIDES

Drug	Dosage and Administration	Nursing Considerations
Tobramycin sulfate (Nebcin)	*Adults:* 3 mg/kg/day, IM or IV, in three equal doses every 8 hr Life-threatening infections: up to 5 mg/kg/day, IM or IV, in three or four equal doses *Pediatric:* 6 to 7.5 mg/kg/day in three to four equal divided doses (2 to 2.5 mg/kg every 8 hr, or 1.5 to 1.9 mg/kg every 6 hr) *Neonates* (1 week or less): maximum of 4 mg/kg/day, IM or IV, every 12 hr *Impaired renal function:* initially 1 mg/kg/day	This drug is used to treat severe infections caused by susceptible organisms. For IV infusion, dilute in 50 to 100 ml of 0.9% NS or 5% DW (less volume for children) and administer in 20 to 60 minutes.

(Continued from page 653)

Indications

- It is used to treat tinea (ringworm) infections of the skin, hair, and nails (*e.g.*, tinea pedis—athlete's foot; tinea capitis—scalp ringworm; tinea cruris—groin ringworm; and tinea unguium—nail fungi).
- It is more effective for chronic fungal infections.
- The drug should not be used for systemic fungal infections.

Adverse Effects and Contraindications

- Skin rashes and photosensitivity reactions may occur.
- Headache (severity usually decreases during the course of therapy), dizziness, and mental confusion are possible.
- Oral thrush can result from monilial overgrowths.
- The leukopenia that can occur usually reverses itself during the course of therapy.
- Patients with liver damage or acute porphyria should not receive this drug.

Dosage and Administration

- *Adults:* Administer 250 to 500 mg of ultramicrosize or 500 mg to 1 g of microsize, orally per day. It frequently is given in divided doses at 6-hr intervals.
- *Pediatric:* The usual dosage is 5 mg ultramicrosize or 10 mg microsize/kg/day.

Nursing Considerations

- Milk and other fatty foods enhance absorption of the drug.
- This drug antagonizes warfarin anticoagulants, and it may be necessary to increase the dosage of the anticoagulant.
- Barbiturates antagonize griseofulvin, and the dosage of the antimicrobial may need to be increased.
- Patients should be encouraged to shampoo their hair and cut their hair and nails frequently *to assist the drug therapy.*
- Blood counts and renal and hepatic function tests should be done periodically (see LAB).
- Giving the drug after meals may prevent gastrointestinal problems.
- Duration of therapy may range from several weeks to several months.

MICONAZOLE NITRATE (MICATIN, MONISTAT)

Actions

- This drug is a fungicidal against *Candida albicans* and similar species.

Indications

- It is used topically to treat vulvovaginal candidiasis, tinea pedis, tinea cruris, tinea corporis, and tinea versicolor.
- Parenterally, it is used to treat severe systemic fungal infections (*e.g.*, coccidioidomycosis, candidiasis).
- Bladder instillations are used to treat susceptible urinary tract infections.

Adverse Effects and Contraindications

- Tachycardia and cardiac arrhythmias can occur from rapid IV injection.
- Localized burning, itching, and irritation may occur.
- Pelvic cramps, hives, and headaches have been reported.
- IV use also has produced nausea, vomiting, diarrhea, and thrombocytopenia.

Dosage and Administration

- *Adult:* Usually, 200 to 3600 mg/day, IV, is divided into three infusions.
- *Pediatric:* Administer 20 to 40 mg/kg/day, IV, in divided doses.
- Intravaginal: Use 1 applicator/day in vagina at bedtime for 7 days. This may be repeated if necessary.
- Topical: Cover affected area morning and evening.
- Bladder instillation: Instill 200 ml of a 10 mg/200 ml solution.

Nursing Considerations

- Infections caused by dermatophytes (tineas) may require about 1 week of treatment. Tinea pedis (athlete's foot) usually is treated for 1 month.
- IV administration should be over 30 to 60 minutes. The drug is diluted in at least 200 ml of 5% DW or 0.9% NS.

NYSTATIN (MYCOSTATIN, NILSTAT)

Actions

- This is both fungistatic and fungicidal against a wide variety of yeasts and yeastlike fungi.

Indications

- It is used topically to treat monilial infections of the skin, mucous membranes of the mouth (thrush), and the vagina.
- Orally, it is used to prevent superinfections (from increased fungi of the intestine) when tetracyclines or other broad-spectrum antimicrobials are taken. High-risk patients (*e.g.,* diabetic patients or patients on steroids or antineoplastic drugs) may benefit from this type of prophylactic use.

Adverse Effects and Contraindications

- Diarrhea and epigastric distress may occur after large oral doses.
- Hypersensitivity reactions to topical application are rare.

Dosage and Administration

- *Adults*
  1. 500,000 to 1,000,000 units of the oral tablet, tid
  2. 400,000 to 600,000 units of the oral suspension, qid
  3. One to two vaginal tablets (100,000 units each) deposited high in the vagina
  4. Topical cream, ointment, and powder available containing 100,000 u/g
- *Pediatric:* 400,000 to 600,000 units of oral suspension, qid
- *Infants:* 200,000 units, qid
- *Premature and low birth weight:* 100,000 units, qid

Nursing Considerations

- Nystatin should be kept in light-resistant containers.
- Fixed dosage combinations (nystatin and another antibiotic contained in the same tablet or capsule) usually are not as effective in preventing intestinal moniliasis as when the drugs are taken separately because the dosage of nystatin is too small.
- The drug is available in combination with corticosteroids (Myconef, Mycolog, Florotic) and tetracycline (Terrastatin).

CEPHALOSPORINS

Actions

- These drugs are bactericidal and interfere with bacterial cell-wall synthesis.

Indications

- They may be used to treat infections from many gram-positive cocci and gram-negative bacilli because they have a broad-spectrum of activity.

- However, the penicillins are usually the first choice in treating gram-positive infections because they are safer and less expensive (see PH, Penicillins).
- One advantage that cephalosporins have over many of the penicillins is that they are not inactivated by penicillinase (an enzyme that destroys some penicillins). But they are inactivated by cephalosporinase—a closely related enzyme.

Adverse Effects and Contraindications

- A positive Coombs' test may develop when large doses are given, and hemolytic anemia can occur.
- Reversible renal tubular necrosis has occurred.
- Pain and sterile abscesses at injection sites may result; also, thrombophlebitis may occur following IV administration.
- Skin rashes may occur in patients with a history of penicillin allergy.

Dosage, Administration, and Nursing Considerations

- See Table 7-3.
- At times, cephalosporins are used to treat infections when the patient is allergic to the penicillins. However, these drugs are similar in chemical structure to penicillin, and it is possible that the patient could be cross-sensitive. Observe the patient very carefully for adverse effects.
- Anaphylactic reactions to cephalosporins are rare.
- For long-term therapy, for use of large doses, or for patients with impaired kidney function, blood counts should be monitored.
- Cephalosporins may produce false-positive glucose determinations when certain agents are used for urine testing (*e.g.*, Clinitest).
- Watch carefully for superinfections (black tongue, sore mouth, vaginal or rectal itching, loose stools, vaginal discharge).
- Therapy for beta-hemolytic streptococcal infections should continue for at least 10 days as a precaution against development of rheumatic fever.

CHLORAMPHENICOL (CHLOROMYCETIN, CHLOROPTIC, OPHTHOCHLOR)

Actions

- The drug is primarily bacteriostatic, but it may be bactericidal in certain species or at higher concentrations.
- It interfers with protein synthesis of bacterial ribosomes.

(*Text continues on page 668*)

TABLE 7-3 CEPHALOSPORINS

Drug	Dosage and Administration	Nursing Considerations
Cefaclor (Ceclor)	*Adults*: 250 to 500 mg, orally, every 8 hr, up to a maximum of 4 g daily *Pediatric*: 20 to 40 mg/kg/day, orally, in divided doses every 8 hr, up to a maximum of 1 g daily	This drug treats infections of the upper and lower respiratory tract, urinary tract, and skin. It is also effective for otitis media caused by *Hemophilus influenzae, Escherichia coli, Proteus mirabilis.*
Cefadroxil (Duricef, Ultracef)	1 to 2 g, orally, in single dose or every 12 hr Doses for patients with renal impairment—modified according to creatinine clearance	This drug treats urinary tract infections caused by *E. coli, P. mirabilis,* and *Klebsiella.* It is used to treat skin infections caused by staphylococci and streptococci. It is effective against Group A beta-hemolytic streptococcal pharyngitis. Nausea is the most frequent side-effect and can be diminished by giving the drug with food.
Cefamandole nafate (Mandol)	*Adults*: 500 mg to 1 g, IM or IV, every 4 to 8 hr; for life-threatening infections, up to 2 g, IV, every 4 hr *Pediatric*: 50 to 100 mg/kg/day, IM or IV, in divided doses every 4 to 8 hr up to a maximum of 150 mg/kg/day, but not to exceed the maximum adult dose	This treats serious infections of the respiratory, biliary, and urinary tracts, skin, bones and joints, peritonitis, and septicemia.

PH

(continued)

TABLE 7-3 CEPHALOSPORINS

Drug	Dosage and Administration	Nursing Considerations
Cefazolin sodium (Ancef, Kefzol)	*Adults:* 250 mg to 1.5 g, IM or IV, every 6 to 8 hr, depending on the severity of infection, up to a maximum of 12 g/day Gonorrhea: 2 g, IM, with 1 g probenecid *Pediatric:* 25 to 50 mg/kg/day, IM or IV, divided into three or four equal doses, up to a maximim of 100 mg/kg/day Patients with renal impairment: dosage adjustments based on BUN and creatinine clearance	This is used to treat severe infections of the urinary and biliary tracts, skin, and bone. It may be used for bacteremia and endocarditis. Also, it is given prophylactically before high-risk surgeries (*e.g.*, open-heart). With probenecid, it treats uncomplicated gonorrhea in pregnant patients allergic to the penicillins.
Cefotaxime sodium (Claforan)	*Adult:* 1 g, IM or IV, every 6 to 8 hr *Perioperative:* 1 g, IV, 30 to 90 min preoperatively, during surgery, and within 2 hr following surgery *Pediatric (1 month to 12 years)* 1. Less than 50 kg: 50 to 180 mg/kg/day, IM or IV, divided into four to six equal doses 2. 50 kg or more: usual adult dose 3. *Neonates (birth to 1 month)* 0–1 week: 50 mg/kg, IV, every 12 hr 1–4 weeks: 50 mg/kg, IV, every 8 hr Maximum daily dose: 12g	This drug treats serious infections of the lower respiratory and genitourinary tracts, skin, bones and joints, and central nervous system. It also is used to treat bacteremia/septicemia, and peritonitis. It also may be given perioperatively for high-risk surgeries. Most common adverse effects have been local reactions following IM or IV injection.

Cefoxitin sodium (Mefoxin)	*Adults:* 1 to 2 g, IM or IV, every 6 to 8 hr, up to a maximum of 12 g/day *Gonorrhea:* 2 g, IM, with 1 g probenecid *Perioperative:* 2 g, 30 to 60 min preoperatively, and 2 g every 6 hr for 24 hr *Pediatric (3 months and older):* 80 to 160 mg/kg/day, IM or IV, divided into four to six equal doses, up to a maximum of 12 g/day *Perioperative:* 30 to 40 mg/kg, IM or IV, at the same intervals as for adults	This treats serious infections of the genitourinary tract, lower respiratory tract, skin, bones and joints, septicemia, and peritonitis. It may be given prophylactically before high-risk surgery. It is used to treat penicillinase-producing *Neisseria gonorrhoeae* (PPNG) and gonococcal infections resistant to penicillin or tetracycline.
Ceftizoxime sodium (Cefizox)	*Adults:* 1 or 2 g every 8 to 12 hr (up to a maximum of 12 g/day). Reduced dosages for patients with impaired renal function	This treats infections of the lower respiratory tract, urinary tract, intra-abdomen, skin and skin structures, bones and joints. It also is used for septicemia and uncomplicated gonorrhea.
Cefuroxime sodium (Zinacef)	*Adults:* 750 mg to 1.5 g, IM or IV, every 8 hr up to a maximum of 9 g/day *Gonorrhea:* 1.5 g, IM, with 1 g probenecid *Perioperative:* 1.5 g, IV, 30 to 60 min preoperatively, and 750 mg every 8 hr if procedure is prolonged *Pediatric (3 months and older):* 50 to 100 mg/kg/day divided every 6–8 hr	This drug treats serious infections of the genitourinary tract, lower respiratory tract, skin, septicemia, and meningitis.

(continued)

TABLE 7-3 CEPHALOSPORINS

Drug	Dosage and Administration	Nursing Considerations
Cephalexin (Keflex)	*Adults:* 1 to 4 g, orally, daily in divided doses *Pediatric:* 25 to 50 mg/kg/day in four equally divided doses	This is used for follow-up therapy for patients treated with parenteral cephalosporins. It treats respiratory and urinary tract infections. It is used for infections of the middle ear, skin, soft tissue, and bone. Oral suspensions and pediatric drops (100 mg/ml) should be refrigerated after reconstitution.
Cephalothin sodium (Keflin, Neutral)	*Adults:* 500 mg to 1 g, IM or IV, every 4 to 6 hr, up to a maximum of 12 g/day *Perioperative:* 1 to 2 g, IV, 30 to 60 min preoperatively, during surgery, and every 6 hr for 24 hr *Intraperitoneal:* up to 6 mg/100 ml of dialysis fluid *Pediatric:* 80 to 160 mg/kg/day, IM or IV, in divided doses	This treats severe infections of the gastrointestinal, urinary, and respiratory tracts, bones, joints, soft tissue, and skin. It also is used to treat septicemia, endocarditis, and meningitis. It may be given prophylactically before high-risk surgery. It is used intraperitoneally for bacterial peritonitis. IM injection is not recommended because it causes intense pain and induration.

Cephapirin sodium (Cefadyl)	*Adults:* 500 mg to 1 g, IM or IV, every 4 to 6 hr, up to a maximum of 12 g/day *Impaired renal function:* 7.5 to 15 mg/kg every 12 hr *Pediatric (over 3 months):* 40 to 80 mg/kg/day, IM or IV, in four equally divided doses	This treats serious infections of the respiratory and urinary tracts, and the skin. It also is used for osteomyelitis, septicemia, and endocarditis.
Cephradine (Anspor, Velosef)	*Adults:* 250 to 500 mg, orally, every 6 hr or 500 mg to 1 g orally every 12 hr, up to a maximum of 6 g/day *IM or IV:* 500 mg to 1 g every 6 hr, up to a maximum of 8 g/day *Pediatric (over 1 yr):* 6.25 to 25 mg/kg, orally, every 6 hr in divided doses, up to a maximum of 4 g/day *IM or IV:* 12.5 to 25 mg every 6 hr up to a maximum of 8 g/day	This treats serious infections of the urinary and respiratory tracts, skin, and otitis media. Oral cephradine is not destroyed by gastric acid, and food may delay absorption.

(*Continued from page 662*)

Indications

- It is used to treat severe infections when other antibiotics are ineffective or are contraindicated.
- It is effective against *Salmonella, H. influenzae,* Rocky Mountain spotted fever, *Chlamydia,* and *Mycoplasma.*
- Regimens for patients with cystic fibrosis include this drug, and it also is used topically for skin, eye, and external auditory canal infections.

Adverse Effects and Contraindications

- Chloramphenicol should not be used prophylactically, for the treatment of minor infections, or with other drugs that produce bone marrow depression.
- Use cautiously in patients with impaired liver or kidney function, with intermittent porphyria, or in children.
- Bone marrow depression may be dose related and reversible (*e.g.,* leukopenia, thrombocytopenia, reduced Hgb anemia) or non-dose related and irreversible (*e.g.,* agranulocytosis, aplastic anemia, leukemia).
- Nausea, vomiting, and diarrhea may occur.
- Optic neuritis and optic nerve atrophy have been reported.
- Headache, depression, and mental confusion are possible.

Dosage and Administration

- *Adults:* 12.5 mg/kg every 6 hr, IV (sodium succinate preparation); 50 mg/kg/day orally in four equally divided doses every 6 hr, up to a maximum of 100 mg/kg/day
- *Pediatric:* 50 mg/kg/day, orally, in four equally divided doses every 6 hr
  1. Full-term infants over 2 weeks old: up to 50 mg/kg/day, orally, in four equally divided doses
  2. Infants up to 2 weeks old and children with immature metabolic function: 25 mg/kg/day, orally, in four equally divided doses
- Topical cream: 1% rubbed into affected area three or four times/day after cleansing
- Ophthalmic ointment: 1%, small strip in lower conjunctival sac every 3 to 6 hr
- Ophthalmic solution: (0.16, 0.25, 0.5%) 1 or 2 gtt every 1 hr to 6 hr
- Otic solution: 0.5%, 2 or 3 gtt in affected ear, tid, at 6- to 8-hr intervals

Nursing Considerations

- Take with a full glass of water at least 1 hr before or 2 hr after a meal.
- Baseline CBC, platelets, serum iron, and reticulocytes should be done prior to therapy and repeated periodically during therapy.
- Monitor patients carefully for signs of sore throat, fever, fatigue, unusual bruising, and any evidence of superinfection.

CLINDAMYCIN HYDROCHLORIDE (CLEOCIN HYDROCHLORIDE)

Actions

- This drug suppresses bacterial protein synthesis by binding to bacterial ribosomes.

Indications

- It is used to treat serious infections when less toxic alteratives cannot be used.
- It is effective against some anaerobic streptococci and aerobic gram-positive cocci.
- Topical preparations are used for acne vulgaris.

Adverse Effects and Contraindications

- Abdominal pain, nausea, vomiting, and diarrhea have occurred. In some cases, the diarrhea has progressed to a severe colitis, which may be fatal.
- Hypersensitivity reactions such as mild to moderate skin rashes are the most frequently reported adverse reactions. Rarely, anaphylactoid reactions and erythema multiforme have occurred.
- Blood dyscrasias, jaundice, and abnormal liver function test results are possible.
- Use cautiously for patients with a history of kidney, liver, or gastrointestinal disease. Patients with a history of regional enteritis or ulcerative colitis should not use clindamycin.

Dosage and Administration

- *Adults:* 150 to 450 mg, orally, every 6 hr
  1. Clindamycin phosphate: 300 to 600 mg, IM or IV, every 6 to 8 hr, up to 2700 mg/day
- *Pediatric (over 1 month old):* 8 to 25 mg/kg/day, orally, divided into three or four equal doses (Clindamycin Palmitate Hydrochloride, Cleocin Pediatric)

2. *IM or IV:* 15 to 40 mg/kg/day divided into three or four equal doses, or 350 to 450 mg/M^2/day

- Topical: apply twice daily

Nursing Considerations

- Clindamycin capsules should be taken with a full glass of water.
- Intravenous infusion should not exceed 1200 mg/hr. The concentration should be 6 mg/ml or less, and run in no faster than 30 mg/minute.
- Hypotension has occurred following IM injections.
- Severe diarrhea or colitis can occur several weeks after therapy has stopped. Observe for watery stools, or blood, pus, or mucus in the stools.

ERYTHROMYCINS

Actions

- Erythromycin can be either bacteriostatic or bactericidal, depending on the size of the dose and the infecting pathogen. It interferes with protein synthesis.

Indications

- It is a safe substitute for penicillin in patients who are allergic to it.
- It is effective against gram-positive cocci and is used to treat problems such as streptococcal pharyngitis, pneumococcal pneumonia and meningitis, and subacute bacterial endocarditis.
- Because the incidence of toxicity is very low, erythromycin frequently is given to children.
- It also is used for some gram-negative urinary tract infections when the urine is kept alkaline (by administering sodium bicarbonate).

Adverse Effects and Contraindications

- Occasionally it causes nausea, vomiting, diarrhea, abdominal discomfort, and cramps.
- The estolate ester of erythromycin has produced an allergic hepatitis characterized by jaundice, fever, and abdominal pain.
- Skin and other hypersensitivity reactions have occurred.
- Superinfection by resistant bacteria and fungi can develop. The drug is then discontinued.

- Patients with impaired liver function or a history of hepatic disease should use erythromycin preparations cautiously.

Dosage, Administration, and Nursing Considerations

- See Table 7-4
- Patients on long-term therapy, especially those receiving the estolate, should have periodic tests of liver function.
- The erythromycin base usually is administered before meals. The acid-resistant coatings keep the drug from being inactivated.

LINCOMYCIN HYDROCHLORIDE (LINCOCIN)

Actions

- This drug is bacteriostatic or bactericidal, depending on the concentration and sensitivity of the organism.
- It suppresses bacterial protein synthesis.

Indications

- It is used for serious infections (caused by gram-positive pathogens, and some anaerobes) in patients allergic or resistant to the penicillins.

Adverse Effects and Contraindications

- Patients sensitive to clindamycin, those with untreated monilial infections, and those with impaired liver function should not receive this drug.
- Use cautiously for patients with respiratory, gastrointestinal, or renal disease.
- Diarrhea occurs frequently, and acute colitis or pseudomembranous colitis may occur up to several weeks after therapy with lincomycin. Encourage patients to report changes in bowel frequency and elevated temperature.
- Glossitis, stomatitis, nausea, and vomiting may occur.
- Blood dyscrasias and skin rashes have been reported.
- Rare instances of hypotension and cardiac arrest have occurred after too rapid intravenous infusion.

Dosage and Administration

- *Adults*
  1. 500 mg, orally, every 6 to 8 hr
  2. 600 mg, IM, every 12 to 24 hr
  3. 600 mg to 1 g, IV, every 8 to 12 hr

TABLE 7-4 ERYTHROMYCINS

Drug	Dosage and Administration	Nursing Considerations
Erythromycin (E-Mycin, Erythrocin)	*Adults:* 250 mg, orally, every 6 hr (range, 1 to 4 g/day) *Pediatric:* 30 to 50 mg/kg/day, orally, in four equally divided doses (The dosage may be doubled for more severe infections.) Ophthalmic ointment 5 mg/g: Apply 1 or more times daily. Topical ointment 1% to 2%: Apply bid or tid.	Absorption is best when taken on an empty stomach. However, the drug may be taken with meals to help prevent GI side-effects.
Erythromycin estolate (Ilosone)	*Adults:* 250 mg, orally, every 6 hr (up to 4 g or more/day) *Pediatric:* 30 to 50 mg/kg/day, orally, in divided doses (The dosage may be doubled for more severe infections.)	It is available in tablets, chewable tablets, capsules, drops, and suspension. Observe carefully for cholestatic hepatitis syndrome (malaise, nausea, vomiting, abdominal cramps, jaundice, fever, and headache).
Erythromycin ethylsuccinate (E.E.S., E-Mycin, Pediamycin)	*Adults:* 400 mg, orally, every 6 hr (up to 4 g or more/day); may give 100 mg, IM, at 4- to 8-hr intervals (5 to 8 mg/kg/day) *Pediatric:* 30 to 50 mg/kg/day, orally, in four equally divided doses (The dosage may be doubled for more severe infections.)	Oral forms are available as tablets, chewable tablets, and suspension. Patients 2 years of age or older can take this drug without regard to meals.

Erythromycin gluceptate (Ilotycin Gluceptate)	*Adults and Pediatric:* 15 to 20 mg/kg/day IV; up to 4 g/day for severe infections Continuous infusion is preferable. It also may be administered intermittently over 20 to 60 minutes, usually at 6-hr intervals.	Thrombophlebitis has been associated with infusion of large doses. Tests of hearing and hepatic function are recommended.
Erythromycin lactobionate (Erythrocin Lactobionate—I.V.)	*Adults and Pediatric:* 15 to 20 mg/kg/day IV; up to 4 g/day may be given for severe infections. Continuous infusion is preferable. It may also be administered intermittently over 20 to 60 minutes, usually at 6-hr intervals.	Large IV doses have been associated with hearing difficulty and thrombophlebitis at the site. Tests of hepatic function are advised for patients on long-term therapy.
Erythromycin stearate (Erythrocin Stearate, SK-Erythromycin)	*Adults:* 250 mg, orally, every 6 hr, up to 4 g/day or more *Pediatric:* 30 to 50 mg/kg/day, orally, in four equally divided doses. (The dosage may be doubled for more severe infections.)	Optimum blood levels are achieved when the drug is given on an empty stomach.

PH

- *Pediatric (over 1 month)*
  1. 30 to 60 mg/kg, orally, divided into three or four equal doses
  2. 10 mg/kg, IM, every 12 to 24 hr
  3. 10 to 20 mg/kg/day, IV, divided equally and infused every 8 to 12 hr
- The maximum recommended dose is 8 g.

Nursing Considerations

- One gram of Lincocin IV should be diluted in at least 100 ml of D_5W and infused over a period of at least 1 hr.
- Drug should be stopped immediately if diarrhea develops.
- Absorption is best when the oral preparation is taken on an empty stomach.

PENICILLINS

Actions

- The penicillins are bactericidal drugs that inhibit the synthesis of the bacterial cell wall.
- Because the cell walls of the bacteria differ from those of mammalian cells, the penicillins exhibit a high degree of selective toxicity (*e.g.,* they are not toxic to the human cells).

Indications

- See Table 7-5

Adverse Effects and Contraindications

- Allergic or hypersensitivity reactions are very common with the penicillins. They range from all types of skin eruptions and rashes to *anaphylactic shock.*
- Diarrhea, nausea, and vomiting may occur.
- Phlebitis and thrombophlebitis have resulted from intravenous administration of the penicillins.
- Muscular twitching or convulsions may result from large doses.
- Intravenous forms of penicillin are either sodium or potassium salts. When large doses are used, electrolyte imbalances can occur. Particular care should be used if the patient's kidney function is impaired.

Dosage, Administration, and Nursing Considerations

- See Table 7-5
- Taking a complete drug history of the patient is of crucial importance because of the high incidence of allergic reactions.

- Most forms of oral penicillin are affected by gastric acid. (Penicillin V Potassium, USP, Pen-Vee-K is an exception.) Therefore, most oral penicillins should be given at least 1 hour before meals or 2 to 3 hours after meals.
- The kidneys efficiently filter out, excrete, and secrete the penicillins into the tubules. Probenecid (Benemid) blocks the secretion of the penicillin into the tubules and keeps the drug in the blood and tissues for longer periods.
- Intravenous forms of penicillin can be very irritating to the veins and can cause phlebitis and thrombophlebitis. The medication should be well diluted and run in slowly.
- Carbenicillin and gentamicin frequently are used together to fight serious infections. The two drugs should never be mixed together because they may inactivate each other.

POLYMYXINS

Actions

- These are bactericidal drugs that bind to lipid phosphates in bacterial membranes. The change in permeability permits leakage of cytoplasm.

Indications

- They are used to treat severe acute infections of the bloodstream, meninges, and urinary tract caused by gram-negative organisms.
- Topically, and in combination with other drugs, polymixins treat superficial infections of the eye, ear, mucous membrane, and skin.

Adverse Effects and Contraindications

- Neurotoxicity occurs, especially in patients with impaired renal function. Dizziness, ataxia, paresthesias, dysphasia, ototoxicity, convulsions, and coma are possible.
- Neuromuscular blockage with respiratory depression or arrest has occurred with the first dose, and as long as 45 days after therapy has been started.
- Nephrotoxicity is usually reversible but may progress even after drug has been discontinued.
- Topical use may cause local irritation and burning.
- Intramuscular injections can cause severe pain and thrombophlebitis may occur at the intravenous site.
- Use cautiously in patients with impaired kidney function and myasthenia gravis.

(*Text continues on page 683*)

TABLE 7-5 PENICILLINS

Drug	Indications	Dosage and Administration	Nursing Considerations
Amoxicillin (Amoxil, Polymox, Trimox, Wymox)	Same as those for ampicillin	*Adults and Pediatric (over 20 kg):* 250 to 500 mg, orally, every 8 hr Gonorrhea: 3 g (with 1 g probenecid) *Pediatric (under 20 kg):* 20 to 40 mg/kg/day, orally, in equally divided doses every 8 hr	Amoxicillin may be given without regard to meals. Unused portions of the reconstituted suspension must be discarded after 14 days. It is inactivated by penicillinase. It produces higher serum levels than ampicillin and is more expensive.
Ampicillin (Omnipen, Polycillin) Ampicillin sodium (Omnipen-N, Polycillin-N)	Broad-spectrum antibiotic effective against streptococcal, staphylococcal, pneumococcal, and meningococcal organisms Also, treatment of some strains of gonorrhea, syphilis, hemophilus, *E. coli, Proteus, Salmonella,* and *Shigella* For prophylaxis of bacterial endocarditis	*Adults and Pediatric (over 20 kg):* 250 to 500 mg, orally, every 6 hr *Pediatric (under 20 kg):* 50 to 100 mg/kg/day in equally divided doses at 6- to 8-hr intervals *Ampicillin sodium* 1. *Adults and Pediatric (over 40 kg):* 250 to 500 mg, IM or IV, every 6 hr 2. *Pediatric (under 40 kg):* 25 to 50 mg/kg/day in equally divided doses every 6 to 8 hr *Gonorrheal urethritis:* 500 mg, IM or IV, at 8- to 12-hr intervals, × 2	Food hampers absorption of the drug. Unused portions of the reconstituted suspension must be discarded after 14 days. Rashes must be carefully inspected to determine if they are nonallergic or a hypersensitivity reaction. Superinfections are common. Observe for black, furry tongue, oral lesions, and rectal or vaginal itching and discharge. If diarrhea occurs, drug-induced colitis must be ruled out. It is inactivated by penicillinase.
Azlocillin sodium (Azlin)	Same as those for ampicillin Primarily indicated to treat strains of *Pseudomonas* that are resistant to other broad-spectrum penicillins (*e.g.,* in respiratory and urinary tracts, bones and joints, skin, and septicemia)	*Adults:* for serious infections, 200–300 mg/kg/day, IV, in four to six divided doses (usually 3 g every 4 hr), up to a maximum of 24 g/day	It is inactivated by penicillinase. It frequently is used with an aminoglycoside to destroy *Pseudomonas.* Therapy continues for 10–14 days, but difficult infections (*e.g.,* osteomyelitis) may require longer treatment.

			The drug usually is mixed in 50 to 100 ml of a compatible IV solution and administered piggyback over 30 minutes.
Bacampicillin hydrochloride (Spectrobid)	Same as those for ampicillin	*Adults and Pediatric (over 25 kg):* 400 mg, orally, every 12 hr; severe infections: 800 mg every 12 hr; acute gonorrhea: 1.6 g orally with 1 g probenecid	It is inactivated by penicillinase. It may be given without regard to food.
Carbenicillin disodium (Geopen)	Derived from penicillin G, but has a broader range of antibacterial activity Especially effective against gram-negative infections from *Pseudomonas, Proteus, E. coli, N. gonorrhoeae*	*Adults:* 1 to 2 g, IM or IV, every 6 hr 1. Serious infections: 200 mg/kg/day, IV 2. Severe systemic infections: 300 to 500 mg/kg/day, IV 3. Gonorrhea: 4 g, IM, divided between two sites with 1 g probenecid orally 30 min before injection 4. Maximum: 40 g/day *Pediatric:* 1. Urinary tract infections: 50 to 200 mg/kg/day, IM or IV 2. Severe systemic infections: 400 to 600 mg/kg/day, IV 3. Infants under 1 week old: 200 mg/kg/day in divided doses every 12 hr, over 1 week old; 300 to 400 mg/kg/day in divided doses every 6 to 8 hr	Patients with impaired renal function are susceptible to both neurotoxicity and nephrotoxicity. Bleeding tendency may occur 12 to 24 hr after therapy is started. Observe patients closely, especially if kidney dysfunction is present. Each gram of carbenicillin contains approximately 5.2 to 6.5 mEq of sodium. Observe closely for electrolyte imbalances.

(continued)

TABLE 7-5 PENICILLINS

Drug	Indications	Dosage and Administration	Nursing Considerations
Carbenicillin indanyl sodium (Geocillin)	Similar to those for carbenicillin disodium, but not used in systemic infections Prostatitis and acute and chronic infections of the urinary tract caused by gram-negative organisms	One to two tablets (382 to 764 mg), orally, every 6 hr	It is best taken with a full glass of water on an empty stomach. Each gram of the drug contains approximately 1 mEq sodium. Observe for electrolyte imbalances. Patients may not tolerate the drug because of nausea, unpleasant taste, dry mouth, and furry tongue.
Cloxacillin sodium (Cloxapen, Tegopen)	Used primarily to treat infections caused by penicillinase-producing staphylococci and penicillin-resistant staphylococci	*Adults and Pediatric (over 20 kg):* 250 to 500 mg, orally, every 6 hr *Pediatric (under 20 kg):* 12.5 to 25 mg/kg, orally, every 6 hr	Food hampers drug absorption. The oral reconstituted solution is stable if refrigerated for 14 days.
Cyclacillin (Cyclapen-W)	Same as those for ampicillin	*Adults:* 250 to 500 mg, orally, every 6 hr *Pediatric (over 20 kg):* 250 mg orally every 6 hr; *(under 20 kg):* 125 mg orally every 6 hr, up to a maximum of 2 g/day.	Absorption is slower when food is present. After reconstitution, the suspension is stable for 14 days if refrigerated.
Dicloxacillin (Dynapen, Veracillin)	Used primarily to treat infections caused by penicillinase-producing staphylococci and penicillin-resistant staphylococci	*Adults and Pediatric (over 40 kg);* 125 to 250 mg, orally, every 6 hr *Pediatric (under 40 kg):* 3 to 6 mg/kg, orally, every 6 hr	Food reduces drug absorption. After reconstitution, suspension is stable for 14 days if refrigerated.

Methicillin sodium (Celbenin, Staphcillin)	Used primarily to treat infections caused by penicillinase-producing staphylococci	*Adults:* 1 g every 4 to 6 hr, IM; 1 g every 6 hr, IV, in 0.9% sodium chloride at 10 ml/min *Pediatric:* 25 mg/kg, IM, every 6 hr	Patients may experience interstitial nephritis 2 to 4 weeks after starting therapy. Observe for fever, anorexia, oliguria, hematuria, and cloudy urine.
Mezlocillin sodium (Mezlin)	Broad-spectrum antibiotic active against many gram-negative and gram-positive organisms, both aerobic and anaerobic Treats susceptible respiratory, urinary, skin, gynecologic, and abdominal infections, and septicemia	*Adults:* depending on severity of infection, 200 to 300 mg/kg, IV, divided in equal doses every 4 to 6 hr; also may be given IM; up to maximum of 24 g/day *Pediatric* 1. One month to 12 years: 50 mg/kg, IM or IV, every 4 hr (300 mg/kg/day) 2. Dosage for newborns—based on age and weight	One gram of mezlocillin is mixed in 50 to 100 ml of D_5W or 0.9% NS and infused piggyback over a period of 30 minutes.
Nafcillin sodium (Nafcil, Unipen)	Primarily used to treat infections caused by penicillinase-producing staphylococci	*Adults* 1. 250 mg to 1 g every 4 to 6 hr, orally 2. 500 mg every 4–6 hr, IM 3. 500 mg to 1 g every 4 hr, IV *Pediatric* 1. 25 to 50 mg/kg/day in four divided doses, orally 2. 25 mg/kg, bid, IM 3. 50 mg/kg/day in four equally divided doses, IV *Neonates* 1. 10 mg/kg, orally, tid or qid 2. 10 mg/kg, IM, bid	Food interferes with absorption of oral nafcillin. IV injection should be made directly into the vein or into the tubing of a running IV infusion. Dilute with 15 to 30 ml of sterile water or isotonic sodium chloride for injection and give over a 5- to 10-min period. Nafcillin contains approximately 3 mEq of sodium per gram.

(continued)

TABLE 7-5 PENICILLINS

Drug	Indications	Dosage and Administration	Nursing Considerations
Oxacillin sodium (Prostaphlin, Bactocil)	Same as those for dicloxacillin	*Adult and Pediatric (over 40 kg):* 250 mg to 1 g every 4 to 6 hr, PO, IM, or IV; for severe infections up to 20 g/day, IM or IV *Pediatric (under 40 kg):* 50 to 100 mg/kg every 6 hr, PO, IM, or IV	Oral oxacillin should be given with a full glass of water on an empty stomach. Oral solution is stable for 14 days after reconstitution if refrigerated. Each gram of oxacillin contains approximately 3.1 mEq of sodium. Observe for hepatic dysfunction with IV oxacillin.
Penicillin G potassium (Aqueous penicillin G, K-Cillin, Penicillin G) Penicillin G sodium	Used to treat streptococcal infections such as acute pharyngitis, tonsillitis, scarlet fever, and subacute bacterial endocarditis Also used in patients on a prophylactic basis if they have mitral valve disease and will be undergoing such procedures as dental extractions or surgery, or cystoscopy Used to treat *staphylococcal* infections, but only after the laboratory has indicated that the organism is more sensitive to it than to one of the other types of penicillins	*Adults and Pediatric (over 12 yr)* 1. 200,000 to 500,000 u, orally, every 6 to 8 hr 2. One to 20 million u daily, IM or IV (up to 80 million u/day for serious infections) *Pediatric (under 12 yr):* 1. 25,000 to 90,000 u/kg/day, orally, in three to six divided doses 2. 50,000 to 250,000 u/kg/day, IM or IV, in four to six divided doses	It is inactivated by penicillinase. Penicillin G potassium contains approximately 1.7 mEq of potassium and 0.3 mEq of sodium/million units. Penicillin G sodium contains approximately 2 mEq of sodium/million units. Oral penicillin should be taken on an empty stomach. Allergy to penicillin is unpredictable and severe hypersensitivity reactions may occur rapidly. Observe patients carefully, especially when using parenteral preparations. It can inhibit platelet aggregation, and patients should be observed for bleeding.

	Pneumococcal pneumonia responds to penicillin G, especially if treatment is begun early. Usually, the IM route is used (penicillin G procaine) *Meningococcal meningitis* responds to large doses given intravenously. Although resistant strains of gonorrhea have developed, penicillin G is still effective when given in large doses (4.8 million units of penicillin G procaine given IM, usually divided into two or more sites). It also is used to treat syphilis.		
Penicillin G benzathine (Bicillin, Permapen)	Same as those for Penicillin G potassium Used in the prophylaxis of rheumatic fever	*Adults and Pediatric (over 12 yr)* 1. 400,000 to 600,000 u, orally, every 4 to 6 hr 2. 1.2 to 2.4 million u, IM, as a single dose Rheumatic fever prophylaxis: 1.2 million units IM monthly *Pediatric (under 12 yr)* 1. 25,000 to 90,000 u/kg/day, orally, in three to six equally divided doses 2. 600,000 to 1.2 million units, IM, as a single dose, to 1.2 million units monthly	Because this drug is absorbed so slowly after IM injection, there is a great risk of severe and prolonged reactions. Select IM sites with great care and aspirate *carefully* to be sure you are not giving the medication in a vein. Arterial occlusion and cardiac arrest have occurred.

PH

(continued)

TABLE 7-5 PENICILLINS

Drug	Indications	Dosage and Administration	Nursing Considerations
Penicillin G procaine suspension (Duracillin A.S., Wycillin)	Same as those for penicillin G potassium when low but prolonged concentrations are effective (*e.g.*, uncomplicated pneumonia, gonorrhea, and syphilis)	*Adults:* 600,000 to 1.2 million units, IM, daily Uncomplicated gonorrhea: 4.8 million units, IM, divided into two injection sites with 1 g probenecid orally 30 minutes before injection Syphilis: 600,000 u, IM, daily for 8 to 15 days *Pediatric:* 500,000 to 1 million u/M^2/day, IM	Procaine reduces the pain of the injection, but some patients are sensitive to it. Inadvertent IV injection has resulted in death. Aspirate carefully.
Penicillin V (V-Cillin) Penicillin V potassium (Penicillin VK, Pen-Vee-K)	Treats mild to moderate infections caused by streptococci, pneumococci, and staphylococci	*Adults and Pediatric (over 12 yr):* 125 to 500 mg, orally, every 6 to 8 hr *Pediatric (under 12 yr):* 15 to 50 mg/kg/day, orally, in three to six equally divided doses	It is inactivated by penicillinase. Each 125 mg = 200,000 units. Food may enhance absorption.
Ticarcillin disodium (Ticar)	Treats serious systemic infections, especially those caused by gram-negative organisms (*e.g.*, *Pseudomonas, Proteus,* and *E. coli*)	*Adults and Pediatric (over 40 kg):* 150 to 300 mg/kg/day, IV, in divided doses every 3, 4, or 6 hr *Pediatric (under 40 kg):* 150 to 200 mg/kg/day in divided doses every 4 to 6 hr *Neonates (over 2 kg):* 100 mg/kg, IM, or as a 10- to 20-minute IV infusion initially, then 75 mg/kg every 4 hr	Gentamycin or tobramycin exhibits synergistic action with ticarcillin for certain strains of *Pseudomonas.* However, they cannot be mixed in the same infusion fluid. It may be given IM but should not exceed 2 g per injection site. Infusions should run from 30 min to 2 hr. It can inhibit platelet aggregation, and patients should be observed for bleeding.

Dosage, Administration, and Nursing Considerations

- See Table 7-6.
- Before initiating parenteral therapy, electrolytes and renal function studies should be done. They should be monitored at regular intervals during therapy.
- Renal toxicity may occur even with therapeutic doses. Urine output should be maintained at 1500 ml in 24 hr.
- Other nephrotoxic and neurotoxic drugs should not be used concurrently.

SULFONAMIDES

Actions

- When administered in the usual dosage range, these drugs are primarily bacteriostatic.
- They prevent bacterial cells from using one of the B complex vitamins, para-aminobenzoic acid (PABA), that inhibits the formation of folic acid. Therefore, the bacteria cannot grow and reproduce.
- These drugs may be divided according to the duration of their action: short acting, intermediate, long acting, and ultralong acting.

Indications

Because more effective bactericidal drugs are available (*e.g.*, penicillins and aminoglycosides), the sulfonamides are not used frequently to treat common infections. Sensitivity testing should be done because many organisms have become resistant to the sulfonamides. However, they continue to be useful when patients are allergic to the first-choice antibiotics and in the following conditions:

- Acute and chronic urinary tract infections (UTI) caused by gram-negative bacteria *(e.g., E. coli)*: usually, a short-acting sulfonamide (*e.g.,* sulfisoxazole) is used to treat uncomplicated acute UTIs, and an intermediate-acting sulfonamide (*e.g.,* sulfamethoxazole with trimethoprim) may be used for chronic UTIs.
- Sulfamethoxazole with trimethoprim is used for patients with chronic obstructive pulmonary disease (COPD) when they develop infections of the respiratory tract and, at times, to prevent these infections.
- Patients with a history of rheumatic fever who are allergic to penicillin use sulfisoxazole to prevent recurrences of the rheumatic fever.
- Ulcerative colitis may be treated with sulfasalazine. It also is used to prevent relapses.

TABLE 7-6 POLYMYXINS

Drug	Dosage and Administration	Nursing Considerations
Colistimethate sodium (Coly-mycin M Parenteral)	*Adults and Pediatric:* 2.5 to 5 mg/kg/day divided into two to four doses, IM or IV Direct intermittent IV: ½ daily dose given over 3 to 5 minutes every 12 hr Continuous IV infusion: ½ daily dose given over 3 to 5 minutes; add the remaining half to the compatible solution and give 1 to 2 hr after the initial dose at the rate of 5 to 6 mg/hr.	Severe, resistant, acute and chronic urinary tract infections caused by some gram-negative organisms may respond to colistimethate.
Colistin sulfate, polymyxin E (Coly-Mycin S for Oral Suspension)	*Pediatric:* 5 to 15 mg/kg/day, orally, divided into three doses at 8-hr intervals Each 5 ml of suspension contains 25 mg of colistin base.	It is used to treat diarrhea in infants and children. It is available with hydrocortisone and neomycin (Coly-Mycin S Otic) for treatment of ear infections.

Polymyxin B sulfate (Aerosporin)	*Adults and Pediatric:* 25,000 to 30,000 u/kg/day, IM, in divided doses; 15,000 to 25,000 u/kg/day, IV, divided and given every 12 hr *Infants:* up to 40,000 u/kg/day, IM or IV *Intrathecal:* over 2 yr of age, give 50,000 u daily for 3 to 4 days, then qod for at least 2 weeks after negative CSF cultures. For children under 2 yr of age, give 20,000 units, qd, for 3 or 4 days, followed by 25,000 u, qod, for at least 2 weeks after negative CSF cultures. *Ophthalmic:* 1 to 3 gtt of 0.1% to 0.25% (10,000 to 25,000 u)/ml every hr, gradually increasing dosage intervals *Otic:* 3 or 4 gtt in affected ear, tid or qid	This drug is available with neomycin and hydrocortisone (Cortisporin); with neomycin (Statrol Ophthalmic); with neomycin and gramicidin (Neosporin); with lidocaine (Lidosporin Otic); with oxytetracycline (Terramycin w/Polymixin B Sulfate); and with bacitracin zinc (Polysporin).

- Occasionally, they are used to treat *Shigella* and *Salmonella* infections, but sensitivity testing must be done because many strains are now resistant to the sulfonamides.
- Topical preparations, silver sulfadiazine and mafenide acetate, are used adjunctly in the treatment of severe burns. The purpose is to prevent local sepsis and septicemia from such organisms as *Staphylococcus, Streptococcus,* and *Pseudomonas.*
- Sulfonamides may be combined with other drugs to treat malaria, nocardiosis, actinomycosis, and histoplasmosis.
- Some strains of gonorrhea and chancroid are sensitive to the sulfonamides.

Adverse Effects and Contraindications

- Nausea, vomiting, and abdominal discomfort are the most frequent side-effects.
- Crystalluria (especially from the long-acting sulfonamides) can result in hematuria, oliguria, anuria, and uremia. This precipitation of crystals of the drug out of the urine in the kidneys is less frequent now because many of the available preparations are highly soluble in acid urine.
- Rarely, blood dyscrasias occur (*e.g.,* agranulocytosis, thrombocytopenia, aplastic anemia, and hemolytic anemia).
- Allergic reactions range from skin rashes and eruptions to anaphylactic shock. Drug fever and Stevens-Johnson syndrome have occurred.
- Some patients may become photosensitive.
- Mafenide acetate, when applied to burns covering over 50% of the body surface, may cause metabolic acidosis. Toxic reactions and subsequent damage can involve almost every organ and system in the body.
- These drugs should be used cautiously for patients with impaired kidney or liver function and in those with blood dyscrasias.
- Pregnant women near term, nursing mothers, and infants less than one month old should not receive sulfonamides.

Dosage, Administration, and Nursing Considerations

- See Table 7-7.

- Although crystalluria occurs less frequently now, the patient should be instructed to force fluids while taking sulfonamides. Urine output should be measured, and the patient should take enough fluids to produce a minimum of 1200 ml of urine in 24 hr.
- Observe the patient for skin and mucosal blisters with bleeding centers that could indicate the development of Stevens-Johnson syndrome.

- Monitor the patient for clinical indications of blood dyscrasia (*e.g.*, rash, sore throat, purpura, paleness, jaundice).
- Patients receiving a sulfonamide with phenazopyridine (*e.g.*, *Azo-Gantrisin)* should be informed that their urine will become orange-red in color.
- When the sulfonamides are given with other drugs that also deplete the bacteria's sources of folic acid, a synergistic effect occurs that increases the antibacterial activity. Trimethoprim is such a drug. Bactrim and Septra are commonly used combinations.
- Sulfonamides and some oral hypoglycemics (the sulfonylurea type) interact and can cause severe hypoglycemia.
- Sulfonamides potentiate *oral anticoagulants* and may produce hemorrhage.

TETRACYCLINES

Actions

- When administered in the usual dosage range, these drugs are primarily bacteriostatic.

Indications

Because many tetracycline-resistant bacteria have emerged, these broad-spectrum drugs are generally not the first choice for treating common bacterial infections. However, when sensitivity studies indicate that the tetracyclines are effective, and if the patient is sensitive to the penicillins, these drugs may be used. They also are used to treat the following:

- They are recommended for prevention of acute respiratory infections in patients with chronic obstructive pulmonary disease (COPD) (see MSN, Respiratory).
- The tetracyclines are effective for treating "viral" pneumonia caused by *Mycoplasma pneumoniae*. (This organism is not a true virus.)
- Common urinary tract and venereal infections may be sensitive to the tetracyclines. However, these drugs are especially useful for treating the chlamydiae infections (*e.g.*, lymphogranuloma venereum; psittacosis—parrot fever; and trachoma—a chronic eye infection).
- Rickettsial diseases such as Rocky Mountain fever and typhus respond to the tetracyclines. (Usually, large doses are given IV.)
- Cholera and brucellosis can be treated effectively with these drugs.
- They are used systemically and topically to treat acne.
- Eye infections may be treated with the tetracyclines.

TABLE 7-7 SULFONAMIDES

Drug	Dosage and Administration	Nursing Considerations
Mafenide acetate (Sulfamylon)	Apply topically and aseptically once or twice daily in a layer 1/16 inch thick.	This is used for second- and third-degree burns to prevent sepsis. The cream contains 85 mg of mafenide base per gram. Patients may need an analgesic to diminish pain during application.
Silver sulfadiazene (Silvadene)	Apply the 0.1% ointment topically and aseptically once or twice daily in a layer 1/16 inch thick.	This drug prevents and treats sepsis in second- and third-degree burns.
Sulfacetamide sodium (Bleph 10 Liquifilm, Sodium Sulamyd Ophthalmic, Sulf-10, Sulfacel-15, Sebizon Lotion)	*Ophthalmic solution 10%, 15%, 30%:* Initially, give 1 to 2 gtt in lower conjunctival sac every 1 to 2 hr during the day. *Ophthalmic ointment 10%:* Apply ½ to 1 inch in the lower conjunctival sac every 6 hr and at bedtime. *Skin lotion 10%:* Apply the lotion to affected area two to four times daily.	Ophthalmic preparations treat conjunctivitis, corneal ulcers, and superficial ocular infections. Topical preparation treats scaly dermatoses, seborrheic dermatitis, and other bacterial skin infections.
Sulfadiazine (Microsulfon)	*Adults:* Initially, 2 to 4 g followed by 2 to 4 g/day, orally, in three to six equally divided doses *Pediatric (over 2 months):* Initially, 75 mg/kg followed by 150 mg/kg/day, orally, in four to six equally divided doses Rheumatic fever prophylaxis: 0.5 to 1 g daily, orally	This is a short-acting sulfonamide.

Sulfamethizole (Microsul, Sulfstat, Urifon, Thiosulfil)	*Adults:* 0.5 to 1 g, orally, tid or qid *Pediatric (over 2 months):* 30 to 45 mg/kg/day, orally, divided into four doses	This is a short-acting sulfonamide used primarily in the treatment of acute and chronic urinary tract infections.
Sulfamethoxazole (Gantanol, Methoxal)	*Adults:* Initially, 2 g followed by 1 g, bid or tid, orally *Pediatric (over 2 months):* Initially, 50 to 60 mg/kg, orally, then 25 to 30 mg/kg, bid, at 12-hr intervals, up to a maximum of 75 mg/kg/day	This is an intermediate-acting sulfonamide. It is available with trimethoprim (Cotrimoxazole, Bactrim, Septra) to enhance the antibacterial effect. It also is available with phenazopyridine (Azo Gantanol) to relieve dysuria.
Sulfasalazine (Azulfidine, Sulfadyne)	*Adults:* Initially, 1 to 2 g daily, orally, then 3 to 4 g daily in equally divided doses. The maintenance dosage is 2 g daily orally in divided doses. *Pediatric:* 40 to 60 mg/kg/day, orally, in three to six divided doses. Maintenance dosage is 30 mg/kg/day in four divided doses.	This drug treats ulcerative colitis and mild regional enteritis. Skin and alkaline urine may become orange-yellow in color. The drug should be taken after eating if possible.
Sulfisoxazole (Gantrisin)	*Adults:* Initially, 2 to 4 g, orally, followed by 4 to 8 g/day divided into four to six doses *Pediatric (over 2 months):* Initially, 75 mg/kg/day, orally. The maintenance dosage is 150 mg/kg/day orally, divided into four to six doses.	This is a short-acting sulfonamide.

PH

Adverse Effects and Contraindications

- Frequently they cause nausea, and occasionally diarrhea and vomiting.
- The tetracyclines may discolor children's teeth because they bind with calcium in bones and teeth. Also, fetal skeletal development may be retarded, and bone growth may be slowed temporarily in young children. Pregnant women and young children should avoid the tetracyclines, especially for long-term use.
- Patients taking these drugs can experience photosensitivity, especially if they have a history of it. Skin rashes do occur, but less frequently than with the penicillins.
- Tetracyclines are hepatotoxic and can cause fatty degeneration of the liver. Patients with impaired kidney function should receive a reduced dose.
- Outdated or degraded drugs have caused kidney tubule impairment with acidosis, proteinuria, and glycosuria.
- Superinfections are fairly common and range from moniliasis to severe staphylococcal enterocolitis.
- Prolonged IV use may lead to thrombophlebitis.

Dosage, Administration, and Nursing Considerations

- See Table 7-8.
- Age, exposure to light, extreme heat, and humidity can cause the tetracyclines to undergo toxic changes. Always store these drugs properly and check for expiration dates.
- Patients receiving these drugs should avoid direct sunlight and keep their skin covered.
- Do not administer the tetracyclines with antacids or iron because the drugs will combine with metal ions and will not be absorbed.
- Avoid giving the tetracyclines (except doxycycline and minocycline) with milk or other dairy products because the drug will join with the calcium. Giving tetracyclines 1 hr before meals or 2 hr to 3 hr after meals will prevent the possibility of drug–food interactions.
- The tetracyclines may delay blood coagulation.
- Superinfections such as candidiasis occur most often in diabetic, debilitated, or pregnant patients and in those receiving corticosteroids.

TUBERCULOSTATICS

Nursing Considerations

- A variety of drugs are now available that are effective against *Mycobacterium tuberculosis* (see MSN, Respiratory system).

- Long-term chemotherapy (often up to 2 years) is necessary.
- Usually, a combination therapy, using two or three drugs concurrently, is necessary to prevent resistant forms of the bacteria from developing.
- The most common reason for treatment failure is that the patients do not take their medication for the prescribed length of time.
- The following individuals may need drug therapy (usually isoniazid) on a preventive basis:
  1. Infants born to mothers with active tuberculosis
  2. Other household members where tuberculosis has been diagnosed
  3. Individuals whose skin tests have changed recently from negative to positive (recent converters), and those who have had an inactive, untreated infection for many years
  4. Patients who have a *positive skin test* and a *low resistance* to infection also may receive isoniazid, for example:
     a. Those on prolonged therapy with corticosteroids
     b. Those treated for leukemia or Hodgkin's disease
     c. Patients with poorly controlled diabetes
     d. Children with measles or whooping cough
- Antituberculosis drugs are available free of charge from most health departments throughout the country.
- Therapeutic response to therapy is indicated by a feeling of well-being, improved appetite, decreased cough and sputum, negative sputum cultures, and improved chest x-rays.

AMINOSALICYLATE SODIUM (PAS SODIUM, TEEBACIN)

AMINOSALICYLIC ACID (PAS, PARA-AMINOSALICYLIC ACID)

Actions

- When used alone, it has a relatively weak bacteriostatic effect against *Mycobacterium* tuberculosis by preventing folic acid synthesis.
- However, when used with other drugs (*e.g.,* isoniazid or streptomycin) it can decrease the rate at which resistance develops and can potentiate the effects of the other drugs.

PH

Indications

- This drug is used in combination with other drugs (*e.g.,* isoniazid or streptomycin) to treat pulmonary tuberculosis, miliary tuberculosis, tuberculous meningitis, renal tuberculosis, and bone and joint tuberculosis.

TABLE 7-8 TETRACYCLINES

Drug	Dosage and Administration	Nursing Considerations
Demeclocycline hydrochloride (Declomycin, DMCT)	*Adults:* 150 mg, orally, every 6 hr, or 300 mg every 12 hr *Gonorrhea:* Initially, 600 mg, orally, followed by 300 mg every 12 hr for 4 days (total 3 g) *Pediatric (over 8 yr):* 6 to 12 mg/kg/day, orally, divided into two to four doses	More frequent photosensitivity reactions are seen than with other tetracyclines.
Doxycycline hyclate (Vibramycin, Vibra-Tabs)	*Adults:* On day 1, 100 mg, PO, every 12 hr, then 100 mg every day or 50 mg every 12 hr IV: On day 1, 200 mg, IV, given in one or two infusions, then 100 to 200 mg/day, IV, depending on the severity of the infection *Pediatric (over 8 yr, 45 kg and under):* 4.4 mg/kg, orally or IV, on day 1 as a single dose or divided into two doses, then 2.2 to 4.4 mg/kg/day as a single dose or divided into two doses	This drug requires smaller and less frequent doses than most tetracyclines. IV doxycycline should not be used in children under 8 yr old.
Methacycline hydrochloride (Rondomycin)	*Adults:* 150 mg every 6 hr, or 300 mg every 12 hr, orally *Pediatric:* 6 to 12 mg/kg/day, orally, in two to four equally divided doses	

Minocycline hydrochloride (Minocin)	*Adults:* 200 mg, orally or IV, followed by 100 mg every 12 hr *Pediatric (over 8 yr):* 4 mg/kg orally followed by 2 mg/kg every 12 hr	This drug is active against some strains of staphylococci that are resistant to other tetracyclines. Photosensitivity is rare.
Oxytetracycline (Terramycin) Oxytetracycline hydrochloride (terramycin)	*Adults* 1. 250 to 500 mg, orally, every 6 to 12 hr 2. 100 mg, IM, every 8 to 12 hr (maximum 250 mg every 12 hr) 3. 250 to 500 mg, IV, every 12 hr (maximum 500 mg every 6 hr) *Pediatric* 1. 25 to 50 mg/kg/day, orally, in four equal doses 2. 15 to 25 mg/kg/day, IM, in two or three divided doses 3. 10 to 20 mg/kg/day, IV, in two divided doses	No single IM injection should exceed 250 mg.
Tetracycline and tetracycline hydrochloride (Achromycin-V, Cyclopar, Tetracyn)	*Adults* 1. 250 mg, orally, every 6 hr 2. 250 mg, IM, every 24 hr, or 300 mg/day in divided doses every 8 to 12 hr 3. 250 to 500 mg, IV, every 12 hr *Pediatric (over 8 yr)* 1. 25 to 50 mg/kg/day, orally, in two to four equal doses 2. 15 to 25 mg/kg/day, IM, divided and given in two or three equal doses 3. 12 mg/kg/day, IV, divided into two doses	Children weighing more than 40 kg should receive the adult dose. Frequent stools from local irritation by the drug usually occur early in therapy. When the frequent stools are a result of superinfection, the drug should be discontinued.

PH

Adverse Effects and Contraindications

- Frequently it causes anorexia, nausea, vomiting, cramps, and diarrhea.
- Patients with peptic ulcer should not receive PAS.
- Occasionally, skin eruptions, sore throat, fever, and blood dyscrasias occur.
- Liver damage and goiter are rare.
- The sodium and potassium salts should be used cautiously in patients with electrolyte imbalances or kidney or cardiac impairment.
- Patients with blood dyscrasias, impaired renal or hepatic function, gastric ulcer, or goiter should use these drugs cautiously.

Dosage and Administration

- Aminosalicylate Sodium
  1. *Adults:* 14 to 16 g/day in two or three divided doses
  2. *Pediatric:* 275 to 420 mg/kg/day in three or four divided doses
- Aminosalicylic Acid
  1. *Adults:* 10 to 12 g/day, orally, in two or three divided doses
  2. *Pediatric:* 200 to 300 mg/kg/day, orally, in three or four divided doses

Nursing Considerations

- See Tuberculostatics, Nursing Considerations.
- Food and antacids may help reduce the gastrointestinal irritation.
- Sodium, potassium, and calcium salts of this drug are available. These derivatives may cause less gastric irritation. Avoid the sodium derivative if the patient is on a sodium-restricted diet.
- Hypersensitivity reactions can result in nephritis, pancreatitis, and hepatic damage. Monitor for abrupt increases in temperature, malaise, fatigue, enlarged spleen and lymph nodes, sore throat, joint pains, and headache.
- Patients should check with their physician before taking any new prescription or OTC drugs. Interactions are frequent.

CAPREOMYCIN SULFATE (CAPASTAT SULFATE)

Actions

- This is a secondary agent bacteriostatic against *Mycobacterium* tuberculosis.

Indications

- It is used to treat pulmonary tuberculosis when primary agents are not effective or cannot be tolerated.

Adverse Effects and Contraindications

- This drug is ototoxic and nephrotoxic and should not be used with other medications that have the same potential (*e.g.*, aminoglycosides, potent diuretics).
- Large doses can result in skeletal muscle weakness and respiratory arrest.
- Blood dyscrasias, rash, fever, and hypokalemia have been reported.
- Use cautiously for patients with renal or hepatic disease, myasthenia gravis, parkinsonism, or auditory impairment.

Dosage and Administration

- *Adults:* 1 g daily, IM, given for 60 to 120 days, followed by 1 g 2 or 3 times/week. The maximum dosage is 20 mg/kg/day.

Nursing Considerations

- See Tuberculostatics, Nursing Considerations.
- Injections should be made into a large muscle mass.
- During therapy, patients should receive audiometric measurements, tests of vestibular function, CBC, SMA-12, renal and liver function studies, and serum potassium level tests.

CYCLOSERINE (SEROMYCIN)

Actions

- This is a broad-spectrum antibiotic similar to streptomycin. It inhibits cell wall synthesis in *Mycobacterium* tuberculosis and some gram-positive and gram-negative bacteria.

Indications

- It is used with other tuberculostatic drugs to treat pulmonary and extrapulmonary tuberculosis when primary agents are not effective.

Adverse Effects and Contraindications

- Neurotoxic reactions such as headache, tremors, convulsions, dizziness, depression, confusion, aggression, paresthesias, and peripheral neuropathy have been reported.

- Congestive heart failure, arrhythmias, and anemias have occurred.
- Use cautiously for patients with a history of depression, psychoses, epilepsy, alcoholism, and renal impairment.

Dosage and Administration

- *Adults:* Initially, give 250 mg, orally, bid (at 12-hr intervals) for 2 weeks, then 500 mg to 1 g daily in divided doses, monitored by blood levels. The maximum dosage is 1 g/day.

Nursing Considerations

- See Tuberculostatics, Nursing Considerations.
- Prevent gastrointestinal irritation by taking the drug after meals.
- The risk of convulsive seizures increases with the use of alcohol.

ETHAMBUTOL HYDROCHLORIDE (MYAMBUTOL)

Actions

- This has a good bacteriostatic effect against *Mycobacterium* tuberculosis, but it usually is used in combination with another drug because resistance develops rapidly.

Indications

- It is used in combination with other drugs (*e.g.*, isoniazid or streptomycin) to treat pulmonary tuberculosis (both primary and chronic relapsing cases), miliary tuberculosis, tuberculous meningitis, renal tuberculosis, and bone and joint tuberculosis.
- It frequently replaces the aminosalicylic acid because it causes less gastric irritation.

Adverse Effects and Contraindications

- Optic neuritis, resulting in loss of visual acuity, peripheral vision, and color discrimination, is the most serious side-effect.
- Skin eruptions, joint pains, headache, gastric distress, mental confusion, and anaphylactoid reactions also occur.
- Patients with impaired kidney function should receive a reduced dose.
- Do not give to children under 13 years old.

Dosage and Administration

- The usual adult oral dosage is 15 mg/kg in a single daily dose. To treat relapses, 25 mg/kg per day is given.

Nursing Considerations

- See Tuberculostatics, Nursing Considerations.
- Patients on long-term therapy should have their vision checked before beginning treatment and at monthly intervals. If changes are significant, the drug must be discontinued.
- A decreased ability to distinguish red and green is an early indication of optic toxicity.
- Renal and hepatic function, blood counts, and serum uric acid should be checked periodically during therapy.

ETHIONAMIDE (TRECATOR-SC)

Actions

- This drug inhibits bacterial peptide synthesis, and is bacteriostatic or bactericidal (depending on concentration and organism) against *Mycobacterium* tuberculosis and other *Mycobacterium* strains.

Indications

- It is used with other tuberculostatic drugs to treat pulmonary and extrapulmonary tuberculosis when primary agents are not effective.
- It also is used to treat dapsone-resistant lepromatous leprosy.

Adverse Effects and Contraindications

- Gastrointestinal distress possibly caused by CNS stimulation is dose related and frequent (*e.g.*, anorexia, nausea, vomiting, diarrhea, and stomatitis).
- Mental depression, hallucinations, dizziness, convulsions, paresthesias, optic neuritis, and olfactory disturbances have been reported.
- Severe postural hypotension, alopecia, impotence, goiter, jaundice, hypoglycemia, superinfections, and joint pains have occurred.
- Use cautiously for patients with hepatic impairment and diabetes mellitus.

Dosage and Administration

- *Adults:* 0.5 to 1 g/day, orally, in one to three equally divided and spaced doses
- *Pediatric:* 12 to 15 mg/kg/day, orally, in three or four divided doses, up to a maximum of 750 mg/day

Nursing Considerations

- See Tuberculostatics, Nursing Considerations.
- Take the drug with food to minimize gastrointestinal distress.
- Renal and liver function should be monitored during therapy.
- Diabetic patients are especially prone to hepatotoxicity.

ISONIAZID (INH, ISONICOTINIC ACID HYDRAZINE, PANAZID)

Actions

- This is the single most effective bacteriostatic drug for treating and preventing tuberculosis.
- Resistance develops when it is used alone.

Indications

- It is used in combination with other drugs (*e.g.*, PAS or streptomycin) to treat pulmonary tuberculosis (both primary and chronic relapsing cases), miliary tuberculosis, tuberculous meningitis, renal tuberculosis, and bone and joint tuberculosis.
- This is also the drug of choice for preventing tuberculosis (see PH, Tuberculostatics, Nursing considerations, for a list of individuals who would receive INH for this reason).

Adverse Effects and Contraindications

- Patients most likely to experience toxic effects are those who take high doses, inactivate the drug slowly, or are hypersensitive to it.
- Severe and sometimes fatal hepatitis may develop.
- Peripheral neuropathy occurs (*e.g.*, muscle weakness, numbness, tingling).
- Blood dyscrasias have been reported.
- Central nervous system effects include convulsive seizures, hallucinations, and mental depression.
- A patient may experience postural hypotension and difficulty in urinating.
- Use cautiously in patients with convulsive disorders, diabetes, active liver disease, and impaired kidney function.

Dosage and Administration

- *Adults:* 5 mg/kg/day, orally or IM (up to 300 mg). Preventive dosage: 300 mg/day, orally
- *Pediatric:* 10 to 20 mg/kg/day, orally or IM, depending on the severity of infection. Preventive dosage: 10 mg/kg/day (up to 300 mg total)

Nursing Considerations

- Monitor liver function at monthly intervals, and observe for nausea, vomiting, and jaundice (see LAB).
- This drug may cause a deficiency of pyridoxine (vitamin B_6). A supplement is recommended for adolescents and malnourished patients.
- INH is best taken on an empty stomach.
- It is available in combination with pyridoxine (P-I-N Forte) and with rifampin (Rifamate).

PYRAZINAMIDE

Actions

- Pyrazinamide is a tuberculostatic drug chemically similar to niacin.
- It interferes with renal capacity to concentrate and excrete uric acid, thus resulting in hyperuricemia.

Indications

- It is used to treat advanced tuberculosis before surgery.
- It also is used on a short-term basis when primary agents are not effective.

Adverse Effects and Contraindications

- Hepatotoxicity, decreased plasma prothrombin, gout, and elevated serum uric acid have occurred.
- Headache, photosensitivity, aggravation of peptic ulcer, difficulty in urination, anemia, and fatal hemoptysis have been reported.
- Use cautiously when impaired liver or kidney function are present, with a history of diabetes mellitus, gout, or peptic ulcer, or acute intermittent porphyria.

Dosage and Administration

- *Adults:* 25 to 30 mg/kg/day, orally, in three or four divided doses, up to a maximum of 3 g/day

Nursing Considerations

- See Tuberculostatics, Nursing Considerations.
- Monitor closely for liver toxicity and gout. If they occur, the drug should be discontinued.

RIFAMPIN (RIFADIN, RIMACTANE)

Actions

- It is bacteriostatic against *Mycobacterium* tuberculosis by suppressing RNA synthesis.
- Resistance develops easily when it is used alone.

Indications

- It is used in combination with other drugs (*e.g.*, isoniazid or ethambutol) to treat pulmonary tuberculosis. It also is used to treat miliary tuberculosis, tuberculous meningitis, renal tuberculosis, and bone and joint tuberculosis.
- Asymptomatic carriers of meningococci are treated with this drug to prevent spreading the meningitis in high-risk situations.

Adverse Effects and Contraindications

- The drug causes abnormalities in liver-function tests, high serum bilirubin, and jaundice.
- Use cautiously in patients with liver disease and alcoholism.
- Nausea, vomiting, cramps, diarrhea, and anorexia can occur.
- Thrombocytopenia and leukopenia may develop.

Dosage and Administration

- *Adults*
  1. Pulmonary tuberculosis: 600 mg/day, orally, as a single dose
  2. Meningococcal carriers: 600 mg/day, orally, for 4 days
- *Pediatric*
  1. Pulmonary tuberculosis: 10 to 20 mg/kg/day, orally, up to a maximum of 600 mg/day
  2. Meningococcal carriers: 10 to 20 mg/kg/day for 4 days

Nursing Considerations

- See Tuberculostatics, Nursing Considerations.
- Liver function studies should be done periodically (see LAB).
- Rifampin interacts with anticoagulant drugs (see PH, Cardiovascular system). Prothrombin times should be checked daily because the dose of the anticoagulant may need to be increased (see LAB).
- Rifampin-isoniazid combination drugs are available, but they usually are more expensive than the use of the drugs separately. However, the combinations provide greater convenience for the patients.

- The drug should be taken on an empty stomach.
- Urine, feces, sputum, sweat, and tears may be red-orange in color.
- Rifampin hastens the metabolism of oral contraceptives, and an alternative method of contraception should be considered.

STREPTOMYCIN SULFATE

- See PH, Aminoglycosides.

URINARY TRACT ANTISEPTICS

CINOXACIN (CINOBAC)

Actions

- Cinoxacin is a bactericidal agent similar to nalidixic acid.
- It is effective against a variety of gram-negative pathogens.

Indications

- It is used to treat urinary tract infections caused by susceptible organisms.

Adverse Effects and Contraindications

- Headache, dizziness, and insomnia can occur.
- Nausea, vomiting, and diarrhea have been reported.
- Rash, edema, photophobia, and tinnitus are possible.

Dosage and Administration

- 1 g/day orally in two to four doses for 7 to 14 days

Nursing Considerations

- This drug may be taken with food to reduce gastrointestinal distress.

METHENAMINE HIPPURATE (HIPREX)

METHENAMINE MANDELATE (MANDELAMINE)

Actions

- When the urine is acid, formaldehyde is released and exerts a bactericidal effect.
- This drug contributes to the acidification of the urine.

Indications

- It is used to suppress or eliminate bacteria in the urine in cases of pyelonephritis, cystitis, and other chronic urinary tract infections.
- It may be used on a long-term basis because there is a low incidence of resistance and it is low in toxicity.

Adverse Effects and Contraindications

- Occasionally, patients experience gastrointestinal distress.
- Rarely, skin rashes occur.
- High doses may cause dysuria, hematuria, and crystalluria.
- Do not give to patients with renal insufficiency or hepatic disease.
- Do not give if the patient's urine cannot be acidified.
- Do not give concurrently with sulfonamides because an insoluble precipitate may form with formaldehyde in the urine.

Dosage and Administration

- *Adults and Pediatric (over 12 yr)*
  1. Hiprex: 1 g, orally, bid
  2. Mandelamine: 1 g, orally, qid, after meals and at bedtime
- *Pediatric (6 to 12 yr)*
  1. Hiprex: 0.5 to 1 g, orally, bid
  2. Mandelamine: 0.5 g, orally, qid
- *Pediatric (under 6 yr)*
  1. Mandelamine: 18.4 mg/kg, qid

Nursing Considerations

- It may be necessary to acidify the patient's urine by using such drugs as ascorbic acid, sodium acid phosphate, or ammonium chloride.
- Because the bactericidal effects depend on the release of formaldehyde in the urine, it is questionable whether a patient with a Foley catheter would benefit from the use of this drug since the catheter keeps the bladder empty.
- The gastrointestinal distress may be alleviated by giving the drug after meals or by using the enteric-coated form.
- Monitor urine pH during therapy and maintain it at 5.5 or below.
- Alkaline-producing foods should be used in limited amounts (*e.g.*, vegetables, milk, peanuts, and fruits).
- Fruits that contribute to an acid urine are cranberries, plums, and prunes.

METHENAMINE, PHENYL SALICYLATE, METHYLENE BLUE, BENZOIC ACID, ATROPINE SULFATE, AND HYOSCYAMINE (URISED)

Actions

- In an acid urine, methenamine hydrolyzes into formaldehyde, thus providing mild antiseptic activity.
- Methylene blue and benzoic acid are antiseptics that potentiate the action of methenamine.
- Phenyl salicylate is an antipyretic and mild analgesic.
- Atropine and hyoscyamine relax smooth muscle spasms.

Indications

- The drug is used to treat cystitis, urethritis, and trigonitis caused by organisms that produce or maintain an acid urine and are susceptible to formaldehyde.
- It relieves lower urinary tract discomfort caused by diagnostic procedures or inflammation.

Adverse Effects and Contraindications

- Patients with glaucoma, urinary bladder neck obstruction, pyloric or duodenal obstruction, or cardiospasm should not use Urised.
- The dosage should be decreased if the patient experiences dry mouth, flushing, or difficulty in urination.
- Discontinue the drug if the patient experiences rapid pulse, dizziness, or blurring of vision.

Dosage and Administration

- *Adults:* Give 2 tablets, orally, qid.
- *Pediatric: (12 yr or older):* Reduce dosage in proportion to age and weight.

Nursing Considerations

- Urine may become blue to blue-green.
- Patients should not use sulfonamides concurrently because insoluble precipitates may form with formaldehyde in the urine.
- Monitor urine pH during therapy and maintain it at 5.5 or below.
- Alkaline-producing foods should be taken in limited amounts (*e.g.*, vegetables, milk, peanuts, and fruits).
- Acidifying drugs may be taken (*e.g.*, ascorbic acid and ammonium chloride).
- Fruits that contribute to an acid urine are cranberries, plums, and prunes.

NALIDIXIC ACID (NEGGRAM)

Actions

- This is bactericidal against some gram-negative organisms *(e.g., Proteus, Klebsiella, E. coli)*. It is ineffective against *Pseudomonas*.

Indications

- It can treat urinary tract infections caused by susceptible organisms.

Adverse Effects and Contraindications

- Nausea, vomiting, and diarrhea are common.
- Dizziness, visual disturbances, and muscle weakness have been reported. Overdosage can produce intracranial hypertension, convulsions, and 6th cranial nerve palsy.
- Rash, fever, photosensitivity, joint pain, and swelling may occur.
- Use cautiously with renal or hepatic disease, epilepsy, or severe cerebral arteriosclerosis.

Dosage and Administration

- *Adults:* Initially, 1 g, qid, orally, for 1 or 2 weeks, then 500 mg, qid, for prolonged therapy.
- *Pediatric (3 months to 12 years):* Initially, 55 mg/kg/day, orally, in four equally divided doses, then 33 mg/kg/day for prolonged therapy.

Nursing Considerations

- Infants, children, and the elderly are particularly susceptible to CNS adverse effects.
- For prolonged therapy, renal and hepatic function tests and blood counts are recommended.

NITROFURANTOIN (FURADANTIN, MACRODANTIN)

Actions

- This drug exerts bactericidal effects against gram-negative and gram-positive organisms.

Indications

- It is used to treat cystitis, pyelitis, and pyelonephritis.
- It frequently is used in cases of chronic urinary tract infections because resistance seldom develops.

Adverse Effects and Contraindications

- When used to treat acute infections, the large doses can cause nausea, vomiting, and diarrhea.
- Headache, dizziness, drowsiness, and peripheral neuropathy may occur.
- It may produce various types of skin rashes.
- Pregnant women (especially near term) and young infants should not receive this drug.
- Do not give to patients with impaired kidney function because the drug accumulates to toxic levels in nervous tissue.
- Hemolytic anemia has occurred in patients who lack the enzyme glucose 6-phosphate dehydrogenase, and in young infants whose enzyme systems are immature.
- It may cause pulmonary reactions manifested by dyspnea, chest pain, cough, fever, and chills. Onset may be sudden or after prolonged therapy.

Dosage and Administration

- *Adults:* 50 to 100 mg, orally, qid
- *Pediatric (over 3 months):* 5 to 7 mg/kg/day, orally, divided into four equal doses

Nursing Considerations

- Nitrofurantoin causes a yellow-brown discoloration of the urine.
- When taken on a long-term basis, the patient may take a single daily dose at bedtime. The patient should empty his or her bladder before taking the drug because the urine stored during the night will have a higher concentration of the drug.
- The absorption of Macrodantin is slower, and its excretion is somewhat less, than that of Furadantin.
- Peripheral neuropathy may be severe and irreversible. Monitor for muscle weakness, tingling, and numbness.

PHENAZOPYRIDINE HYDROCHLORIDE (PYRIDIUM)

Actions

- The drug has a weak bacteriostatic action, but it is used for its topical anesthetic effects.

Indications

- It is used to relieve bladder irritation and to reduce the burning, urgency, and frequency that occurs with urinary tract infections and following endoscopic procedures.

Adverse Effects and Contraindications

- Occasionally, the drug causes gastrointestinal discomfort.
- Overdoses may lead to kidney and liver toxicity and blood dyscrasias.
- Patients with impaired kidney function should not receive this drug.

Dosage and Administration

- *Adults:* 200 mg, orally, tid
- *Pediatric:* 12 mg/kg/day in three divided doses

Nursing Considerations

- Patients should be told that their urine will become orange-red in color.
- It is available in fixed combination with methenamine mandelate (Azolate, Azo Mandelamine, Uritral), sulfamethizole (Microsul-A, Thiosulfil-A), sulfamethoxazole (Azo Gantanol), and sulfisoxazole (Azo Gantrisin).

ANTINEOPLASTICS

OVERVIEW

Chemotherapy, or the use of drugs to treat cancer, can accomplish three things: regression of the neoplasm, prolongation of life, and palliation (alleviation of symptoms without curing). This mode of therapy has limitations: long-term remissions are not possible in many instances; resistance to drugs emerges; and the drugs lack selective toxicity, *i.e.*, they also damage normal cells. Choice of drugs and dosage is highly individualized. The aim is to destroy the maximum number of cancer cells with minimal toxicity to normal tissues. Normal cells most susceptible to damage are those with a naturally high rate of proliferation (*e.g.*, bone marrow, mucosal lining of the gastrointestinal tract, and hair-follicle cells of the scalp).

Combinations of two or more drugs frequently are used (see Table 7-14 on page 724). The advantages over single-drug therapy are that resistance can be delayed or prevented, and that the combinations are frequently more effective. It is common to give the drugs intermittently in high doses, rather than in small, daily doses. This allows time for the bone marrow to recover. Individual dosages usually are computed according to total body surface. Therefore, accurate weights are very important. Drug dosages must be checked carefully because some are ordered in micrograms, and others in milligrams. Drug names may also be similar.

The patient receiving antineoplastic drugs should not use any over-the-counter preparations without the approval of his or her physician. Unwanted drug interactions must be avoided.

Patients who are still in their reproductive years should understand that these medications can cause permanent sterility and could be damaging to a developing fetus. (See MSN, Oncology nursing consideration.)

ALKYLATING AGENTS

Actions

- These drugs interfere with cell division by binding DNA molecules together. The damage occurs during mitosis.

Indications

- See Table 7-9.

Adverse and Toxic Effects

- See Table 7-9.

Dosage, Administration, and Nursing Considerations

- See Table 7-9.
- Almost all alkylating agents cause nausea and vomiting, frequently on a long-term basis. Good antiemetic control is essential (see PH).
- Secondary malignancies (*e.g.,* of the urinary bladder) have developed.
- Pregnant and nursing women should not use these drugs.
- Sterility can result and may be permanent.
- Use cautiously in patients with impaired liver and kidney function.
- See MSN, Oncology nursing considerations.

PH

ANTIMETABOLITES

Actions

- These drugs resemble essential amino acids. They compete with the amino acids on the DNA molecule and interfere with the manufacturing of proper proteins.

Indications

- See Table 7-10.

(*Text continues on page 714*)

TABLE 7-9 ALKYLATING AGENTS

Drug	Indications	Adverse and Toxic* Effects	Dosage and Administration	Nursing Considerations
Busulfan (Myleran)	Palliative treatment of chronic myelogenous (myeloid, myelocytic, granulocytic) leukemia	BMD; interstitial pulmonary fibrosis (rare); hyperpigmentation; hyperuricemia	*Adults:* for remission induction give 4 to 8 mg/day orally. Maintenance (when remission shorter than 3 months): 1 to 3 mg/day, orally *Pediatric:* 60 mcg/kg/day, orally, or 1.8 mg/m^2/day	When total leukocyte count has declined to approximately 15,000/mm^3, the drug should be withheld because the leukocyte count can continue to fall for more than a month after busulfan is withdrawn.
Dacarbazine (DTIC-Dome)	Malignant melanoma; sarcoma; Hodgkin's lymphoma	BMD; flu-like syndrome; N/V; metallic taste in mouth; pain at injection site; VESICANT*	2–4.5 mg/kg/day for 10 days, q4 weeks; or 250 mg/M^2/day for 5 days, IV, q3 weeks	N/V is controlled by limiting food 4–6 hours prior to treatment and slow infusion of the drug. Infiltration may be treated with an ice compress. Protect the drug from light.
Nitrogen Mustards				
Chlorambucil (Leukeran)	CLL; ovarian tumor; Hodgkin's lymphoma	Dose-related BMD; mild N/V; dermatitis	*Adults:* Initially, 0.1–0.2 mg/kg/day for 3–6 weeks; Maximum maintenance dosage:	Clinical examination and blood studies should be done at least every 2 weeks.

			0.1 mg/kg/day, PO *Pediatric:* 0.1–0.2 mg/kg/day or 4.5 mg/m^2/day, PO	
Cyclophosphamide (Cytoxan, CTX, Neosar)	Lymphomas: breast, lung (small cell), and ovarian; leukemias	BMD (7–14 days after dose); alopecia; N/V; liver dysfunction; pulmonary fibrosis; hemorrhagic cystitis*	*Adults:* 1–5 mg/kg/day, PO, or induction of 40–50 mg/kg, IV, in divided doses over 2–5 days. Maintenance dosage: 10–15 mg/kg q7–10 days, 3–5 mg/kg twice a week, or 1.5–3 mg/kg/day, IV *Pediatric:* Induction of 2–8 mg/kg or 60–250 mg/m^2 q day for 6 or more days, PO Maintenance dosage is 2–5 mg/kg or 50–150 mg/M^2, PO, twice a week. Induction IV is the same as PO Maintenance IV is 10–15 mg/kg q 7–10 days, or 30 mg/kg q 3–4 weeks.	The patient should drink plenty of fluids and empty bladder frequently. The drug may interfere with normal wound healing. This drug is immunosuppressive. Therefore, the patient is susceptible to chicken pox and herpes zoster.

PH

(continued)

TABLE 7-9 ALKYLATING AGENTS

Drug	Indications	Adverse and Toxic* Effects	Dosage and Administration	Nursing Considerations
Mechlorethamine hydrochloride (Nitrogen mustard; Mustargen)	Hodgkin's lymphomas; bronchogenic carcinoma; CLL; CML	BMD; severe N/V; mucositis; stomatitis; diarrhea; alopecia; VESTICANT*	0.4 mg/kg as a single dose or 0.1–0.2 mg/kg, IV, in two to four divided doses *Intracavitary:* 0.2–0.4 mg/kg	Wear gloves when preparing and administering solution. Extravasation may be treated with sodium thiosulfate solution and ice compresses. Profound immunosuppression occurs. Meticulous mouth care is essential. Encourage increased fluid intake to prevent hyperuricemia.
Melphalan (Alkeran)	Breast, ovarian, and testicular; melanoma; multiple myeloma	BMD; stomatitis; alopecia; hypersensitivity	6 mg daily, PO, for 2–3 weeks Maintenance is instituted after 4–5 weeks at 2 mg/day.	Dosage adjustments are based primarily on blood counts. The patient may be susceptible to infection and hyperuricemia.

Nitrosoureas				
Carmustine (BCNU, BiCNU)	CNS tumors; multiple myeloma; lymphomas breast tumors	BMD (dose limiting, may be cumulative), stomatitis; pain during infusion; N/V; hepatotoxicity*; pulmonary fibrosis; nephrotoxicity*	200 mg/m^2 q 6 weeks as a single dose, or 100 mg/m^2 on two successive days	Repeat only if platelets are above 100,000/mm^3, and leukocytes are above 4,000/mm^3. Watch for signs of infection and bleeding. Report jaundice, dark urine, pruritus, light stools.
Lomustine (CCNU)	CNS tumors; Hodgkin's lymphoma: multiple myeloma; GI, lung, and prostate tumors	BMD (cumulative and long); stomatitis/ulceration; N/V (may be severe); nephrotoxicity*	*Adults and Pediatric:* 130 mg/m^2 as a single dose q 6 weeks, PO	Repeat only if platelets are above 100,000/mm^3 and leukocytes are above 4,000/mm^3. Inspect the oral cavity and provide meticulous mouth care.
Streptozocin (Streptozotocin Zanosar)	Hodgkin's lymphoma; pancreatic, and colon-rectal tumor	BMD; N/V; diarrhea; hypoglycemia; renal* or hepatic* toxicity	500 mg/m^2, IV, daily for 5 days every 6 weeks, or 1000–1500 mg/m^2 weekly until maximum benefit or toxicity	Serial determinations of urinary protein are valuable in detecting early renal effects.

Key: BMD = bone marrow depression; N/V = nausea/vomiting; CLL = chronic lymphocytic leukemia, and CML = chronic myelocytic leukemia.
*Indicates toxic effect

TABLE 7-10 ANTIMETABOLITES

Drug	Indications	Adverse and Toxic* Effects	Dosage and Administration	Nursing Considerations
Cytarabine (ARA-C, Cytosar, Cytosine arabinoside)	AML; ALL; CML	N/V (limited to administration time); rash; stomatitis; BMD; liver*/renal* damage	*Adults and Pediatric:* 200 mg/m^2/day continuous IV for 5 days; repeat q 2 weeks. *Intrathecal* (IT): 5–75 mg/m^2 q 2–7 days; Maintenance therapy 1–1.5 mg/kg, IM or SC, at 1 to 4-weeks intervals	Higher doses are better tolerated if they are given by rapid IV injection. However, premedication with antiemetics is usually necessary. Meticulous mouth care is very important. The patient may need increased fluids and allopurinol to prevent hyperuricemia.
5-Fluorouracil (5-FU)	Tumors of the breast; GI tract, pancreas, ovary, liver, and bladder	BMD; stomatitis/ulceration; N/V; alopecia; diarrhea; hyperpigmentation of the skin	Administration is *highly individualized:* 12 mg/kg, IV, for 4 days; if *no* toxicity is seen, give 6 mg/kg on the 6th, 8th, 10th, and 12th days. Maintenance therapy: If no toxicity is seen, repeat at 1-month intervals following the last IV dose.	If the patient is obese, the dosage may be determined by *ideal* weight. Ice compresses should be used if extravasation occurs. Inspect mouth daily and give or monitor mouth care.

Mercaptopurine (6-MP, Purinethol)	ALL; CML; AML	N/V (mild); rash; stomatitis; BMD; hepatic*	*Adults and Pediatric (over 5 years):* 2.5 mg/kg in single or divided doses, PO Maintenance therapy: 1.5–2.5 mg/kg/day	Allopurinol may be given to treat or prevent hyperuricemia. It retards metabolism of 6-MP and, therefore enhances antineoplastic acitivity and toxicity. Reduce the dose to 1/3 to1/4 of the usual dose.
Methotrexate (Amethopterin, MTX, Folex, Mexate)	Head and neck tumors; ALL; lung, breast, cervix, testicular, and ovarian tumors; sarcoma; (also used to treat unresponsive, severe psoriasis)	BMD; stomatitis; GI ulceration; diarrhea; some N/V; liver* and kidney* toxicity	*Highly individualized:* 15–50 mg/m^2, orally, 1 to 2 times per week. 20–50, mg/m^2/week, IV or IM, 10–15 mg/m^2, IT, every 2 to 5 days. High dose: 100 mg/m^2 to 10 g/m^2 every 1 to 3 weeks	*Leucovorin* rescue must be given with high-dose MTX. Hydration with sodium bicarbonate ($NaHCO_3$) also may be necessary. Inspect mouth. Report patchy necrotic areas or a black, furry tongue.
Thioguanine (6-thioguanine, TG)	AML; ALL; CML	BMD; mild N/V; stomatitis (usually dose related); jaundice*	2 mg/kg/day PO	Observe the patient's skin and sclera for jaundice.

Key: BMD = bone marrow depression; N/V = nausea/vomiting, AML = acute myelocytic leukemia, ALL = acute lymphocytic leukemia; CLL = chronic lymphocytic leukemia; and CML = chronic myelocytic leukemia.

*Indicates toxic effect

Adverse and Toxic Effects

- See Table 7-10.

Dosage, Administration, and Nursing Considerations

- See Table 7-10.
- Pregnant and nursing women should not use these drugs.
- Sterility can result and may be permanent.
- Use cautiously in patients with impaired liver and kidney function.
- Stomatitis can be an early sign of toxicity. Report cracked lips, white patches, and erythema of buccal membranes.
- In the plasma, portions of methotrexate are bound to serum albumin. The following drugs can displace methotrexate and increase its potential for toxicity: salicylates (aspirin and aspirin products), sulfonamides, phenytoin (Dilantin), phenylbutazone, tetracycline, chloramphenicol, and para-amino benzoic acid. They should not be given at the same time as the methotrexate.
- Response to methotrexate may be decreased by vitamin supplements containing folic acid.
- See MSN, Oncology nursing considerations.

NATURAL PRODUCTS

Actions

- Antibiotics interfere with RNA transcription and DNA synthesis.
- The enzyme L-asparaginase deprives malignant cells of the L-asparagine they need to meet their metabolic needs.
- Plant alkaloids stop cell division at metaphase and prevent synthesis of DNA.

Indications

- See Table 7-11.

Adverse and Toxic Effects

- See Table 7-11

Dosage, Administration, and Nursing Considerations

- See Table 7-11
- Pregnant and nursing women should not use these drugs.
- Sterility can result and may be permanent.

(*Text continues on page 718*)

TABLE 7-11 NATURAL PRODUCTS

Drug	Indications	Adverse and Toxic* Effects	Dosage and Administration	Nursing Considerations
Antibiotics				
Bleomycin	Tumors of the testicles, head and neck, cervix, lung, esophagus, and genitourinary tract; Hodgkin's lymphoma	Fever and chills (4–6 hours after dose); hypotension; rash; alopecia; stomatitis; pulmonary fibrosis* (dose limiting)	5–30 u/m^2, IV/IM/SC, 1 to 2 times per week	Patients over 70 years old or those who have received over 400 u are at greatest risk for developing pulmonary complications. Chest x-rays should be done every 1–2 weeks. Assess for dyspnea and fine rales. Patients with testicular tumors or Hodgkin's lymphomas usually demonstrate improvement within 2 weeks.
Dactinomycin (Actinomycin D, Cosmegen)	Choriocarcinoma; Ewing's sarcoma; Wilm's tumor; Rhabdomyosarcoma; lung tumor	BMD; N/V (severe); stomatitis; diarrhea	Intravenous medication should not exceed 15 μg/kg, or 400–600 μg/m^2, qd, for 5 days. *Adults:* 0.5 mg/day for 5 days, q 4–6 weeks *Pediatric:* 0.015 mg/kg/day for 5 days, q 4–6 weeks	Ice compresses can be used to treat extravasation. Severe, sometimes fatal, toxic effects occur with high frequency (2 days to 2 weeks after therapy). Inspect the patient's mouth carefully and provide mouth care. Observe for hyperuricemia.

(continued)

TABLE 7-11 NATURAL PRODUCTS

Drug	Indications	Adverse and Toxic* Effects	Dosage and Administration	Nursing Considerations
Daunorubicin (Daunomycin Cerubidine)	Acute leukemias	BMD/ N/V; stomatitis; alopecia; fever; cardiotoxicity*; hepatotoxicity*; vesicant*	30–60 mg/m^2, IV, for 3 days, or once weekly	The drug may impart a red color to the urine for 1–2 days after therapy. Extravasation can cause severe tissue necrosis. Monitor carefully for symptoms of congestive heart failure. Inspect mouth daily and give meticulous mouth care. Monitor for symptoms of hyperuricemia.
Doxorubicin (Adriamycin)	Tumors of the breast, lung, ovary; sarcoma; lymphoma; acute leukemias; tumors of the thyroid, and stomach	N/V BMD; alopecia; stomatitis; radiosensitizer; impaired hepatic function*; cardiomyopathy* (may be irreversible); vesicant*	60–75 mg/m^2, IV, q 21 days, or 30 mg/M^2 for 3 days (maximum cumulative dosage is 400–550 mg/m^2)	Patients receiving more than 550 mg/m^2 are at high risk for developing cardiotoxicity. Extravasation must be treated immediately to minimize tissue damage and necrosis. The drug may impart a red color to the urine 1–2 days after therapy.
Mitomycin (Mitomycin-C, MTC, Mutamycin)	Tumors of the head and neck, breast, cervix, pancreas, stomach, colon and bladder; advanced lung tumors	BMD; N/V (severe); stomatitis; diarrhea; alopecia; pruritis; vesicant*	2 mg/m^2, IV, for 5 days; after two drug-free days, repeat 2 mg/m^2 for 5 days; the cycle may be repeated q 6–8 weeks.	Observe carefully for extravasation. Inspect the patient's mouth carefully and provide meticulous mouth care.

Enzymes				
L-Asparaginase (Elspar)	ALL; AML; lymphoma	Anorexia; lethargy; confusion; mild N/V; hypoproteinemia; Anaphylaxis*	As a single agent, 200 IU/kg/day for 28 days; or 1,000 IU/kg/day for up to 10 days in combination with vincristine and prednisone	*Never* leave the patient alone during an infusion. Have emergency equipment immediately available. When given concurrently or immediately before a course of prednisone and vincristine, the toxicity potential is increased.
Plant Alkaloids				
Vinblastine sulfate (Velban, VLB)	Hodgkin's lymphoma; tumors of the head and neck, breast, and testicles	Mental depression; BMD (cumulative); N/V; diarrhea; vesicant*	*Adults:* initial dose, 3.7 mg/m^2, IV *Pediatric:* initial dose, 2.5 mg/m^2, IV May be given q 7 days and increased according to the WBC count (not to go below 3000 $cells/mm^3$)	Hyaluronidase has been used to treat extravasation. Blood counts must be monitored carefully.
Vincristine sulfate (Oncovin)	ALL; tumors of the breast and testicles, sarcoma; Hodgkin's lymphoma; neuroblastoma; Wilms' tumor; Rhabdomyosarcoma	N/V; alopecia; neurotoxicities* (may be irreversible); severe constipation and ileus; IADH syndrome (high urinary sodium excretion, hyponatremia, dehydration, hypotension)	*Adults:* 1.4 mg/m^2, IV, q week *Pediatric:* 2 mg/m^2, IV, q week Highly individualized and frequently used in combination therapy	Hyaluronidase has been used to treat extravasation. Observe for tingling and numbness of the extremities, which may precede loss of deep-tendon reflexes, muscle weakness and footdrop, hoarseness, ptosis, and double vision.

Key: BMD = bone marrow depression; N/V = nausea/ vomiting; ALL = acute lymphocytic leukemia; and AML = acute myelocytic leukemia.
*Indicates toxic effect

PH

(*continued from page 714*)

- Use cautiously in patients with impaired liver and kidney function. Cardiovascular and pulmonary disease also increase the hazards.
- See MSN, Oncology nursing considerations.

MISCELLANEOUS PRODUCTS

Indications

- See Table 7-12.

Adverse and Toxic Effects

- See Table 7-12.

Dosage, Administration, and Nursing Considerations

- See Table 7-12
- Pregnant and nursing women should not use these drugs.
- Sterility can result from the antineoplastic drugs and may be permanent.
- Use cautiously in patients with impaired liver and kidney function.
- See MSN, Oncology nursing considerations.

HORMONES/ADRENOCORTICOSTEROIDS

Actions

- Estrogens, progestins, and androgens act by biologic antagonism.
- Steroids suppress immune response, potentiate other agents, and affect cell energy.

Indications

- See Table 7-13.

Adverse and Toxic Effects

- See Table 7-13.

Dosage, Administration, and Nursing Considerations

- See Table 7-13.
- See MSN, Oncology nursing considerations.

COMBINATION CHEMOTHERAPY

- Some examples of commonly used combinations of chemotherapeutic agents are listed in Table 7-14, page 724.

CARDIOVASCULAR SYSTEM

ADRENERGICS (SYMPATHOMIMETICS)

Actions

- These drugs mimic the actions of epinephrine or norepinephrine at receptor sites in the sympathetic nervous system.
- They may displace natural norepinephrine from storage sites.
- There are three major receptor types: alpha, beta, and dopaminergic. When stimulated, these receptors do the following:
  1. Alpha receptors cause vasoconstriction and uterine and sphincter contractions.
  2. $Beta_1$ receptors (mostly in the heart) increase the rate and force of myocardial contractions and the rate of atrioventricular node conduction.
  3. $Beta_2$ receptors (mainly in the bronchi, blood vessels, and uterus) produce bronchodilation, vasodilation, and uterine relaxation.
  4. Dopaminergic receptors (primarily in splanchnic blood vessels) produce dilation of these vessels.

Indications

- See Table 7-15.

Adverse and Toxic Effects

- See Table 7-15.

Dosage, Administration, and Nursing Considerations

- See Table 7-15
- Concurrent use of adrenergics and digitalis may produce ectopic pacemakers and other arrhythmias.

(Text continues on page 730)

TABLE 7-12 MISCELLANEOUS PRODUCTS

Drug	Actions and Indications	Adverse and Toxic* Effects	Dosage and Administration	Nursing Considerations
Allopurinol (Zyloprim)	This drug reduces the production of uric acid. It is used to prevent or treat hyperuricemia caused by rapid destruction of cells by antineoplastic agents.	Skin rash; N/V; diarrhea; blood dyscrasias; BMD; drowsiness	600–800 mg, PO, for 2–3 days or longer (maximum of 800 mg/day) *Pediatrics:* under 6 yr—50 mg, tid; 6–10 yr—100 mg, tid	High fluid intake should accompany the allopurinol. Untreated hyperuricemia can produce renal calculi and tissue urate deposits. Discontinue the drug at the first sign of skin rash; severe hypersensitivity may follow.
Cisplatin (cis-DDP, Platinol)	This acts most like an alkylating agent. It is used to treat testicular, ovarian, head and neck, breast, bladder, cervical and prostate tumors; Hodgkin's lymphoma; melanoma; and osteogenic sarcoma.	Severe N/V; minimal BMD; peripheral neuropathy; nephrotoxic* anaphylaxis; ototoxicity*, fluid accumulation in lungs	*Testicular:* 20 mg/m^2, IV, for 5 days; repeat every 3 weeks *Ovarian:* 50 mg/m^2, IV, once every 3 weeks, or 100 mg/m^2, IV, once every 4 weeks *Bladder:* 50 to 70 mg/m^2, IV, once every 3 to 4 weeks	Vigorous hydration (1–2 liters of fluid for 8–12 hr prior to treatment, and then continued for 24 hours following the drug) and the use of furosemide or mannitol concurrently are recommended to prevent nephrotoxicity. *Accurate* intake and output must be maintained to avoid fluid overload. Report output of less than 100 ml/hr. Children who receive repeated doses of cisplatin are especially susceptible to ototoxicity.

Leucovorin calcium (citrovorum factor, folinic acid, Wellcovorin)	This prevents serious toxocity by protecting normal cells from the action of folic acid antagonists such as methotrexate. Treatment is called "leucovorin rescue."	Allergic sensitization (urticaria, pruritus, rash, wheezing)	The dosage is dependent on the dose of methotrexate, *e.g.*, 10–15 mg/m^2 q 6 hr for 1 to 3 days. It is to be given in amounts equal to the weight of the antagonist given.	Plasma methotrexate levels may be used to determine dosage and duration of therapy. To be effective as an antidote for overdosage of folic acid antagonists, it should be given within one hour if possible.
Procarbazine hydrochloride (Matulane)	This drug is similar to the antimetabolites. It is used in Hodgkin's lymphoma; multiple myeloma; bronchogenic tumor; and malignant melanoma.	N/V; BMD; diarrhea; stomatitis; anorexia; alopecia; peripheral neuropathy; headache; depression; MAO inhibitor* action	*Adults:* Begin at 2–4 mg/kg/day (to the nearest 50 mg) for 1 week, then 4–6 mg/kg/day until the maximum response is obtained or the WBC count is less than 4,000/mm^3 or the platelet count is less than 100,000/mm^3. After recovery from hematologic toxicity, maintain at 1–2 mg/kg/day. *Pediatric:* There is limited use of this drug. The following is a guideline only. Administer 50 mg, qd, for 1 week, then 100 mg/m^2 (to the nearest 50 mg) until hematologic toxicity or the maximum reponse is obtained. After recovery, maintain at 50 mg/day.	Give with meals. Antabuse-like reaction may occur when used with alcohol. Hypertensive crises may occur if used with sympathomimetic drugs (OTC nose drops, cough medicines, epinephrine, amphetamine) or tricyclic antidepressants. Foods high in tyramine should be avoided (e.g., ripe cheeses, and yogurt).

Key: BMD = bone marrow depression; N/V = nausea/vomiting.

PH

TABLE 7-13 HORMONES/ADRENOCORTICOSTEROIDS

Drug	Indications	Adverse and Toxic* Effects	Dosage and Administration	Nursing Considerations
Androgens				
Fluoxymesterone (Halotestin)	Tumors of the breast (in postmenopausal women)	Some N/V; anorexia; libido changes; hot flashes; virulization; hypercalcemia*; hepatotoxicity*	10–30 mg/day, PO, in divided doses	Urge early reporting of voice change (hoarsening or deeping) and hirsutism.
Testosterone (Oreton, Testolin, Testrone)	Tumors of the breast (in postmenopausal women)	Same as those for fluoxymesterone, plus sodium and water retention (especially in the elderly)	Short acting: 100 mg, 3 times a week, IM Long acting: 200–400 mg, IM, every 2 to 4 weeks	Considerations are the same as those for fluoxymesterone. IM injections should be made deep into gluteal muscles. Diuretic therapy may be needed. Hypercalcemia may indicate progression of bone metastasis. Immobilized patients are at higher risk for developing hypercalcemia.
Estrogens				
Diethylstilbestrol (Stilbestrol, DES)	Tumors of the breast and prostate	Fluid retention; some N/V; libido changes; feminization in males; uterine bleeding	Breast: 15 mg/day, PO Prostate: 1–3 mg/day, PO	Feminine characteristics (in males) will disappear with termination of therapy.

Tamoxifen citrate (Nolvadex)	Tumors of the breast	Some nausea; fever; slightly decreased WBC count; facial hair growth; hypercalcemia	10–20 mg, PO, twice daily (morning and evening)	Objective response may require 4–10 weeks of therapy, or longer if there is bone metastasis.
Progestins				
Medroxyprogesterone acetate (Depo-Provera)	Endometrial, breast, renal cell, and prostate tumors	Fluid retention; breakthrough uterine bleeding	400–1,000 mg/week, IM	IM injections may be painful. Monitor sites for evidence of sterile abscesses.
Megestrol acetate (Megace, Pallace)	Endometrial and breast tumors	Same as those for medroxyprogesterone acetate; also deep vein thrombophlebitis	40–320 mg/day, PO, in divided doses	Monitor for breathing distress characteristic of asthma.
Steroids				
Dexamethasone (Decadron)	Metastatic breast tumors; CNS tumors; lymphomas; ALL; CLL; Hodgkin's lymphoma; multiple myeloma	Increased appetite; Cushing-type changes; GI irritation; immunosuppression; fluid/electrolyte imbalances; hypertension; osteoporosis	*Highly individualized:* 5–150 mg/day Decadron and prednisone may be given PO Solu-Cortef may be given IM or IV.	Increases or decreases in dosage should be made gradually. A salt-restricted, potassium-rich diet may be needed Monitor signs and symptoms of infection and wound healing.
Hydrocortisone sodium succinate (Solu-Cortef)	Same as those for dexamethasone	Same as those for dexamethasone	Same as those for dexamethasone	Same as those for dexamethasone
Prednisone (Meticorten, Deltasone)	Same as those for dexamethasone	Same as those for dexamethasone	Same as those for dexamethasone	Same as those for dexamethasone

Key: N/V = nausea/vomiting.
*Indicates toxic effect

PH

TABLE 7-14 EXAMPLES OF COMBINATION CHEMOTHERAPY REGIMENS

Carcinoma	Abreviations	Drug Names
Breast cancer	CMF	Cytoxan, methotrexate, 5-FU*
	CAF	Cytoxan, adriamycin, 5-FU
	CMFVP	Cytoxan, methotrexate, 5-FU, vincristine, prednisone
Lung cancer	VAC/CAV	Vincristine, adriamycin, cytoxan
	MACC	Methotrexate, adriamycin, cytoxan, CCNU†
	BACON	Bleomycin, adriamycin, CCNU, oncovin, mustargen
Hodgkin's lymphoma	MOPP	Mustargen, oncovin, prednisone, procarbazine
	MVPP	Mustargen, velban, prednisone, procarbazine
	ABVD	Adriamycin, bleomycin, velban, DTIC‡
Non-Hodgkin's lymphoma	CHOP	Cytoxan, adriamycin, oncovin, prednisone
	COP	Cytoxan, oncovin, prednisone
	CVP	Cytoxan, vincristine, prednisone
	CHOP-BLEO	Cytoxan, adriamycin, oncovin, prednisone, bleomycin

	C-MOPP	Cytoxan, oncovin, prednisone, procarbazine
	COMA	Cytoxan, oncovin, methotrexate, Ara-C§
Leukemia	POMP	Prednisone, oncovin, methotrexate, 6-mercaptopurine
	DOAP	Daunomycin, oncovin, Ara-C, prednisone
Malignant melanoma	BVD	BCNU,‖ vincristine, DTIC
Sarcomas	VAC	Oncovin, adriamycin, cytoxan
	VCR-MTX	Oncovin, methotrexate
	CY-VA-DIC	Cytoxan, oncovin, adriamycin, DTIC
Gastrointestinal	FAM	5-FU, adriamycin, mitomycin C
	5-FU-MeCCNU-VCR	5-FU, methylCCNU, oncovin

*5-FU = 5-fluorouracil.
†CCNU = lomustine, CeeNU
‡DTIC = dacarbazine
§Ara-C = cytarabine.
‖BCNU = carmustine, BiCNU

PH

TABLE 7-15 ADRENERGICS

Drug	Actions and Indications	Adverse Effects and Contraindications	Dosage and Administration	Nursing Considerations
Dobutamine hydrochloride (Dobutrex)	This drug stimulates $beta_1$ receptors of the heart. It increases myocardial contractility and cardiac output. It can produce mild increases in heart rate and blood pressure (BP). It is used to increase BP and cardiac output in severely decompensated states, such as heart failure and cardiogenic shock.	Tachycardia and hypertension occur in about 10% of patients. Dobutamine should never be used for patients with idiopathic hypertrophic subaortic stenosis (IHSS). Use cautiously for patients with atrial fibrillation, hypertension, continuing hypotension, or hypovolemia. There is still question as to whether dobutamine could increase the area of a myocardial infarction.	The patient's weight must be known to determine the accurate dosage. The usual range is 2.5 to 10 μg/kg/min, IV. Toxic levels are about 15 μg/kg/min.	ECG and BP should be monitored continuously during administration. Swan-Ganz catheter may be used to monitor pulmonary artery wedge pressure. A digitalis preparation may be used before administration in patients with atrial fibrillation and a rapid ventricular response. Using a consistent method of mixing the dobutamine will minimize errors. One example is to mix a 250-mg vial in 250 ml of D_5W, giving 1 mg per ml. An IV pump with microdrip tubing should be used. The patient must be weaned from the medication gradually and must be watched carefully for signs of heart failure (see MSN, Cardiovascular). Drug interactions 1. The actions of dobutamine may be antagonized by beta-blocking drugs. (Dobutamine stimulates beta receptors.)

				2. Dobutamine must be piggybacked to the main IV line because sodium bicarbonate (administered to treat metabolic acidosis) would inactivate it.
Dopamine hydrochloride (Intropin)	This drug stimulates beta receptors of the heart. It strengthens cardiac contractility and increases cardiac output. Blood flow to peripheral vascular beds decreases and mesenteric flow increases. It is used to treat cardiogenic shock following a myocardial infarction, septicemic shock, and shock from congestive heart failure.	Hypertension and increased heart rate are common side-effects. Overdose can cause ectopic heartbeats, tachycardia, anginal chest pains, or dyspnea. Decreasing the infusion rate may correct these. Tachyarrhythmias and hypovolemia should be corrected before adminstering dopamine. Nausea, vomiting, and headache also may occur.	The patient's weight must be known to determine accurate dosage. Mix a 5-ml vial (40 mg/ml) in 500 ml of D_5W giving 400 μg/ml. The initial infusion rate is usually 2 to 5 μg/kg/min and is adjusted according to the individual's BP, urine flow, and cardiac output. There are also vials of dopamine available with 80 mg/ml and 160 mg/ml.	Dopmaine has certain advantages over other vasoconstrictors. It dilates mesenteric and renal blood vessels and often increases urine output. It causes less peripheral vasoconstriction, and myocardial oxygen consumption is comparatively low. BP and apical and radial pulse should be monitored q 10 min. Because of the constant care required, these patients are usually placed in an intensive-care unit. An IV pump and microdrip tubing should be used. If extravasation occurs, infiltration of the area with phentolamine (Regitine) may dilate the constricted blood vessels and prevent tissue damage. Dopamine should be discontinued gradually.

(continued)

TABLE 7-15 ADRENERGICS

Drug	Actions and Indications	Adverse Effects and Contraindications	Dosage and Administration	Nursing Considerations
Epinephrine (Adrenalin)	Epinephrine imitates all actions of the sympathetic nervous system, except those on the arteries of the face and sweat glands. Because of rapid bronchodilation and vasoconstriction effects, epinephrine is useful in treating acute asthmatic attacks and anaphylactic shock. In cardiac arrest and complete heart block, epinephrine can speed and strengthen cardiac contractions. When used topically, it exerts a hemostatic effect in epistaxis. The ophthalmic preparation is used in the management of simple (open-angle) glaucoma. When combined with local anesthetics, it prolongs local effect and delays systemic absorption.	Overdose causes a rapid rise in BP and may lead to severe headache and intracranial hemorrhage. Severe, rapid arrhythmias can occur. Smaller doses may cause tachycardia, dyspnea, pallor, palpitations, feelings of anxiety, fear, and dizziness. It usually is not given to patients with diabetes, angina pectoris, hypertension, and hyperthyroidism.	It is available in 1:1000 solutions for SC, IM and intracardiac use. The usual dosage range is 0.2 to 1 ml (mg). Start small and increase the dosage if required. 1. *Pediatric:* 0.01 mg/kg or 0.3 mg/m^2, to a maximum of 0.5 mg, SC, repeated every 4 hr, as required for bronchial asthma 2. *Cardiac resuscitation:* 0.5 ml (0.5 mg) diluted to 10 ml with NaCl injection, given either IV or intracardially	Epinephrine is extremely potent. Prepare dosages with great care. Always check the type of solution, concentration, dosage, and route. Rotate injection sites to avoid vascular constriction. Possible drug interactions are extensive.

	Nasal and ocular decongestion occur with topical preparations.			
Isoproterenol hydrochloride (Isuprel)	This drug increases cardiac output by increasing cardiac contractility and heart rate. It relaxes smooth muscle, especially that of the bronchi and gastrointestinal tract. It can treat some cardiac arrhythmias, such as standstill, and excessively slow rhythms, such as that caused by digitalis toxicity. Because it dilates blood vessels, it is useful in treating septic shock when vasoconstriction is excessive. It relieves bronchial spasms to provide symptomatic treatment of chronic bronchopulmonary disorders (*e.g.*, asthma and COPD) (see MSN, Respiratory).	Do not give in the presence of rapid arrhythmias because tachycardia and heart palpitations can occur. When administering to treat shock, slow or discontinue the infusion if the pulse goes above 110. Prolonged use may cause the parotid glands to swell. Overdosages may lead to arrhythmias, an elevation followed by a fall in BP, severe bronchoconstriction, cardiac arrest, and sudden death (especially following excessive use of aerosols). Headache, flushing, sweating, tremors, and nervousness also may occur.	The dosage varies according to the problem under treatment. For IV infusion, mix 5 ml of 1:5000 solution in 500 ml of D_5W. The sublingual dosage is 10 to 15 mg qid It also is available in solutions for nebulization and oral inhalation. *Pediatric:* Dosage 5–10 mg, three or four times daily, sublingual, up to a maximum of 30 mg/day	Check BP and apical and radial pulse during administration. For IV administration, an IV pump and microdrip tubing should be used. Saliva and sputum may appear pink after oral inhalation. Propranolol and other beta blockers may antagonize the effects of isoproterenol.

(*continued from page 719*)

- Patients receiving both adrenergics and monamine oxidase (MAO) inhibitors may experience a hypertensive crisis.
- Diuretics and some antihypertensives can interfere with the effects of adrenergics.
- Serious arrhythmias can occur if epinephrine and isoproterenol are administered concurrently.
- When adrenergics are administered intravenously, use an IV pump and microdrip tubing. Watch carefully for extravasation.
- Caution patients not to use OTC asthma medications or decongestants without checking with their physician.

ANTIANEMICS

CYANOCOBALAMIN INJECTION (VITAMIN B_{12})

Actions

- Vitamin B_{12} is a hematopoietic substance (forms blood cells).
- It counteracts glossitis (smooth, sore, ulcerated tongue).
- It decreases gastrointestinal (GI) symptoms such as constipation or diarrhea.
- Vitamin B_{12} can prevent damage to the spinal cord and other central nervous system (CNS) areas (*e.g.*, numbness, tingling, and muscle incoordination decreases).

Indications

- It is used to treat pernicious anemia, a lack of intrinsic factor, and inability to absorb vitamin B_{12}.
- It replaces vitamin B_{12} in patients who have had their entire stomach or portions of it removed.
- It also is used in vitamin B_{12} absorption (Schilling) test.

Adverse Effects and Contraindications

- Toxic reactions to vitamin B_{12} are rare, but thrombosis, hypokalemia, congestive heart failure, and pulmonary edema have been reported.
- Patients who have optic nerve damage or who are hypersensitive to cobalt should not receive vitamin B_{12}.

Dosage and Administration

- An average course of treatment for pernicious anemia would be 30 to 100 μg, qd, for 1 week, then one to three times weekly until remission is achieved. This is followed by 100 μg per month for the rest of the patient's life.

- Vitamin B_{12} can be given SC or IM.
- *Pediatric:* Administer 100-μg doses up to a total of 1–5 mg over 2 or more weeks; the maintenance dosage is 60 μg/month.

Nursing Considerations

- Emphasize that the medication is treating, not curing, the anemia, and that the therapy cannot be discontinued.
- The patient or a family member should be taught to give the injections, which will result in the dual benefits of self-sufficiency and lower cost.

FOLIC ACID (FOLVITE)

Actions

- A member of the vitamin-B complex, folic acid is essential for cell division in all types of tissue.

Indications

- It is used to treat individuals with deficiencies: *e.g.,* patients with malnutrition from alcoholism, advanced age, or poverty; food faddists; women with several successive pregnancies; and patients on long-term anticonvulsant therapy.

Adverse Effects and Contraindications

- Adverse effects are rare.
- Folic acid is contraindicated in patients with pernicious anemia because it masks the symptoms and makes diagnosis difficult.

Dosage and Administration

- A maintenance dosage of 1 mg, PO, daily is usually adequate.

IRON

Actions

- Iron is needed by all body cells and is essential in the body's red blood cells to form the hemoglobin (Hb) responsible for oxygen and carbon dioxide transportation.

Indications

- Iron is used to prevent and treat iron-deficiency anemias in susceptible individuals: 6-month-old infants to 2-year-old children, adolescents (especially female), pregnant women in the second and third trimester, women with heavy menstrual flow, and GI bleeders.

Adverse Effects and Contraindications

- Iron can cause varying degrees of epigastric distress: nausea, vomiting, or abdominal cramps (with either diarrhea or constipation).
- Overdose can result in corrosion of the lining of the stomach and intestine, with black, tarry stools; weak, rapid pulse; and hypotension sufficient to produce shock.
- The IM preparation can cause *anaphylactic shock,* and should be used very cautiously if liver function is impaired. Iron administration parenterally also can cause vomiting, chills, fever, headache, joint pain, and urticaria.
- Caution also should be used in the presence of GI disorders (*e.g.,* ulcers), and in patients receiving repeated transfusions.

Dosage and Administration

- Ferrous sulfate (Feosol): The usual daily dosage is one to four 300-mg tablets. The pediatric dosage is 120 to 600 mg daily for children 6–12 years old, and 75 to 225 mg for children under 6 years of age.
- Ferrous gluconate (Fergon): The usual daily dosage is 1 capsule (435 mg), yielding 50 mg of elemental iron. The pediatric dosage is 100 to 300 mg, three times daily for children 6 to 12 years old, and 100 to 300 mg daily in divided doses for children under 6 years of age.
- Iron-Dextran injection (Imferon): The total dosage is calculated using the following formula:

$$0.3 \times \text{weight in lb} \times \frac{(100 - \text{Hb g/dl} \times 100)}{14.8} = \text{mg of iron}$$

- Begin therapy with an IM test dose of 0.5 ml. If no adverse reaction occurs, give the total calculated amount following this schedule of maximum doses:
  1. Infants under 10 lb: 0.5 ml (25 mg of iron)
  2. Children under 20 lb: 1.0 ml (50 mg of iron)
  3. Patients under 110 lb: 2.0 ml (100 mg of iron)
  4. Patients over 110 lb: 5.0 mg (250 mg of iron)
- Iron dextran can be administered intravenously to avoid the pain and discoloration of IM injections. Use only the Imferon brand,

and the 2-ml and 5-ml ampules *without* preservatives. Mix with 500 ml to 1,000 ml of normal saline. Observe for allergic reactions by running the solution in slowly (10 gtt/min) for about 10 minutes to 15 minutes, then increase the rate to no more than 60 gtt/min.

Nursing Considerations

- Giving more iron than the situation warrants is useless and also can be harmful. The intestines regulate the amount absorbed, which is usually enough to replace the daily loss (about 10% to 15% of ingested iron).
- Oral iron is absorbed best from an empty stomach, but it can be very irritating. Begin giving the medication on a full stomach, and gradually reduce the amount of food taken with it.
- Liquid preparations can stain teeth. Dilute the liquid and have the patient drink it through a straw.
- Iron given IM can produce staining, soreness, and inflammation. It should be given deep IM, only in the muscle of the upper, outer quadrant, using the Z-track technique (see PH, Drug therapy).
- Inform patients that their stools may be black and tarry, even with normal doses. Otherwise they may think they are bleeding.
- To reduce the risk of phlebitis when giving the Imferon IV, do not mix with D_5W. If possible, do not let the infusion run over 5 hours.

ANTIARRHYTHMICS

- Also see beta-adrenergic blockers and calcium-channel blockers.

DISOPYRAMIDE PHOSPHATE (NORPACE)

Actions

- This is a type 1 antiarrhythmic drug similar to procainamide and quinidine.
- Norpace decreases the rate of ectopic pacemakers and the rate of impulse conduction in the atrial and ventricular muscle.
- It does not significantly alter conduction through the atrioventricular (AV) node.

Indications

- It is used to suppress premature ventricular contractions (PVCs) and ventricular tachycardia.

Adverse Effects and Contraindications

- Bradycardia or tachycardia can occur.
- Severe hypotension may develop.

- This drug is not recommended for patients with heart block.
- Patients also may experience atropine-like side-effects, such as mouth dryness, constipation, and blurred vision. It may be unsafe for patients with glaucoma, prostatic hypertrophy, or myasthenia gravis.
- Use cautiously for patients with congestive heart failure (CHF) because severe hypotension and cardiogenic shock could result.
- Rarely, ventricular tachycardia or fibrillation has occurred.

Dosage and Administration

- The usual PO dosage is 100 to 150 mg, q 6 hr (600 mg/day).
- If the patient is less than 110 lb, the dosage is 100 mg q 6 hr (400 mg/day).

Nursing Considerations

- Always check the patient's BP and apical and radical pulse before giving the drug.
- Be alert to your patient's reports of fainting, dizziness, weakness, and pulse changes.
- Monitor intake and output, especially for patients with impaired renal function or prostatic hypertrophy.
- Concurrent use of alcohol can produce additive hypoglycemic and hypotensive effects.
- Patients with atrial fibrillation or flutter are usually digitalized prior to Norpace therapy.
- Concurrent use of anticholinergics is not recommended. Advise patients against using OTC medications without checking with their physician.

LIDOCAINE (XYLOCAINE)

Actions

- Lidocaine depresses excessive automaticity and, therefore, PVCs.
- It does not depress conduction, so there is less likelihood of heart block or ventricular, ectopic rhythms.
- It does not depress contractility, so CHF is less likely.
- It also acts as a local anesthetic.

Indications

- Lidocaine is useful for rapid control of PVCs in patients during acute myocardial infarction and cardiac surgery, and thus helps to prevent ventricular tachycardia.

- Ventricular arrhythmias resulting from digitalis toxicity also respond well to lidocaine.

Adverse Effects and Contraindications

- Lidocaine can produce bradycardia and hypotension.
- Drowsiness is usually the first central nervous system (CNS) effect, but excitation may follow. Paresthesias also can occur.
- Lidocaine should not be used with severe heart block.
- Reports of convulsions are common.

Dosage and Administration

- To ensure accurate dosage, the patient's weight must be known.
- The usual bolus IV dose is 1 mg/kg.
- In emergency situations, a bolus of 50 to 100 mg is given IV push at an approximate rate of 20 to 50 mg/minute. Then, 1 g is mixed in 500 ml of D_5W for administration, piggyback to the main IV line, and delivered at a rate of 1 to 4 mg/minute (20 to 50 μg/kg/minute).
- Because *fluid overload* is always a danger, mixing *2 g* in *500 ml* may be indicated because the patient would receive less fluid. The use of microdrip tubing and an infusion pump also is indicated.
- Never give more than 200 to 300 mg during a one-hour period.

Nursing Considerations

- Monitor BP and apical and radial pulse very carefully.
- Lidocaine must be administered by IV injection. It goes quickly to the myocardium and other organs with a rich blood supply, but the infusion must continue for relatively long periods to maintain effective levels. The patient must be weaned from it gradually.
- Anticonvulsants and barbiturates can increase the metabolism of lidocaine. Therefore, higher doses of the lidocaine may be needed.
- The risk of CHF is increased when the following drugs are used with lidocaine: phenytoin, procainamide, propranolol, quinidine, and disopyramide.
- Only lidocaine hydrochloride without preservatives or epinephrine and specifically labeled for IV use should be used for IV injection or infusion.

PHENYTOIN SODIUM (DILANTIN)

Actions

- Phenytoin's antiarrhythmic activity is similar to procainamide and quinidine.

- It suppresses automaticity in ectopic pacemakers and actually may increase the rate at which impulses are conducted through the AV node and Purkinje's fibers.

Indications

- It is used to treat the arrhythmias caused by digitalis toxicity such as atrial tachycardia with block, and premature ventricular systoles.
- It is more effective against ventricular than atrial arrhythmias.

Adverse Effects and Contraindications

- Bradycardia and hypotension can occur.
- Phenytoin should not be given in advanced heart block.
- Nausea, vomiting, and constipation occur.
- Gingival hyperplasia (overgrowth of gum tissue) is common.
- Hirsutism, skin rashes, and megaloblastic anemia occur.
- Excessive doses cause lethargy, slurred speech, and a staggering gait. Patients also experience double vision, dizziness, and headache.
- Overdose results in coma, apnea, and death.
- Cardiac arrest can occur from rapid IV administration.

Dosage and Administration

- An average oral maintenance dosage is 200 to 400 mg, qd (*e.g.*, 100 mg, qid).

Nursing Considerations

- Monitor BP and apical and radial pulse carefully.
- Heart block or bradycardia may be reversed with IV administration of atropine.
- Patients metabolize phenytoin at different rates, so blood levels should be checked to monitor the drug for effectiveness and toxicity.
- Giving phenytoin during or after meals will minimize the gastric distress.
- Patients receiving this drug for long periods may need folic acid to prevent anemia.
- The following drug interactions occur with phenytoin:
  1. The action of phenytoin is potentiated by aspirin, chloramphenicol, sulfonamides, and anticoagulants.
  2. The action of phenytoin is inhibited by alcohol, barbiturates, and sedatives.

3. Phenytoin induces metabolism of quinidine, and may reduce the antiarrhythmic effect.
4. Phenytoin inhibits the action of steroids and digitalis.

- See PH, Neurological system.

PROCAINAMIDE HYDROCHLORIDE (PRONESTYL HYDROCHLORIDE)

Actions

- Procainamide is similar to quinidine. Parenteral administration, however, is considered to be somewhat safer than that with quinidine.
- It depresses ectopic pacemakers and slows conduction in the atrium and ventricle.

Indications

- It is used to control PVCs and ventricular tachycardia, especially following myocardial infarction, cardiac surgery, and digitalis toxicity.
- It also is used for atrial fibrillation and paroxysmal atrial tachycardia.

Adverse Effects and Contraindications

- Hypotension can occur, especially following IV administration.
- Gastrointestinal disturbances, such as anorexia, nausea, and vomiting, occur.
- Agranulocytosis has occurred with long-term use of the drug.
- Prolonged oral administration can produce signs and symptoms resembling the syndrome of lupus erythematosus. If the antinuclear antibody test (ANA) becomes positive, the drug should be discontinued. Agranulocytosis and the lupus syndrome are rare, but very serious.
- The drug should not be given to patients with myasthenia gravis or complete heart block.

Dosage and Administration

- For ventricular tachycardia, give a total daily dosage of 50 mg/kg at 3-hour intervals.
- The maintenance dose for atrial arrhythmias is 0.5 g to 1 g, every 4 to 6 hr.

Nursing Considerations

- Monitor BP, especially during IV administration. Apical and radial pulse also should be checked.

- Observe for clinical signs of lupus (*e.g.*, fever, arthritis, or pleuritic pain).
- Observe for clinical signs of decreased white blood cell (WBC) count, *e.g.*, sore throat or upper respiratory infections.

QUINIDINE

Actions

- Quinidine preparations can be considered a prototype of other antiarrhythmic drugs.
- These preparations depress automaticity, especially in the latent or ectopic (non-sinoatrial node) pacemakers, giving the sinoatrial node a chance to regain control, or at least causing a decrease in heart rate.
- They can delay conduction, which worsens heart block.
- Contractility also may be decreased, but usually not to a serious extent.

Indications

- It is used to prevent and treat both atrial and ventricular arrhythmias.
- One of its main uses is to prevent recurrences of atrial tachycardia, fibrillation, or flutter following conversion to a normal sinus rhythm (NSR) by electric shock or other drugs.

Adverse Effects and Contraindications

- GI symptoms, especially diarrhea, are very common.
- Hypotension can occur.
- A common toxic effect is the development of AV block. This can result in asystole, PVCs, ventricular tachycardia, or fibrillation.
- Quinidine also can cause or worsen CHF.
- Thrombocytopenia can occur as a hypersensitivity reaction.
- Quinidine is contraindicated in patients with heart block.

Dosage and Administration

- Quinidine sulfate (Quinidex): The usual maintenance dosage is 200 mg to 300 mg, PO, tid, or qid. It is absorbed readily from the GI tract.
- Quinidine gluconate: This usually is given IM. The initial dose is from 300 mg to 500 mg.

Nursing Considerations

- Always check the patient's BP and apical and radial pulse before giving the drug. Notify the physician of any significant decrease.

- Quinidine can prolong the patient's prothrombin time (PT) and potentiate anticoagulants. Observe for signs of bleeding.
- To maintain therapeutic blood levels, the drug should be evenly spaced (*e.g.*, q 6 hr rather than qid). Check with the physician before withholding *any* dose.
- Quinidine can potentiate the effects of antihypertensives and diuretics and can cause excessive hypotension.
- Serum digoxin levels can more than double rapidly when quinidine is added. Digoxin levels should be checked, and it may be necessary for the physician to lower the dose of digoxin.
- Toxic reactions to quinidine are most likely to occur in patients with liver disease, renal insufficiency, or CHF.
- Embolization from dislodgement of atrial mural emboli is a risk when reverting to a sinus rhythm from long-standing fibrillation.

ANTICOAGULANTS

Nursing Considerations

- Observe for bleeding (*e.g.*, in the stool, urine, nose, vagina, gums, or as indicated by any abnormal bruising). Patients may need soft toothbrushes and stool softeners. Use an electric razor rather than a blade. Test the patient's urine and stool for occult blood.
- The patient should always carry an ID card or wear a bracelet stating the medications he or she is receiving.
- Remind patients to inform their other doctors and dentists that they are receiving anticoagulants when they go for treatment. They also should notify their physician if they become ill, especially with a fever or diarrhea.
- Emphasize the importance of periodic blood tests.
- Advise patients to avoid activities such as contact sports that could lead to injury and bleeding.
- Caution patients *not* to take any new medications or to stop taking previously prescribed or OTC drugs without notifying their physician. OTC drugs such as aspirin and cold products with antihistamines can interact with serious consequences.

HEPARIN SODIUM

Actions

- This drug prevents the formation of new blood clots.
- It affects circulating factors in the bloodstream in an immediate, rapid fashion to prevent clot formation. It has a short duration of action.
- Heparin sodium cannot dissolve preexisting clots.

Indications

- Heparin sodium is used to treat venous thromboembolism (from thrombophlebitis), pulmonary embolism, and thromboembolism from heart disease (*e.g.,* myocardial infarction, atrial fibrillation, CHF, and mitral valve disease, which can produce cerebral emboli from intramural thrombi).
- It usually is given in the acute stages when rapid effects are required.
- It may be used prophylactically following major surgery to prevent deep vein thrombosis.
- Heparin is also used for disseminated intravascular clotting (DIC).
- Heparin usually is given prior to oral anticoagulant therapy.

Adverse Effects and Contraindications

- *Hemorrhage* is the main adverse effect.
- Hypersensitivity reactions, such as chills, fever, and urticaria, have been reported.
- Patients also have experienced asthma, rhinitis, lacrimation, and anaphylactoid reactions.
- Intravenous doses of heparin have produced acute, reversible thrombocytopenia.
- Long-term therapy with high doses has produced osteoporosis and suppression of renal function.
- Heparin should not be used in the following conditions: history of blood disorders; peptic ulcer; ulcerative colitis; GI carcinoma; recent head injury; liver, kidney, or biliary disease; or following surgery on the CNS. Also, it should not be used in patients who cannot cooperate to take the proper dosages and receive the necessary follow-up care (*e.g.,* laboratory work).

Dosage and Administration

- The dosage is determined by laboratory results. A partial thromboplastin time (PTT) usually is used.
- The patient's PTT should be maintained at one and one-half to two times the control for the anticoagulation to be effective.
- Heparin must be administered parenterally. Three methods are used: continuous infusion—usually considered the most effective method because it maintains a constant blood level; intermittent IV injection through a heparin lock; and intermittent SC injection.

Nursing Considerations

- See PH, Anticoagulants, Nursing considerations.
- A baseline PTT should be drawn before therapy is started.

- When a patient is receiving an intermittent form of heparin, blood samples to check PTT must be timed *carefully*. Usually, the blood is drawn 30 min to 1 hr *before* the next dose. That dose of heparin usually is given; then, the physician is notified of the lab results before other doses are administered. A change in dosage may be indicated.
- Heparin is considered most effective when administered through continuous infusion; however, this is also the most dangerous method. Monitor the IV carefully, place on a IV pump, and use microdrip tubing.
- Heparin comes in prefilled Tubex syringes. The size remains the same even though the doses differ (*e.g.*, a 100-unit Tubex is the same size as a 10,000-unit Tubex). Check *carefully*. Be very careful when mixing heparin in the IV bottle so that you will be administering the proper dose. The following is one method of mixing:

$$\frac{20{,}000 \text{ units heparin}}{500 \text{ ml } D_5W} = 40 \text{ units/ml}$$

- To maintain the patency of the heparin lock, check for blood return, observe closely for signs of infiltration (*e.g.*, redness, swelling, pain), inject heparin slowly, and flush tubing completely.
- When using a heparin lock to administer other medications, flush with normal saline before and after to avoid interactions. Heparin flush is done following the second normal saline.
- When removing a heparin lock, be sure to apply firm pressure for 5 minutes. Then return to check for bleeding.
- To minimize bruising from heparin administered SC: do not draw back on the syringe, do not massage the area; apply firm pressure following injection; instruct the patient not to scratch the area. Although the SC tissue of the abdomen has been the common site for injection, heparin can be given into any SC tissue.
- Heparin's antagonist is *protamine sulfate*.
- Intramuscular injections and arterial punctures should be avoided unless absolutely necessary.
- The effectiveness of heparin is diminished in the elderly.

WARFARIN SODIUM (COUMADIN)

Actions

- Warfarin sodium prevents the formation of new blood clots.
- Coagulation factors: It interferes with Factor II (liver synthesis of prothrombin) and Factors VII, IX, and X to prevent clot formation.
- It requires 1 day to 4 days to become effective, and usually is started while the patient is still receiving heparin.

Indications

- It is used to treat venous thromboembolism (from thrombophlebitis), pulmonary embolism, and thromboembolism from heart disease (*e.g.*, myocardial infarction, atrial fibrillation, CHF, and mitral valve disease, which can produce cerebral emboli from intramural thrombi).
- Use for long-term therapy when rapid action is not required.

Adverse Effects and Contraindications

- *Hemorrhage* is the main adverse effect.
- Other side-effects are infrequent, but include the following: alopecia, urticaria, dermatitis, fever, nausea, diarrhea, and a reaction consisting of hemorrhagic infarction and necrosis of the skin.
- Warfarin usage in the elderly must be monitored carefully.
  1. Ninety-eight percent of warfarin is bound to plasma proteins. Even small changes in the degree of protein binding can produce *large* changes in the concentration of free drug in the circulation.
  2. Females and the elderly usually require smaller doses.
  3. Patients in CHF are at greater risk for hemorrhage (possibly the result of liver dysfunction).
  4. Absorption may be slow and erratic.
  5. The elderly frequently experience vitamin K deficiencies if their nutritional status is poor or if they have chronic disease. The chance of hemorrhage, therefore, is increased.
  6. The elderly are at a greater risk for drug interactions because they take more drugs more frequently than other age groups.
- Warfarin should not be used in the following conditions: history of blood disorders; peptic ulcer; ulcerative colitis; GI carcinoma; recent head injury; liver, kidney, or biliary disease; or following surgery on the CNS. Also, it should not be used in patients who cannot cooperate to take the proper dosages and receive the necessary follow-up care (*e.g.*, laboratory work).

Dosage and Administration

- The dosage is determined by the lab results. A PT usually is used.
- A patient's PT should be maintained at two to two and one-half times the control (the control is usually 11 to 13 seconds).
- The average initial loading, or priming, dose is 40 to 60 mg, orally.
- The maintenance dosage range usually is 5 to 10 mg, orally, qd

Nursing Considerations

- See PH, Anticoagulants, nursing considerations.
- Drug interactions: Chloral hydrate, Atromid S, Butazolidin, quinidine, salicylates (*e.g.*, aspirin and aspirin products), oral hypogly-

cemics, sulfonamides, and broad-spectrum antibiotics can potentiate oral anticoagulants. Antacids, barbiturates, estrogens (*e.g.*, birth control pills), thiazides, and other diuretics can reduce the patient's response to oral anticoagulants.

- Oral anticoagulants should be taken at the same time each day. This aids in maintaining consistent blood levels. In the hospital situation, 6 P.M. is a convenient time because the PT usually is drawn in the morning. This gives the nurse adequate time to contact the physician with the results in case a dosage change is indicated.
- Warfarin's antagonist is vitamin K (see PH, Cardiovascular, hemostatic).
- Other oral anticoagulants are dicumarol, phenprocoumon (Liquamar), warfarin potassium (Athrombin-K), anisindione (Miradon), and phenindione (Hedulin).

ANTIHYPERTENSIVES

Nursing Considerations

- Monitor BP daily (more frequently if the patient's condition indicates).
- To help patients avoid orthostatic hypotension, instruct them to rise slowly from a sitting or lying position. They should not stand perfectly still for long periods of time because blood may pool in their legs. Weakness or dizziness usually can be alleviated by having them lie down for a few minutes.
- Sudden omissions of medications can cause rapid rise in BP, and as a result there is a severe crisis for the patient.
- A stepped-care approach to therapy is now recommended (see Table 7-16). Therapy is initiated with a small dosage of a step-1 drug. The dosage is increased as necessary, and other drugs are added sequentially as needed.
- An advantage of the stepped-care threapy is the synergistic interaction that can occur between various agents. Smaller doses of individual drugs may be necessary, thus reducing the incidence and severity of side-effects.
- Adverse effects may be a dose-limiting factor before the maximum dosage has been reached.
- Lack of response to therapy always should be investigated before proceeding to a successive treatment step. Factors to consider are the following:
  1. Poor adherence to therapy
  2. Insufficient dosage with current drugs
  3. Weight gain or excessive sodium intake
  4. Concurrent use of competing drugs that interfere with the action of the antihypertensives (*e.g.*, vasopressor decongestants, appetite suppressants, oral contraceptives)

TABLE 7-16 STEPPED-CARE THERAPY FOR HYPERTENSION

Step	Drug Category	Examples*	Implications
1	Diuretic	Hydrochlorothiazide (Hydrodiuril) (Also seen as HCTZ)	Thiazide diuretics are usually the drugs of choice. Loop diuretics (*e.g.*, furosemide [Lasix]) may be selected for certain patients. Potassium-sparing agents may be indicated.
+			Hypokalemia, hyperuricemia, and hyperglycemia are all possible with diuretic therapy.
2	Adrenergic-blocking agent	Atenolol (Tenormin), clonidine (Catapres), methyldopa (Aldomet), metoprolol (Lopressor), nadolol (Corgard), prazosin (Minipress), propranolol (Inderal), reserpine (Serpasil)	Prazosin may be used as a step-3 drug if it has not been added in step 2.
+			Fatigue or lethargy, depression, and sexual dysfunction may be experienced.
3	Vasodilator	Hydralazine (Apresoline)	This type of drug may increase heart rate and cardiac output and should be used concurrently with an adrenergic-blocking agent.
+			
4	Additional adrenergic blocking agent	Guanethidine (Ismelin)	These agents may cause orthostatic hypotension, diarrhea, or impaired ejaculation.

*Many other drugs are currently on the market. This is a sample of commonly used agents.

- Advise all patients to notify their physician before using OTC preparations for coughs, colds, or allergies. Many contain sympathomimetic agents that can increase BP.
- Elderly patients may be more sensitive to sympathetic inhibition and volume depletion than younger individuals. Cardiovascular reflexes may be impaired and hypotension is a definite consideration. Treatment should be started with smaller than usual doses, and increased with great caution (smaller increments at longer intervals).
- The elderly can experience isolated systolic hypertension that may be resistant to treatment. The risks and benefits of treatment must be considered on an individual basis.

BETA-ADRENERGIC BLOCKERS

- See Beta-adrenergic blockers section, page 752.

CAPTOPRIL (CAPOTEN)

Actions

- Captopril inhibits the angiotensin converting enzyme, thereby blocking the conversion of angiotensin I to angiotensin II.
- It decreases total peripheral resistance.
- It also reduces aldosterone secretion with less sodium and water retention.

Indications

- Captopril is used primarily when BP is refractory to treatment with standard multidrug regimens (See Table 7-16).
- It also is used when side-effects of beta blockers or vasodilators are unacceptable to the patient, or when these agents are contraindicated because of concurrent pathologic conditions.

Adverse Effects and Contraindications

- Proteinuria has occurred and may lead to the nephrotic syndrome. Prior existence of renal disease increases the risk.
- Neutropenia/agranulocytosis has been reported, especially in patients with renal impairment or an autoimmune collagen disorder (*e.g.,* systemic lupus erythematosus).
- Although the incidence of mental depression, cardiac depression, impotence, fatigue, and orthostatic hypotension appears to be less than with other antihypertensives, they do occur.
- Rash (often with pruritus), photosensitivity, angioedema of the face and mucous membranes of the mouth, and laryngeal edema have been reported.

- Hypotension is a risk for patients on diuretic therapy, those on dietary salt restriction or dialysis, and those experiencing excessive vomiting, diarrhea, or perspiration.
- A reversible loss of taste perception (dysgeusia) also has occurred.

Dosage and Administration

- Therapy usually is started with 25 mg, PO, tid.
- After 1 week to 2 weeks the dosage may be increased to 50 mg, PO, tid.
- Evaluate in one week to two weeks. If necessary, small doses of a thiazide diuretic may be added.
- At 1- to 2-week intervals, the diuretic may be increased. For further BP control, captopril may be increased to 100 mg, tid, and then to 150 mg, tid.
- The maximum daily dosage is 450 mg.

Nursing Considerations

- See PH, Antihypertensives, nursing considerations.
- Administer captopril one hour before meals.
- Patients should be told to report signs of infection (*e.g.,* sore throat, fever). WBC counts and differentials should be done before starting therapy, at 2-week intervals for about 3 months, and periodically thereafter.
- Observe for volume depletion caused by decreased fluid intake, diaphoresis, vomiting, and diarrhea.
- Urinary protein determinations (*e.g.,* dip stick on first morning urine) should be done prior to therapy, at monthly intervals for about nine months, and periodically thereafter.
- *If* possible, previous antihypertensive therapy should be discontinued one week prior to administering captopril.

CLONIDINE HYDROCHLORIDE (CATAPRES)

Actions

- This drug centrally mediates a decrease in sympathetic discharge by stimulating alpha-adrenergic receptors.
- It decreases heart rate and cardiac output.

Indications

- It is used to treat hypertension usually in combination with a diuretic and other antihypertensive agents (See Table 7-16).

- It also is used as prophylaxis for migraine, and to treat dysmenorrhea and opiate withdrawal.

Adverse Effects and Contraindications

- Frequent occurrences include dry mouth, sedation, drowsiness, constipation, dizziness, headache, weakness, and fatigue.
- Gastrointestinal distress, postural hypotension, bradycardia, CHF, urinary retention, and mental depression also have been related to clonidine use.

Dosage and Administration

- Maintenance dosage for hypertension treatment is 0.1 mg to 0.2 mg, two to four times daily, PO.

Nursing Considerations

- See Antihypertensives, nursing considerations.
- Lowering the BP gradually is important, especially for elderly patients.
- The drug should be withdrawn gradually, over a period of 2 days to 4 days.

HYDRALAZINE HYDROCHLORIDE (APRESOLINE HCl)

Actions

- This drug directly dilates vascular smooth muscle, especially the arterioles.
- It reduces peripheral vascular resistance and increases renal and cerebral blood flow.

Indications

- It is used to treat essential hypertension, usually in combination with other antihypertensives (see Table 7-16).

Adverse Effects and Contraindications

- Patients may experience headache, tachycardia, anginal chest pain, orthostatic hypotension, nausea, vomiting, and diarrhea.
- Discontinue the medication if the patient develops signs and symptoms of systemic lupus erythematosus (*e.g.*, fever and joint pains).
- Patients with coronary artery or mitral valve disease should not receive hydralazine.

Dosage and Administration

- Depending on the severity of the patient's problem, the dosage can range from 40 mg to 200 mg, PO, daily, in divided doses.
- A usual IV dose is 10 mg to 40 mg, repeated as necessary.
- *Pediatric Dosage:* Initially, give 0.75 mg/kg or 25 mg/m^2 daily in four divided doses, PO. This may be increased gradually up to 7.5 mg/kg daily.

Nursing Considerations

- See PH, Antihypertensives, nursing considerations.
- A lupus erythematosus (LE) cell preparation is indicated if patient develops arthralgia, fever, chest pain, and malaise.

METHYLDOPA (ALDOMET)

Actions

- Methyldopa reduces transmissions of impulses by adrenergic nerves.
- It decreases peripheral resistance, but it does not decrease kidney perfusion or cardiac output.

Indications

- Methyldopa may be used alone for moderate hypertension, but it usually is given with a diuretic (See Table 7-16).
- This drug is preferred for patients with renal insufficiency.

Adverse Effects and Contraindications

- Drowsiness is common, especially when therapy is first started.
- Orthostatic hypotension is possible.
- Mouth dryness, depression, and nightmares may occur.
- Hypersensitivity reactions involving the liver, blood, and skin (*e.g.,* hepatitis and hemolytic anemia) have been reported.
- Patients may experience a drug-induced fever within about 3 weeks of starting the drug.
- Patients with active liver disease should not receive methyldopa.

Dosage and Administration

- The usual adult dosage is 500 mg to 2 g, PO, qd, in divided doses.
- *Pediatric Dosage:* The usual dosage is 10 mg/kg up to 65 mg/kg/24 hours, given in two to four divided doses, orally.
- It also may be given IV.

Nursing Considerations

- See PH, Antihypertensives, nursing considerations.
- A baseline blood count should be done before therapy is begun to detect the presence of anemia. Blood counts should be repeated periodically to monitor the patient for hemolytic anemia.
- A direct Coombs' test should be done before therapy, and then at 6 months and 12 months. Patients with a positive direct Coombs' test may develop hemolytic anemia.
- Monitor liver function during therapy, especially when unexplained fever occurs, to detect hypersensitivity reactions.

PRAZOSIN HYDROCHLORIDE (MINIPRESS)

Actions

- This drug acts as an alpha-adrenergic blocking agent.
- It reduces total peripheral vascular resistance.

Indications

- It is used to treat hypertension, usually in combination with a diuretic and other antihypertensive agents (See Table 7-16).

Adverse Effects and Contraindications

- Frequent adverse effects include dizziness, headache, drowsiness, fatigue, weakness, nausea, and palpitations.
- Syncope with sudden loss of consciousness can occur, especially with rapid increases in dosage, with the addition of another antihypertensive agent, or when initiating therapy with a dosage greater than 1 mg.

Dosage and Administration

- The initial dosage is usually 1 mg, two to three times daily, PO.
- The maintenance dosage is a *gradual* increase to 20 mg/day in divided doses.

Nursing Considerations

- See PH, Antihypertensives, nursing considerations.

RESERPINE (SERPASIL)

Actions

- Reserpine partially blocks transmission of impulses from sympathetic (adrenergic) nerves.

- It produces gradual drops in BP.
- It also slows the heart rate and reduces cardiac output.

Indications

- It is used for chronic essential hypertension (mild to moderate severity). Usually, it is combined with a diuretic (See Table 7-16).

Adverse Effects and Contraindications

- Patients may experience nasal congestion and stuffiness, drowsiness, weakness, fatigue, and severe mental depression.
- Do not give if there is a history of suicidal tendencies or epilepsy.
- Use cautiously for patients with a history of peptic ulcer or ulcerative colitis.

Dosage and Administration

- The usual adult dosage is 0.25 to 0.5 mg, PO, qd, for 1 week to 2 weeks.
- The maintenance dosage is 0.1 to 0.25 mg daily.

Nursing Considerations

- See PH, Antihypertensives, nursing considerations.

SODIUM NITROPRUSSIDE (NIPRIDE)

Actions

- This drug produces peripheral vasodilation by acting directly on vascular smooth muscle.
- It lowers arterial BP, slightly increases heart rate, and mildly decreases cardiac output and peripheral vascular resistance.

Indications

- It is used in hypertensive crises for short-term, rapid reduction of BP.

Adverse Effects and Contraindications

- Nausea, abdominal pain, nasal stuffiness, diaphoresis, headache, dizziness, restlessness, apprehension, palpitations, and muscle twitching usually are associated with a too-rapid reduction in BP.
- Overdosage produces profound hypotension, metabolic acidosis, absence of reflexes, and loss of consciousness.

Dosage and Administration

- The average dose is 3μg/kg/minute, IV. The dose may range between 0.5 to 10 μg/kg/minute, IV.

Nursing Considerations

- Solutions must be freshly prepared using sterile 5% dextrose in water, and used no later than 4 hours after reconstitution. Nipride is *not* for direct IV injection.
- Promptly wrap the container with an opaque material, such as aluminum foil, to protect the drug from light.
- An infusion pump should be used for precise measurement of flow rate.
- Nipride can be used concomitantly with oral antihypertensives.

THIAZIDES

- See PH.

ATROPINE SULFATE

Actions

- Anticholinergics interfere with the action of acetylcholine and cholinergic drugs.
- They decrease GI muscle tone and motility, and in large doses they decrease secretion of gastric acid and digestive enzymes (*e.g.*, pepsin).
- They reduce the tone and motility of the ureters and the bladder wall, and they increase bladder sphincter tone.
- Large doses may accelerate the heart rate; small doses may slow it.
- Ocular effects include mydriasis (dilation of pupil) and cycloplegia (paralysis of accommodation).
- Anticholinergics cause a decrease in sweating, salivation, and nasal and bronchial secretions, and also abnormal skeletal muscle tone.

Indications

- It is used to treat GI disorders such as peptic ulcer, gastritis, and spastic colon.
- It also is used in symptomatic treatment of Parkinson's disease.
- It counteracts bradycardia and partial heart block by increasing the heart rate.
- It can abolish vagal reflexes in cardiac arrest.

- It is used in diagnostic eye examinations.
- Frequently, it is included in preoperative medications to reduce salivation and bronchial secretions.

Adverse Effects and Contraindications

- Common side-effects include dryness of the mouth and blurring of the vision.
- The tachycardia often produced is undesirable in cardiac disorders. Hypertension or hypotension may occur.
- Constipation and urinary retention can occur.
- Do not give to patients with prostatic hypertrophy, narrow-angle glaucoma, or severe ulcerative colitis.

Dosage and Administration

- The usual adult dose is 0.4 mg to 0.6 mg, PO, SC, IV, or IM, and may be repeated every 4 hours to 6 hours.
- The usual pediatric dose is 0.01 mg/kg, PO, SC, IM, or IV, and may be repeated every 4 hours to 6 hours.
- Sterile ophthalmic solutions and ointments are available for eye examinations.

Nursing Considerations

- Oral atropine usually is given 30 minutes before meals.
- A paradoxic bradycardia may follow IV atropine, but it usually lasts only 1 minute to 2 minutes.

BETA-ADRENERGIC BLOCKERS

Actions

- These agents inhibit $beta_1$ receptors in cardiac muscle, resulting in decreases in cardiac contractility, cardiac output, and myocardial oxygen consumption.
- They depress automaticity of the sinus node and ectopic foci.
- They slow conduction through the AV node, resulting in a decreased heart rate.
- These drugs also inhibit $beta_2$ receptors in bronchial and vascular smooth muscle, resulting in bronchoconstriction and bronchospasm, peripheral vasoconstriction, and increased peripheral vascular resistance.
- Plasma renin activity or renin secretion is suppressed by these agents.
- They may potentiate hypoglycemic response in diabetic patients following insulin administration.

Indications

- See Table 7-17.

Adverse Effects and Contraindications

- Beta blockers should be used cautiously in patients with heart failure or left ventricular dysfunction, diabetes, hyperthyroidism, chronic obstructive pulmonary disease, asthma, or peripheral vascular disease.
- They may cause hypotension, heart failure, and arrhythmias such as bradycardia and heart block.
- Beta blockers may increase the frequency or intensity of anginal attacks if the dosage is decreased or withdrawn suddenly.
- Alteration in the level of consciousness, confusion, agitation, fatigue, and mental depression can occur.
- Allergic and hematologic reactions are possible.
- Gastrointestinal distress and either hyper- or hypoglycemia have been reported.
- Beta blockers may decrease peripheral circulation.

Dosage, Administration, and Nursing Considerations

- See Table 7-17.
- Nonselective beta blockers exert their antagonizing effects equally at both $beta_1$ (cardiac) and $beta_2$ (peripheral) receptor sites. Examples of nonselective beta blockers are nadolol, pindolol, propranolol, and timolol.
- Atenolol and metoprolol are considered to be cardioselective when given in low doses because they preferentially block $beta_1$ receptors. These drugs may be preferred for individuals with COPD or asthma to avoid bronchoconstriction.
- Beta blockers should be withdrawn gradually (decreasing the dose over 1 week to 2 weeks) to avoid precipitating anginal attacks, severe arrhythmias, or MI.
- Beta blockade may increase the risks of surgical procedures and general anesthesia.
- In the elderly, the hypotension frequently results in dizziness and confusion.
- If the apical rate is below 60 beats/minute, notify the physician before administering these drugs.
- Encourage patients to wear warm clothing during cold weather, to avoid prolonged exposure to cold, and not to smoke.

CALCIUM

- See PH, Endocrine system, calcium.

TABLE 7-17 BETA-ADRENERGIC BLOCKERS

Drug	Indications	Dosage and Administration	Nursing Considerations
Atenolol (Tenormin)	Hypertension	50 to 100 mg, PO, qd	It is cardioselective at lower doses
Metoprolol (Lopressor)	Hypertension	Initial therapy, 50 mg, PO, bid; usual maintenance dosage 100 mg, PO, bid (up to 450 mg daily)	Some patients require doses tid to maintain satisfactory control.
Nadolol (Corgard)	Angina; hypertension	*Angina:* initially, 40 mg, PO, qd; maintenance, 80–240 mg, PO, qd *Hypertension:* initially, 40 mg, PO, qd; maintenance, 80–320 mg, PO, qd	Blood pressure and apical pulse rate should be used as guides to dosage. Protect the drug from light.
Pindolol (Visken)	Hypertension	Initially, 10 mg, PO, bid, or 5 mg tid; average dose, 15–30 mg, PO, qd, up to a maximum of 60 mg, PO, qd	

Propranolol (Inderal, Inderide, Inderal LA)	Angina; hypertension, arrhythmias; hypertrophic cardiomyopathy; pheochromocytoma; migraine; myocardial infarction (MI) prophylaxis	*Angina:* initially, 10–20 mg, PO, tid or qid, before meals and at bedtime; average dosage: 160 mg/day *Hypertension:* 160–480 mg, qd, in four divided doses up to a maximum of 640 mg, qd *Arrhythmias:* 10–30 mg, tid or qid, before meals and at bedtime, PO; for life-threatening arrhythmias, give 1–3 mg, IV (never more than 1 mg/min). Give the second dose after 5 min.	Adverse reactions are most frequent following IV administration, but the elderly and those with impaired renal function are also at risk. Multiple drug interactions are possible. Inderide is a combination drug that contains both propranolol and hydrochlorothiazide.
Timolol (Blocadren) (Timoptic as an antiglaucoma agent)	Hypertension; MI prophylaxis	*Hypertension:* initially, 10 mg, PO, bid; maintenance, 20–40 mg, qd, with a maximum of 60 mg, qd, in two divided doses *MI prophylaxis:* 10 mg, PO, bid	For secondary prevention, therapy should be started within 1 week to 4 weeks after acute MI.

CALCIUM CHANNEL BLOCKERS

Actions

- These drugs reduce myocardial oxygen demand by inhibiting the flow of calcium ions into the myocardial cells during depolarization.
- Muscle cell contraction becomes less forceful.
- They affect smooth muscle cells of coronary arteries, resulting in coronary artery dilation. Perfusion to the myocardium is improved.
- Peripheral arterioles are dilated and afterload (the arterial pressure against which the left ventricle must pump during systole) is reduced.

Indications

- See Table 7-18.

Adverse Effects and Contraindications

- Hypotension may occur, especially with the concurrent use of antihypertensives.
- Increased frequency or severity of anginal pain can occur, especially when the calcium channel blocker is started or increased, or when abrupt withdrawal of a beta blocker has occurred.
- Congestive heart failure is rare, but the risk increases with concurrent use of a beta blocker.
- Verapamil may cause bradycardia, heart block, and sinus arrest.
- Use cautiously for patients with preexisting heart block, hypotension, or sick sinus syndrome (unless a functioning ventricular pacemaker is present).

Dosage, Administration, and Nursing Considerations

- See Table 7-18.
- Sublingual nitroglycerin may be taken as required during therapy with the calcium channel blockers.

DIGITALIS PREPARATIONS

Actions

- Digitalis increases the strength of myocardial contraction (positive inotropic effect) and slows the heart rate (negative chronotropic effect).

Indications

- Digitalis is used to treat CHF. The increased contractility allows the ventricles to empty more completely, and the slower heart rate allows for more complete filling.
- In atrial fibrillation, digitalis does not usually convert the heart to a normal sinus rhythm (NSR), but it does keep the ventricles from being overstimulated.
- It can be used to treat atrial flutter and paroxysmal atrial tachycardia (PAT), and in some cases, it may convert the heart to a NSR.
- For elderly or cardiac patients, digitalis may be given prophylactically before the stress of major surgery.

Adverse Effects and Contraindications

- Digitalis toxicity is the main problem with this drug.
- Early signs of digitalis toxicity are anorexia followed by nausea and vomiting.
- Drowsiness, fatigue, and headache also are common.
- Vision may be blurred, and patients may see colors (*e.g.*, yellow and green).
- The most serious effects are the *cardiac effects;* digitalis can produce almost any type of *arrhythmia.* Examples are partial or complete heart block, premature atrial contractions (PACs), PVCs, and ventricular fibrillation.
- Use cautiously in renal insufficiency, hypokalemia, premature and immature infants, elderly or debilitated patients.

Dosage and Administration

- It has been common practice to start a patient on digitalis therapy by the process called *digitalization.* This refers to giving priming, or loading, doses first, followed by a daily maintenance dose to replace what the body excretes.
- Rapid digitalization (especially IV) is dangerous and should be reserved for patients with severe CHF (specifically, pulmonary edema) and very rapid ventricular rates from atrial arrhythmias.
- Slower digitalization is safer and more common now. This method uses smaller doses at longer intervals. (It may take about a week to digitalize a patient.)
- See Table 7-19

Nursing Considerations

- See Table 7-19
- The following are predisposing factors to digitalis toxicity: a low serum potassium (K^+), especially from concurrent use of diuret-

(*Text continues on page 762*)

TABLE 7-18 CALCIUM CHANNEL BLOCKERS

Drug	Indications	Dosage and Administration	Nursing Considerations
Diltiazem (Cardizem)	Exertional angina; angina at rest caused by coronary artery spasm (Prinzmetal's)	Initially, give 30 mg, qid, before meals and at bedtime. Increase gradually to 240 mg, qd, PO, in divided doses.	Additive effects on cardiac conduction may occur with concomitant use of beta blockers or digitalis.
Nifedipine (Procardia)	Exertional angina; angina at rest caused by coronary artery spasm (Prinzmetal's)	Initially, give 10 mg, PO tid. The usual effective dosage range is 10–20 mg, PO, tid, and is established by titration. The maximum dosage is 180 mg, qd.	Nifedipine also has been given sublingually by piercing the capsule and squirting the liquid center under the tongue. Patients may develop pedal edema and need a diuretic.

Verapamil (Calan, Isoptin)	Supraventricular tachyarrhythmias such as atrial fibrillation and atrial flutter; exertional angina; angina at rest caused by coronary artery spasm (Prinzmetal's) or unstable angina (crescendo)	Initially, give 80 mg, PO, every 6 to 8 hours. The total daily dosage ranges from 240 to 480 mg. Isoptin (for IV injection) should be given slowly, over at least a 2-minute period. *Adults:* Initially, give 5–10 mg (0.075–0.15 mg/kg) as an IV bolus over a 2-minute period. Repeat dose: Give 10 mg 30 minutes after the first dose. *Elderly:* Administer the drug over at least a 3-minute period. *Pediatric* 1. 0–1 year old: 0.1 to 0.2 mg/kg over 2 minutes 2. 1–15 years old: 0.1 to 0.3 mg/kg over 2 minutes. If necessary, repeat the same dose 30 minutes later.	Concurrent use of quinidine is not recommended because severe hypotension may result. Observe closely for digitalis toxicity in patients receiving both a digitalis preparation and verapamil.

TABLE 7-19 DIGITALIS PREPARATIONS

Drug	Dosage and Administration	Nursing Considerations
Digitoxin (Crystodigin)	*Adults* 1. Slow digitalization: 0.2 mg, bid for four days, followed by a maintenance dose 2. Maintenance dosage: 0.5 to 0.3 mg, qd *Pediatric* 1. Premature and immature infants require careful titration. 2. Under one year of age: 0.045 mg/kg 3. One year to two years of age: 0.04 mg/kg 4. Over two years of age: 0.03 mg/kg (0.75 mg/m^2) 5. Total dose should be divided into three, four, or more portions, with 6 hours or more between doses. 6. Maintenance dosage: $\frac{1}{10}$ of the digitalizing dose	Digitoxin is absorbed almost totally from the GI tract. It binds to serum albumin and is released slowly. Therefore, it takes longer to become effective and stays in the body longer. It is metabolized in the liver, but most is reabsorbed into the bloodstream. Therefore, digitoxin may be considered preferable if the patient has kidney disease.

Digoxin (Lanoxin)	*Adults and children 10 years and older* 1. Digitalizing dosage: 1–1.5 mg, PO, in divided portions at 6- to 8-hr intervals, or 0.5–1 mg, IV, in divided doses over 24 hours 2. Maintenance dosage: 0.125–0.5 mg, PO, qd *Pediatric:* digitalizing dose 1. Total doses are divided into two or more doses PO, and given every 6 to 8 hr, or three or more doses IV and given every 4 to 8 hr. 2. Premature infant: 0.02–0.035 mg/kg, PO, or 0.015–0.025 mg/kg IV 3. Full term infant: 0.025–0.035 mg/kg, PO, or 0.02–0.03 mg/kg, IV 4. 1–24 months: 0.035–0.06 mg/kg, PO, or 0.03–0.05 mg/kg, IV 5. 2–5 yr: 0.03–0.04 mg/kg, PO, or 0.025–0.035 mg/kg, IV 6. 5–10 yr: 0.02–0.035 mg/kg, PO, or 0.015–0.03 mg/kg, IV 7. Over 10 yr: 0.01–0.015 mg/kg, PO, or 0.008–0.012 mg/kg, IV 8. Maintenance dosage: usually 20% to 35% of digitalizing dosage	Digoxin usually is 55% to 75% absorbed from the GI tract. It circulates freely and diffuses easily, and therefore becomes effective quickly. It is relatively unchanged by the liver, and is excreted unchanged by the kidneys; therefore, kidney disease can drastically reduce excretion. Be sure digoxin blood levels are drawn *before* the daily dose is given. Slow infusion of Lanoxin Injection or Injection Pediatric is preferable to bolus administration. It can be mixed with 0.9% sodium chloride or 5% dextrose and administered over a period of 5 minutes or longer.

(Continued from page 757)

ics (therefore, a patient's electrolytes should always be checked both before he or she is started on digitalis and during the course of the therapy); pathologic conditions, especially of the kidneys, liver, and heart (interferes with metabolism and excretion); old age (slower body functions); IV administration of digitalis and rapid digitalization; and drug interactions.

- The following drugs, when given with digitalis, may increase the risk of toxicity: quinidine; diuretics that cause potassium loss (*e.g.*, thiazides and furosemide); amphotericin B; intravenous calcium and glucose; propantheline; and verapamil.
- The following drugs could interfere with the action of digitalis: barbiturates; antacids; phenytoin; phenylbutazone; rifampin; sulfasalazine; kaolin-pectin mixtures; cholestyramine; colestipol; metoclopramide; and neomycin.
- Correct dosage is extremely important because there is only a small range between therapeutic and toxic dosages.
- Check apical rate for a full minute before giving each dose. If the rate is below 60, hold the dose and notify the physician.
- Digitalis toxicity can be diagnosed partially by laboratory results. Safe levels are considered to be 0.8 nanogram to 1.6 nanograms per milliliter of serum (a nanogram [ng] is one-billionth of a gram). Patients usually experience symptoms if the level of digitalis is over 2 ng.
- Digitalis toxicity can easily occur while the patient is at home. Good teaching in the hospital can help prevent this.

HEMOSTATIC AGENTS

PHYTONADIONE (VITAMIN K, MEPHYTON, AQUA-MEPHYTON)

Actions

- Phytonadione controls bleeding and is involved in the synthesis of Factors II (prothrombin), VII, IX, and X in the liver.

Indications

- It is used as an antidote to oral anticoagulant therapy.
- It can be used to treat newborns who may lack vitamin K, patients with liver disease, and those who cannot absorb vitamin K.

Adverse Effects and Contraindications

- Gastric upset and headache have occurred following oral doses.
- Pain, hematoma, and erythematous rash have occurred at injection sites.

- Following IV use, hypersensitivity and anaphylaxis have been reported.

Dosage and Administration

- The usual oral adult dose is 2.5 mg to 10 mg.
- The usual IM or SC dose is 0.5 mg to 10 mg.
- The usual IV dose is 0.5 to 10 mg, given at a rate of 1 mg/minute (for emergency use only).
- For hemorrhagic disease of newborns, the prophylactic dose is 0.5 mg to 1 mg IM following delivery. The treatment dose is 1 mg to 2 mg, IM or SC.

Nursing Considerations

- Overdosage of phytonadione is treated with heparin.
- Severe reactions (including death) have occurred during and immediately after IV injection.

POTASSIUM SUPPLEMENTS

Actions

- Potassium, a predominately intracellular ion, maintains the excitability of nerves and muscles, and is essential for normal renal function and enzyme activity.
- Potassium is also necessary to maintain a normal acid-base balance.

Indications

- It is given to treat hypokalemia (low serum potassium levels) resulting from the following: vomiting, diarrhea, and suction drainage; use of potassium-excreting diuretics and corticosteroids; diabetic ketoacidosis; uremia; cardiac arrhythmias resulting from digitalis toxicity; and administration of potassium-free IV fluids.

Adverse Effects and Contraindications

- Patients can experience nausea, vomiting, diarrhea, and abdominal discomfort from oral potassium supplements.
- Hyperkalemia (high serum potassium levels) can result from treatment with both oral or intravenous preparations. Symptoms include paresthesias of extremities; flaccid paralysis; listlessness; mental confusion; weakness; hypotension; and cardiac arrhythmias, including heart block and cardiac arrest.

Dosage and Administration

- Potassium bicarbonate (K-Lyte)
  1. Each effervescent tablet contains 25 mEq of potassium.
  2. The tablets should be dissolved in 4 ounces of cold water, and the solution should be sipped slowly (over 5 to 10 minutes).
  3. A usual adult dosage is one tablet taken one to two times daily with meals.
  4. The pediatric dosage is 1 to 3 mEq/kg daily in divided doses.
- Potassium chloride (Kay Ciel)
  1. Fifteen milliliters of the elixir contain 20 mEq of potassium. Each powder packet contains 20 mEq of potassium.
  2. Both the elixir and the powder should be mixed with 4 ounces of cold water or juice, and taken after meals.
  3. A usual adult dosage is 20 mEq twice daily.
- Potassium chloride injection
  1. Potassium is very irritating to the veins and should never be given by IV push. No more than 40 mEq is usually added to 1 liter of fluid. Avoid adding the medication to partially empty bottles.
  2. The usual adult dosage is 50 to 100 mEq per 24 hr.
  3. The maximum pediatric dosage is 3 mEq/kg or 40 mEq/m^2 per 24 hr; the maximum pediatric infusion rate is 0.02 mEq/kg/minute.
- Potassium gluconate (Kaon)
  1. Each sugar-coated (not enteric-coated) tablet contains 5 mEq of potassium.
  2. The usual adult dosage is two tablets, four times a day (after meals and at bedtime).
  3. The pediatric dosage is 20 to 40 mEq/m^2 daily in divided doses.

Nursing Considerations

- Frequent serum potassium levels must be done to determine if adequate and safe dosages of potassium are being administered.
- Slow-release tablets (*e.g.*, Slow-K) have been associated with intestinal and gastric ulceration and bleeding. They should be used only when patients cannot tolerate the other preparations or refuse to use them.
- KCl is *never* administered by IV push as a bolus, IM, or in concentrated amounts.
- Foods rich in potassium include avocados, broccoli, carrots, fruits (especially apricots, bananas, grapefruits, melons, oranges,

prunes), lima beans, peanut butter, potatoes, nuts, whole grain cereals, instant coffee, cocoa, and molasses. Increased amounts of these foods could lead to hyperkalemia if the individual is receiving a potassium supplement.

SODIUM BICARBONATE ($NaHCO_3$)

Actions

- Sodium bicarbonate replaces bicarbonate ions and restores the buffering capacity of the body in acidosis.
- It neutralizes gastric acid to form sodium chloride, carbon dioxide, and water. It acts rapidly and briefly.

Indications

- $NaHCO_3$ corrects metabolic acidosis resulting from diabetes mellitus, cardiac arrest, shock, or vascular collapse.
- It increases the solubility of sulfonamides and the effectiveness of aminoglycosides.
- It promotes renal excretion of barbiturate and salicylate overdosage.
- Heart-burn and indigestion are relieved by $NaHCO_3$.
- Topical pastes or soaks relieve itching and minor skin irritations.

Adverse Effects and Contraindications

- Prolonged therapy with sodium bicarbonate is contraindicated.
- Use cautiously for individuals with hypertension, heart disease, renal insufficiency, or peptic ulcer.
- Oral preparations can produce gastric distention and flatulence.
- Systemic alkalosis, electrolyte imbalance, renal calculi, and impaired renal function are possible.

Dosage and Administration

- For cardiac arrest, administer 200 to 300 mEq as the 7.5% or 8.4% solution rapid IV bolus in divided doses (*e.g.*, 50 mEq q 5 minutes). Further doses are based on results of arterial blood-gas analysis.
- For metabolic acidosis, give 2 to 5 mEq/kg, IV, over a 4- to 8- hour period. Infants up to 2 years old may receive 8 mEq/kg/day as a 4.2% solution.
- For alkalinization of urine, the usual dosage is 300 mg to 1.8 g, PO, one to four times daily before meals and at bedtime.

Nursing Considerations

- Routine use of sodium bicarbonate (baking soda) as an antacid is not recommended because of the systemic effects.
- Urinary pH should be monitored as a guide to dosage for urinary alkalinization.
- Severe tissue damage has occurred with extravasation.

THROMBOLYTICS

Actions

- These drugs dissolve formed clots by accelerating the formation of plasmin by activation of plasminogen. Plasmin is responsible for clot lysis.

Indications

- Thrombolytics are used to treat pulmonary embolism, deep vein thrombosis, arterial thrombosis and embolism, coronary artery thrombosis, and arteriovenous cannulae occlusion.
- They reduce damage to myocardial tissue during acute myocardial infarction (investigational use).

Adverse Effects and Contraindications

- Thrombolytics should not be used concurrently with heparin or other anticoagulants because of the high risk of hemorrhage.
- Individuals with recent cerebrovascular accidents, central nervous system hemorrhage, or other active internal bleeding should not receive these drugs.
- Use cautiously in patients who have had recent major surgery, obstetric delivery, organ biopsy, puncture of a noncompressible vessel, or in those who have advanced liver disease.
- Hemorrhage is a major adverse effect.
- Febrile complications occur that resemble serum sickness.
- Extravasation may cause local ulceration.
- Allergic reactions are rare but range in severity from minor breathing difficulties to anaphylaxis.

Dosage and Administration

- Dosage may differ according to the problem under treatment. It is common to administer a loading dose followed by maintenance doses.
- *Streptokinase (Kabikinase, Streptase):* Initially, 250,000 IU are infused in a peripheral vein over 30 min. Then, 100,000 IU/hr are

given for 24 hours to 72 hours (depending on the problem and patient response). Streptokinase also may be given as an intracoronary artery infusion or intracannula.

- *Urokinase (Abbokinase, Breokinase):* Initially, 4,400 IU/kg are given IV at a rate of 90 ml/hr over 10 min. Then, 4,400 IU/kg/hr are infused at a rate of 15 ml/hr for 12 hours. Urokinase usually is used in the treatment of pulmonary embolism, but it also may be used for IV catheter clearance.
- See the *Physicians' Desk Reference* (*PDR*) or the package insert for the product for specific reconstitution and administration directions.

Nursing Considerations

- Urokinase is similar in action to streptokinase, but it is much more expensive.
- When the body itself destroys a blood clot, the venous valves adjacent to the clot also may be destroyed. This action can lead to a "postphlebitic syndrome" that has a high mortality rate. Prompt treatment with thrombolytics may prevent this.
- Thrombolytic therapy is monitored by clinical response and laboratory values. Tests that are used include thrombin times, fibrinogen levels, partial thromboplastin times, and fibrin split product titers.
- For the best response, thrombolytics should be used within a week of the onset of symptoms, optimally within the first 72 hours. Duration of therapy should not exceed 72 hours.
- Thrombolytic therapy usually is followed by anticoagulant therapy with heparin to prevent the formation of more clots. Then, oral anticoagulation is started.
- Some patients may be resistant to streptokinase as a result of an immune response. Antibodies may have formed from past streptococcal infections. If thrombin time or other lysis parameters are still less than 1.5 times the normal control values after 4 hours of therapy, it should be discontinued.

VASODILATORS

NITRATES

Actions

- The nitrates relax all types of smooth muscle, especially coronary arteries, and lead to vasodilation.
- Vasodilation increases blood flow, but it also may decrease blood pressure. Blood flow increases only to healthy vessels or to the

collateral circulation because diseased coronary vessels cannot dilate.

- Nitrates also reduce the work load on the heart because blood can pool in the extremities.

Indications

- Nitrates are used to treat angina pectoris (See MSN, Cardiovascular). The nitrates may stop an existing attack, prevent an attack just before physical activity, or reduce the total number of attacks per day.

Adverse Effects and Contraindications

- Nitrates can cause postural hypotension (*e.g.,* dizziness, weakness, and fainting), throbbing headache, flushing, nausea, and vomiting.
- Nitrate syncope, a severe shocklike reaction, also can occur.
- These drugs usually are not given during the acute phase of a myocardial infarction.
- Use cautiously in patients with glaucoma because the drug can cause an increase in intraocular pressure.

Dosage and Administration

- Isosorbide dinitrate (Isordil, Sorbitrate): The sublingual dose range is 2.5 mg to 10 mg. The oral dose range is 5 mg to 30 mg, tid or qid. The drug peaks in 2 minutes to 5 minutes (sublingually), and its action lasts 1 hour to 2 hours.
- Nitroglycerin (NTG): The usual dose range is 0.15 mg to 0.6 mg, sublingually. It may be repeated every 5 minutes for a total of three doses. This is a rapid-acting nitrate and should peak in 2 minutes to 3 minutes. Its prophylactic effect lasts 5 minutes to 15 minutes.
- Nitroglycerin, topical (Nitro-Dur, Transderm-Nitro): These products are prepared patches that are applied to the skin of the chest or proximal portion of the extremities.
    1. Nitro-Dur is available in 5-cm^2, 10-cm^2, 15-cm^2, 20-cm^2, and 30-cm^2 systems containing 26 mg, 51 mg, 77 mg, 104 mg, and 154 mg respectively, of nitroglycerin. A system releases approximately 0.5 $mg/cm^2/24$ hr. The initial starting dose is a 10-cm^2 system. A patch may be left in place for up to 24 hours. An old patch should be removed when applying a new one.
    2. Transderm-Nitro is available in 5-cm^2, 10-cm^2, 20-cm^2 and 30-cm^2 systems. Therapy usually is started with a Transderm-Nitro 5-cm^2 system.

- *Nitroglycerin, topical (Nitro-Bid, Nitrol):* These products are ointments applied to the skin, usually in 1-inch to 2-inch areas. They can be applied to the chest, abdomen, arms, and legs.
  1. The ointment should be spread and then covered with a 4-inch × 6-inch piece of plastic wrap. Taping all sides increases the water content of skin, and increased hydration promotes absorption of the ointment. Wipe off any old ointment before applying a new dose.
  2. The drug is effective up to several hours for sustained prophylaxis.

Nursing Considerations

- If the patient has not obtained relief from angina within 15 minutes when using a rapid-acting nitrate, notify his or her physician.
- When applying topical preparations, do not touch the ointment with your fingers. Spread it with the measuring paper provided. Your fingers could absorb it, and you could experience side-effects of the drug.
- Tablets should be kept in the original dark bottle, tightly closed, in a relatively cool place. Remove the cotton from the bottle because it may absorb some of the drug. A potent tablet should produce a brief stinging or burning sensation when placed under the tongue.
- The patient should sit or lie down after taking the tablet to counteract postural hypotension.
- Taking alcohol with a nitrate can intensify the hypotension and bring on nitrate syncope.
- Patients can develop tolerance to nitrates. Be sure to determine if a patient is obtaining the same degree of relief as before.
- Patients usually keep NTG at their bedside, but you are still responsible for recording the time, the number of tablets, and the relief obtained.

NITROGLYCERIN, INTRAVENOUS (TRIDIL, NITRO-BID, NITROSTAT, NITROL)

Actions

- It is used to relax vascular smooth muscle.
- It promotes peripheral pooling of blood and decreases venous return to the heart. Therefore, preload (left ventricular end-diastolic pressure) is reduced.
- Systemic vascular resistance and afterload (arterial pressure) are reduced by arteriolar relaxation.
- NTG decreases myocardial oxygen consumption.

- It reduces systolic, diastolic, and mean arterial blood pressures.
- Heart rate may increase with the drug.

Indications

- It is used to control blood pressure in perioperative hypertension. (Frequently, it is used during coronary artery bypass graft surgery.)
- It can treat CHF associated with acute MI.
- It relieves angina pectoris in patients who have not responded to organic nitrates or beta blockers.
- NTG produces controlled hypotension during surgical procedures.

Adverse Effects and Contraindications

- The most frequent adverse reaction is headache.
- Tachycardia, nausea, vomiting, restlessness, palpitations, abdominal pain, and dizziness also occur.
- Overdosage may result in severe hypotension and reflex tachycardia.
- Patients with increased intracranial pressure, constrictive pericarditis, hypotension, or hypersensitivity to nitroglycerin should not receive this drug.

Dosage and Administration

- Each milliliter of Tridil contains 5 mg of NTG.
- Mixing 5 ml of Tridil (25 mg NTG) in 250 ml of D_5W or normal saline produces 100 μg NTG/ml.
- For patients on restricted fluid volume, mixing 10 ml Tridil (50 mg NTG) in 250 ml of D_5W or normal saline gives 200 μg NTG/ml.
- The initial dose usually is 5 μg/minute delivered through an infusion pump. Titration is adjusted according to the clinical situation and is usually in increments of 5 μg/minute, with increases every 3 minutes to 5 minutes, until some response is noted.

Nursing Considerations

- Several preparations of intravenous nitroglycerin are now available. Their concentration, dilution, dosage, and administration instructions differ. Check each product's directions carefully.
- NTG adheres easily to many plastics. Solutions should be mixed only in glass containers and the accompanying administration set (Tridilset) should be used.

- Keep any additional tubing needed for the infusion pump to a minimum and no other medications should be added to the NTG solution or through the tubing and needle.
- Headache from the vasodilation can be relieved by reducing the infusion rate (if possible) or by administering acetaminophen or other analgesics.
- Propranolol may be used to counteract the sinus tachycardia.
- Observe the patient closely for thrombophlebitis at the peripheral IV site. The site may need to be changed.
- Patients should be weaned gradually from the IV NTG to prevent a return of pretherapy symptoms or cardiovascular distress.
- Oral or topical vasodilators may be initiated prior to weaning, and the weaning should begin during the peak effectiveness of these drugs.

ENDOCRINE SYSTEM

ADRENOCORTICOSTEROIDS

Actions

- Important pharmacologic effects of steroid drug action are anti-inflammatory, antiallergic, antipyretic, and antistress.

Indications

- Replacement therapy for adrenocortical insufficiency
- Rheumatoid arthritis and osteoarthritis
- Collagen diseases (*e.g.*, lupus erythematosus)
- Severe or incapacitating allergic problems
- Chronic obstructive pulmonary disease (COPD)
- Skin disorders (*e.g.*, psoriasis, erythema multiforme)
- Cerebral edema
- Severe acute and chronic inflammatory processes of the eye
- Blood dyscrasias (*e.g.*, hemolytic anemia)
- Neoplastic diseases (*e.g.*, lymphocytic leukemia)
- Gastrointestinal diseases (*e.g.*, exacerbations of ulcerative colitis)
- Nephrotic syndrome

Adverse Effects and Contraindications

- Cushing's-type symptoms (*e.g.*, moon face, buffalo hump, hirsutism, edema) (See MSN, Endocrine.)

- Delayed wound healing
- Peptic ulcer
- Amenorrhea
- Reduced resistance to infections
- Thrombophlebitis (with possible embolism)
- Headache
- Mood changes (*e.g.*, euphoria, depression, insomnia)
- Osteoporosis
- Increased blood glucose
- Suppression of growth in children
- Cataracts, glaucoma, and damage to the optic nerve resulting from prolonged use
- Caution *must* be used when administering steroids to patients with infections (including a history of tuberculosis), osteoporosis, diabetes, hypertension, peptic ulcer, acute heart and kidney disease, emotional problems, and thrombophlebitis, and to women in the first trimester of pregnancy.
- See Table 7-20 for dosage, administration, and nursing considerations.
- See Table 7-21 for a listing on *topical* corticosteroids.

Dosage and Administration

- Whenever possible, steroids that act at local sites (*e.g.*, joints, eyes, lungs) are used to help reduce systemic toxicity.
- The physician will always attempt to determine the *smallest dosage* that will relieve the symptoms, and then reduce that dosage (*e.g.*, during remission).
- Using massive dosages for short periods is acceptable treatment in emergency situations (*e.g.*, anaphylactic shock or adrenal crisis).
- Another measure used to reduce systemic toxicity is an intermittent dosage schedule. For example, the total daily dosage may be taken with the morning meal, or the total dosage for 2 days may be taken qod with the morning meal.
- Steroids are best given between 7 A.M. and 8 A.M. This is when the body's own production of glucocorticoids is highest (between 6 A.M. and 9 A.M.). Fewer side-effects will occur because there will be less suppression of the hypothalamus, pituitary and adrenals.
- Dosages for all preparations are *highly* individualized.

Nursing Considerations

- Help patients to understand that steroids cannot cure or prevent progress of their diseases. They are used to minimize symptoms.

(Text continues on page 777)

TABLE 7-20 ADRENOCORTICOSTEROIDS

Drug	Dosage and Administration	Nursing Considerations
Beclomethasone diproprionate (Beclovent, Vanceril)	See PH, Respiratory system.	
Betamethasone (Celestone)	0.6 to 7.2 mg/day, PO or 0.5 to 9 mg/day, IM or IV. May be given intrabursal or intra-articular	
Cortisone acetate (Cortistan, Pantisone)	*Adults:* Initially, 25 to 300 mg/day, PO or IM, as single or divided doses *Pediatric* 1. 2.5 to 10 mg/kg, PO, or 20 to 300 mg/m^2 per day in four divided doses 2. 700 μg to 5 mg/kg, IM, or 20 to 150 mg/m^2, qd or bid	Alternate day therapy may decrease growth retardation in children.
Dexamethasone (Decadron)	0.75 to 9 mg/day, PO, in two to four divided doses	It also is available in IM, intra-articular, topical, intranasal, and inhalation preparations.
Fludrocortisone acetate (Florinef)	Addison's disease: 0.1 mg, PO, daily (ranges: 0.1 mg, three times/week to 0.2 mg daily) Salt-losing adrenogenital syndrome: 0.1 to 0.2 mg/day, PO	During prolonged therapy, electrolytes should be monitored.

(continued)

TABLE 7-20 ADRENOCORTICOSTEROIDS

Drug	Dosage and Administration	Nursing Considerations
Hydrocortisone (Cortef, Cortisol) Hydrocortisone sodium succinate (Solu-Cortef)	PO: 20 to 240 mg daily IM: ⅓ to ½ oral dose every 12 hr IV: 20 to 240 mg daily SC: 20 to 240 mg daily Intra-articular, intralesional: 25 to 50 mg Retention enema: 100 mg, hs, for 21 days Rectal suppository: one suppository two or three times daily, or two suppositories twice daily	Multiple preparations of hydrocortisone are available. Check carefully that the preparation is appropriate for the desired route of administration.
Methylprednisolone (Medrol) Methylprednisolone acetate (Depo-Medrol) Methylprednisolone sodium succinate (Solu-Medrol)	Oral: 4 to 48 mg/day in single or divided doses Intra-articular: 4 to 80 mg IV: 10 to 500 mg; may be repeated every 6 hr, prn IM: 10 to 40 mg; may be repeated every 6 to 24 hr, prn	Check the preparation carefully to be sure it is appropriate for the desired route.

Paramethasone acetate (Haldrone)	*Adults:* Initially, 2 to 24 mg, PO, in divided doses, then decrease to maintenance dose of 1 to 8 mg/day *Pediatric:* 58 to 800 μg/kg/day	At high doses (above 15 mg/day), the urinary excretion of calcium and nitrogen is increased significantly
Prednisolone	*Adult* 1. 5 to 60 mg/day, PO 2. 4 to 60/mg/day, IM or IV 3. 2 to 60 mg weekly, intra-articular *Pediatric* 1. 140 μg to 2 mg/kg/day, PO, in divided doses 2. 40 to 250 μg/kg, qd or bid, IM or IV	It also is available in ophthalmic and otic dosage forms
Prednisone (Deltasone, Meticorten)	*Adults:* Initially, 5 to 60 mg/day, PO, in single or divided doses, then gradually reduce to lowest effective maintenance level (5 to 20 mg/day) *Pediatric:* 2 mg/kg/day, PO, then reduce	Administer after meals and at bedtime. Periodic serum potassium levels are recommended.
Triamcinolone (Aristocort, Kenacort) Triamcinolone diacetate (Aristocort)	Initially, 8 to 32 mg, PO, daily	It also is available for SC, intra-articular, IM, intralesional, and topical use.

TABLE 7-21 TOPICAL ADRENOCORTICOSTEROIDS

Drug	Dosage and Administration
Amcinonide (Cyclocort)	0.1% cream and ointment: Apply two to three times daily.
Betamethasone (Uticort)	Apply a thin film to the affected area, one to three times daily.
Desoximetasone (Topicort)	Apply a small amount of cream (0.25%, 0.05%) bid.
Dexamethasone sodium phosphate (Decadron)	0.1% cream: Apply sparingly to the affected area, two or three times/day.
Diflorasone diacetate (Florone)	Apply a small amount of ointment (0.05%), one to three times/day.
Fluocinolone acetonide (Fluonid, Synemol, Synalar)	Apply in a thin layer over the affected area, two to four times daily. The 0.2% cream should be used only for a short time and should not exceed 2 g/day.
Fluorometholone (Oxylone)	Apply 0.025% cream, one or two times/day.
Flurandrenolide (Cordran)	*Adults* 1. Cream, lotion, ointment, 0.025% to 0.05%: Apply bid or tid. 2. Tape, 0.004 mg/cm^2: Apply qd or bid at 12-hr intervals. *Pediatric* 1. Ointment or cream, 0.025%: Apply qd or bid; 0.05%, apply qd. 2. Tape: Apply qd.
Halcinonide (Halciderm, Halog)	*Adults:* Cream, ointment (0.025% or 0.1%), solution (0.1%), apply bid or tid. *Pediatric:* Apply once daily.
Hydrocortisone Prednisolone	Apply a thin film or spray to affected area two to four times/day. *Adults:* Apply three to four times/day. *Pediatric:* Apply once or twice/day.
Triamcinolone (Aristocort, Kenalog)	Apply a thin layer two to four times/day.

SUCRALFATE (CARAFATE)

Actions

- Sucralfate forms an ulcer-adherent complex that covers the ulcer site and protects it from acid, pepsin, and bile salts.

Indications

- It is used to treat duodenal ulcers on a short-term basis (up to eight weeks).

Adverse Effects and Contraindications

- Constipation is the most frequent adverse effect.
- Dry mouth, skin rash, nausea, diarrhea, and dizziness may occur.

Dosage and Administration

- Give 1 g, PO, qid, 1 hour before each meal and hs.

Nursing Considerations

- Antacids may be used for pain relief, but should not be taken within 0.5 hr before or after sucralfate.
- Sucralfate decreases tetracycline absorption.

GENITOURINARY SYSTEM

ANDROGENS

Actions

- Androgens control development and maintenance of male secondary sexual characteristics.
- They restore and maintain positive nitrogen balance.
- They can reduce excretion of chloride, nitrogen, phosphorus, potassium, and sodium in males and in some females.
- Bone, hair, skeletal muscle, and skin growth are stimulated by androgens.
- These agents increase erythropoiesis and promote vascularization and darkening of the skin.
- Large doses suppress male gonadotropic secretion.
- They antagonize the effects of estrogen excess on female breast and endometrium.

TABLE 7-30 ANDROGENS

Drug	Dosage and Administration	Nursing Considerations
Danazol (Danocrine)	Endometriosis: 400 mg, bid, PO, for 3 to 6 mo Fibrocystic breast disease: 100 mg to 400 mg, bid, PO	It is used as palliative treatment for endometriosis when alternative therapy cannot be used.
Dromostanolone propionate (Drolban)	100 mg, IM, three times/week	It is used as palliative therapy in advanced metastatic breast cancer in women 1 to 5 yr postmenopausal.
Fluoxymesterone (Halotestin)	Male hypogonadism and climacteric: 2 to 10 mg/day, PO Metastatic carcinoma of female breast: 15 to 30 mg daily, PO, in divided doses Postpartum breast engorgement: 2.5 mg, PO, at start of active labor, then 5 to 10 mg/day in divided doses for 4 to 5 days	Administer with food.
Methyltestosterone (Android, Oreton Methyl)	Replacement therapy: 10 to 40 mg/day, PO, in divided doses after therapy with IM testosterone Postpartum breast engorgement: 80 mg/day, PO, for 3 to 5 days Breast cancer: 200 mg/day, PO Buccal preparation: One-half of the oral dose	
Testolactone (Teslac)	250 mg, PO, qid	It is used for palliative antineoplastic therapy.
Testosterone (Oreton, Testrone)	Replacement therapy: 10 to 25 mg, IM, two or three times weekly Postpartum breast engorgement: 25 to 50 mg, IM, daily for 3 or 4 days Metastatic breast cancer: 100 mg, IM, three times weekly	

Indications

- Androgens are used to treat male sex hormone deficiency states: cryptorchidism, hypogonadism, impotence, and male climacteric.
- They are given for palliation for androgen-responsive inoperable breast cancer in patients, 1 year to 5 years postmenopausal.
- Refractory anemias and osteoporosis are treated with androgens.
- They can reverse protein loss after burns, debilitating disease, extensive surgery, and prolonged immobilization.

Adverse Effects and Contraindications

- Women of child-bearing potential and those who are pregnant or lactating should not use androgens.
- Males with prostatic or breast cancer and those with benign prostatic hypertrophy should avoid androgen use.
- Androgens also are contraindicated for patients with impaired cardiac, renal, or hepatic systems, or those with hypercalcemia.
- Both sexes may experience increased libido, skin flushing, acne, leukopenia, sodium and water retention, nausea, vomiting, anorexia, diarrhea, hypercalcemia with renal calculi (especially in immobilized patients), and jaundice.
- Postpubertal males may experience testicular atrophy, decreased ejaculatory volume, azoospermia, impotence, epididymitis, and priapism.
- Females may experience suppression of ovulation, lactation, or menstruation. They may develop virilism (hoarseness or deepening of voice), hirsutism, clitoral enlargement, regression of breasts, and male-pattern baldness.

Dosage, Administration, and Nursing Considerations

- See Table 7-30
- Intake, output, and weight should be monitored daily during initial therapy.
- Diuretics may be used to control sodium and water retention.
- Serum calcium and cholesterol levels should be checked periodically during therapy.
- Therapeutic response in patients with breast cancer may take up to 3 months.
- Androgens interact with anticoagulants to enhance the anticoagulant effects. Dosage may need to be reduced.
- The high doses recommended for treatment of metastatic breast cancer in women frequently cause virilism. These patients need a great deal of emotional support. If no response is achieved after 3 months, therapy usually is discontinued (see PH, antineoplastics).

DINOPROSTONE (PGE_2, PROSTIN E_2)

Actions

- Dinoprostone is a prostaglandin that acts directly on myometrium and other smooth muscle to stimulate contractions in a gravid uterus in the early weeks of gestation.

Indications

- It is used for the termination of a pregnancy from the 12th week through the second trimester.
- It is used to evacuate the uterine contents in the management of missed abortion or intrauterine fetal death (up to 28 weeks).
- It manages benign hydatidiform mole.

Adverse Effects and Contraindications

- Dinoprostone should not be used to manage intrauterine fetal death during the third trimester.
- Use cautiously for patients with cardiovascular, hepatic, or renal disease; cervicitis or acute vaginitis; asthma; epilepsy; anemia; or diabetes mellitus.
- Headache, nausea, vomiting, fever, diarrhea, and chills may occur.

Dosage and Administration

- Insert one suppository (20 mg) high into the vagina. Repeat at 3- to 5-hr intervals until abortion occurs. The maximum dosage is 240 mg.

Nursing Considerations

- Warm the suppository to room temperature prior to use.
- Patients may need antiemetics and antidiarrheals before using dinoprostone to minimize gastrointestinal side-effects.

DIURETICS

Nursing Considerations

- Diuretics can remove sodium, potassium, hydrogen, chloride, and bicarbonate; therefore, all types of electrolyte and acid-base imbalances can occur.
- Monitor serum electrolytes.
- Observe patients for signs of muscle cramps, weakness, fatigue, anorexia, thirst, mental confusion, and vomiting.

- Accurate intake and output measurements must be recorded by either the nurse or the patient. This does not require a physician's order and is a nursing responsibility.
- The patient should be weighed daily, at the same time and on the same scale, while wearing the same type of clothing. Usually, weights are taken before breakfast.
- Examine the patient for signs of edema (see MSN, Cardiovascular).
- Diuretics should be administered early in the day so that the patient's sleep is not interrupted. Once-a-day diuretics can be administered at 8 A.M. or 10 A.M.; twice-a-day diuretics can be given at 8 A.M. and 2 P.M.
- To avoid injury to your patients, carefully determine the type of assistance they will need. The urinal, bedpan, and call light should be within reach. If a patient is independently ambulatory, be sure that extra furniture will not be in the way if he or she must make a hurried trip to the bathroom.
- Many diuretics result in a loss of potassium, so patients may require a potassium supplement. However, some patients can replace the loss by eating potassium-rich foods (*e.g.*, bananas, tomatoes, citrus fruits and juices, and whole milk).
- Because of the potassium loss that occurs with most diuretic therapy, patients receiving digitalis are more likely to develop toxicity.
- Patients receiving lithium should not use diuretics because of the danger of lithium intoxication.
- Diuretics can potentiate the action of antihypertensives. Reduction in dosage of the antihypertensive may be necessary and beneficial.

CARBONIC ANHYDRASE INHIBITORS

Actions

- These agents inhibit the enzyme carbonic anhydrase.
- In the eye, the secretion of aqueous humor is reduced, resulting in a decrease in intraocular pressure.
- In the kidneys, bicarbonate is lost, which results in the excretion of sodium, potassium, and water.

Indications

- These drugs are used to reduce intraocular pressure in chronic open-angle glaucoma, secondary glaucoma and, preoperatively, in acute closed-angle glaucoma.
- They are used with anticonvulsant drugs and provide additional control of grand mal and petit mal seizures.

- They are used to treat drug-induced edema, and can reduce edema resulting from congestive heart failure.

Adverse Effects and Contraindications

- Paresthesias (tingling and numbness of the extremities, especially the fingers, toes, and lips) can occur.
- Drowsiness and confusion may occur.
- Metabolic acidosis can result from the accumulation of hydrogen and chloride ions in relation to the excretion of bicarbonate ions.
- Hypersensitivity reactions are possible (*e.g.,* fever, rash, and blood dyscrasias).
- Crystalluria and renal calculi are possible.
- Patients with low sodium and potassium levels should not receive carbonic anhydrase inhibitors.
- Do not give these agents to patients with anuria.
- They are contraindicated for patients with kidney and liver disease.
- Use carbonic anhydrase inhibitors cautiously for patients with chronic obstructive pulmonary disease because these drugs may aggravate acidosis.
- Pregnant women, especially in the first trimester, should avoid all diuretics.

Dosage and Administration

- Acetazolamide (Diamox)
  1. For congestive heart failure: Usually, a dose of 250 mg to 375 mg is given PO, every other day (alternating with another diuretic).
  2. For chronic open-angle glaucoma: The usual dosage is 250 mg to 1 g per day, PO, in divided doses.
  3. For acute closed-angle glaucoma: Preoperative treatment is usually 250 mg, PO, q 4 hr. For rapid relief of intraocular pressure, the IV route is used (Acetazolamide sodium, Diamox Parenteral).
  4. For epilepsy: The usual range is 250 mg to 1 g, PO, daily in divided doses. Therapy may begin with 250 mg, PO, daily, and is increased as needed.
  5. For drug-induced edema: The usual range is 250 mg to 375 mg, PO, once daily for 1 day or 2 days, alternating with a day of rest.
  6. *Pediatric:* For glaucoma and epilepsy, give 10 to 15 mg/kg/day in divided doses q 6 hr; as a diuretic, give 5 mg/kg once daily.

Nursing Considerations

- See PH, Diuretics, nursing considerations.
- Brand interchange is not recommended for carbonic anhydrase inhibitor products.
- These drugs may cause substantial increases in blood glucose levels.
- Because these drugs cause alkalinization of the urine, excretion of other drugs may be decreased (*e.g.,* amphetamines, quinidine). They may increase the excretion of lithium.

LOOP OR HIGH-CEILING DIURETICS

Actions

- Loop diuretics inhibit reabsorption of sodium and chloride in the ascending loop of Henle, and possibly in both the proximal and distal tubules.
- They cause a greater degree of diuresis than most other diuretics.

Indications

- They are used to relieve edema associated with congestive heart failure, renal disease, and cirrhosis of the liver.
- Intravenous forms are used in acute pulmonary edema.
- These diuretics reduce blood pressure when used alone or with other antihypertensives.

Adverse Effects and Contraindications

- They can produce serious fluid and electrolyte imbalances (*e.g.,* hypokalemia, or low serum potassium levels).
- Sudden, massive diuresis can precipitate cardiovascular collapse or blood clot formation.
- Ototoxicity may occur, especially in patients with impaired kidney function, resulting in hearing loss, tinnitus, and vertigo.
- Mild diarrhea may occur. However, ethacrynic acid can produce profuse, watery diarrhea, which necessitates discontinuance of the drug.
- Elevations of blood glucose and serum uric acid may precipitate diabetes and gout.
- Do not give to patients with anuria.
- Use cautiously for patients with advanced cirrhosis of the liver. The electrolyte imbalances may lead to hepatic coma and death.

TABLE 7-31 LOOP OR HIGH-CEILING DIURETICS

Drug	Dosage and Administration	Nursing Considerations
Bumetanide (Bumex)	The usual total daily dosage is 0.5 mg to 2 mg, PO, as a single dose. The maximum daily dosage is 10 mg. Usually, the initial dosage IM or IV is 0.5 to 1 mg.	This drug has a rapid onset and short duration of action. Intravenously, the drug should be given over a period of 1 minute to 2 minutes. One milligram of Bumex produces diuretic action approximately equivalent to 40 mg of furosemide. It does not appear to exhibit cross-sensitivity with furosemide.
Ethacrynic acid (Edecrin)	The usual adult daily dosage is 50 to 200 mg, PO. Treatment usually is started with 50 mg, PO, after breakfast, and gradually is increased by 25 mg or 50 mg as needed. The maximum dosage is usually 200 mg twice daily.	

	In emergencies, 50 to 100 mg of *sodium ethacrynate* may be administered IV. *Pediatric:* Usually, 25 mg, PO, is given initially. The IV route is not recommended.	
Furosemide (Lasix)	The usual adult daily dosage is 20 to 80 mg, PO. Dosage may be increased carefully (20 to 40 mg every 6 to 8 hr) to a maximum of 600 mg per day. In emergencies, 20 to 40 mg of furosemide may be given IM or IV. Intravenous injection should be given slowly (over 1 minute to 2 minutes). A second dose may be administered 2 hr after the first. *Pediatric:* Usually, 2 mg/kg, PO, is given as a single dose. It may be increased by 1 to 2 mg/kg every 6 to 8 hr. Also, 1 mg/kg, IM or IV, may be given.	If high-dose parenteral therapy is necessary, furosemide may be mixed with isotonic saline, lactated Ringer's solution, or 5% dextrose. The pH of the solutions should be above 5.5. The rate should not exceed 4 mg/min. The smallest dose necessary to produce a gradual weight loss of 1 to 2 lb per day is recommended.

Dosage, Administration, and Nursing Considerations

- See Table 7-31.
- See PH, Diuretics, nursing considerations.
- Ethacrynic acid can displace warfarin from plasma proteins, so it may be necessary to reduce the dosage of the warfarin. Monitor the patient's prothrombin time (PT).
- Furosemide competes with salicylates for renal excretion. Therefore, the salicylates may reach toxic levels in the body.
- Excessive dehydration is most likely to occur in the elderly. Thrombi, emboli, or circulatory collapse are possible.
- Do not give with other ototoxic drugs.

OSMOTIC DIURETICS

Actions

- These nonelectrolytes are given in quantities that are sufficient to ensure that only a small amount can be reabsorbed by the renal tubules. The rest remains in the tubules and acts (by osmosis) to keep water from leaving the tubules. Thus, the volume of urine produced is increased.
- When in the bloodstream, osmotic diuretics draw fluid from the extravascular spaces into the plasma.

Indications

- Osmotic diuretics are used to prevent renal failure in situations in which glomerular filtration is reduced severely, for example, when patients have been severely injured and burned, have undergone heart surgery, or have had transfusion reactions.
- They can reduce elevated intracranial and intraocular pressure. Therefore, these diuretics are useful during neurosurgery and in treating head injuries, and prior to surgery for acute closed-angle glaucoma or detached retina.

Adverse Effects and Contraindications

- Disorientation, confusion, and headache are possible.
- Nausea and vomiting can occur.
- Give cautiously to patients with severely impaired kidney, liver, or cardiac function.
- Dehydrated patients or those with active intracranial bleeding should not receive osmotic diuretics.
- Extravasation of the fluid into the surrounding tissue causes irritation and possible tissue necrosis.
- Convulsions and anaphylaxis have been reported with *mannitol.*

- These diuretics are not indicated for use with chronic edema.
- Do not give to patients with anuria.

Dosage, Administration, and Nursing Considerations

- See Table 7-32.
- Osmotic diuretics usually are indicated for use in short-term therapy.
- See PH, Diuretics, nursing considerations.

POTASSIUM-SPARING DIURETICS

Spironolactone (Aldactone)

Actions

- Spironolactone blocks the action of aldosterone in the distal portion of the renal tubule.
- Increased amounts of sodium and water are excreted, and potassium is retained.

Indications

- Spironolactone assists in the management of primary hyperaldosteronism.
- It is used adjunctively to relieve the edema of congestive heart failure and the nephrotic syndrome when other diuretics do not produce a satisfactory response.
- It relieves the edema and ascites of cirrhosis of the liver.
- When used in combination with other drugs, it can manage essential hypertension.
- It can be used to treat hypokalemia (low potassium) levels when other measures do not produce a satisfactory response, and is used on a prophylactic basis for patients receiving digitalis.

Adverse Effects and Contraindications

- Potassium retention resulting in hyperkalemia may occur. The high potassium levels can precipitate cardiac arrhythmias and arrest.
- Excessive loss of sodium (hyponatremia) can result in dryness of the mouth, thirst, lethargy, and drowsiness.
- Spironolactone is a steroid that can cause gynecomastia, deepening of the voice, hirsutism, irregular menses or amenorrhea, and impotence.
- Do not give to patients with anuria.
- It may produce lethargy, fatigue, and mental confusion.

TABLE 7-32 OSMOTIC DIURETICS

Drug	Dosage and Administration	Nursing Considerations
Glycerin (Glycerol, Glyrol, Osmoglyn)	Usually, 1 to 1.5 g/kg of 50% to 75% solution, PO, 1 to 1.5 hr prior to surgery for glaucoma, retinal detachment, or cataract extraction Sterile anhydrous glycerin: 1 or 2 gtt in the eye every 3 to 4 hr to reduce corneal edema	Glycerin suppositories may be used in adults and children to relieve constipation. Lemon and glycerin swabs are not recommended for mouth care because of the drying effect of the glycerin.
Isosorbide (Ismotic)	Initially, 1.5 g/kg, PO; usual range: 1 to 3 g/kg, two to four times a day	This drug reduces intraocular pressure prior to and following surgery for glaucoma and cataracts.
Mannitol (Osmitrol)	Acute renal failure: 50 to 100 g of 5% to 25% solution, IV Elevated intraocular or intracranial pressure: 1.5 to 2 g/kg, IV, as a 15% to 25% solution over 30 to 60 minutes Acute chemical toxicity: 100 to 200 g, IV A test dose of 0.2 g/kg of 15%, 20%, or 25% solution infused over 3 to 5 minutes may be given to produce urine flow of 30 to 50 ml/hr.	The IV rate usually is adjusted according to urine output (at least 30 to 50 ml/hr). If output is not adequate, accumulation can cause pulmonary edema and water intoxication.
Urea (Ureaphil)	*Adults:* 1 to 1.5 g/kg, IV, of 30% solution to infuse slowly over 1 to 2.5 hours, up to a maximum of 120 g/24 hr (rate not to exceed 4 ml/min) *Pediatric* 1. 2 yr and older: 0.5 to 1.5 g/kg, IV 2. Up to 2 yr: 0.1 to 0.5 g/kg, IV	The solution must be prepared fresh for each patient and the unused portion discarded.

Dosage and Administration

- For edema: The usual adult dosage is 25 mg, qid, PO. After 5 days, if the response is inadequate, a diuretic that acts in the proximal renal tubule may be added.
- For essential hypertension: The usual adult dosage is 50 to 100 mg per day, PO, in divided doses. Frequently, it is given with antihypertensives and other diuretics.
- For hypokalemia: The usual adult dosage is 25 to 100 mg per day, PO.
- For primary hyperaldosteronism: The usual adult and pediatric dosage is 100 to 400 mg per day, PO.
- *Pediatric:* The usual dosage is 1.5 to 3.3 mg/kg daily in four divided doses, PO.

Nursing Considerations

- See PH, Diuretics, nursing considerations.
- When spironolactone is used, all potassium supplements usually are discontinued, and a diet high in potassium is discouraged.
- Diabetics, the elderly, and patients with impaired kidney function are at greatest risk for developing hyperkalemia.
- Only one potassium-sparing diuretic should be used at a time because of the danger of hyperkalemia.
- It is available in combination with hydrochlorothiazide (Aldactazide).

Triamterene (Dyrenium)

Actions

- Triamterene acts on the distal portion of the renal tubule to block sodium-potassium and sodium-hydrogen exchange mechanisms.

Indications

- It reduces the edema of congestive heart failure, the nephrotic syndrome, and cirrhosis of the liver.
- The drug relieves steroid-induced edema.
- It also aids in preventing hypokalemia, thereby reducing the danger of toxicity in patients taking digitalis.

Adverse Effects and Contraindications

- Potassium retention resulting in hyperkalemia can occur. The high potassium levels can precipitate cardiac arrhythmias and arrest.

- Excessive loss of sodium (hyponatremia) can result in dryness of the mouth, thirst, lethargy, and drowsiness.
- Diarrhea, nausea, and vomiting can occur.
- Weakness, headache, rash, and photosensitivity are possible.
- Blood dyscrasias have been reported.
- Do not give to patients with anuria.
- Use cautiously in patients with impaired liver and kidney function.
- Hypotension and mental confusion are possible, especially in elderly patients.

Dosage and Administration

- The usual, adult daily dosage is 100 to 200 mg, PO (frequently given 100 mg twice daily after meals). It may be given qod.
- The usual pediatric dosage is 2 to 4 mg/kg, PO, in divided doses, qd or qod.

Nursing Considerations

- See PH, Diuretics, nursing considerations.
- When triamterene is used, all potassium supplements usually are discontinued, and a diet high in potassium is discouraged.
- Diabetics, the elderly, and patients with impaired kidney function are at greatest risk for developing hyperkalemia.
- Only one potassium-sparing diuretic should be used at a time because of the danger of hyperkalemia.
- Monitor blood counts for evidence of blood dyscrasias.
- It is available in combination with hydrochlorothiazide (Dyazide).
- The drug should be given with or after meals to prevent or minimize nausea.

SULFONAMIDES

- See Thiazides for actions, adverse effects, and contraindications.
- See Table 7-33 for indications, dosage, administration, and nursing considerations.
- See PH, Diuretics, nursing considerations.

THIAZIDES

Actions

- Thiazides block active tubular reabsorption of chloride and sodium in the ascending loop of Henle.
- They can reduce elevated blood pressure.

TABLE 7-33 SULFONAMIDE DIURETICS

Drug	Indications	Dosage and Administration	Nursing Considerations
Chlorthalidone (Hygroton)	This is used to treat the edema of congestive heart failure (CHF), renal disease, and hepatic cirrhosis, and also to treat severe hypertension.	*Adult diuretic:* 50 to 100 mg, qd, or 100 to 200 mg, qod, PO *Adult antihypertensive:* Initially, 25 mg, PO, qd *Pediatric:* 2 mg/kg or 60 mg/m^2, PO, three times/week	It is available in combination with reserpine (Regroton) and with clonidine (Combipres). Serum calcium levels should be monitored to detect hypercalcemia.
Metolazone (Diulo, Zaroxolyn)	This treats edema of CHF and renal disease. Alone and in combination, it is used to manage hypertension.	*CHF:* Initially, 5 to 10 mg, PO, qd *Renal failure:* 5 to 20 mg, qd *Hypertension:* Initially, 2.5 to 5 mg, PO, qd	Alcohol potentiates the orthostatic hypotension produced by metolazone.
Quinethazone (Aquamox, Hydromox)	This drug treats edema of CHF, hepatic cirrhosis, and renal disease. It assists in managing hypertension.	50 to 100 mg, PO, qd or bid, up to a maximum of 200 mg/day in divided doses	It is available in combination with reserpine (Hydromox-R).

Indications

- Thiazides can reduce the edema of congestive heart failure, cirrhosis, and renal dysfunctions.
- They relieve drug-induced edema from steroid and estrogen therapy.
- They are given to reduce hypertension. In mild hypertension they may be used alone, or for more severe hypertension, they can be given concurrently with other antihypertensive drugs.
- In some patients with diabetes insipidus, they produce a more concentrated urine.

Adverse Effects and Contraindications

- Hypokalemia (low serum potassium levels) is a common electrolyte imbalance resulting from thiazide therapy.
- Serum glucose levels may rise, resulting in the symptoms of diabetes mellitus.
- Blood levels of uric acid may rise, precipitating an attack of gout.
- Patients with severe liver or kidney disease should use the thiazides cautiously. Hepatic coma or kidney failure are possible.
- Do not give to patients with anuria.
- Anorexia, nausea, vomiting, diarrhea, or constipation can occur.

Dosage, Administration, and Nursing Considerations

- See Table 7-34
- See PH, Diuretics, nursing considerations.
- Older patients are more likely to experience orthostatic hypotension and hypokalemia.
- Patients should check with physician before using OTC medications because many contain sodium and potassium and could contribute to electrolyte imbalances.

ESTROGENS

Actions

- Estrogen controls the development and maintenance of female secondary sexual characteristics.
- Normal menstrual cycles during reproductive years are controlled by estrogen.
- Development of endometrial lining is promoted by estrogen.
- Estrogen induces sodium and fluid retention.
- Estrogen stimulates uterine motility.

- Bone resorption rate, which is accelerated at menopause, is decreased by estrogen.
- Prolonged therapy blocks function of anterior pituitary.

Indications

- These agents treat natural or surgical menopausal symptoms.
- Estrogens can treat female hypogonadism and atrophic vaginitis.
- They also suppress lactation.
- They can prevent and treat postmenopausal osteoporosis.
- Palliation for advanced prostatic carcinoma and inoperable breast cancer in women at least 5 years postmenopause can be provided by estrogens.
- Synthetic estrogen can be used as emergency postcoital contraceptive and is combined with progestins in many oral contraceptives.

Adverse Effects and Contraindications

- Estrogens should not be used when there is a known or suspected pregnancy, for estrogenic-dependent neoplasms, for patients with thromboembolitic disorders, undiagnosed abnormal genital bleeding, history of gallbladder or thyroid disease, or blood dyscrasias.
- Use cautiously in adolescents and in patients with endometriosis, hypertension, hypercalcemia, asthma, epilepsy, migraine headaches, jaundice, mental depression, family history of breast or genital tract neoplasm, or dysfunction of the cardiac, renal, or hepatic systems.
- Nausea, vomiting, diarrhea, bloating, and thirst have occurred.
- Skin rash, acne, loss of scalp hair, hirsutism, chorea, and intolerance to contact lenses have been reported.
- Females experience breast secretion, changes in menstrual patterns and flow, spotting, reactivation of endometriosis, increase in size of existing fibroids, and vaginal candidiasis.
- Males may experience gynecomastia, feminization, impotence, and testicular atrophy.
- Hypercalcemia, hypertension, fluid and water retention, weight gain or loss, thromboembolitic disorders, fatigue, leg cramps, and changes in libido are also possible.

Dosage, Administration, and Nursing Considerations

- See Table 7-35.
- Intake, output, and weight should be monitored daily during initial therapy.

(Text continues on page 834)

TABLE 7-34 THIAZIDE DIURETICS

Drug	Dosage and Administration	Nursing Considerations
Bendroflumethiazide (Naturetin)	*Adult* 1. *Diuretic:* Initially, 2.5 to 10 mg, PO, qd or bid, once qod, or once qd for 3 to 5 days/week; maintenance dosage, 2.5 to 5 mg qd, once qod, or once qd 3 to 5 days/week 2. *Antihypertensive:* Initially, 5 to 20 mg/day, PO, as a single dose or in two divided doses; maintenance dosage, 2.5 to 15 mg/day as a single dose or in two divided doses *Pediatric* 1. *Diuretic:* Initially, up to 400 μg/kg, PO, as a single dose or in two divided doses; maintenance dosage—50 to 100 μg/kg, qd 2. *Antihypertensive:* Initially, 100 to 400 μg/kg, PO, as a single dose or in two divided doses; maintenance dosage, 50 to 300 μg/kg as a single dose or in two divided doses	It is available with potassium chloride (Naturetin W-K) and with rauwolfia serpentina (Rauzide). The diuretic action lasts longer than 18 hr. This permits longer intervals between doses and helps reduce the problems of electrolyte imbalance.

Benzthiazide (Aquapres, Hydrex)	*Adult* 1. *Diuretic:* 25 to 100 mg, PO, bid, qod, or qd for 3 to 5 days/week 2. *Antihypertensive:* 25 to 100 mg, bid PO *Pediatric:* 0.3 to 1.3 mg/kg, PO, tid	
Chlorothiazide (Diuril)	*Adult* 1. *Diuretic:* 0.5 to 1 g, qd or bid, PO or IV 2. *Antihypertensive:* Initially, 0.5 to 1 g, bid, PO; maintenance dosage, up to 2 g daily (determined by BP) *Pediatric* 1. Under 6 mo: Up to 30 mg/kg/day, PO, divided into two doses 2. 6 mo to 2 yr: 125 to 375 mg/day, PO, divided into two doses 3. 2 to 12 yr: 375 mg to 1 g/day, PO, divided into two doses	The intravenous form is chlorothiazide sodium (Diuril sodium). Do not give SC or IM because it is extremely irritating. Observe carefully for extravasation. Some patients achieve good results by using Diuril 3 to 5 days/week.
Cyclothiazide (Anhydron)	*Adult* 1. *Diuretic:* Initially, 1 to 2 mg, PO, qd; maintenance dosage, 1 to 2 mg, qod, or two or three times/week 2. *Antihypertensive:* 2 mg, PO, qd; may increase to 2 mg, bid or tid *Pediatric:* 0.02 to 0.04 mg/kg/day, PO	

(continued)

TABLE 7-34 THIAZIDE DIURETICS

Drug	Dosage and Administration	Nursing Considerations
Hydrochlorothiazide (Esidrex, HydroDiuril, Oretic)	*Adults* 1. *Diuretic:* Initially, 25 to 100 mg, PO, qd or bid; maintenance dosage, 25 to 100 mg, qd or intermittently 2. *Antihypertensive:* Initially, 75 mg, PO, qd; maintenance dosage, 25 to 100 mg, qd *Pediatric:* 2.2 mg/kg/day, PO, in two divided doses	
Hydroflumethiazide (Diucardin, Saluron)	*Adults* 1. *Diuretic:* Initially, 50 mg, PO, qd or bid; maintenance dosage, 25 to 200 mg in divided doses, qd, qod, or three to five times/week	It is available with reserpine (Salutensin).

	2. *Antihypertensive:* Initially, 50 mg, PO, bid (adjusted according to BP); maintenance dosage, 50 to 100 mg, qd or bid, up to a maximum of 200 mg daily *Pediatric:* 1 mg/kg or 30 mg/m^2, qd	
Methyclothiazide (Aquatensen, Enduron)	*Adults* 1. *Diuretic:* 2.5 to 5 mg, PO, qd, or three to five times/week 2. *Antihypertensive:* 2.5 to 10 mg, PO, qd *Pediatric:* 0.05 to 0.2 mg/kg, qd	It is available with reserpine (Diutensen-R), with pargyline (Eutron), and with deserpidine (Enduronyl).
Trichlormethiazide (Diurese, Metahydrin, Naqua)	*Adults* 1. *Diuretic:* Initially, 1 to 4 mg, PO, qd or bid; maintenance dosage, 1 to 4 mg, qd 2. *Antihypertensive:* 2 to 4 mg, qd, as a single dose or divided into two doses *Pediatric:* 0.07 mg/kg, PO, qd	It is available with reserpine (Metatensin, Naquival).

TABLE 7-35 ESTROGENS

Drug	Dosage and Administration	Nursing Considerations
Chlorotrianisene (Tace)	Prostatic cancer: 12 to 25 mg, PO, daily Postpartum breast engorgement: 12 mg, PO, qid for 7 days, or 72 mg, bid, for 2 days Female hypogonadism: 12 to 25 mg, PO, daily for 21 days followed by IM progesterone; next cycle begins on day 5 of induced uterine bleeding Menopause: 12 to 25 mg/day, PO for 30 days; may be repeated Atrophic vaginitis: 12 to 25 mg/day, PO, for 30 to 60 days	This is less suitable for cyclic therapy than the shorter-acting estrogens.
Dienestrol (DV, Estraguard)	Intravaginal cream (0.01%): one or two applicators/day for 1 week to 2 weeks; then, one-half original dose one to three times/week for 1 week or 2 weeks Vaginal suppository (0.7 mg): one or two daily for 1 week to 2 weeks, then one qod for 1 week to 2 weeks	This can be used for atrophic vaginitis and kraurosis vulvae associated with menopause. Administration at bedtime increases absorption.
Diethylstilbestrol (Stilbestrol, DES)	Estrogen deficiency: 0.2 to 0.5 mg/day, PO, (3 weeks on, followed by 1 week of rest) Postpartum breast engorgement: 5 mg, PO, qd to tid, for a total dosage of 30 mg	DES has a strong teratogenic potential and may cause vaginal or cervical cancer in offspring if the mother uses DES during pregnancy.

	Breast carcinoma (palliation): 15 mg/day, PO Prostatic carcinoma (palliation): 1 to 3 mg/day, PO Postcoital contraception: 25 mg, PO, bid for 5 days Vaginal suppository: 0.1 to 0.5 mg, qd or bid, for 10 to 14 days	
Diethylstilbestrol diphosphate (Stilphostrol)	50 to 200 mg, PO, tid 250 to 500 mg, IV, once or twice weekly as a maintenance dose	It is used in advanced stages of prostatic cancer when tolerance to other estrogens has developed.
Estradiol (Estrace)	1 to 2 mg/day, PO, on a cyclic schedule (3 weeks on, followed by 1 week of rest)	Patients have experienced systemic effects from excessive use of estrogen creams, and there is no scientific evidence that they are more effective for dry skin than simple emollients.
Estradiol cypionate (Depo-Estradiol)	Menopause: 1 to 5 mg, IM, repeated in 3 to 4 weeks Hypogonadism: 1.5 to 2 mg, IM, each month	
Estradiol valerate (Delestrogen)	Menopause or atrophic vaginitis: 10 to 20 mg, IM, every 4 weeks Prostatic carcinoma: 30 mg or more, IM, every 1 week to 2 weeks Postpartum breast engorgement: 10 to 25 mg, IM, one time at the end of the first stage of labor	

(continued)

TABLE 7-35 ESTROGENS

Drug	Dosage and Administration	Nursing Considerations
Estrogens, conjugated (Premarin)	Menopause: 0.3 to 1.25 mg/day, PO, cyclically adjusted to lowest possible maintenance dose Female hypogonadism: 2.5 to 7.5 mg/day, PO, in divided doses for 20 days, followed by 10 days of rest; dosage adjusted and progestin added according to bleeding pattern Atrophic vaginitis or kraurosis vulvae: 0.3 to 1.25 mg/day, PO Breast cancer (palliation): 10 mg, PO, tid for at least 3 mo Prostatic cancer (palliation): 1.25 to 2.5 mg, PO, tid Vaginal cream: 2 to 4 g/day on a cyclic schedule	Large doses used in the treatment of breast or prostate cancer increase the risk of nonfatal myocardial infarction, pulmonary embolism, and thrombophlebitis.
Estrogens, esterified (Estratab)	Menopause: 1.25 mg/day orally on a cyclic schedule Female hypogonadism: 2.5 to 7.5 mg/day, PO, in divided doses for 20 days, followed by 10 days of rest Prostatic carcinoma: 1.25 to 2.5 mg, PO, tid, for several weeks, then about one-half of the dose for maintenance Breast carcinoma: 10 mg, PO, tid for 2 to 3 mo	These are the same estrogens as those in conjugated form, but they are in different proportions.

Estrone estrogenic substance	Menopause: 0.1 to 0.5 mg, IM, two or three times/week Female hypogonadism: 0.5 to 2 mg week/IM Prostatic carcinoma (palliation): 2 to 4 mg, IM, two or three times/week	Preparations have either a water or oil base. Warm oily solutions to room temperature until clear before giving.
Estropipate (Estrone sulfate)	Menopause: 0.625 to 5 mg/day, PO, on a cyclic schedule Female hypogonadism: 1.25 to 7.5 mg/day, PO, for 21 days, followed by 8 to 10 days of rest; may add progestin Atrophic vaginitis and kraurosis vulvae: 2 to 4 g/day of vaginal cream on a cyclic schedule	
Ethinyl estradiol (Estinyl)	Menopause: 0.02 to 0.05 mg/day, PO, on a cyclic schedule Postpartum breast engorgement: 0.5 to 1 mg daily for 3 days, then gradually decreased to 0.1 mg after 7 days Female hypogonadism: 0.05 mg, one to three times/day, PO, for 2 weeks, followed by 2 weeks of progestin (for 3 to 6 mo) Breast cancer: 1 mg, PO, tid Prostatic cancer: 0.15 to 0.2 mg, PO, qd	
Quinestrol (Estrovis)	Initially, 100 μg, PO, qd for 7 days Maintenance: 100 μg, PO, once a week, beginning 2 weeks after starting treatment	

(continued from page 825)

- Diuretics may be used to control sodium and water retention, and blood pressure should be monitored.
- Serum calcium levels should be checked periodically during therapy.
- Estrogens frequently are administered on a cyclic schedule to mimic natural menses (*e.g.,* 3 weeks on and 1 week off).
- Take oral estrogens with food to minimize nausea.
- Male patients should be reassured that impotence and feminization are reversible after therapy is stopped.

MAGNESIUM SULFATE (EPSOM SALTS)

Actions

- Parenterally, it depresses the CNS as well as smooth, skeletal, and cardiac muscle.
- Excessive doses produce vasodilation.
- Orally, it retains fluid by osmosis, which causes colon distention, increases water content of feces, and mechanically stimulates bowel activity.

Indications

- The parenteral form controls seizures in toxemia of pregnancy, epilepsy, acute nephritis, hypomagnesemia, and hypothyroidism.
- It replaces magnesium in acute deficiencies and is part of total parenteral nutrition (TPN) regimens.
- Topically, it reduces edema, inflammation, and itching.
- Orally, it relieves acute constipation and prepares the bowel for intestinal x-rays.

Adverse Effects and Contraindications

- It should not be used in patients with myocardial damage or heart block.
- Patients with nausea, vomiting, fecal impaction, or intestinal obstruction or perforation should not use the oral preparation.
- Use cautiously in the presence of renal dysfunction or other CNS-depressant or neuromuscular-blocking drugs.
- Symptoms of hypermagnesemia include flushing, extreme thirst, hypotension, confusion, depressed or absent reflexes, flaccid paralysis, hypothermia, complete heart block, circulatory collapse, and respiratory paralysis.
- Repeated use as a laxative may result in electrolyte imbalance (including hypocalcemia) and dehydration.

Dosage and Administration

- The usual oral dosage is 5 to 15 g.
- Intramuscularly, 1 g to 5 g of a 25% to 50% solution are given.
- One to 4 g are given IV as a 10% or 20% solution. The rate should not exceed 1.5 ml/min of 10% solution, or its equivalent for other concentrations.
- Topically, hot or cold compresses are made with a 25% to 50% solution.

Nursing Considerations

- Monitor blood pressure and pulse rate every 10 min to 15 min during IV administration.
- Intake and output also should be monitored carefully during parenteral administration.
- Newborns whose mothers received magnesium sulfate within a few hours of delivery may experience respiratory and neuromuscular depression.
- Foods rich in magnesium are whole grain cereals, most green leafy vegetables, bananas, and legumes.

ORAL CONTRACEPTIVES (ESTROGEN-PROGESTIN COMBINATIONS)

Actions

- See PH, Estrogens and progestins for actions of the individual components.
- These agents produce contraception by preventing ovulation.
- The female reproductive tract becomes resistant to sperm penetration and zygote implantation.

Indications

- They are used to prevent conception.
- They also can be used to treat hypermenorrhea and endometriosis.

Adverse Effects and Contraindications

- Oral contraceptives (OCs) should not be used during pregnancy or lactation.
- Other contraindications include personal or family history of breast cancer or estrogen-dependent carcinomas, history or existence of thrombophlebitis or thromboembolic disorders, cardio-

vascular or cerebral vascular disease, hepatic neoplasm or dysfunction, or undiagnosed abnormal genital bleeding.

- Women who are 40 years old and over, and adolescents with incomplete epiphyseal closure should not use OCs.
- OCs should be used cautiously in patients with depression, hypertension, migraines, renal disease, asthma, convulsive disorders, gallbladder disease, rheumatic diseases, diabetes, or varicosities.
- Estrogen excess may produce nausea, bloating, hypertension, migraine headache, breast fullness, edema, or menstrual tension.
- Estrogen deficiency can result in hypomenorrhea or breakthrough bleeding.
- Progestin excess may produce hypomenorrhea, breast regression, vaginal candidiasis, increased appetite, weight gain, depression, fatigue, acne, hair loss, or hirsutism.
- Progestin deficiency can result in amenorrhea or breakthrough bleeding.
- Thromboembolitic disorders, jaundice, diarrhea, constipation, urinary tract infections, optic neuritis, papilledema, and an increased risk of congenital anomalies also have been reported.

Dosage and Administration

- In the 21-day schedule, day 1 is the first day of menstrual bleeding. Starting on day 5, one tablet is taken PO every day for 20 or 21 days. Withdrawal bleeding usually occurs 2 days or 3 days after the last tablet is taken, and the cycle is resumed 7 days after cessation of medication.
- In the 28-day schedule the package may contain seven inert or iron tablets to permit continuous, daily pill taking during the entire 28 days.

Nursing Considerations

- Users of OCs who smoke heavily and who are over 35 years old are at greater risk for serious cardiovascular adverse effects than are nonsmokers.
- During the first week of the *initial* cycle, a back-up method of birth control should be used.
- Tablets should be taken at the same time each day.
- The size and shape of contact lenses, if worn by the patient, may need to be changed because of changes in ocular contour and lubricant quality of tears.
- Estrogen-dominant preparations include Enovid-E, Norinyl, Ortho-Novum 2 mg, and Ovulen.

- Progestin-dominant preparations include Loestrin, Lo/Ovral, Norlestrin, and Ovral.
- Other products that contain an intermediate or low ratio of estrogens and progestins are Brevicon, Modicon, Nordette, Ovcon, and Ortho-Novum.

OXYTOCICS

Actions

- Oxytocics produce phasic uterine contractions that are characteristic of normal delivery.
- They promote milk ejection reflex (letdown) in nursing mothers and facilitate flow during the period of breast engorgement.

Indications

- These agents are used to initiate or improve uterine contraction at term after the cervix is dilated and presentation of the fetus has occurred.
- They also can be used to manage inevitable, incomplete, or missed abortion.
- The drugs can control postpartum hemorrhage and promote postpartum uterine involution.
- Oxytocics are used to induce labor in cases of erythroblastosis fetalis, eclampsia, preeclampsia, and maternal diabetes.
- Letdown reflex in nursing mothers is stimulated by oxytocic drugs.

Adverse Effects and Contraindications

- Oxytocics should be used only in carefully selected patients and are contraindicated for significant cephalopelvic disproportion, unfavorable fetal presentations, obstetric emergencies that favor surgical intervention, fetal distress when delivery is not imminent, prematurity, placenta previa, previous surgery of the uterus (including cesarean section), grand multiparity, or in a primipara patient over 35 years of age.
- The mother may experience uterine hypertonicity, tetanic contractions, uterine rupture, anaphylactic reactions, postpartum hemorrhage, cardiac arrhythmias, nausea, vomiting, and hypertension.
- Antidiuretic hormone (ADH) effects include severe water intoxication, hyponatremia, hypotension, arrhythmias, edema, and cardiovascular collapse.

TABLE 7-36 OXYTOCICS

Drug	Dosage and Administration	Nursing Considerations
Ergonovine maleate (Ergotrate maleate)	0.2 mg (1 ml), IM or IV, every 2 to 4 hr, up to a maximum of five doses 0.2 to 0.4 mg, PO, every 6 to 12 hr, until danger of atony passes (about 48 hr)	It prevents or reduces postpartum and postabortal hemorrhage caused by uterine atony. An IM injection may be given to the mother as the infant is born, and in 2 to 5 min produces contractions that separate the placenta and prevent blood loss. The IV route is used for emergencies only.
Methylergonovine maleate (Methergine)	0.2 mg, PO, tid or qid, in puerperium for maximum of 1 week 1 ml (0.2 mg), IM, every 2 to 4 hr, prn, after delivery of anterior shoulder, after delivery of placenta, or during puerperium 1 ml (0.2 mg), IV, given slowly over 1 min *only* in emergencies	This prevents or reduces postpartum and postabortal hemorrhage caused by uterine atony.
Oxytocin injection (Pitocin) Oxytocin nasal solution	Stimulation or induction of labor 1. One to 2 mu/min (0.001 to 0.002 units/min IV); gradually increased by 1 to 2 mu/min until contractions simulate normal labor Postpartum uterine bleeding 1. 10 to 40 u, IV, added to 1000 ml of nonhydrating diluent at a rate needed to control uterine atony 2. 5 to 10 u, IM, after delivery of placenta Milk letdown: One spray into one or both nostrils, 2 to 3 min before nursing (40 u/ml)	

- The fetus may experience bradycardia and other arrhythmias, hypoxia, intracranial hemorrhage, trauma from rapid passage through the pelvis, neonatal jaundice, and death.

Dosage, Administration, and Nursing Considerations

- See Table 7-36.
- The mother and fetus must be monitored carefully throughout IV administration of oxytocics.
- Oxytocics should never be given by more than one route at a time.

PROGESTINS

Actions

- Progestins transform the endometrium from a proliferative to secretory state.
- They suppress pituitary gonadotropin secretion and block follicular maturation and ovulation.
- With estrogen, they promote mammary gland development without causing lactation.
- They stimulate endocervical secretion of glycogen and thick mucus.
- Spontaneous contraction of the uterus is prohibited by progestins.

Indications

- They are used to treat secondary amenorrhea, functional uterine bleeding, and endometriosis.
- They also provide fertility control as Progestasert, or in combination with estrogens.

Adverse Effects and Contraindications

- Progestins should not be used in patients with breast or genital malignancy, thrombophlebitis or thromboembolic disorders, impaired liver function, or undiagnosed vaginal bleeding.
- They are contraindicated during the first four months of pregnancy and for nursing mothers.
- They should be used cautiously in patients with cardiac or renal dysfunction, diabetes mellitus, epilepsy, migraine, asthma, or severe depression.
- Benign and malignant mammary nodules, masculinization of female fetus, amenorrhea, breakthrough bleeding, and changes in libido have been reported.

- Loss of vision, diplopia, depression, and migraine headaches have occurred.
- Thromboembolitic disorders and pulmonary embolus are possible.
- Patients also have experienced acne, alopecia, hirsutism, fatigue, rash, edema, chloasma, candidiasis, and jaundice.

Dosage, Administration, and Nursing Considerations

- See Table 7-37
- Monitor blood pressure, fluid retention, and weight during therapy.
- Progestin preparations have a teratogenic potential.

RITODRINE HYDROCHLORIDE (YUTOPAR)

Actions

- This drug stimulates $beta_2$ receptors in uterine smooth muscle.
- It reduces the intensity and frequency of uterine contractions.

Indications

- It is used to manage premature labor in selected patients.

Adverse Effects and Contraindications

- This drug should not be used prior to the 20th week of pregnancy, or if continuation of pregnancy would be hazardous to the mother and fetus.
- Patients with cardiac arrhythmias, hypertension, asthma, diabetes mellitus, and mild-to-moderate preeclampsia should not receive this drug.
- Patients may experience altered maternal and fetal heart rates and maternal blood pressure, especially following IV infusion.
- Temporary hyperglycemia, arrhythmias, tremor, headache, nausea, vomiting, restlessness, anxiety, and pulmonary edema have been reported.

Dosage and Administration

- Usually, 0.1 mg/min (0.33 ml/min) IV is administered with a constant rate infusion pump. Gradually increase the dose by 0.05 mg/min every 10 min until adequate uterine relaxation is achieved. It may continue for 12 hr after contractions cease.
- Orally, 10 mg are given every 2 hr for the first 24 hr (start 30 min prior to terminating the infusion). Then, 10 mg to 20 mg are given every 4 hr to 6 hr. Maximum dosage is 120 mg/day.

Nursing Considerations

- To prepare the IV solution, add 150 mg of ritodrine to 500 ml of D_5W or normal saline solution for a concentration of 0.3 mg/ml.
- During infusion, the patient should lie on her left side to reduce the risk of hypotension.

Rho (D) IMMUNE GLOBULIN (HUMAN) (RhoGAM)

Actions

- This drug suppresses the specific immune response of Rh-negative individuals to Rh-positive red blood cells.
- It prevents hemolytic disease in the newborn.

Indications

- It is used for postpartum women with Rh-negative blood who deliver a baby with Rho (D)-positive or D^u-positive blood.
- The drug should be given to women with Rh-negative blood after an abortion or ectopic pregnancy, unless the father or the products of conception are shown conclusively to be Rh negative.
- It also is given to women with Rh-negative blood who have an amniocentesis or experience other abdominal trauma that results in fetal cells entering the maternal circulation.

Adverse Effects and Contraindications

- Reactions are infrequent, mild, and mostly confined to the area of injection.
- There are no known contraindications for use of RhoGAM.

Dosage and Administration

- Postpartum prophylaxis: Administer the contents of one vial, IM, within 3 days of delivery.
- Antepartum prophylaxis: Administer the contents of one vial, IM, at approximately 28 weeks. This *must* be followed by one vial, IM, within 3 days of delivery.
- Amniocentesis, miscarriage, abortion, ectopic pregnancy (at or beyond 13th week of gestation): Administer the contents of one vial, IM.

Nursing Considerations

- One vial of RhoGAM will completely suppress the immune response to 15 ml of Rh-positive red blood cells.

TABLE 7-37 PROGESTINS

Drug	Dosage and Administration	Nursing Considerations
Hydroxyprogesterone caproate (Delalutin, Pro-Depo)	Amenorrhea: 375 mg, IM; may follow with cyclic therapy Advanced uterine adenocarcinoma: 1 to 7 g/week, IM; stop at relapse or after 12 weeks of therapy Test for endogenous estrogen production: 250 mg, IM; may repeat in 4 weeks	
Medroxyprogesterone acetate (Depo-Provera)	Abnormal uterine bleeding or secondary amenorrhea: 5 to 10 mg/day, PO, for 5 to 10 days, beginning on the 16th or 21st day of the menstrual cycle Endometriosis: 30 mg/day, PO, or 150 mg, IM, every 3 mo Menopause: 10 mg, PO, for 5 to 7 days during the third week of estrogen administration Endometrial and renal carcinoma: 400 to 1000 mg, IM, weekly	Monitor IM injection sites for sterile abscesses.
Megestrol acetate (Megace)	Breast carcinoma: 40 mg, PO, qid Endometrial carcinoma: 40 to 320 mg, PO, qd, in divided doses	This is used for palliation for advanced carcinoma of the breast or endometrium. Therapy should continue for at least 2 months to determine the effectiveness.

Norethindrone (Norlutin)	Amenorrhea: 5 to 20 mg, PO, on days 5 through 25 of the menstrual cycle Endometriosis: 10 mg, PO, qd for 2 weeks; increase gradually to 30 mg/day Progestin-only contraception: 0.35 mg, PO, qd of the first day of the menstrual flow, and then qd Norethindrone acetate: about one-half of the norethindrone dosage	
Norgestrel (Ovrette)	0.075 mg (one tablet), PO, qd, every day of the year, beginning on the first day of menstruation	This is a progestin-only contraceptive (mini-pill).
Progesterone (Progestasert)	Amenorrhea: 5 to 10 mg, IM, for 6 to 8 consecutive days Functional uterine bleeding: 5 to 10 mg, IM, qd, for 6 days. Intrauterine contraception (Progestasert): Delivery of 65 μg/day progesterone into uterine cavity for one year	The intrauterine contraception may result in endometritis, spontaneous abortion, septic abortion, septicemia, perforation of uterus and cervix, pelvic infection, ectopic pregnancy, pregnancy, amenorrhea, and anemia.

PH

MUSCULOSKELETAL SYSTEM

ACETAMINOPHEN (DATRIL, LIQUIPRIN, TEMPRA, TYLENOL)

Actions

- Analgesic and antipyretic

Indications

- Acetaminophen can relieve mild to moderate pain.
- It may be preferred to aspirin in the following:
  1. Patients who easily experience gastrointestinal irritation
  2. Gout patients receiving drugs to promote excretion of uric acid
  3. Patients on anticoagulants or those with hemorrhagic disorders
  4. Patients who are allergic to the salicylates

Adverse Effects and Contraindications

- There are few side-effects from ordinary doses.
- Rarely, renal damage, hemolytic anemia, and methemoglobinemia (a part of hemoglobin is changed and oxygen cannot be transported) have occurred.
- Drug should be discontinued if skin redness, itching, or urticaria occur.
- Liver damage, especially in children, can occur with normal therapeutic doses.
- Massive overdose may lead to death from acute hepatic necrosis, hypoglycemia, or metabolic acidosis.

Dosage and Administration

- *Adults:* Administer 300 mg to 650 mg, PO or rectally, every 4 hr as needed. Maximum dosage is 2.6 g/day, and self-administration is intended for short-term use only.
- *Pediatric:* Administer every 4 hr to 6 hr as needed, PO or rectally. Maximum dosage is 5 doses/24 hr or for 5 days.
  1. *6 to 12 yr:* 150 to 325 mg up to a maximum of 1.2 g/day.
  2. *3 to 6 yr:* 120 mg, up to a maximum 480 mg/day
  3. *1 to 3 yr:* 60 mg to 120 mg
  4. *Under 1 yr:* 60 mg (highly individualized)

Nursing Considerations

- Combination OTC drugs that include acetaminophen are BromoSeltzer, Excedrin, Trigesic, and Vanquish.
- Acetaminophen is available with codeine as Empracet and Percocet.
- It is available with butabarbital as Phrenilin.
- Acetylcystein (Mucomyst) (see PH, Respiratory) is an antidote for acetaminophen toxicity when given PO, if used within 16 hr after the poisoning.

ALLOPURINOL (LOPURIN, ZYLOPRIM)

Actions

- Allopurinol reduces the production of uric acid by inhibiting the biochemical reactions immediately before its formation. Its action is not antagonized by salicylates.

Indications

- Allopurinol reduces hyperuricemia in both primary and secondary gout.
- It reduces the recurrence of uric acid stone formation.
- It is used to prevent renal calculi, uric acid nephropathy, and tissue urate deposits in patients with leukemias, lymphomas, and malignancies, who are receiving antineoplastic drugs or radiation therapy that elevate serum uric acid levels.

Adverse Effects and Contraindications

- Discontinue allopurinol at the first sign of skin rash or other adverse effects. Severe hypersensitivity reactions may follow a skin rash.
- Patients may experience nausea, vomiting, and diarrhea.
- Blood dyscrasias have occurred in patients receiving allopurinol. Concurrent administration of other drugs that have the potential of causing blood dyscrasias usually is involved.
- Drowsiness occurs occasionally.
- Use cautiously in patients with liver or renal dysfunction, a history of peptic ulcer or lower intestinal disease, or bone marrow depression.
- Allopurinol should not be used for the initial treatment of acute gouty attacks.

Dosage and Administration

- *Adults*
  1. Gout: Administer 100 mg, PO, initially, and increase by 100 mg at weekly intervals. Maximum dosage is 300 mg/day as a single dose.
  2. Secondary hyperuricemia: Administer 200 mg to 800 mg, PO, daily for 2 or 3 days or longer. Maximum dosage is 800 mg/day. Doses over 300 mg/day are divided and given after meals.
- *Pediatric*
  1. *(6 to 10 yr):* Administer 100 mg, PO, three times/day.
  2. *(Under 6 yr):* Administer 50 mg, PO, three times/day.

Nursing Considerations

- Serum uric acid levels are used to determine appropriate maintenance doses of allopurinol.
- Liver and kidney functions should be monitored during therapy.
- Caution patients against driving if the medication causes drowsiness.
- Allopurinol may precipitate attacks of gout when treatment is started. Usually, maintenance doses of colchicine (0.5 mg, bid) are given as a prophylactic measure.
- Patients receiving allopurinol should drink enough fluid to produce two liters of urine daily. Another measure to prevent calculi is the use of urinary alkalinizers (*e.g.,* sodium bicarbonate).
- Oral iron salts should not be taken with allopurinol because the iron may be deposited in the liver.
- Allopurinol can prolong the half-life of anticoagulants. Monitor prothrombin times carefully.
- The doses of mercaptopurine (antileukemic drug) and azathioprine (an immunosuppressant) should be reduced by one-third to one-fourth when allopurinol is added. Otherwise, severe bone marrow depression results.

ASPIRIN (ACETYLSALICYLIC ACID, A.S.A., ECOTRIN, EMPIRIN)

Actions

- Analgesic; antipyretic; anti-inflammatory; inhibits platelet aggregation; and prolongs bleeding time

Indications

- Aspirin reduces fever.
- It relieves mild to moderate pain (*e.g.*, in joints and muscles, with headache).
- It reduces inflammation.
- Aspirin can be given to prevent coronary thrombosis and cerebral or pulmonary embolism.
- It also relieves pain associated with osteoarthritis.

Adverse Effects and Contraindications

- Nausea, vomiting, *gastrointestinal (GI) bleeding,* and ulceration can occur.
- Mild toxicity produces tinnitus (ringing in ears), visual blurring, drowsiness, and mental confusion.
- Acute toxicity produces severe *acid-base imbalances,* especially in children, *convulsions, coma,* and *respiratory failure.*
- Aspirin also may produce skin rashes and wheezing.
- Children with chickenpox or any other viral infection should not receive aspirin products because of the association with Reye's syndrome.
- Patients with gout, hemorrhagic disorders, renal or hepatic dysfunction, or a history of GI ulceration should use aspirin cautiously.
- Postoperative patients and children with fever and dehydration also should be cautious with aspirin use.

Dosage and Administration

- *Adults*
  1. Analgesic and antipyretic: 325 mg to 650 mg (5 to 10 grains), PO or by rectal suppository, every 4 to 6 hr, prn
  2. Arthritis and rheumatic disorders: 2.6 to 5.2 g/day, PO, in divided doses
  3. Acute rheumatic fever: Up to 7.8 g/day, PO, in divided doses
  4. Thromboembolitic disorders: 80 to 650 mg, PO, qd or bid
- *Pediatric:* 1.5 g/m^2/day, PO, in divided doses
- *OTC use:* Maximum of five doses/day, or no more than 5 consecutive days

Nursing Considerations

- To minimize GI irritation, give aspirin with meals, milk, snacks, or antacids.
- In small doses, aspirin can interfere with probenecid and uric acid excretion.
- Aspirin may potentiate the action of oral anticoagulants.

- Salicylates are the most common cause of accidental poisoning among children.
- Some surgeons recommend abstaining from the use of aspirin products for 2 weeks prior to elective surgery to minimize the risk of bleeding.
- Ecotrin is enteric-coated aspirin that is designed to reduce GI irritation. However, elderly patients and other high-risk individuals may experience occult bleeding.
- Effervescent aspirin preparations such as Alka-Seltzer have a high sodium content and are not recommended for patients on a restricted sodium intake.
- Aspirin is available in many combination products:
  1. Aspirin and maalox (Ascriptin)
  2. Aspirin, antacid, acetaminophen, caffeine (Vanquish)
  3. Aspirin and caffeine (Anacin)
  4. Aspirin, acetaminophen, salicylamide, caffeine (Excedrin)
- Presently, more than 500 aspirin-containing compounds are available.

COLCHICINE

Actions

- Colchicine inhibits the migration of granulocytes into the inflamed area.
- It is thought to decrease lactic acid production by the leukocytes, thereby decreasing urate crystal deposits and subsequent inflammation.

Indications

- Colchicine is used to prevent and treat acute attacks of gout.

Adverse Effects and Contraindications

- Nausea, vomiting, or diarrhea can occur with therapeutic doses.
- Prolonged therapy may cause bone marrow depression with agranulocytosis, thrombocytopenia, and aplastic anemia. The drug is not indicated for more than 5 days to 7 days.
- Use cautiously in elderly and debilitated patients, or in those with cardiovascular, renal, hepatic, or GI impairment.
- Mental confusion, peripheral neuritis, respiratory failure, and convulsions have been reported.

Dosage and Administration

- Acute gouty attack: Initially, give 1 or 1.2 mg, PO, then 0.5 or 0.6 mg every hr or every 2 or 3 hr until the pain is relieved or GI symptoms appear. The IV dose is 1 mg to 3 mg initially, followed by 0.5 mg every 6 hr until the pain is relieved or GI symptoms appear.

- Prophylaxis: For mild to moderate cases, give 0.5 to 2 mg, PO, every night or every other night. For severe cases, administer 0.5 to 1.8 mg, PO, daily.

Nursing Considerations

- Monitor blood counts for signs of bone marrow depression.
- The oral drug should be taken with food or milk.
- IV colchicine should be diluted only with sterile water for injection and administered over a 3- to 5-minute period.
- Severe tissue irritation and nerve damage can occur from extravasation.
- Colchicine is available with probenecid (Colbenemid, Robenecid with colchicine).

NONSTEROIDAL ANTI-INFLAMMATORIES (NSAID)

Actions

- The agents reduce inflammation, possibly by inhibiting prostaglandin synthesis.
- They possess analgesic and antipyretic properties.
- They prolong bleeding time and may inhibit platelet aggregation.

Indications

- They are used to relieve symptoms of acute and chronic rheumatoid arthritis and osteoarthritis.

Adverse Effects and Contraindications

- GI effects are most frequent. They include nausea, heartburn, diarrhea, vomiting, and constipation.
- Dizziness, headache, nervousness, depression, and tinnitus can occur.
- Patients have experienced rashes, decreased appetite, and fluid retention.
- Use cautiously for patients with a history of GI disease because ulceration and bleeding have been reported. Patients with hematologic defects also should use these drugs cautiously.
- Patients with cardiovascular disease should use these drugs cautiously because of the fluid retention that can occur.
- Blurred or diminished vision and changes in color vision have been reported with some NSAID.

- Anaphylactoid reactions have occurred in patients with aspirin hypersensitivity.

Dosage, Administration, and Nursing Considerations

- See Table 7-38
- Patients receiving prolonged or high-dose therapy should receive baseline and periodic evaluations of hemoglobin, hepatic and renal function, and ophthalmic and auditory examinations.
- Both aspirin and alcohol may increase the risk of GI ulceration and bleeding tendencies, and should be avoided while patients are using NSAID.
- Because NSAID may prolong bleeding time, patients should inform their dentist, surgeon, or other health-care provider that they are taking these drugs.
- Therapeutic effects may take up to about 3 weeks to become evident, and are characterized by relief of joint pains and stiffness, reduced joint swelling, increased grip strength, and improved mobility.
- Patients should be cautioned to take care when driving or performing other hazardous activities because these drugs may cause drowsiness and dizziness.
- Fluid retention and edema should be monitored, especially in patients with cardiac decompensation.

PHENYLBUTAZONE (BUTAZOLIDIN)

Actions

- Anti-inflammatory, analgesic, antipyretic, uricosuric

Indications

- Phenylbutazone relieves symptoms of rheumatoid arthritis and ankylosing spondylitis in patients unresponsive to other treatments.
- It also relieves acute gout attacks not controlled by colchicine.

Adverse Effects and Contraindications

- This drug produces a *high* incidence of side-effects.
- Edema, nausea, vomiting, stomatitis, rash, and dizziness occur.
- Hemorrhage, peptic ulcer, and ulceration of the bowel are possible.
- Bone marrow depression has occurred, leading to serious blood dyscrasias (*e.g.,* leukopenia, thrombocytopenia, and agranulocytosis).

- Hyperglycemia, thyroid hyperplasia, and severe acid-base imbalances have been reported.
- Blurred vision, optic neuritis, retinal hemorrhage and detachment, hearing loss, and tinnitus may occur.
- Patients with a history of cardiac, liver, or renal disorders, peptic ulcer, or blood dyscrasias should not receive this drug.
- Toxic effects also may include hepatitis, hypertension, or renal and liver necrosis.

Dosage and Administration

- Rheumatoid arthritis: Administer 300 to 600 mg, PO, tid or qid, initially. Maintenance dosage is 400 mg/day.
- Acute gout and gouty arthritis: Administer 400 mg, PO, initially, followed by 100 mg every 4 hr.
- Phenylbutazone generally is considered for short-term therapy.

Nursing Considerations

- Take immediately before or after meals or with milk.
- The following drug interactions occur with phenylbutazone:
  1. It potentiates the action of warfarin.
  2. It potentiates the hypoglycemic effects of insulin and oral hypoglycemic drugs.
  3. It potentiates the sulfonamides.
  4. Increased incidence of nephrotoxicity or increased ulcerogenic effects may occur when used with other anti-inflammatory agents.
- Because of the high risk of severe, fatal, toxic reactions in patients over 60 years old, the treatment period should be limited to one week.
- Phenylbutazone may precipitate an acute, asthmatic attack.

PROBENECID (BENEMID)

Actions

- Probenecid inhibits tubular reabsorption of urate.
- It increases urinary excretion of uric acid.
- The drug also inhibits tubular secretion of penicillin and cephalosporin antibiotics, and increases their plasma levels.

Indications

- It is used to treat hyperuricemia associated with gout and gouty arthritis.

TABLE 7-38 NONSTEROIDAL ANTI-INFLAMMATORY DRUGS (NSAID)

Drug	Dosage and Administration	Nursing Considerations
Fenoprofen calcium (Nalfon)	*Analgesic:* 200 mg, PO, every 4 to 6 hr, prn *Arthritis:* 300 to 600 mg, PO, qid, up to maximum of 3.2 g/day	
Ibuprofen (Motrin, Rufen)	300 to 600 mg, PO, tid or qid, up to a maximum of 2.4 g/day	It has also been used as an analgesic for dysmenorrhea.
Indomethacin (Indocin)	*Rheumatoid arthritis:* 25 mg, PO, bid or tid, and if tolerated, increased by 25 mg at weekly intervals up to a maximum of 150 to 200 mg/day *Acute gouty arthritis:* 50 mg, PO, tid, until pain is tolerable, then rapid weaning of the patient from the drug	It is used for palliative therapy in moderate to severe arthritic conditions that have not responded to other therapy. It also is used for dysmenorrhea and to close patent ductus arteriosus in the neonatal period. Elderly individuals have a high incidence of adverse effects. The drug may mask signs and symptoms of latent infections.
Naproxen (Naprosyn) Naproxen sodium (Anaprox)	*Musculoskeletal pain:* 250 to 375 mg, PO, of naproxen (275 mg for naproxen sodium), bid, up to a maximum of 1000 mg for naproxen, (1100 mg for naproxen sodium) *Acute gout:* 750 mg naproxen, PO, followed by 250 mg every 8 hr until attack subsides *Juvenile arthritis:* 10 mg/kg/day, PO, in two divided doses	Naproxen sodium contains about 25 mg (1 mEq) of sodium and is absorbed more rapidly than naproxen. Naproxen may have an advantage over some other NSAID because of the bid administration schedule.

	Dysmenorrhea: 500 mg, PO (550 mg for naproxen sodium), followed by 250 mg every 6 to 8 hr (275 mg for naproxen sodium)	
Piroxicam (Feldene)	20 mg, PO, qd	The single daily dose administration is convenient and easier to remember than multiple-dose therapy.
Sulindac (Clinoril)	*Arthritis and ankylosing spondylitis:* 150 mg, PO, bid, up to a maximum of 400 mg/day *Acute painful shoulder, gouty arthritis:* 200 mg, PO, bid, for 7 to 14 days, and then reduced dosage	It has the advantage of bid administration.
Tolmetin sodium (Tolectin, Tolectin DS)	*Adults:* 400 mg, PO, tid, initially Maintenance: 1. Rheumatoid arthritis: 600 to 1800 mg/day in divided doses, up to a maximum of 2000 mg/day 2. Osteoarthritis: 600 to 1600 mg/day, up to a maximum of 1600 mg/day *Pediatric (2 yr and older):* 1. Juvenile rheumatoid arthritis: 20 mg/kg/day, PO, in divided doses 2. Maintenance: 15 to 30 mg/kg/day	It may be used alone or in combination with corticosteroids or gold.

- It is used to maintain elevated and prolonged levels of the penicillins and cephalosporins, when indicated.

Adverse Effects and Contraindications

- Nausea, vomiting, headache, and urinary frequency have occurred.
- Nephrotic syndrome and hepatic necrosis are possible.
- Hypersensitivity reactions such as anaphylaxis, dermatitis, and fever have been reported.
- It may precipitate attacks of gout and increase the formation of uric acid stones.
- Probenecid should not be used within 2 to 3 weeks of an acute gouty attack or to treat hyperuricemia secondary to cancer chemotherapy.

Dosage and Administration

- Adults
  1. Gout therapy: 0.25 g, PO, bid, for 1 week, followed by 0.5 g, bid
  2. Penicillin or cephalosporin therapy: 0.5 g, PO, qid
  3. Gonorrhea: 1 g, PO, concurrently with an acceptable antibiotic.
- Pediatric (2 to 14 yr):
  1. Penicillin or cephalosporin therapy: 25 mg/kg, PO, initially, followed by 40 mg/kg/day in four divided doses

Nursing Considerations

- Therapy with probenecid may precipitate an attack of gout. If this occurs colchicine usually is given. It is available in combination as ColBenemid.
- Uric acid tends to crystallize out of an acid urine. Patients should drink enough fluid to produce 2 liters of urine daily. Three to 7.5 g of sodium bicarbonate given daily can maintain an alkaline urine.
- Probenecid increases plasma levels of methotrexate. The dosage of methotrexate should be reduced, and serum levels should be monitored.
- Salicylates should not be used with probenecid because they antagonize the uricosuric action of probenecid.
- Probenecid may potentiate the action of oral hypoglycemics. Blood glucose levels should be monitored.
- Plasma levels of indomethacin usually increase when probenecid is given concurrently.

SKELETAL MUSCLE RELAXANTS

Actions

- These agents produce skeletal muscle relaxation by depressing nerve transmission through multisynaptic pathways in the central nervous system (CNS), and possibly by a sedative effect.

Indications

- They are used to relieve skeletal muscle spasm, stiffness, and pain in musculoskeletal disorders.
- They also relieve spasticity and rigidity in cerebral palsy.

Adverse Effects and Contraindications

- These drugs may cause drowsiness, dizziness, headache, depression, and insomnia.
- Allergic reactions such as skin rash, asthma, fever, and anaphylactic shock may occur.
- Nausea, vomiting, constipation, and diarrhea are possible.

Dosage, Administration, and Nursing Considerations

- See Table 7-39.
- These drugs should be used cautiously with alcohol or other CNS depressants because of the possible additive effects.
- Rest and physical therapy are used concurrently with the medication.

NEUROLOGIC SYSTEM

AGENTS FOR AFFECTIVE DISORDERS

ANTIDEPRESSANTS

Monoamine Oxidase Inhibitors

Actions

- These agents inhibit the enzyme monoamine oxidase (MAO).
- They produce antidepressant activity.

Indications

- They are used to treat depressed patients who do not respond to tricyclic antidepressants or electroconvulsive therapy. They also are used in phobic anxiety states.

TABLE 7-39 SKELETAL MUSCLE RELAXANTS

Drug	Dosage and Administration	Nursing Considerations
Baclofen (Lioresal)	Start therapy at a low dosage, increase gradually until optimal effect is achieved (usually between 40–80 mg/day PO) Sample titration schedule 5 mg, tid, for 3 days 10 mg, tid, for 3 days 15 mg, tid, for 3 days 20 mg, tid, for 3 days Maximum dosage: 20 mg, qid	This drug is not recommended for children. Transient drowsiness is the most common adverse reaction. Dizziness, weakness, fatigue, nausea, and hypotension also have been reported. Abrupt withdrawal of the drug should be avoided, if possible. (Hallucinations and seizures have occurred.) It can be used to relieve spasticity from multiple sclerosis and some spinal cord injuries.

Carisoprodol (Rela, Soma)	350 mg, PO, qid	This drug has a low incidence of toxicity. Extreme weakness, temporary loss of vision or diplopia, and confusion may occur. It is available with aspirin (Soma Compound) and with codeine and aspirin (Soma Compound w/Codeine).
Chlorzoxazone (Paraflex)	*Adults:* 250 to 500 mg, PO, tid or qid up to a maximum of 750 mg, tid or qid. *Pediatric:* 20 mg/kg/day, PO, in three or four divided doses	Urine may appear orange or purplish-red in color. It also is available with acetaminophen (Parafon Forte, Miflex).
Cyclobenzaprine (Flexeril)	Usual adult dosage: 10 mg, PO, tid Maximum dosage: 60 mg daily	It should be used only for short periods (up to 2 or 3 weeks). Cyclobenzaprine is closely related to the tricyclic antidepressants (see PH, Neurological) and also may have atropine-like actions (see PH, Cardiovascular).

Adverse Effects and Contraindications

- Postural hypotension is a frequent side-effect. Patients may experience weakness, dizziness, and faintness.
- Other autonomic side-effects include hypertension, dryness of the mouth, blurred vision, constipation, difficulty in urination, impotence, and sweating.
- Effects on the CNS include euphoria, hyperactivity and hyperreflexia, confusion, hallucinations, delirium, tremors, and convulsions.
- Patients also may experience skin rashes, photosensitivity, edema, and weight gain.
- Do not give these drugs to patients with severely impaired liver or kidney function, congestive heart failure, or pheochromocytoma.

Dosage and Administration

- *Isocarboxazid (Marplan):* The initial dosage is 30 mg, PO, daily, in single or divided doses. The maintenance dosage is 10 mg to 20 mg daily.
- *Phenelzine sulfate (Nardil):* The initial dosage is 15 mg given three times a day. The dosage is titrated gradually until the maximum benefit is achieved. The patient may be maintained on 15 mg daily or every other day.
- *Tranylcypromine sulfate (Parnate):* The initial dosage is 10 mg, bid. (The maximum dosage is 30 mg, qd.) Following improvement, the dosage is reduced to the lowest effective maintenance level.

Nursing Considerations

- The numerous potential drug interactions are a major deterrant to the use of MAO inhibitors. They are not recommended for use in children or the elderly.
- MAO inhibitors potentiate the activity of sympathomimetic substances and can produce a hypertensive crisis.
    1. Drugs in this category are amphetamines, methyldopa, levodopa, dopamine, tryptophan, epinephrine, and norepinephrine. OTC preparations to treat colds and hay fever and reducing preparations also contain sympathomimetics.
    2. Foods high in tyramine include cheese, beer, chianti wine, pickled herring, chicken livers, yeast extract, sour cream, raisins, bananas, avocados, chocolate, and soy souce.
- Excessive caffeine intake also can precipitate a hypertensive crisis.
- The use of MAO inhibitors with CNS depressants and general anesthesia can lead to circulatory collapse and death. MAO inhibitors should be discontinued at least 10 days before elective surgery.

- The use of MAO inhibitors with other psychotropics decreases the margin of safety.
- MAO inhibitors should not be given concurrently (*e.g.*, pargyline hydrochloride—Eutonyl; phenelzine sulfate—Nardil; and tranylcypromine—Parnate), or with the dibenzazepines (*e.g.*, desipramine hydrochloride—Norpramin; and imipramine hydrochloride—Tofranil). The combination can result in hypertensive crisis, fever, convulsions, coma, and circulatory collapse. A 14-day interval should occur between discontinuing one of these days and starting therapy with another.
- The hypertensive crisis seen with MAO inhibitors is frequently treated with 5 mg of phentolamine, administered intravenously at a slow rate.
- Patients receiving MAO inhibitors should have their liver function monitored.
- The risk of suicide may increase as the patient's depression is relieved.

Tricyclic Antidepressants

Actions

- These drugs potentiate the action of norepinephrine by blocking neuronal re-uptake.
- They increase the release of norepinephrine by blocking alpha-adrenergic receptor sites that control norepinephrine release.

Indications

- They are used to relieve symptoms of depression and anxiety.
- Tricyclic antidepressants also are used to treat enuresis and neurogenic bladder.

Adverse Effects and Contraindications

- Autonomic side-effects include dry mouth, blurred vision, constipation, difficulty in urinating, postural hypotension, localized sweating, impotence, nausea, and vomiting.
- Early CNS effects are drowsiness and fatigue. Patients also may experience restlessness, agitation, mania, confusion, hallucinations, tremors, and convulsions.
- Numbness, tingling of the extremities, and ringing in the ears can occur.
- Hypersensitive patients may develop skin rashes, photosensitivity, jaundice, and agranulocytosis.
- Cardiovascular problems include hypertension, tachycardia, myocardial infarction, arrhythmias, precipitation of congestive heart failure, and stroke.
- Weight gain is possible.

- Patients with glaucoma or an enlarged prostate should not receive tricyclics.
- Use cautiously for patients with a history of liver, kidney, or cardiovascular disease.

Dosage and Administration

- *Amitriptyline hydrochloride (Elavil):* Oral dosages range from 25 mg to 300 mg per day, but most patients respond to 75 mg per day (25 mg, tid).
- For maintenance therapy, 40 mg to 100 mg per day may be sufficient, and is taken in a single dose, preferably at bedtime.
- *Doxepin hydrochloride (Sinequan):* Oral dosages range from 25 mg to 300 mg daily, depending on the severity of the depression or anxiety.
- *Imipramine hydrochloride (Tofranil):* The usual adult oral dosage is 150 mg per day, but it may range from 25 mg to 300 mg.
- Imipramine also is used to treat childhood enuresis in children 6 year old and older. Initially, 25 mg is given PO 1 hour before bedtime. The dosage may be increased, but it should not exceed 2.5 mg/kg/day.

Nursing Considerations

- Tricyclic antidepressants should not be given with MAO inhibitors. The combination can result in hypertensive crisis, fever, convulsions, coma, and circulatory collapse. A 14-day interval should occur between discontinuing one of these drugs and beginning therapy with another.
- Patients should be cautioned against driving and operating machinery, because these drugs cause drowsiness and impair alertness.
- Tricyclics can enhance the CNS-depressant effects of alcohol.
- The risk of suicide may increase as the patient's depression begins to resolve.

Lithium Carbonate (Lithane, Lithonate)

Actions

- Lithium carbonate alters sodium transport in muscle and nerve cells, and affects the metabolism of catecholamines.
- The specific mechanism for treating mania is unknown.

Indications

- It is used to treat manic episodes of manic-depressive illness.
- It prevents or reduces the intensity of further episodes.

Adverse Effects and Contraindications

- Use *cautiously* in patients with cardiovascular or kidney disease, low serum sodium levels, and dehydration, and in those receiving diuretics. In these instances, the risk of lithium toxicity is very high.
- Initial therapy may produce mild nausea, thirst, and fine hand tremors. These side-effects usually subside, but occasionally they continue throughout therapy.
- Early signs of lithium toxicity include diarrhea, vomiting, drowsiness, muscular weakness, and lack of coordination. These can occur at serum lithium levels below 2 mEq per liter.
- Ataxia, giddiness, tinnitus, blurred vision, and a large amount of dilute urine occur at higher levels.
- Severe toxicity produces the following:
  1. Tremor, twitching, hyperreflexia, and clonic spasms
  2. Restlessness, confusion, convulsive seizures, stupor, and coma
  3. Cardiac arrhythmias, hypotension, and circulatory collapse.

Dosage and Administration

- Acute episodes of mania usually are treated with 600 mg, PO, tid. Serum lithium levels range from 1 to 1.5 mEq per liter.
- Maintenance dosages usually are 300 mg, PO tid or qid. Serum levels should range between 0.6 and 1.2 mEq per liter.

Nursing Considerations

- Lithium toxicity can occur at doses close to therapeutic levels. Serum lithium levels must be monitored closely. Emphasize the importance of follow-up appointments to the patient.
- The blood should be drawn 8 hours to 12 hours after the previous dose.
- The patient's ability to tolerate lithium appears to be greater during acute episodes and to decline during long-term therapy.
- It is very important for the patient to maintain a normal diet, including salt, and to drink adequate fluids (at least 2500 to 3000 ml during initial therapy).
- It may be necessary to temporarily reduce the lithium dosage if the patient develops infection with elevated temperature, diarrhea, or sweating.
- A few patients treated with lithium plus haloperidol have developed an encephalopathic syndrome followed by irreversible brain damage. Observe patients for neurologic toxicity.
- Encourage patients to notify their physicians immediately if they experience symptoms of toxicity (see adverse effects). The drug should be discontinued, and serum levels should be checked.

- Elderly patients may develop toxicity at serum levels tolerated by younger patients. Careful monitoring and lower dosages are indicated.

ANTIANXIETY AGENTS (BENZODIAZEPINES)

CHLORDIAZEPOXIDE HYDROCHLORIDE (LIBRIUM)

Actions

- This drug depresses subcortical levels of the CNS; higher doses depress the cortex.
- It produces calming, mild sedative, mild anticonvulsant, and skeletal muscle relaxant effects.

Indications

- It relieves anxiety and tension in various disease states.
- It also is used to treat withdrawal symptoms of acute alcoholism.
- Preoperative apprehension and anxiety can be managed with this drug.

Adverse Effects and Contraindications

- Drowsiness, ataxia, and confusion occur, especially in the elderly.
- Rarely, patients have experienced skin eruptions, edema, nausea, and constipation.
- Orthostatic hypotension and tachycardia are possible.
- Blood dyscrasias such as agranulocytosis occur occasionally.
- Physical and psychological dependence is possible.
- Use cautiously for patients with impaired liver and kidney function.
- Paradoxical reactions (*e.g.,* excitation) have been reported, as well as hallucinations, depression, and delirium.

Dosage and Administration

- The usual adult dosage for mild to moderate anxiety is 5 mg to 10 mg, PO, three or four times daily.
- Severe anxiety is treated with 20 mg to 25 mg, PO, three or four times daily.
- Alcoholic patients receive 50 mg to 100 mg in repeated doses, IM or IV. The maximum dosage is 300 mg per 24 hours.
- Elderly or debilitated patients receive 10 mg or less, PO, per day. Dosage is increased gradually as tolerance develops.

- The usual pediatric, (over 6 yr) dosage is 5 mg, PO, two to four times daily. It may be increased to 10 mg, two to three times daily.

Nursing Considerations

- Blood counts and liver and kidney function should be monitored in patients receiving long-term therapy.
- Patients should be cautioned against driving or operating machinery because of the drowsiness that can occur.
- Chlordiazepoxide may potentiate the actions of other CNS depressants, such as barbiturates, narcotic analgesics, and alcohol.
- Patients with suicidal tendencies may require protective measures.
- Elderly patients are especially vulnerable to renal dysfunction from cumulative effects.

CLORAZEPATE DIPOTASSIUM (TRANXENE)

Actions

- Clorazepate dipotassium depresses subcortical levels of the CNS; higher doses depress the cortex.
- It produces calming, mild sedation, mild anticonvulsant, and skeletal muscle relaxant effects.

Indications

- It is used to treat anxiety disorders and anxiety associated with chronic disease.
- It provides symptomatic relief in acute alcohol withdrawal.
- As adjunctive therapy, it helps to manage partial seizures.

Adverse Effects and Contraindications

- Drowsiness, ataxia, blurred vision, and mental confusion occur, especially in elderly patients.
- Hypotension, insomnia, and headache are possible.
- Use cautiously in patients with impaired liver and kidney function.
- It is not recommended for children or patients with acute narrow-angle glaucoma.
- Physical and psychological dependence are possible.

Dosage and Administration

- The usual adult dosage for relief of anxiety is 30 mg, PO, daily, but it may range from 15 mg to 60 mg.

- Elderly patients should begin therapy with a reduced dose: 7.5 mg to 15 mg, PO, daily.
- For symptomatic relief of acute alcohol withdrawal, the maximum total daily dosage is 90 mg.
- Initial therapy in seizure control for children 9 years to 12 years is 7.5 mg, PO, bid.
- Initial therapy in seizure control for patients over 12 years is 7.5 mg, PO, tid.

Nursing Considerations

- Blood counts and liver and kidney function should be monitored in patients receiving long-term therapy.
- Patients should be cautioned against driving or operating machinery because of the drowsiness that can occur.
- Clorazepate may potentiate the actions of other CNS depressants, such as barbiturates, narcotic analgesics, and alcohol.
- Patients with suicidal tendencies may require protective measures.

DIAZEPAM (VALIUM)

Actions

- Diazepam possesses antianxiety, anticonvulsant, and skeletal muscle relaxant properties.

Indications

- It is used to relieve anxiety and tension in transient situational disturbances, functional or organic disorders, and psychoneurotic states.
- In acute alcohol withdrawal, diazepam relieves acute agitation, tremors, and delirium tremens.
- Large parenteral doses reduce muscle spasticity in cerebal palsy and athetosis, and control recurring convulsions in status epilepticus, tetanus, and other seizure states.
- It produces sedation preoperatively and prior to cardioversion, gastroscopy, and esophagoscopy.
- It relieves skeletal muscle spasticity and spasm.

Adverse Effects and Contraindications

- Frequent side-effects include drowsiness, fatigue, and ataxia.
- Hypotension, tachycardia, urinary retention, constipation, and tardive dyskinesia are possible.

- Physical and psychological dependence are possible.
- Use cautiously in patients with impaired liver and kidney function.
- Paradoxical reactions (*e.g.*, excitation, hallucinations, and rage) sometimes occur, and necessitate discontinuing the drug.
- Do not give to patients with acute narrow-angle glaucoma.

Dosage and Administration

- The usual adult dosage for anxiety and muscle spasm is 2 mg to 10 mg, PO, two to four times daily.
- Alcoholic withdrawal may require 10 mg, PO, three or four times daily.
- Elderly or debilitated patients usually receive 2 mg, PO, one or two times daily.
- The usual pediatric (over 6 months of age) dosage is 1 to 2.5 mg, three to four times daily
- For control of convulsions and acute agitation in adults, repeated doses of 5 mg to 10 mg are given IM or IV every 3 to 4 hours.
- Do not mix or dilute diazepam with other solutions or drugs.
- For IV administration, take at least 1 minute for each 5 mg (1 ml) given. The maximum single dose is 30 mg. In children, take at least 3 minutes, and do not exceed 0.25 mg/kg.
- If direct IV injection is not possible, give slowly through infusion tubing as close as possible to the vein insertion.

Nursing Considerations

- Caution patients against driving or operating machinery because of the drowsiness that can occur.
- Diazepam may potentiate the actions of other CNS depressants, such as barbiturates, narcotic analgesics, and *alcohol*.
- Blood counts and liver function should be monitored in patients receiving long-term therapy.
- Patients with suicidal tendencies may require protective measures.
- Patients on prolonged therapy should be weaned from the drug to avoid withdrawal symptoms.

LORAZEPAM (ATIVAN)

Actions

- Lorazepam depresses subcortical levels of the CNS; higher doses depress the cortex.
- It produces calming, mild sedative, mild anticonvulsant, and skeletal muscle relaxant effects.

Indications

- The oral form is used to relieve anxiety and tension.
- The intravenous or intramuscular form is used as a preanesthetic, to produce sedation, relief of anxiety, and decreased ability to recall events related to the surgery.

Adverse Effects and Contraindications

- The most frequent adverse effect is sedation, followed by dizziness, weakness, and unsteadiness.
- Restlessness, confusion, hallucinations, hypertension, or hypotension also may occur.
- Use cautiously in elderly and debilitated patients and in patients with renal, hepatic, or gastrointestinal disorders.
- Physical and psychological dependence is possible.
- Children under 12 and patients with acute narrow-angle glaucoma should not receive lorazepam.

Dosage and Administration

- The usual adult dosage range is 2 to 6 mg/day in divided doses, with the largest dose at bedtime.
- Elderly patients should begin therapy with 1 to 2 mg/day in divided doses.
- For premedication, give 0.05 mg/kg, IM, at least 2 hours before surgery (maximum dose, 4 mg).
- The IV form is given by direct injection into the vein or IV tubing; the rate should not exceed 2 mg/minute.

Nursing Considerations

- Caution patients against driving or operating machinery because of the drowsiness that can occur.
- Lorazepam may potentiate the action of other CNS depressants, such as barbiturates, narcotic analgesics, and *alcohol.*
- Blood counts and liver function should be monitored in patients receiving long-term therapy.
- Patients with suicidal tendencies may require protective measures.
- Intra-arterial injection may produce spasm of the artery resulting in gangrene. Amputation may be required.
- Elderly patients on lorazepam are particularly susceptible to upper gastrointestinal disease.
- Patients on prolonged therapy should be weaned from the drug to avoid withdrawal symptoms.

OXAZEPAM (SERAX)

Actions

- Oxazepam depresses subcortical levels of the CNS; higher doses depress the cortex.
- It produces calming and mild sedation.

Indications

- Oxazepam relieves anxiety and tension associated with a wide range of emotional disturbances.
- It controls acute withdrawal symptoms in chronic alcoholism.

Adverse Effects and Contraindications

- Drowsiness, dizziness, confusion, and headache are usually infrequent and mild.
- Paradoxic reactions, nausea, hypotension, and skin rash also have occurred infrequently.
- Children under 6 years of age and patients with acute narrow-angle glaucoma should not receive oxazepam.
- Use cautiously in the elderly and debilitated, and in patients with chronic obstructive pulmonary disease, or impaired kidney and liver function.
- Physical and psychological dependence are possible.

Dosage and Administration

- For anxiety, administer 10 mg to 30 mg, three or four times daily.
- For alcohol withdrawal, give 15 mg to 30 mg, three to four times daily.
- For elderly patients, start with 10 mg, three times daily.

Nursing Considerations

- Oxazepam has a shorter duration of action than other benzodiazepines.
- Caution patients against driving or operating machinery because of the drowsiness that can occur.
- Oxazepam may potentiate the action of other CNS depressants, such as barbiturates, narcotic analgesics, and *alcohol.*
- Blood counts and liver function should be monitored in patients receiving long-term therapy.
- Patients with suicidal tendencies may require protective measures.

- Patients on prolonged therapy should be weaned from the drug to avoid withdrawal symptoms.

ANTICHOLINESTERASE AGENTS

Actions

- These drugs inhibit the action of acetylcholinesterase at the junctions of cholinergic nerve endings. Acetylcholine accumulates at cholinergic receptor sites.
- They also produce miosis, increased tone of intestinal and skeletal muscles, constriction of bronchi and ureters, slower pulse rate, and stimulation of salivary and sweat glands.
- They stimulate voluntary muscle fibers.

Indications

- These drugs are used to prevent and treat postoperative abdominal distention and urinary retention.
- They provide symptomatic control and differential diagnosis in myasthenia gravis.
- See PH, Ophthalmic preparations.

Adverse Effects and Contraindications

- Cholinergic crisis occurs with overdose, and can include any or all of the following effects.
- Salivation and fasciculations (small, local, involuntary muscular contractions visible under the skin) are common.
- Abdominal cramps, diarrhea, involuntary or difficult defecation, or micturition also occur.
- Hypotension, bradycardia, respiratory depression, dyspnea, and diaphoresis are possible.
- Lacrimation, miosis, and blurred vision may occur.

Dosage and Administration

- *Ambenonium chloride (Mytelase)*
  1. Adults: Usually, 5 to 25 mg, PO, three or four times daily is adequate, but as much as 50 mg to 75 mg per dose may be required.
  2. Pediatric: Initially, give 0.3 mg/kg/24 hr in divided doses. Up to 1.5 mg/kg/24 hr divided into three or four doses may be required.
  3. It is approximately six times more potent than neostigmine bromide, and is used in patients with bromide sensitivity.

- *Edrophonium chloride (Tensilon)*
  1. This drug has a short duration of action and is used in differential diagnosis of myasthenia gravis.
  2. Adults: Prepare 10 mg in a tuberculin syringe. Inject 2 mg within 15 seconds to 30 seconds; if no reaction occurs after 45 seconds, inject the remaining 8 mg. The test may be repeated after 30 minutes.
  3. Pediatric: For children up to 75 lb, give 1 mg, IV. If no response is seen after 45 seconds, the dose may be titrated up to 5 mg. For children over 75 lb, give 2 mg IV. If no response is seen after 45 seconds, the dose may be titrated up to 10 mg. For infants, the recommended dose is 0.5 mg.
- *Neostigmine bromide (Prostigmin)*
  1. Initially, administer 15 to 30 mg, PO, three or four times daily. The maintenance dosage range is 15 to 375 mg, PO, daily, depending on the patient's needs and tolerance.
  2. Neostigmine methylsulfate is the injectable form. To treat abdominal distention or urinary retention, give 0.5 to 1 mg, SC or IM.
- *Pyridostigmine bromide (Mestinon)*
  1. Adults: Administer 60 mg to 1.5 g, PO, daily, spaced according to requirements and response. For the timespan tablets, give one to three 180-mg tablets once or twice daily, at least 6 hours apart.
  2. Pediatric: Administer 7 mg/kg/24 hr, PO, divided in five or six doses.

Nursing Considerations

- Atropine is used as an antidote for drug-induced bradycardia. Check pulse rates before giving the drug to bradycardic patients.
- GI side-effects usually occur early in therapy, and can be reduced by taking the drug with milk or food.
- Regulation of the dosage interval is very difficult. The patient or patient's family should be encouraged to keep accurate records of drug response to assist in dosage regulation.
- Respiratory depression may appear abruptly. Monitor carefully for apprehension, restlessness, increased respirations, tachycardia, and elevated blood pressure.
- Therapy is life-long, and patients and their families need a great deal of support.

ANTICONVULSANTS

Nursing Considerations

- Status epilepticus can result if anticonvulsant therapy is discontinued abruptly. Gradual weaning is necessary.

- Combinations of two or more drugs may be necessary to provide adequate control of seizures.
- Most drugs are started at low doses and are increased gradually until seizures are controlled or side-effects develop.
- The patient's understanding of his illness and the drug therapy is extremely important because failure to take the drugs is the most frequent cause of treatment failure.

CARBAMAZEPINE (TEGRETOL)

Actions

- Carbamazepine reduces the number and severity of seizures.
- It reduces synaptic transmission within the trigeminal nucleus.
- It also has sedative, antidepressant, anticholinergic, and muscle relaxant actions.

Indications

- It is used to treat grand mal, psychomotor epilepsy, and mixed seizures.
- It relieves symptoms of trigeminal neuralgia (tic douloureux).

Adverse Effects and Contraindications

- It should not be used if the patient is sensitive to tricyclic compounds, if hematologic reactions to other drugs have occurred, or if the patient is receiving MAO inhibitors.
- Use cautiously for patients with cardiac, hepatic, renal, or collagen disease.
- The most serious adverse reactions involve the hemopoietic system (aplastic anemia, agranulocytosis, thrombocytopenia, and leukopenia), the integumentary system (Stevens-Johnson syndrome, erythema multiforme, and aggravation of disseminated lupus erythematosus), and the cardiovascular system (congestive heart failure, hypertension, arrhythmias, and thrombophlebitis).
- The most frequent adverse reactions (especially in the beginning of therapy) are dizziness, drowsiness, unsteadiness, nausea, and vomiting.
- Jaundice, urinary retention, impotence, and eye (lens) opacities also have occurred.

Dosage and Administration

- *Adults and pediatric (over 12 yr) with epilepsy:* Initially, give 200 mg, PO, bid. The usual maintenance dosage is 800 to 1200 mg daily in divided doses.

- *Pediatric (6 to 12 yr) with epilepsy:* Administer 100 mg, PO, bid, and gradually increase to tid or qid. The maintenance dosage is 400 to 800 mg daily (maximum: 1000 mg).
- *Adults with trigeminal neuralgia:* Initially, give 100 mg, bid. The usual maintenance dosage is 200 to 800 mg, qd.

Nursing Considerations

- Baseline data obtained before starting therapy are extremely important and should include complete blood count, liver function, BUN, urinalysis, ECG, and an eye examination.
- Blood studies should be performed weekly during the first month, and monthly for at least 2 or 3 years.
- Instruct patients to watch for signs of hematologic problems: fever, sore throat, malaise, tendency to bruise or bleed, and unusual fatigue.
- Elderly patients may have difficulty tolerating this drug, and may show evidence of confusion and agitation.
- See PH, Anticonvulsants, nursing considerations.

CLONAZEPAM (CLONOPIN)

Actions

- This is similar to other benzodiazepines and has strong anticonvulsant activity.

Indications

- Clonazepam is used to treat Lennox-Gastaut syndrome (petit mal variant), and akinetic and myoclonic seizures.
- It reduces absence seizures (petit mal) in patients who do not respond to the succinimides, *e.g.,* Zarontin.

Adverse Effects and Contraindications

- Use cautiously in patients with renal disease, chronic obstructive pulmonary disease, and several coexisting seizure disorders.
- Patients with hepatic disease or acute narrow-angle glaucoma should not receive this drug.
- Both physical and psychological dependence may occur, especially with high-dose or long-term therapy.
- The most frequent adverse effect is CNS depression. Drowsiness, ataxia, and behavior problems are common.
- Depression, hallucinations, headache, aphasia, and coma have been reported.

- Increased appetite and salivation, nausea, constipation, and diarrhea have occurred.
- Respiratory congestion and depression, and heart palpitations may occur.

Dosage and Administration

- *Adults:* Give 1.5 mg/day divided in three doses. Side-effects may be dose limiting. The maximum dosage is 20 mg/day.
- *Pediatric (up to 10 yr):* Administer 0.01 to 0.03 mg/kg/day. The maximum dosage is 0.05 mg/kg/day in three divided doses. Maintenance dosage is 0.1 to 0.2 mg/kg/day in three doses.

Nursing Considerations

- After 3 months, anticonvulsant activity frequently declines and dosage adjustment is necessary.
- Patients should avoid alcohol and other CNS depressants, as well as OTC medications.
- See PH, Anticonvulsants, nursing considerations.

DIAZEPAM (VALIUM)

- See PH, Antianxiety agents.

ETHOSUXIMIDE (ZARONTIN)

Actions

- Ethosuximide reduces the frequency of attacks by depressing motor cortex and by elevating the CNS threshold to stimuli.

Indications

- It is used to manage absence (petit mal) epilepsy.

Adverse Effects and Contraindications

- Patients frequently experience gastrointestinal symptoms including anorexia, nausea, vomiting, weight loss, and diarrhea.
- Leukopenia, aplastic anemia, and agranulocytosis have occurred.
- Drowsiness, dizziness, headache, and ataxia have been reported.
- Disturbances of sleep, night terrors, and aggressiveness are more common in patients with previous psychological abnormalities.
- Also reported are urticaria, Stevens-Johnson syndrome, and systemic lupus erythematosus.

Dosage and Administration

- *Adults and pediatric (over 6 yr):* The usual dosage is 250 mg, PO, bid. The maximum dosage is 1.5 g/day.
- *Pediatric (3–6 yr):* The usual pediatric dosage is 250 mg/day. The maximum dosage is 1 g/day.

Nursing Considerations

- Baseline blood, liver, and renal studies should be done before starting therapy, and repeated periodically during therapy.
- Ethosuximide may impair mental and physical abilities.
- See PH, Anticonvulsants, nursing considerations.

PHENOBARBITAL (LUMINAL)

- See PH, Barbiturates.

PHENYTOIN (DILANTIN)

Actions

- Phenytoin reduces the number and severity of epileptic attacks.

Indications

- The oral form is used to treat grand mal and other major motor seizures and psychomotor epilepsy.
- Parenterally, phenytoin may be used to treat status epilepticus and to control rapid cardiac arrhythmias, and it may be used prior to neurosurgical procedures to prevent seizures during surgery.

Adverse Effects and Contraindications

- Nausea, vomiting, and constipation occur.
- Gingival hyperplasia (overgrowth of gum tissue) is common.
- Hirsutism, skin rashes, and megaloblastic anemia may occur.
- Excessive doses cause lethargy, slurred speech, and staggering gait. Also, double vision, dizziness, and headache occur.
- Overdose results in coma, apnea, and death.
- Cardiac arrest can occur from rapid intravenous administration.
- Phenytoin may be withdrawn gradually before or during a pregnancy for patients with mild, infrequent seizures. However, the danger of hypoxia to the fetus following a major seizure may be an indication for continuing the drug.
- Use cautiously in patients with bradycardia, heart block, impaired hepatic or renal function, hypotension, heart failure, diabetes, and the elderly.

Dosage and Administration

- The usual initial PO dosage is 100 mg, tid, but it may be increased to 600 mg per day.
- Intravenous phenytoin is injected slowly (maximum 50 mg/min) in doses of 150 mg to 250 mg. It should be given IV push because it is not soluble when mixed.
- It also may be given IM (100 mg to 200 mg), but it can cause tissue necrosis and sterile abscesses.
- The usual pediatric dosage is 4 to 8 mg/kg/day, PO, divided into two or three doses. As an intravenous anticonvulsant, give 5 mg/kg as a single dose or divided into two doses.

Nursing Considerations

- Patients metabolize phenytoin at different rates, so blood levels should be drawn to monitor the drug for effectiveness and toxicity.
- Giving phenytoin during or after meals will minimize the gastric distress.
- Patients receiving this drug for long periods may need folic acid to prevent anemia.
- The following drug interactions occur with phenytoin:
    1. The action of phenytoin is potentiated by aspirin, sulfonamides, and anticoagulants.
    2. The action of phenytoin is inhibited by alcohol, antihistamines, barbiturates, and sedatives.
    3. Phenytoin decreases the action of quinidine.
    4. Phenytoin inhibits the action of steroids and digitalis.
- The patient's urine may turn pink or red to red-brown.
- Avoid mixing any other drugs with parenteral phenytoin sodium. Precipitates can occur.
- Elderly or debilitated patients may require lower than usual doses.
- Advise the patient to inform his or her dentist that he or she is receiving phenytoin. Treatment for gingival hyperplasia may be needed.
- Hepatic, renal, and blood tests should be done prior to therapy, and repeated monthly.
- See PH, Anticonvulsants, nursing considerations.

PRIMIDONE (MYSOLINE)

Actions

- Primidone is related to phenobarbital and reduces the frequency and severity of seizures.

- It increases the metabolism of vitamin D, and may impair calcium, folic acid, and vitamin B_{12} metabolism and utilization.

Indications

- It is used to control cortical, focal, psychomotor, and grand mal seizures.

Adverse Effects and Contraindications

- Use cautiously in patients sensitive to barbiturates, with COPD, hepatic or renal disease, and porphyria.
- Ataxia and vertigo are experienced most frequently.
- Nausea, anorexia, vomiting, fatigue, emotional disturbances, diplopia, and impotence also have been reported.

Dosage and Administration

- *Adults and pediatric (over 8 yr):* Initially, give 100–125 mg/day and gradually increase over 10 days to 250 mg, tid. The maximum dosage is 2 g daily, divided into two to four doses.
- *Pediatric (under 8 yr):* Initially, give 50 mg/day and gradually increase over 10 days to 125 to 250 mg, tid. The maximum dosage is 1 g daily, divided into two to four doses.

Nursing Considerations

- Drowsiness and dizziness frequently disappear as therapy continues.
- Observe for signs and symptoms of folic acid deficiency.
- Patients should avoid alcohol, other CNS depressants, and OTC medications during therapy.
- Blood levels of primidone and phenobarbital should be monitored during therapy.
- See PH, Anticonvulsants, nursing considerations.

TRIMETHADIONE (TRIDIONE)

Actions

- Trimethadione reduces the frequency and severity of seizures.

Indications

- It is used to control petit mal seizures refractory to other drugs.

Adverse Effects and Contraindications

- Use cautiously in patients with severe hepatic or renal disease, blood dyscrasias, and diseases of the retina and optic nerve.

- Nausea, vomiting, and abdominal pain have been reported.
- Drowsiness, fatigue, vertigo, headache, grand mal seizures, and personality changes may occur.
- Blood dyscrasias and severe forms of erythema multiforme are possible.
- Fatal nephrosis, lupus, hepatitis, and a myasthenia gravis-like syndrome are rare but serious adverse effects.

Dosage and Administration

- *Adults:* 300 to 600 mg, three or four times daily
- *Pediatric:* 300 to 900 mg in three or four equally divided doses

Nursing Considerations

- Complete blood count, differential, and urinalysis are recommended at monthly intervals.
- Seizures may increase temporarily at the beginning of therapy. A record of the number, duration, and time should be kept.
- Trimethadione has great potential for toxicity.
- See PH, Anticonvulsants, nursing considerations.

VALPROIC ACID (DEPAKENE)

Actions

- This drug reduces the number and severity of seizures.

Indications

- It can be used to manage simple (petit mal) and complex absence seizures.
- It may relieve tardive dyskinesia in patients on long-term antipsychotic drug therapy.

Adverse Effects and Contraindications

- Use cautiously in patients with bleeding disorders, hepatic or renal disease, angina pectoris, or recent myocardial infarction.
- Valproic acid usually is used with other anticonvulsants, and the following adverse effects may be the results of combined drug therapy:
  1. Patients frequently experience nausea, vomiting, and indigestion. Diarrhea, constipation, and both weight gain and loss have been reported.
  2. Sedation is frequent, but ataxia, headaches, and diplopia are rare.

3. Depression, aggression, and hyperactivity have occurred.
4. Thrombocytopenia, pancreatitis, and hyperglycemia are possible.

Dosage and Administration

- Initially, give 15 mg/kg/day, PO. The maximum dosage is 60 mg/kg/day.
- Total daily dosage should be divided if it exceeds 250 mg.
- The syrup contains 250 mg per 5 ml.

Nursing Considerations

- To avoid gastric irritation, the drug should be taken with meals.
- Valproic acid may cause a false-positive result when testing for urine ketones.
- OTC medications should be avoided, especially those containing aspirin, allergy medications, and sedatives.
- Platelet counts, bleeding times, and liver function should be monitored periodically during treatment.
- Light-colored stools, diarrhea, jaundice, vomiting, and rash may be signs of impending liver failure, and should be reported to the physician immediately.
- See PH, Anticonvulsants, nursing considerations.

ANTIPARKINSONISM AGENTS

AMANTADINE HYDROCHLORIDE (SYMMETREL)

Actions

- This drug may assist in the release of dopamine from neuronal storage sites.
- As a virostatic agent, it inhibits the penetration of the virus into the host cell.

Indications

- It is used to treat idiopathic and postencephalitic parkinsonism.
- It relieves drug-induced extrapyramidal reactions.
- Elderly persons who develop parkinsonism in association with cerebral arteriosclerosis can be treated with this drug.
- It can be given to prevent and treat respiratory tract infections caused by influenza A virus strains.

Adverse Effects and Contraindications

- Use cautiously in patients with a history of seizure disorders, psychoses, congestive heart failure, renal or hepatic impairment, or cerebral arteriosclerosis.
- Depression, congestive heart failure, orthostatic hypotension, urinary retention, and psychosis are the most frequent serious adverse effects.
- Hallucinations, confusion, anxiety, and ataxia also have been reported.
- Anorexia, nausea, and constipation may occur.

Dosage and Administration

- *Adults with Parkinson's disease:* When used alone, give 100 mg, PO, bid. When used with other antiparkinsonism drugs, therapy is initiated with 100 mg, qd.
- Adults with Parkinson's disease or drug-induced extrapyramidal reactions may receive up to 300 mg, PO, qd, in divided doses.
- Prophylaxis and treatment of influenza A
  1. *Adults:* The usual dosage is 200 mg, PO, qd
  2. *Pediatric (1–9 yr):* The usual dosage is 2 to 4 mg/lb/day (4.4 to 8.8 mg/kg/day), and should not exceed 150 mg/day.
  3. *Pediatric (9–12 yr):* Administer 100 mg, PO, bid.

Nursing Considerations

- To be effective in treating influenza, amantadine must be started within 48 hours of the onset of symptoms.
- To avoid insomnia, divided doses frequently are given after breakfast and lunch.
- CNS and psychic disturbances tend to decline when the drug is given in divided doses.
- The drug may reduce akinesia and rigidity, but it seldom effects tremors.

CARBIDOPA-LEVODOPA (SINEMET)

Actions

- The carbidopa inhibits conversion of levodopa to dopamine outside the CNS.
- Therefore, more levodopa reaches the CNS, where it is converted to dopamine and can be used to relieve dopamine deficiencies.

Indications

- See PH, Levodopa, indications.

Adverse Effects, Contraindications

- See PH, Levodopa, adverse effects.
- Anorexia, nausea, and vomiting usually occur less with a combination drug than with levodopa alone because the dosage of levodopa can be decreased.
- The adverse mental and extrapyramidal symptoms may be increased with a combination drug, and may occur sooner and last longer. (For extrapyramidal symptoms, see PH, Psychotropics, phenothiazines, adverse effects.)

Dosage and Administration

- The initial and maximum dosages are usually about one-fourth of the dosage for levodopa alone (see PH, Levodopa, dosage).
- Tablets contain 10 mg of carbidopa and 100 mg of levodopa (10:100); 25 mg carbidopa and 250 mg levodopa (25:250); or 25 mg carbidopa and 100 mg levodopa (25:100). The maximum total daily dosage is eight 25:250 tablets.

Nursing Considerations

- See PH, Levodopa, nursing considerations.
- Remember that the involuntary movements and mental changes are more common than with levodopa alone, and the patient must be observed accordingly.

DIPHENHYDRAMINE HYDROCHLORIDE (BENADRYL)

- See PH, Hypnotics.

LEVODOPA (LARODOPA, DOPAR)

Actions

- Levodopa is converted to dopamine in the blood, peripheral tissues, and CNS.
- Only the levodopa that passes the blood-brain barrier intact can form dopamine in the CNS where it is needed.
- When dopamine deficiency in the CNS is relieved, many patients experience improvement in their parkinsonism symptoms.

Indications

- Levodopa is used to treat the symptoms of Parkinson's disease (see MSN, Neurologic system).

Adverse Effects and Contraindications

- Nausea is the most common side-effect and may be accompanied by anorexia and vomiting.
- Use cautiously in patients with a history of peptic ulcer because levodopa has caused hemorrhage and ulceration.
- Postural hypotension and cardiac arrhythmias occur. Use cautiously in patients with a history of heart disease.
- Involuntary movements of the mouth, face, and head occur. The drug may produce spasms of the trunk and limbs. The "on-off" syndrome (sudden slowing of movement and muscle weakness) occurs with long-term therapy.
- Mental changes occur and may take the form of either hyperactivity and euphoria or depression and drowsiness. Patients with a history of psychiatric problems are especially at risk.
- Levodopa is contraindicated for patients with narrow-angle glaucoma or a history of melanoma, or for those who are taking adrenergic bronchodilators (see PH, Respiratory system).

Dosage and Administration

- The initial dosage usually is 0.5 to 1 g, PO, qd, in divided doses, taken with food. Every 3 days to 7 days, the dosage may be increased by a maximum of 0.75 g; usually, not more than 8 g are taken daily.
- It may take 6 weeks to 8 weeks for the patient to achieve optimum benefits from the drug (*e.g.*, maximum improvements of symptoms with side-effects he or she can tolerate).

Nursing Considerations

- The anorexia, nausea, and vomiting usually disappear after a few months. However, they can be reduced by giving the levodopa with meals, milk, or antacids, and by gradually increasing the dosage.
- The effectiveness of levodopa will be increased by reducing the total amount of protein in the diet.
- The postural hypotension usually disappears. Advise the patient to rise slowly. Elastic stockings may help. Monitor blood pressure and apical and radial pulses. *Antihypertensive* medications may need to be reduced.
- Many of the extrapyramidal symptoms may be relieved by reducing the dosage of levodopa. (For extrapyramidal symptoms, see PH, Psychotropics, phenothiazines, adverse effects.) If the parkinsonism symptoms return, it may be possible to gradually increase the dosage without the return of these neurologic side-effects.

- Observe for depression, suicidal tendencies, hallucinations, and delusions.
- Urine, saliva, and perspiration may darken in color, but this is not harmful.
- Other drug interactions include the following:
  1. The use of pyridoxine (vitamin B_6) with levodopa may cause its conversion to dopamine to occur *before* the drug reaches the brain, thus rendering it ineffective. A multivitamin preparation without vitamin B_6 is available.
  2. Antipsychotic drugs such as the phenothiazines (see PH, Psychotropics) may antagonize the effects of levodopa. If it is necessary to administer both drugs, the patient must be observed for the return of parkinsonism symptoms.

TRIHEXYPHENIDYL HYDROCHLORIDE (ARTANE)

Actions

- This drug reduces skeletal muscle rigidity, and decreases tremor and akinesia.
- It reduces excess sweating and drooling, and produces mild euphoria.
- For other anticholinergic actions, see PH, Atropine sulfate.

Indications

- It relieves symptoms of Parkinson's disease.
- It also is used to treat the parkinsonism-type symptoms produced by some drugs (*e.g.*, the phenothiazines).

Adverse Effects and Contraindications

- About one-half of the patients using trihexyphenidyl experience minor side-effects.
- Frequent side-effects include dry mouth, nausea, vomiting, blurred vision, and constipation. These discomforts can be relieved by reducing the dosage.
- Tachycardia and hypotension also may occur.
- Overdose can produce mental confusion, excitement, disorientation, and psychosis.
- Use cautiously in patients with hypertrophy of the prostate, a tendency for gastrointestinal obstruction, cerebral arteriosclerosis, or cardiovascular disorders.
- It is contraindicated for patients with narrow-angle glaucoma.

Dosage and Administration

- A total daily dosage of 6 to 10 mg, PO, is common.
- Treatment is started initially with 1 mg and is increased by 2 mg every 3 to 5 days. The doses usually are divided and given near meals and at bedtime.

Nursing Considerations

- Dry mouth can be reduced by giving this drug with meals, chewing sugarless gum, sucking on hard candy, or taking frequent sips of water.

ANTIPSYCHOTIC AGENTS (MAJOR TRANQUILIZERS)

PHENOTHIAZINES

Actions

- Phenothiazines sedate and calm patients who are anxious or severely agitated (tranquilizing effect).
- They reduce psychotic patients' hallucinations and delusions, and assist in improving disturbed behavior (antipsychotic effect).
- They control nausea and vomiting (antiemetic effect).
- Both cholinergic and adrenergic effects of the autonomic nervous system are blocked by the phenothiazines.

Indications

- Phenothiazines are used to relieve symptoms of psychosis in schizophrenia, in the manic phase of the manic-depressive psychosis, and in confused, senile patients.
- They also are given to treat toxic psychoses caused by alcohol, amphetamines, and LSD.
- They effectively relieve alcohol withdrawal syndrome.
- The drugs can control postoperative vomiting and assist in preventing vomiting induced by antineoplastic drugs.
- They are used to produce preoperative sedation.

Adverse Effects and Contraindications

- Drowsiness is common, but it may disappear after the first few weeks. Lethargy, fatigue, and weakness also occur.
- Extrapyramidal motor system reactions include the following:
  1. Acute and persistent dyskinesias (*e.g.,* abnormal movements of the extremities and facial disturbances such as lateral jaw movements, sucking and smacking of the lips, and in-and-out tongue movement)

2. Pseudoparkinsonism (*e.g.*, tremor, rigidity, drooling, masklike facial expression, and restlessness)
3. Akinesia (*e.g.*, fatigue and weakness of arms and legs)
4. Akathisia (*e.g.*, motor restlessness)

- Postural hypotension occurs, and the hypotension may progress to a shocklike state. Heart palpitations and cardiac arrest are possible.
- Atropinelike side-effects include dry mouth, blurred vision, constipation, paralytic ileus, urinary retention, and decreased sweating.
- Nasal stuffiness and inhibition of ejaculation result from adrenergic blockage.
- Amenorrhea, false-positive pregnancy tests, gynecomastia, lactation, and a reduction in libido all have occurred.
- Patients may experience weight gain, edema, and increased appetite.
- Phenothiazines can produce hyperglycemia and glycosuria.
- Blood dyscrasias can include leukopenia, agranulocytosis, hemolytic anemia, thrombocytic purpura, and pancytopenia, but occurrences are rare.
- Skin rashes and eruptions, photosensitivity, and jaundice have occurred.
- Long-term therapy may result in skin pigmentation and ocular changes (deposits in the lens and cornea may form opacities).
- Use cautiously for patients with cardiovascular disease, liver disease, chronic obstructive pulmonary disease, blood dyscrasias, peptic ulcer, glaucoma, or epilepsy.
- Phenothiazines are not recommended for use during pregnancy.

Dosage, Administration, and Nursing Considerations

- See Table 7-40.
- Dosage of the phenothiazines is adjusted on an individual basis. The goal is to administer the smallest effective dose.
- These medications should be withdrawn gradually to avoid nausea, vomiting, dizziness, and tremulousness.
- The drugs in this family are closely related chemically. Cross-sensitivity within the family is likely.
- Blood counts and liver function should be monitored, especially for patients on long-term therapy.
- Patients receiving long-term therapy also should have periodic eye examinations to detect opacities and other drug-induced damage to the eyes.
- Observe patients for clinical signs of agranulocytosis, such as sore throat and infection. Patients most commonly develop the problem between the fourth and tenth weeks of therapy.

TABLE 7-40 PHENOTHIAZINES

Drug	Dosage and Administration	Nursing Considerations
Chlorpromazine hydrochloride (Thorazine)	Dosage ranges from 10 mg to 1 g daily; oral administration is most common. *Adults:* maximum, 1 g, PO, daily *Pediatric (5 to 12 yr):* maximum, 75 mg, PO, daily (usually 0.55 mg/kg four times daily) *Pediatric (under 5 yr):* maximum, 40 mg, PO, daily	When using the intramuscular (IM) route, inject slowly, deep into the upper outer quadrant of the buttocks. Patients should remain lying down for ½ hour after the injection because of the possible hypotensive effects. The IV route is reserved for surgery and severe hiccups. Chlorpromazine is the prototype of antipsychotic drugs. Oral concentrate (30 mg/ml and 100 mg/ml), syrup (10 mg/5 ml), and extended release tables are available.
Fluphenazine decanoate (Prolixin)	Dosage ranges from 12.5 to 25 mg, IM or SC, every 1 week to 3 weeks	Fluphenazine may be given either IM or SC. A dry syringe and needle of at least 21 gauge should be used. (The solution may become cloudy if wet needles or syringes are used.)

Fluphenazine (Prolixin)	Dosage ranges from 0.5 mg to 10 mg/day, PO, in divided doses.	Elixir (2.5 mg/ml) and oral solutions (5 mg/ml) are available. The oral concentrate should be diluted in fruit juice, water, milk, or carbonated beverages. It has a higher incidence of extrapyramidal complications and lower frequency of sedative and hypotensive effects.
Thioridazine hydrochloride (Mellaril)	Dosage ranges from 20 to 800 mg, PO, daily. *Adults:* Initially, 25 to 100 mg, PO, tid *Elderly:* Initially, 10 mg, PO, tid *Pediatric (over 2 yrs):* 0.5 to 3 mg/kg/day	It is indicated for severe behavioral problems of children who are combative and explosive. It can be used on a short-term basis to treat hyperactive children.
Trifluoperazine hydrochloride (Stelazine)	Dosage ranges from 2 to 20 mg daily *Adult:* Initially, 1 to 2 mg, PO, bid *Pediatric (6 to 12 yr):* 1 mg, PO, qd or bid Also given IM	It produces more prominent antiemetic and extrapyramidal effects than other phenothiazines.

- The dosages of barbiturates and narcotic analgesics should be cut by one-fourth to one-half when phenothiazines are added.
- Patients should not use alcohol when taking the phenothiazines because of the additive CNS depression.
- The use of atropine with the phenothiazines will potentiate the cholinergic blockade (see atropine sulfate).
- A single daily dose, taken at bedtime, is usually well-tolerated. Dizziness and faintness are less noticeable when the patient is lying down and the drowsiness is desirable.

HALOPERIDOL (HALDOL)

Actions

- Haloperidol antagonizes the neurotransmitter action of dopamine.

Indications

- It is used to treat psychotic disorders.
- The drug can control the tics and vocal utterances of Gilles de la Tourette's syndrome in children and adults.
- Haloperidol reduces behavior problems in children with combative, explosive hyperexcitability.

Adverse Effects and Contraindications

- Extrapyramidal reactions are frequent. They include Parkinson-like symptoms and akathisia. Persistent tardive dyskinesias also may occur. (For extrapyramidal symptoms, see PH, Psychotropics, phenothiazines, adverse effects.)
- Insomnia, restlessness, anxiety, drowsiness, depression, confusion, grand mal seizures, and exacerbation of psychotic symptoms have been reported.
- Tachycardia and hypotension may occur.
- Leukopenia and anemia are usually mild and transient.
- Jaundice and impaired liver function can occur.
- Breast engorgement and lactation, menstrual irregularities, impotence, and increased libido have resulted.
- Hyperglycemia and glycosuria have been produced.
- Gastrointestinal effects include anorexia, constipation, diarrhea, nausea, and vomiting.
- Autonomic reactions such as dry mouth, blurred vision, urinary retention, and diaphoresis occur.
- Laryngospasm and bronchospasm are possible.

- Patients with CNS depression or Parkinson's disease should not take haloperidol.
- Use cautiously for patients with cardiovascular disease or glaucoma, those using anticonvulsants or anticoagulants, and those who have allergies to other drugs.

Dosage and Administration

- The usual dosage range is 1 mg to 15 mg daily, PO or IM.
- Patients with moderate symptoms and elderly patients receive 0.5 to 2.0 mg, two or three times daily. The doses should be evenly spaced to maintain therapeutic blood levels.
- *Pediatric (3 to 12 yr):* The usual dosage is 0.05 to 0.15 mg/kg/day.

Nursing Considerations

- Haloperidol may potentiate the actions of other CNS depressants, such as barbiturates, narcotic analgesics, and alcohol.
- Patients should be cautioned against driving or operating machinery.
- A few patients treated with haloperidol plus lithium have developed an encephalopathic syndrome followed by irreversible brain damage. Observe patients for neurological toxicity.
- The following symptoms may improve with the use of haloperidol: hallucinations, insomnia, hostility, agitation, and delusions.

HYPNOTICS AND SEDATIVES

BARBITURATES

Actions

- Barbiturates depress all parts of the CNS. Small doses produce sedation and a reduction in nervousness and irritability. Larger doses produce hypnosis or sleep.
- Barbiturates also have anticonvulsant action, and in large doses produce anesthesia.
- When administered with an analgesic, barbiturates reduce the patient's emotional response to pain.
- Barbiturates also may reduce inhibitions and produce amnesia.

Indications

- They are used to relieve anxiety and restlessness; to relieve insomnia; as a preoperative medication; to control epileptic seizures and other convulsions; with analgesics, to relieve pain; as an induction anesthetic; and in psychiatry.

Adverse Effects and Contraindications

- The usual adult dosages can produce drowsiness, dizziness, and headache. Some patients (especially the elderly) experience excitation.
- Allergic skin reactions (rashes) and blood dyscrasias (*e.g.*, leukopenia, thrombocytopenia, and agranulocytosis) occur occasionally.
- *Chronic toxicity* (from excessive, long-term dosage) may occur with the following: dizziness, slurred speech, impaired thought and judgment, and disturbances of vision.
- *Acute toxicity* (massive overdose) may occur with the following: confusion, stupor, coma, shock, circulatory collapse, shallow respirations, and respiratory failure.
- Barbiturates are contraindicated for patients with acute intermittent porphyria and COPD.
- Dependence and tolerance do develop.
- Overdose produces respiratory depression and hypotension.

Dosage, Administration, and Nursing Considerations

- See Table 7-41.
- Patients should be cautioned against driving or operating machinery because these drugs reduce alertness.
- Other CNS depressants (*e.g.*, alcohol and analgesics) taken concurrently will potentiate the effects of these drugs. Life-threatening CNS depression can result.
- Barbiturates can alter a person's normal sleep patterns, and this in itself can cause side-effects. The alterations may persist 3 weeks to 5 weeks after the medication is discontinued.
- Barbiturates stimulate liver enzymes and will produce an increase in metabolism of other drugs. These drugs may require a *temporary* increase in dosage to maintain their effectiveness.
- Patients with reduced kidney and liver function and elderly patients may require lower dosages to reduce the chance of toxicity.
- Patients receiving oral anticoagulants should use barbiturates cautiously.

BENZODIAZEPINES

Chlordiazepoxide Hydrochloride (Librium)

- See PH, Antianxiety agents.

Diazepam (Valium)

- See PH, Antianxiety agents.

Flurazepam Hydrochloride (Dalmane)

Actions

- Flurazepam depresses the CNS and produces hypnosis.

Indications

- Flurazepam is used to relieve all types of insomnia.

Adverse Effects and Contraindications

- Drowsiness, dizziness, and motor incoordination (resulting in falls) occur frequently in elderly patients.
- Heartburn, nausea, vomiting, and diarrhea may occur.
- Alcohol and other CNS depressants potentiate the action of flurazepam and can result in serious respiratory depression.
- Physical and psychic dependence and tolerance do develop.
- Use cautiously in patients with impaired liver or kidney function, COPD, or a history of depression and psychoses.

Dosage and Administration

- The usual adult hypnotic dose is 30 mg, PO, at bedtime.
- Elderly or debilitated patients should be started on 15 mg.

Nursing Considerations

- Elderly patients and those with reduced liver and kidney function will have difficulty in metabolizing this drug. Observe carefully for signs that the drug is accumulating in the patient (*e.g.*, daytime drowsiness, sedation, and confusion).

Oxazepam (Serax)

- See PH, Antianxiety agents.

Temazepam (Restoril)

Actions

- Temazepam depresses the CNS and produces hypnosis.

Indications

- It is used to relieve insomnia.

Adverse Effects and Contraindications

- Use cautiously in patients with impaired liver or kidney function, COPD, depression, and in elderly and debilitated patients.

TABLE 7-41 BARBITURATES

Drug	Dosage and Administration	Nursing Considerations
Pentobarbital (Nembutal)	The usual adult sedative dosage is 20 to 30 mg, PO, tid or qid. The usual adult hypnotic dose is 100 mg, PO, at bedtime. For hypnotic effects, 200-mg suppositories are available. The usual pediatric dosage is 30 to 120 mg rectally (determined by weight) for insomnia.	Pentobarbital also may be given IM or IV. Intramuscular injections should be made into a large muscle, such as the gluteus maximus. IV injections should be given over at least one minute. Rapid IV injection can produce respiratory depression, laryngospasm, bronchospasm, and hypotension.
Phenobarbital (Luminal)	The usual adult sedative dosage is 15 to 30 mg, PO, tid or qid. The usual adult hypnotic dose is 100 mg, PO, at bedtime. For convulsive disorders, the adult dosage range is 60 to 250 mg, PO, qd. Phenobarbital is the preferred barbiturate for preventing grand mal seizures.	The parenteral injection (phenobarbital sodium) should not exceed 600 mg/24 hours, and the IV rate should not exceed 60 mg/minute. It frequently is used with phenytoin to treat grand mal, focal motor, and psychomotor epilepsy.

	The pediatric sedative dosage is 2 mg/kg/24 hours. The pediatric hypnotic dose is 3 to 5 mg/kg. The pediatric anticonvulsant dosage is 16 to 50 mg, two or three times daily.	
Secobarbital (Seconal)	The usual adult sedative dosage is 30 to 50 mg, tid. The usual adult hypnotic dose is 100 mg, PO, at bedtime. The hypnotic dose for the rectal suppository is 120 mg or 200 mg. Intravenous dosage ranges from 50 mg to 250 mg (no faster than 50 mg in 15 seconds). It also may be given IM. The pediatric sedative dosage is 6 mg/kg/24 hours. The pediatric hypnotic dose is 3 to 5 mg/kg	Patients receiving IV secobarbital sodium should have their blood pressure, pulse, and respirations monitored every 3 to 5 minutes.

- The most frequent adverse reactions are drowsiness, dizziness, and lethargy.
- Confusion and euphoria may occur.

Dosage and Administration

- The usual adult dose is 30 mg, PO, at bedtime, but elderly and debilitated patients should be started on 15 mg, PO, at bedtime.

Nursing Considerations

- Physical and psychological dependence are possible, especially if the drug is abused.

MISCELLANEOUS

CHLORAL HYDRATE (NOCTEC)

Actions

- Chloral hydrate depresses the CNS, and produces sedation and hypnosis (sleep).

Indications

- It is used to relieve insomnia.

Adverse Effects and Contraindications

- Gastric irritation is common and may lead to nausea and vomiting.
- Alcohol and other CNS depressants potentiate the action of chloral hydrate and may produce serious respiratory depression and cardiac arrhythmias.
- Patients with severe heart, liver, or kidney disease should not use this drug. It may irritate peptic ulcers.
- Patients receiving anticoagulants should use chloral hydrate cautiously because altered metabolism could precipitate bleeding.
- Physical and psychic dependence and tolerance do develop.

Dosage and Administration

- Adult oral dosages for sedation are 250 mg to 500 mg, tid, pc.
- Adult oral hypnotic doses are 500 mg to 1 g at bedtime. Chloral hydrate is also available as a suppository.
- The pediatric hypnotic dose is 50 mg/kg, with a maximum dose of 1 g.

Nursing Considerations

- If the patient is receiving anticoagulants, observe carefully for signs of bleeding.
- Capsules should be taken with a full glass of fluid.

DIPHENHYDRAMINE (BENADRYL)

Actions

- Diphenhydramine is an antihistamine that has the following effects: sedative, antiemetic, antiparkinsonism, and antitussive.

Indications

- It produces sedation and hypnosis in the elderly and may be better tolerated than other hypnotics.
- Diphenhydramine can be used to treat mild parkinsonism in elderly patients.
- It relieves the extrapyramidal symptoms caused by antipsychotic drugs.
- It also prevents and treats motion sickness.
- The drug can relieve allergic reactions from food and pollens and from blood and plasma.
- Parenteral forms are used to treat anaphylaxis (as an adjunct to epinephrine), blood reactions, and other allergic reactions when oral therapy is not possible.

Adverse Effects and Contraindications

- It frequently causes drowsiness.
- Overdoses produce restlessness and confusion. Coma, convulsions, and death occur in children.
- It can cause dryness and thickness of pulmonary secretions, and should be used cautiously in patients with COPD.
- Because of diphenhydramine's atropine-type effects, it is contraindicated for patients with narrow-angle glaucoma and obstructions of the gastrointestinal or genitourinary systems.

Dosage and Administration

- The usual adult oral dosage is 25 mg to 50 mg, three or four times, qd. It may be given IM or IV, up to a maximum of 400 mg qd.
- The usual pediatric dosage is 5 mg/kg/24 hours in four divided doses.

Nursing Considerations

- Because of the drug's sedative effect, driving and operating machinery may be dangerous to the patient.
- Diphenhydramine has additive effects with alcohol and other CNS depressants.
- Monoamine oxidase (MAO) inhibitors (see PH, Psychotropics, antidepressants) potentiate the anticholinergic (drying) effects of antihistamines.
- The antihistaminic activity dries secretions and may assist in reducing drooling for patients with Parkinson's disease.
- Patients with Parkinson's disease who are nervous or who experience insomnia may benefit from the sedative action.

ETHCHLORVYNOL (PLACIDYL)

Actions

- Ethchlorvynol depresses the CNS and produces sedation and hypnosis (sleep).

Indications

- It is used to relieve insomnia if pain and anxiety are not present. It also is used if the patient cannot tolerate barbiturates.

Adverse Effects and Contraindications

- Headache, dizziness, confusion, nausea, and vomiting occur.
- Hypotension and excitation are possible.
- Physical and psychic dependence and tolerance do develop.

Dosage and Administration

- The usual adult hypnotic dose is 500 mg to 1 g, PO, at bedtime.
- For sedative purposes and for elderly patients, doses are lower.

Nursing Considerations

- Because this drug may cause confusion, patients (especially the elderly) should be observed carefully and protected (*e.g.*, by use of side rails).
- Blood pressure should be monitored to detect hypotension.

MEPROBAMATE (EQUANIL, MILTOWN)

Actions

- Meprobamate depresses the CNS in a manner similar to that of barbiturates.

Indications

- It can relieve anxiety and tension.
- It promotes sleep in anxious, tense patients.

Adverse Effects and Contraindications

- Use cautiously for patients with impaired liver and kidney function, convulsive disorders, or a history of suicidal tendencies, and drug or alcohol abuse.
- Drowsiness and ataxia occur frequently.
- Patients also may experience hypotension, tachycardia, arrhythmias, and bronchospasm.
- Anorexia, nausea, vomiting, stomatitis, and diarrhea have been reported.
- Allergic reactions from itching to anaphylaxis have occurred. Blood dyscrasias are rare.

Dosage and Administration

- *Adults:* 400 mg, three or four times, PO, daily, or 600 mg two times daily
- *Pediatric (6 to 12 yr):* 25 mg/kg daily divided into two or three doses

Nursing Considerations

- Lower doses are recommended for elderly and debilitated patients.
- Minimize gastric distress by giving meprobamate with food.
- Physical and psychological dependence does occur.
- *Equagesic* is a combination of meprobamate and aspirin.

OPIUM ALKALOIDS

Actions

- Opium alkaloids relieve pain, produce euphoria, may induce sleep, and depress respirations, constrict the pupil of the eye, depress the cough center, and decrease motility and muscle tone of the gastrointestinal and genitourinary tracts.

Indications

- These drugs can control moderate to severe pain.
- They relieve apprehension and facilitate induction preoperatively.

Adverse Effects and Contraindications

- They frequently cause *constipation;* occasionally, they cause nausea and vomiting.
- Urinary retention may occur, especially if a male patient already has problems with his prostate gland.
- Postural hypotension has been reported.
- *Respiratory depression* occurs, and the patient may need a narcotic antagonist to counteract the depression.
- Patients experience behavioral changes, such as restlessness, excitement, and insomnia.
- Opiates also may produce drowsiness, dizziness, sweating, and flushing.
- Allergic reactions, such as rash and itching, occur.
- *Tolerance* develops, but at different rates for each individual.
- They can produce *physical* and *psychic dependency.*
- Patients with *head* injuries or postoperative *craniotomies* should not receive opiates. Respirations can be depressed, intracranial pressure can increase, and decreased responsiveness resulting from the drug can mask changes in the patient's condition.
- The increased excitation that can occur makes opiates unsafe for patients suffering from *convulsive disorders* and *acute alcoholism.*
- Patients with severe COPD may not be able to tolerate the decreased respirations.
- Patients with *liver disease* may not be able to metabolize these drugs.

Dosage, Administration, and Nursing Considerations

- See Table 7-42.
- When opiates are given before the pain becomes too severe, they are usually more effective.
- Because of decreased ability to metabolize drugs, elderly patients will be more susceptible to adverse effects, and may require less than the usual adult dosage.
- Combining opiates with sedatives or tranquilizers causes a synergistic effect and may allow for a decreased dosage of the opiate.

OPIUM ANTAGONIST

Naloxone Hydrochloride (Narcan)

Actions

- Naloxone hydrochloride displaces the narcotic drugs from the nerve cell receptors.

Indications

- It reverses respiratory depression and hypotension resulting from overdose with opiates and other synthetic narcotics.
- Naloxone is considered capable of diagnosing opiate overdose because it is so effective in reversing the effects.

Adverse Effects and Contraindications

- Severe withdrawal occurs in patients who are physically dependent on narcotics.

Dosage and Administration

- For treating narcotic overdose, 1 ml (0.4 mg) is administered IV, IM, or SC. It may be repeated every 2 minutes to 3 minutes until respiratory function improves.
- Narcotic addicts and patients with postoperative respiratory depression may receive small doses.
- The newborn dosage usually is 0.01 mg/kg, IV, IM, or SC. Again, dosage may be repeated every 2 to 3 minutes.

Nursing Considerations

- Observe patients carefully for signs of narcotic withdrawal (*e.g.*, nausea, vomiting, sweating, and hypertension).
- Maintain an open airway and have resuscitation equipment and personnel available.

SYNTHETIC ANALGESICS

Butorphanol Tartrate (Stadol)

Actions

- Butorphanol tartrate is a CNS depressant that produces analgesia.

Indications

- It relieves moderate to severe pain and prepartum pain.
- It is used as a preoperative or preanesthetic medication.

Adverse Effects and Contraindications

- Use cautiously in patients with cardiovascular, respiratory, renal, or hepatic impairment.
- Patients with gallbladder disease, head injury, increased intracranial pressure, and those who are emotionally unstable or dependent on drugs should use this drug with caution.
- The most frequent adverse effects are sedation, nausea, and sweating.
- Less frequently, headache, vertigo, dizziness, lethargy, and confusion have been experienced.

TABLE 7-42 OPIUM ALKALOIDS

Drug	Dosage and Administration	Nursing Considerations
Codeine	*Adults* 1. Analgesia—15 mg to 60 mg, four times/day 2. Antitussive—10 mg to 20 mg, PO, every 4 to 6 hours *Pediatric* 1. Analgesia—3 mg/kg/day, divided into six doses 2. Antitussive a. 6–12yr: 5 mg to 10 mg, every 4 to 6 hours b. 2–6 yr: 2.5 mg to 5 mg, every 4 to 6 hours	Compared to morphine, codeine causes less respiratory depression, has less dependency potential, and usually causes fewer side-effects. Codeine is the most effective of the opiates for relieving coughing, and is used in many cough preparations. Codeine often is combined with aspirin or acetaminophen (Tylenol) and used to relieve mild-to-moderate pain.
Hydromophone (Dilaudid)	The usual adult dose is 2 mg every 4 to 6 hours, PO, SC, IM, IV. For severe pain, increase the dosage to 3 to 4 mg every 4 to 6 hours. For rectal suppositories (3 mg), administer one every 6 to 8 hours.	Compared to morphine, hydromorphone is more potent, but its effects are shorter.

Morphine sulfate	The usual adult dosage is 10 mg to 30 mg, PO, every 4 hours, or 5 mg to 15 mg every 4 hours, IM or SC. The usual dose is 2.5 to 15 mg in 4 to 5 ml sterile water for injection, administered IV slowly over 4 to 5 minutes. The pediatric dose is 0.1 to 0.2 mg/kg, SC, or 0.05 to 0.1 mg/kg, IV, very slowly.	Morphine is the prototype of the narcotic analgesics. Frequently, it is the drug of choice to relieve chest pain following an acute myocardial infarction. The sedative effects and the peripheral vasodilation make it very effective when used to treat acute pulmonary edema.
Oxycodone hydrochloride (Percodan, Percocet, Tylox)	For adults give one or two tablets every 6 hours as needed. *Pediatric Dosage* 1. 12 yr or older: ½ tablet every 6 hours as needed 2. 6 to 12 yr: ¼ tablet every 6 hours as needed Tylox should not be given to children of any age.	*Percocet—5* is 5 mg oxycodone hydrochloride with 325 mg acetaminophen. *Percodan* is 4.5 mg oxycodone hydrochloride and 0.38 mg oxycodone terephthalate with 325 mg aspirin. *Percodan–Demi* is 2.25 mg oxycodone hydrochloride, 0.19 mg oxycodone terephthalate, and 325 mg aspirin. *Tylox* is 4.5 mg oxycodone hydrochloride, 0.38 mg oxycodone terephthalate and 500 mg acetaminophen.

PH

Dosage and Administration

- The usual adult IM dose is 2 mg (range, 1 to 4 mg) every 3 to 4 hr, prn.
- The usual adult IV dose is 1 mg (range, 0.5 to 2 mg) every 3 to 4 hr, prn.

Nursing Considerations

- It is not recommended for use in children.
- Butorphanol has habit-forming potential.
- Overdosage is treated with naloxone.

Meperidine (Demerol)

Actions

- Meperidine produces analgesia and euphoria, but it is less likely than the opiates to produce sleep.

Indications

- It relieves moderate to severe pain.
- Often it is used preoperatively, especially when combined with a sedative.

Adverse Effects and Contraindications

- Dizziness, nausea, vomiting, sweating, and flushing are common.
- Mental confusion, disorientation, and hypotension occur.
- *Respiratory depression* and *convulsions* may be fatal.
- Tolerance and dependence similar to those that result from morphine develop.
- Patients with *liver dysfunction, increased intracranial pressure,* or *COPD* should not receive meperidine.
- Patients taking such drugs as other narcotic analgesics, sedatives, tranquilizers, alcohol, *MAO* inhibitors, or *tricyclic antidepressants* along with meperidine could have severe reactions (*e.g.,* respiratory depression, hypotension, and profound sedation or coma).

Dosage and Administration

- The usual adult dose range is 50 to 150 mg, PO, SC, or IM, every 3 to 4 hours.
- The usual pediatric dose is 1 to 1.8 mg/kg, IM, SC, or PO, up to 100 mg every 4 hr, prn.

Nursing Considerations

- When patients also are receiving other CNS depressants, the dosage of meperidine should be reduced.
- Dosage should be reduced for elderly patients.

- Postoperative patients who are ambulating (especially for the first few times) may experience postural hypotension and should be protected against injury from falls.

Pentazocine (Talwin)

Actions

- Pentazocine is an analgesic.

Indications

- It relieves moderate to severe pain.
- The oral form often is used to treat chronic pain because of its low potential for producing dependency.

Adverse Effects and Contraindications

- Nausea, vomiting, dizziness, and drowsiness are common.
- Constipation, euphoria, disorientation, and confusion are rare.
- Overdose can produce respiratory depression.
- Use cautiously in patients whose respirations are depressed (*e.g.*, COPD).
- Tolerance and dependency develop, especially with the parenteral forms.

Dosage and Administration

- The usual oral adult dosage is 50 mg, q 3 to 4 hr (not to exceed 600 mg daily).
- The usual IM, SC, or IV adult dosage is 30 mg, q 3 to 4 hr (not to exceed 360 mg daily).

Nursing Considerations

- Subcutaneous injections should be avoided because of possible tissue damage.
- Overdose is counteracted by naloxone (Narcan).
- Oral tablets contain 0.5 mg naloxone, a narcotic antagonist, to eliminate the abuse potential of this dosage form.

Propoxyphene Hydrochloride (Darvon)

Actions

- Propoxyphene hydrochloride is an analgesic.

Indications

- It is used to relieve mild to moderate pain.

Adverse Effects and Contraindications

- Drowsiness, dizziness, and headache may occur.
- Nausea, vomiting, and constipation are possible.

- Both physical and psychic dependence develop if abused.
- Overdose produces *convulsions, coma, circulatory collapse,* and *respiratory failure.*

Dosage and Administration

- The usual adult dosage ranges from 32 to 65 mg, PO, three to four times each day.
- For Darvon-N, the dose ranges from 50 to 100 mg, PO, q 4 hr, prn.

Nursing Considerations

- This drug is widely prescribed and frequently abused.
- When people take propoxyphene with other CNS depressants (*e.g.,* alcohol, sedatives, or tranquilizers), death can result.
- Propoxyphene hydrochloride with acetaminophen is available as Dolacet, Dolene AP, SK-65 APAP, and Wygesic.
- Proproxyphene hydrochloride with aspirin is available as Darvon with A.S.A., and Darvon Compound (also contains aspirin and caffeine).
- Propoxyphene napsylate with acetaminophen is Darvocet-N.
- Propoxyphene napsylate with aspirin is Darvon-N with/A.S.A.

OPHTHALMIC PREPARATIONS

OVERVIEW OF EYE MEDICATIONS

- Know the purpose of eye medications. They are potent, and their specific action may be desired for one eye only.
- Abbreviations are the following: right eye, OD; left eye, OS; and both eyes, OU.
- Different medications may be ordered for each eye.
- Suspensions must be inverted end-to-end and gently rotated to ensure adequate mixing.
- Ophthalmic solutions are sterile and must be protected from contamination and properly stored.
- Eye ointments are placed along the center rim of the lower lid. They will then be "blinked" into the eye.
- To instill eye drops, tilt the patient's head back and instruct him or her to look up. Pull the cheek down with the conjuctiva exposed. Place the drop in the conjunctival fold, not directly onto the cornea or into the lacrimal duct. Avoid touching the patient with the end of the eye-drop bottle.
- To reduce systemic absorption of eye medications, apply gentle pressure on the inner canthus of the eye (nasolacrimal duct) while the drug is being instilled and for a few minutes after instillation.

- If more than one drop is needed, have the patient blink one away before instilling the next one.

ADRENERGICS

- See PH, Cardiovascular, for systemic actions, adverse effects, and nursing considerations.

Actions

- Adrenergics lower the intraocular pressure by decreasing aqueous humor formation and by increasing aqueous outflow.
- They produce brief mydriasis (dilation of the pupil) and vasoconstriction.
- They also relax the ciliary muscle.

Indications

- See Table 7-43.

Dosage, Adminstration, and Nursing Considerations

- See Table 7-43.
- See Overview of eye medications.

ADRENOCORTICOSTEROIDS

- See PH, Endocrine system, for systemic actions, adverse effects, and nursing considerations.

FLUOROMETHOLONE (FML, LIQUIFILM)

Actions

- Fluorometholone reduces inflammation.

Indications

- It is used to manage ocular inflammations.

Adverse Effects

- Increased intraocular pressure may occur, especially in the elderly.
- Excessive use may produce optic nerve damage, cataracts, and glaucoma exacerbation.

Dosage and Administration

- Administer 1 gtt to 2 gtt of 0.1% ophthalmic suspension, tid or qid.

TABLE 7-43 ADRENERGICS (OPHTHALMICS)

Drug	Indications	Dosage and Administration	Nursing Considerations
Epinephrine hydrochloride (Epifrin, Glaucon)	Manages simple (open-angle) glaucoma. It also is an ophthalmic decongestant.	0.1% to 2% solution 1 gtt in the affected eye	Ophthalmic preparations may cause brief stinging or burning of eyes, lacrimation, iritis, and headache. It may cause blurred vision and light sensitivity from the mydriasis. Hypersensitivity may be indicated by edema of lids, itching, and discharge.
Phenylephrine hydrochloride (Ocusol)	It manages wide-angle glaucoma in selected cases. It is used as a mydriatic for ophthalmoscopic examination or surgery.	Ophthalmoscopy 1. *Adults:* 1 gtt of 2.5% or 10% solution 2. *Pediatric:* 1 gtt of 2.5% solution Chronic mydriasis: 1 gtt, two or three times, qd Vasoconstrictor (0.02% to 0.15%): 1 gtt every 3 to 4 hr, PRN	Considerations are the same as those for epinephrine.
Tetrahydrozoline hydrochloride (Murine, Visine)	It can provide symptomatic relief of minor eye irritation and allergies.	1 gtt or 2 gtt of 0.05% solution, OU, two or three times, qd	It may cause transient stinging and headache.

Nursing Considerations

- See Overview of Eye Medications.
- Eye drops are not to be used for an extended period of time.

ANTICHOLINERGICS

ATROPINE SULFATE (BUF-OPTO ATROPINE, ISOPTO ATROPINE)

- See PH, Cardiovascular, for systemic actions, indications, adverse effects, and nursing considerations.

Actions

- Atropine sulfate produces mydriasis and cycloplegia.

Indications

- It is used prior to refraction and to treat anterior uveitis and iritis.

Adverse Effects and Contraindications

- Increased intraocular pressure, blurred vision, and photophobia may occur.
- Cycloplegia (paralysis of the ciliary muscle), edema of eyelids, and chronic conjunctivitis (with long-term use) have been reported.
- Overdosage and continuous use of eye preparations can produce systemic effects of atropine.

Dosage and Administration

- *Adults* (refraction): 1 gtt or 2 gtt of solution, or a small amount of ointment in eyes before refraction
- *Pediatric* (refraction): 1 gtt or 2 gtt of 0.5% solution, or a small amount of ointment in the eyes, bid, for 1 to 3 days prior to examination and before refraction.

Nursing Considerations

- See Overview of Eye Medications.
- Atropine solution usually is instilled one hour before refraction, but the ointment usually takes longer to be effective.
- Systemic absorption of ocular atropine has resulted in some deaths. Infants and children are at the greatest risk, and use of the ointment may be indicated to reduce the systemic absorption.

- Great care also must be taken when administering ocular atropine to elderly patients. Congestive heart failure from tachycardia and glaucoma from increased intraocular pressure are possible. The distorted vision from mydriasis can lead to falls and injury. Urinary retention also may cause problems.

ANTICHOLINESTERASE AGENTS

- See PH, Neurologic, for systemic actions, adverse effects, and nursing considerations.

Actions

- These agents produce intense miosis (excessive contraction of the pupil).
- They decrease intraocular pressure by facilitating outflow of the aqueous humor.
- They also enhance reabsorption of the aqueous humor.

Indications

- Anticholinesterase agents treat open-angle glaucoma and may be used concurrently with a carbonic anhydrase inhibitor (see PH, Genitourinary).
- They are used to manage accommodative esotropia (convergent strabismus), and they may be used following iridectomy.

Adverse Effects and Contraindications

- Ocular pain, lacrimation, and headache may occur.
- Prolonged use can produce lens opacities, iris cysts, and conjunctival thickening.

Dosage and Administration

- Demecarium Bromide (Humorsol)
  1. *Adults* (glaucoma): Administer 1 gtt to 2 gtt of 0.125% or 0.25% solution, twice weekly, up to bid.
  2. *Pediatric* (accommodative esotropia): Initially, instill 1 gtt of 0.125% solution in each eye daily. After 2 to 3 weeks, the dosage is reduced gradually to 1 gtt weekly, and then discontinued.
- Isoflurophate (Floropryl) (0.025% ophthalmic ointment):
  1. *Glaucoma:* Apply a ¼-inch strip in conjunctival sac every 8 to 72 hours.
  2. *Esotropia:* Apply a ¼-inch strip q hs for 2 weeks, then reduced to qod, and then to once a week.

Nursing Considerations

- See Overview of Eye Medications.
- These drugs frequently are used at bedtime to minimize visual disturbances.
- Dermatitis can develop if the drug comes into contact with the skin. Wash the area with copious amounts of water.
- Atropine sulfate may be used as an antidote for systemic toxicity.

BETA-ADRENERGIC BLOCKING AGENTS

- See PH, Cardiovascular, for *systemic* actions, adverse effects, and nursing considerations.

TIMOLOL MALEATE (TIMOPTIC)

Actions

- Timolol maleate appears to reduce the formation of aqueous humor and to increase the outflow.

Indications

- It is used in the treatment of chronic open-angle glaucoma, secondary glaucoma, and ocular hypertension.

Adverse Effects and Contraindications

- Eye irritation, including conjunctivitis and blepharitis, have occurred.
- Some patients experience a slight reduction in heart rate.
- Bronchospasm is rare, but use the drug cautiously in patients with bronchial asthma.
- Use cautiously in patients with severe heart block, heart failure, and sinus bradycardia.

Dosage and Administration

- The usual dosage is 1 gt of a 0.25% or 0.5% solution in each eye, twice daily. As intraocular pressure is controlled, the dosage may be reduced to once daily.

Nursing Considerations

- See Overview of Eye Medications.
- Monitor the heart rate, especially if the patient has a history of heart disease.

- It often is better tolerated than pilocarpine, and it does not cause the dimming and blurring of vision that occurs with the miotics.

CHOLINERGICS—MIOTICS

Actions

- These drugs cause contraction of the ciliary muscle and a decrease in intraocular pressure.
- They increase drainage of fluid into Schlemm's canal.
- They mimic the action of acetylcholine.

Indications

- These medications are used to treat acute narrow-angle and chronic open-angle glaucoma.

Adverse Effects and Contraindications

- Initial use frequently causes stinging, redness, and lacrimation.
- Pupil constriction leads to dimming of vision.
- Contraction of the ciliary muscle causes blurring of vision and nearsightedness (myopia).
- Long-term use can result in iris cysts; lens opacities, which may progress to cataracts; obstruction of the nasolacrimal duct and canal; and allergic reactions.
- Use cautiously in patients with a history of retinal detachment.
- Significant systemic absorption is unlikely with normal dosages. However, systemic absorption could possibly produce the following effects:
    1. Reduced heart rate and lowered blood pressure may result. Use cautiously for patients who had a recent myocardial infarction.
    2. Brochoconstriction and wheezing may occur. Use cautiously for patients with bronchial asthma and other types of chronic obstructive pulmonary disease.
    3. Nausea, vomiting cramps, and diarrhea can occur. Use cautiously for patients with peptic ulcers.
    4. Salivation and sweating have been reported.

Dosage and Administration

- *Carbachol chloride (Cabacel, Isopto-Carbachol):* The usal dosage is 1 gtt or 2 gtt of a 0.75% to 3% solution, administered one to four times a day in the eye.
- *Pilocarpine hydrochloride and nitrate (Pilocar):* The most commonly used solutions range from 0.5% to 4%.

1. Chronic open-angle glaucoma: 1 gtt or 2 gtt of 0.5% to 4% solution instilled in the eye, qid
2. Acute narrow-angle glaucoma: 1 gtt or 2 gtt of a 4% solution every 10 minutes, three or more times

- *Ocusert Pilo-20 or Pilo-40:* This is a plastic disc that is placed in either the upper or lower conjunctival sac and diffuses the pilocarpine into the film of tears over the eye. It delivers either 20 or 40 micrograms (μg) per hour for 7 days.
- Pilocarpine is the most commonly used miotic in the treatment of glaucoma.

Nursing Considerations

- See Overview of Eye Medications.

SILVER NITRATE ($AgNO_3$)

Actions

- Silver nitrate is both a bactericidal and astringent agent.

Indications

- The ophthalmic solution prevents and treats ophthalmia neonatorum.

Adverse Effects and Contraindications

- It produces transient chemical irritation (redness, edema, and discharge).

Dosage and Administration

- Instill 2 gtt of 1% solution in each eye. The drug should contact the whole conjunctival sac for 30 seconds or longer.

Nursing Considerations

- See Overview of Eye Medications.
- Before instilling drops, the eyelids should be cleaned with sterile cotton and sterile water to remove blood, mucus, or meconium.

RESPIRATORY SYSTEM

ADRENOCORTICOSTEROIDS

- See PH, Endocrine system for actions, adverse effects, and nursing considerations.

- See Table 7-44 for indications, dosage, administration, and nursing considerations.

ANTITUSSIVES

CODEINE

- See PH, neurologic system.

DEXTROMETHORPHAN HYDROBROMIDE (BENYLIN DM, HOLD, ROMILAR CF, ST. JOSEPH COUGH SYRUP FOR CHILDREN)

Actions

- It depresses the cough center in the medulla.

Indications

- Dextromethorphan hydrobromide relieves cough spasms in nonproductive coughs due to colds and influenza.
- It is a common ingredient in over-the-counter (OTC) cough preparations.

Adverse Effects and Contraindications

- It should not be used for children under 2 yr of age, or in patients on concurrent MAO inhibitor therapy.
- Use cautiously when asthma or a productive cough is present.
- Adverse effects are rare, but patients may experience dizziness, drowsiness, and anorexia.

Dosage and Administration

- *Adults:* 10 mg to 20 mg, PO, every 4 hr, or 30 mg every 6 to 8 hr
- *Pediatric (6 to 12 yr):* 5 mg to 10 mg, PO, every 4 hr, or 15 mg every, 6 hr to 8 hr
- *Pediatric (2 to 6 yr):* 2.5 mg to 5 mg, PO, every 4 hours, or 7.5 mg every 6 hr to 8 hr

Nursing Considerations

- Encourage fluid to liquify tenacious mucus.

BRONCHODILATORS

ADRENERGICS

- See PH, Cardiovascular system, for actions, indications, and adverse effects.

- See Table 7-45 for dosage, administration, and nursing considerations.

XANTHINES

Actions

- Xanthines relax smooth muscle of the bronchi and bronchioles and of the pulmonary blood vessels.
- They stimulate cardiac muscle and may increase cardiac output.
- They produce diuresis.
- These agents also dilate coronary blood vessels.

Indications

- They are used to treat intermittent and recurring bronchial constriction (*e.g.,* from chronic obstructive pulmonary disease, or COPD), asthma, and acute respiratory distress in children.
- They also are used for the treatment of pulmonary edema.

Adverse Effects and Contraindications

- Gastrointestinal (GI) irritation is common and may cause nausea and vomiting. Intestinal bleeding may occur.
- Restlessness, irritability, and insomnia may result from central nervous system (CNS) stimulation.
- Serious, and at times fatal, cardiac arrhythmias and convulsions occur.
- Use cautiously in patients with severe hypertension, impaired liver or kidney function, and in young children.

Dosage, Administration, and Nursing Considerations

- See Table 7-46.
- There are many OTC bronchodilators available. Patients must be carefully counseled about the side-effects of these drugs. Tolerance develops easily, and patients, therefore, may overdose themselves. Severe hypertension, pulmonary edema, and cardiac arrhythmias can occur. These drugs also contain additives that can dry secretions (antihistamines) and cause sedation.

PH

CROMOLYN SODIUM (DSCG, INTAL)

Actions

- Cromolyn inhibits the release of bronchoconstrictors (histamine and SRS-A) and suppresses an allergic response.

(Text continues on page 919)

TABLE 7-44 ADRENOCORTICOSTEROIDS

Drug	Indications	Dosage and Administration	Nursing Considerations
Beclomethasone dipropionate (Beclovent, Vanceril)	it is used to treat chronic steroid-dependent bronchial asthma Nasal inhalations are used for hay fever and perennial rhinitis (Beconase, Vancenase).	50 μg at valve, delivers 42 μg to the patient *Adults* oral inhalation: two inhalations (84 μg) three to four times daily Maximum: 20 inhalations daily *Pediatric* oral inhalation (6 to 12 yr): one to two inhalations, three to four times daily Maximum: 10 inhalations daily	Allow at least one minute between puffs per treatment. Patients may be weaned from systemic steroids to beclomethasone. During withdrawal/transfer period, patients may experience steroid withdrawal symptoms (muscle and joint pain, depression, lassitude). Inspect oral membranes frequently for candida infection (red, sore membranes with vescicular eruptions).
Hydrocortisone sodium succinate (Solu-cortef)	This is used to treat acute status asthmaticus.	20 to 240 mg/day, IV Dosage depends on severity of the problem and response of the patient.	To prevent withdrawal symptoms and permit adrenals to recover, doses are reduced gradually.

Prednisone (Deltasone, Meticorten)	This is used to treat chronic asthma when bronchodilators and other antiasthmatic drugs cannot stabilize the patient	*Adult:* Initially, 5 to 60 mg/24 hr in single or divided doses; then, gradual reduction by 5 to 10 mg every 4 to 5 days until the lowest effective maintenance level is reached *Pediatric:* 2 mg/kg/24 hr, and then gradually reduced to lowest effective maintenance level	With low maintenance doses, the chance of habituation is reduced and discontinuing the drug is easier. To further reduce the suppressant effect on the pituitary and adrenal glands, an intermittent dosage schedule may be used (*e.g.,* the full daily dosage is given with the morning meal, or the full dosage for 2 days is given qod with the morning meal). Weaning a patient from steroids can be very difficult because the asthmatic symptoms may become worse.

PH

TABLE 7-45 ADRENERGICS (BRONCHODILATORS)

Drug	Dosage and Administration	Nursing Considerations
Ephedrine	*Adult:* (PO, SC, IM, IV slowly) 12.5 to 50 mg, three or four times daily; maximum, 150 mg/24 hr Intranasal (0.5% to 3% solution): 2 to 4 gtt, or a small amount of jelly in each nostril, no more than qid for 3 or 4 days *Pediatric:* 2 to 3 mg/kg/24 hr, divided into four to six doses	Timing of administration and dosage are important in controlling insomnia. Caution patients not to use OTC preparations for coughs, colds, or allergies unless they are approved by their physician.
Epinephrine (Bronkaid Mist, Primatene Mist, Adrenalin)	*Adults:* Parenteral 1:1000 (0.1%) solution—0.2 to 1 ml SC or IM; inhalation 1:100 (1%) solution—by aerosol, nebulizer, or IPPB machine; nasal 1:1000 solution—by drops or spray *Pediatric (over 6 yr):* 1:1000 solution— 0.01 mg/kg per dose, SC, up to six times	A tuberculin syringe may permit greater accuracy in the measurement of parenteral doses. Check the dosage and strength of the solution carefully. Rotate injection sites to prevent tissue necrosis from vasoconstriction. Intranasal solutions can cause rebound congestion and should not be used longer than 3 to 5 days. Epinephrine may increase blood glucose levels.
Isoetharine (Bronkosol, Bronkometer)	Bronkometer delivers 340 μg per metered dose, and one or two inhalations q 4 hr are used.	Repeated excessive use can produce paradoxical airway resistance, tachycardia, headache, nausea, and dizziness.

	In a hand nebulizer, three to seven inhalations of Bronkosol are recommended q 4 hrs	Isoetharine can be alternated with epinephrine, but should not be given concurrently because excessive tachycardia may result.
Isoproterenol (Isuprel, Medihaler-Iso, Norisodrine) (also see PH, cardiovascular)	Metered-dose nebulizer (120 to 250 μg): Use one or two inhalations, four to six times daily at not less than 3- to 4-hour intervals. Metered powder inhaler (10%, 25%): Use one or two inhalations. If necessary, repeat in 5 minutes, and then in 10 minutes after the second dose.	This drug may also be administered by hand-bulb nebulizer, metered aerosol nebulizer, and by an IPPB apparatus. Carefully instruct patients in the use of the appropriate apparatus and dosage (always the lowest effective dose). Rebound bronchospasm may occur when effects of the drug end.
Metaproterenol (Alupent, Metaprel)	*Adults and Pediatric* (over 9 yr): Give 20 mg, PO, every 6 to 8 hr. *Pediatric* (6 to 9 yr): Give 10 mg, PO, every 6 to 8 hr. *Adults by inhalation:* Use two or three inhalations of metered aerosol every 3 to 4 hours, up to a maximum of 12 inhalations daily (0.65 mg in each metered dose).	Long-term use may result in tolerance for the drug.
Terbutaline (Brethine, Bricanyl)	*Adult:* The SC dosage is 0.25 mg. The oral dosage range is from 2.5 mg to 5 mg, tid, at 6-hr intervals. Maximum dosage is 15 mg, qd. *Pediatric* (12 to 15 yr): Administer 2.5 mg, PO, tid, at 6-hr intervals.	Observe dosages carefully. The oral dosage is 2.5 mg, while SC dosage is 0.25 mg. Tolerance develops after a relatively short period of time, so patients should receive regular evaluations.

TABLE 7-46 XANTHINES (BRONCHODILATORS)

Drug	Dosage and Administration	Nursing Considerations
Aminophylline (Aminodur Dura-tabs, Theophylline, Ethylenediamine)	*Adults:* 1. Oral: 500 mg initially; 200 to 315 mg every 6 to 8 hr for maintenance 2. IV: loading dose of 5 to 6 mg/kg over 30 minutes, not to exceed 25 mg/min; maintenance of 0.5 to 0.9 mg/kg/hour with monitoring serum theophylline levels 3. Rectal suppository: 500 mg, one to two times, qd *Pediatric* 1. Oral: 7.5 mg/kg initially; maintenance of 5 or 6 mg/kg every 6 to 8 hr 2. IV: 6 mg/kg in a single dose; maintenance of 20 mg/kg/24 hr divided in four equal doses 3. Rectal suppository: 3 to 5 mg/kg, three or four times daily (at 8-hr intervals)	Monitor blood pressure, pulse, and respirations very carefully, especially during IV administrations. Rapid IV administration can precipitate severe hypotension and circulatory collapse. An IV pump and microdrip tubing should be used. Patients metabolize aminophylline at very different rates. Therefore, a therapeutic dose for one person could produce toxic symptoms in another. Aminophylline levels should be checked every other day. Gastrointestinal absorption can be unpredictable, so aminophylline should be given on an empty stomach. The nausea and vomiting that can occur come from stimulation of the central emetic mechanism in the brain, rather than from local GI irritation. Long-term use of rectal suppositories can produce local irritation and is not recommended. Long-acting forms of oral aminophylline are available for nighttime use.

		Children appear to be more susceptible to the CNS-stimulating effects. Remind patients that coffee, tea, and cola contain xanthines and may increase the risk of adverse effects.
Dyphylline (Dilor, Lufyllin)	*Adults:* 1. Oral: 15 mg/kg every 6 hours 2. IM: 250 to 500 mg at 6-hr intervals *Pediatric* (6 yr and older) 1. 5 to 7 mg/kg daily in divided doses	Serum theophylline levels cannot be used to determine therapeutic doses. It is available in combination with guaifenesin (Dilor-G, Lufyllin-GG).
Oxtriphylline (Choledyl, Choline Theophyllinate)	*Adults:* 200 mg, PO, qid *Pediatric* (2 to 12 yr): 100 mg/ 60 lb, four times a day	This drug is useful in long-term therapy because tolerance develops infrequently.
Theophyllin (Elixophyllin, Slo-Phyllin, Quibron bidCAPS, Theobid, Theo-Dur, Slo-bid)	*Adults:* 100 to 200 mg, PO, every 6 hr, sustained release: 200 to 300 mg, PO, every 12 hr *Pediatric:* 4 to 6 mg/kg, PO, q 6 hr	Oral preparations should be given with a full glass of water. Theophylline levels are used to monitor therapy. Elderly patients frequently experience dizziness, especially early in therapy. Coffee, tea, cola, and many OTC preparations contain xanthines and may increase the risk of adverse effects.

TABLE 7-47 EXPECTORANTS

Drug	Adverse Effects and Contraindications	Dosage and Administration	Nursing Considerations
Guaifenesin (Anti-Tuss, GG-Tussin, Robitussin)	GI upset Drowsiness	*Adult:* 100 to 400 mg, PO, every 3 to 4 hr, maximum: 2.4 g/day *Pediatric* (6 to 12 yr): 50–100 mg every 3 to 4 hr, maximum: 600 mg/day *Pediatric* (3 to 6 hr): 50 mg every 3 to 4 hr, maximum: 300 mg/day	Guaifenesin can interfere with laboratory tests done to determine the presence of excess chemicals in pheochromocytoma and carcinoid syndrome. It is a common ingredient in OTC cough mixtures.
Iodinated glycerol (Organidin)	GI irritation Rash and hypersensitivity Iodism (headache, parotitis, ulcerations of mouth and throat, metallic taste)	*Adult:* 60 mg, PO, qid *Pediatric:* Up to one-half of the adult dosage	It is available as tablets (30 mg), 5% solution (50 mg/ml), and elixir (60 mg/5 ml). Administer all preparations with liquid.
Potassium iodide (KI, SSKI)	Iodine sensitivity may produce skin eruptions similar to acne. Frontal sinus pain and a mumps-like swelling of the parotid gland may occur. GI irritation may result in nausea, vomiting, and diarrhea. Tuberculosis patients should not receive potassium iodide.	*Adult:* 300 to 650 mg, PO, three or four times daily as needed *Pediatric:* 60 to 250 mg, PO, four times daily	SSKI contains 1 g/ml. The oral solution contains 167 mg/5 ml.
Terpin hydrate	High alcohol content (42.5%) may cause gastric irritation.	5 to 10 ml, PO, every 3 to 4 hr	Terpin hydrate may be mixed with codeine.

Indications

- Prophylactically, it is used to treat severe perennial bronchial asthma and may allow reductions in dosage and frequency of bronchodilators, expectorants, antibiotics, or steroids.

Adverse Effects and Contraindications

- Bronchospasm, cough, nasal congestion, pharyngeal irritation, and wheezing have been reported.
- Intal nebulizer solution has produced cough, nasal congestion, nausea, sneezing, and wheezing.
- Do not give to patients with acute asthma or status asthmaticus, or to children under 5 years old.
- Use cautiously for patients with kidney or liver impairment.

Dosage and Administration

- *Adults and Pediatric* (5 yr and older): The contents of one capsule (20 mg) should be inhaled four times daily, using a Spinhaler (turboinhaler).

Nursing Considerations

- Cromolyn must be withdrawn gradually to avoid exacerbation of asthmatic symptoms.

EXPECTORANTS

Actions

- Expectorants stimulate the secretion of the natural lubricating fluid of the lower respiratory tract. This liquifies thick mucus and assists in its expulsion. Coughing becomes productive.

Indications

- Expectorants are used in the treatment of COPD, asthma, bronchitis, colds, and pneumonia.

Adverse Effects and Contraindications

- See Table 7-47.

Dosage, Administration, and Nursing Considerations

- See Table 7-47.
- Patients should be well-hydrated in order to increase the effectiveness of the drug and to reduce GI irritation.

MUCOLYTIC AGENTS

ACETYLCYSTEINE (MUCOMYST)

Actions

- Acetylcysteine reduces the thickness and adhesiveness of pulmonary secretions. Its chemical action breaks up the mucus.

Indications

- It is used to treat COPD, cystic fibrosis, and pneumonia, and used to assist in tracheostomy care.
- It is effective as an antidote for acetaminophen toxicity if used within 24 hr of the poisoning.

Adverse Effects and Contraindications

- Asthmatic patients may experience bronchospasm.
- Acetylcysteine has a wide margin of safety, but it may cause stomatitis, nausea, or rhinorrhea.

Dosage and Administration

- The usual dosage is 1 to 10 ml (20% solution), or 2 to 20 ml (10% solution).
- Usually, it is given by nebulization for about 15 min, tid or qid. It takes 5 to 10 minutes for maximum effects to occur.
- When used as an antidote for acetaminophen toxicity, acetylcysteine is given orally. The initial dose is 140 mg/kg, followed by 70 mg/kg every 4 hours for 17 doses (total of 1,330 mg/kg). If the patient is unconscious, acetylcysteine is given through a nasogastric tube.

Nursing Considerations

- Remember other methods for liquifying secretions (*e.g.,* forcing fluids, using a vaporizer).
- Postural drainage and coughing and deep breathing following the treatment usually are helpful.

NEBULIZATION THERAPY

OVERVIEW

Many of the medications used to treat chronic obstructive pulmonary disease (COPD) and other respiratory problems are delivered through nebulization therapy. In nebulization therapy, the medication is suspended in air in the form of small droplets. Ultrasonic nebulization, which makes use of even smaller drops, is used frequently because the smaller the drops, the more likely they will reach the aveoli. The following types of apparatus are used: hand-held nebulizers, oral inhalers, pump-driven nebulizers, and intermittent positive pressure breathing machines (IPPBs). The following types of drugs are used: bronchodilators, mucolytic agents, antibiotics, and steroids.

Nursing Considerations

- Oral nebulizers vary greatly in the types and strengths of medication used. Patients must be instructed *carefully* so that they will be receiving the smallest, effective dose.
- It is important for patients to avoid overuse of the apparatus and medications because tolerance develops and rebound bronchospasm and adverse cardiac effects can occur.
- When using metered-dose nebulizers, patients should hold the mouthpiece 1 inch to 2 inches from their open mouths. They should exhale through their noses as deeply as possible, then inhale slowly and deeply through their mouths while releasing the dose. They must hold their breath for several seconds, then exhale slowly.
- When using metered-powder inhalers, patients should breathe with normal force and depth.

BIBLIOGRAPHY • Pharmacology

BOOKS

Conrad K, Bressler R: Drug Therapy for the Elderly. St Louis, CV Mosby, 1982
Curren A: Math for Meds, 3rd ed. Seal Beach, Wallcur, 1979
Gilman AG, Goodman L, Gilman A (eds): The Pharmacological Basis of Therapeutics, 6th ed. New York, MacMillan, 1980
Govoni L, Hayes J: Drugs and Nursing Implications, 4th ed. Norwalk, Appleton-Century-Crofts, 1982
Lamy P: Prescribing for the Elderly. Littleton, PSG Publishing, 1980
Oppeneer J, Vervoren T: Gerontological Pharmacology. St Louis, CV Mosby, 1983
Physician's Desk Reference, 39th ed. Oradell, NJ; Medical Economics, 1985
Poe W, Holloway D: Drugs and the Aged. New York, McGraw-Hill, 1980
Raffensperger E, Zusy M, Marchesseault L: Quick Reference to Medical-Surgical Nursing. Philadelphia, JB Lippincott, 1983

JOURNALS

Allen M: Drug therapy in the elderly, Am J Nurs 80:1474, 1980
Brengman S, Burns M: Ritodrine hydrochloride and preterm labor. Am J Nurs 83:537, 1983

Burkle W: What you should know about Tagamet. Nursing '80 10:86, 1980
Butler J, Harrison L: Keeping pace with calcium channel blockers. Nursing '83 13:38, 1983
Chamberlain S: Low-dose heparin therapy. Am J Nurs 80:1115, 1980
Childs B: Insulin infusion pumps. Nursing '83 13:55, 1983
Dickerson J: The pill: A closer look. Am J Nurs 83:1392, 1983
Essig M: Oral antidiabetic agents. Nursing '83 13:58, 1983
Fraulini K, Gorski D: Don't let perioperative medications put you in a spin. Nursing '83 13:26, 1983
Fredholm N, Vignati L, Brown S: Insulin pumps: The patient's verdict. Am J Nurs 84:36, 1984
Fuller E: The effect of antianginal drugs on myocardial oxygen consumption. Am J Nurs 80:250, 1980
Gever L: Acetaminophen overdose. Nursing '80 10:57, 1980
Gever L: New thinking about parenteral iron supplements. Nursing '80 10:60, 1980
Gever L: Reducing the side effects of steroid therapy. Nursing '80 10:59, 1980
Gullatte M, Foltz A: Hepatic chemotherapy via implantable pump. Am J Nurs 83:1674, 1983
Hagen S: Bring help and hope to the patient with Hodgkin's disease. Nursing '83 13:58, 1983
Harris E: Dexamethasone suppression test. Am J Nurs 82:784, 1982
Herget M: For visually impaired diabetics. Am J Nurs 83:1557, 1983
Hill M, Fink J: In hypertensive emergencies, act quickly but also cautiously. Nursing '83 13:34, 1983
Hoeft R, Jones A: Treating metastasis with estramustine phosphate. Am J Nurs 82:828, 1982
Hussar D: New drugs. Nursing '80 10:24, 1980
Johnson G, Johanson B: Beta blockers. Am J Nurs 83:1034, 1983
Kelley M, Mongiello R: Hypertension in pregnancy: Labor, delivery, and postpartum. Am J Nurs 82:813, 1982
Kirilloff L, Tabbals S: Drugs for asthma. Am J Nurs 83:55, 1983
Knott S, Herget M: Teaching self-injection to diabetics: An easier and more effective way. Nursing '84 14:57, 1984
Mattia M, Blake S: Hospital hazards: Cancer drugs. Am J Nurse 83:758, 1983
McDermott J: Ready or not, here comes your patient on lithium, Nursing '83 13:44, 1983
McFadden E, Zaloga G, Chernow B: Hypocalcemia: A medical emergency. Am J Nurs 83:226, 1983
Meissner J, Gever L: Reducing the risks of digitalis toxicity. Nursing '80 10:32, 1980
Meyerowitz B, Watkins I, Sparks F: Quality of life for breast cancer patients receiving adjuvant chemotherapy. Am J Nurs 83:232, 1983
Nursing Update: Tetracyclines. Nursing '84 14:46, 1984
Purcell J, Holder C: Intravenous nitroglycerin. Am J Nurs 82:254, 1982

Resler M, Tumulty G: Glaucoma update. Am J Nurs 83:752, 1983

Rifas E: Teaching patients to manage acute asthma: The future is now. Nursing '83 13:77, 1983

Rossi L, Antman E: Calcium channel blockers: New treatment for cardiovascular disease. Am J Nurs 83:382, 1983

Satterwhite B: What to do when adriamycin infiltrates. Nursing '80 10:37, 1980

Sohn C, Tannerbaum R, Cantwell R, Rogers M: Rescind the risks in administering anticoagulants. Nursing '81 11:34, 1981

Strand C, Clark S: Adult arthritis: Drugs and remedies. Am J Nurs 83:266, 1983

Tannenbaum R, Sohn C, Cantwell R, Rogers M, Hollis R: Angina pectoris: How to recognize it; how to manage it. Nursing '81 11:44, 1981

The 1980 report of the Joint National Committee on detection, evaluation, and treatment of high blood pressure. Arch Intern Med 140:1280, 1980

Todd B: Beta blockers and calcium channel blockers. Geriatric Nurs :228, 1982

Webber-Jones J, Bryant M: Over-the-counter bronchodilators. Nursing '80 10:34, 1980

Young L: Streptokinase therapy. Focus on Critical Care 10:20, 1983

Appendix

CONVERSION TABLES

- Conversion of avoirdupois body weight to metric equivalent
- Conversion of height to metric equivalents
- Equivalent Celsius and Fahrenheit temperature readings

Medical abbreviations and symbols
Regional poison control centers

CONVERSION OF AVOIRDUPOIS BODY WEIGHT TO METRIC EQUIVALENTS

lb	kg	kg	lb
10	4.5	10	22
20	9.1	20	44
30	13.6	30	66
40	18.2	40	88
50	22.7	50	110
60	27.3		
70	31.8		
80	36.4		
90	40.9		
100	45.4		

One pound = 0.454 kilogram.
One kilogram = 2.2 pounds.

CONVERSION OF HEIGHT TO METRIC EQUIVALENTS

Inches	Centimeters
18	46
24	61
30	76
36	91
42	107
48	122
54	137
60	152
66	167

One inch = 2.54 cm.
One cm = 0.3937 inch.

EQUIVALENT CELSIUS AND FAHRENHEIT TEMPERATURE READINGS

Celsius	Fahrenheit
35	95.0
36	96.8
37	98.6
38	100.4
39	102.2
40	104.0
41	105.8

To convert Celsius readings to Fahrenheit, multiply by 1.8 and add 32.
To convert Fahrenheit readings to Celsius, subtract 32 and divide by 1.8.

MEDICAL ABBREVIATIONS AND SYMBOLS

ac before meals
ad lib freely as desired
bid two times a day
c̄ with
C Celsius
c/o complains of
cc cubic centimeter (ml)
DC discontinue
dr dram (measurement), also written ʒ
elix elixir
F Fahrenheit
g gram
gr grain
gtt drop
Hct hematocrit
Hgb (abbreviation); **HB** (symbol) hemoglobin
hs hour of sleep (bedtime)
I and O intake and output
IM intramuscular
IV intravenous
kg kilogram
lb pound
LLQ left lower quadrant (of abdomen)
LUQ left upper quadrant
m minim
mg milligram
ng tube nasogastric tube
noc night
NPO nothing by mouth
O_2 oxygen
OD right eye

OS left eye
OU each eye
oz ounce (also written ℥)
pc after meals
PO by mouth
prn when necessary
PT prothrombin time
PTT partial thromboplastin time
qd every day
qh every hour
qid four times a day
qs quantity sufficient
RLQ right lower quadrant (abdomen)
RUQ right upper quadrant
s̄ without
SC subcutaneously
SG specific gravity
s̄s one-half
stat at once
tid three times a day
$>$ greater than
$<$ less than

POISON CONTROL CENTERS

Arizona	Arizona Poison and Drug Information Center Arizona Health Sciences Center University of Arizona Tucson, AZ 85724 Telephone; 602-626-6016 or 800-362-0101 (statewide)
California	University of California at Davis Medical Center Regional Poison Center 2315 Stockton Boulevard Sacramento, CA 95817 Telephone: 916-453-3692 or 800-852-7221 (northern California)
	San Diego Regional Poison Center University of California Medical Center 225 West Dickinson Street San Diego, CA 92103 Telephone: 619-294-6000
	San Francisco Bay Area Regional Poison Center San Francisco General Hospital Room 1E 86 1001 Potrero Avenue San Francisco, CA 94110 Telephone: 415-666-2845

Colorado	Rocky Mountain Poison Center Denver General Hospital West 8th and Cherokee Streets Denver, CO 80204 Telephone: 303-629-1123 or 800-332-3073 (statewide)
District of Columbia	National Capital Poison Center Georgetown University Hospital 3800 Reservoir Road, N.W. Washington, DC 20007 Telephone: 202-625-3333
Florida	Tampa Bay Regional Poison Control Center Tampa General Hospital Davis Island Tampa, FL 33606 Telephone: 813-251-6995 or 800-282-3171 (statewide)
Illinois	St. John's Hospital Regional Poison Resource Center 800 East Carpenter Springfield, IL 62769 Telephone: 217-753-3330 or 800-252-2022 (statewide)
Indiana	Indiana Poison Center 1001 West Tenth Street Indianapolis, IN 46202 Telephone: 317-630-7351 or 800-382-9097 (statewide)
Iowa	University of Iowa Hospitals and Clinics Poison Control Center Iowa City, IA 52242 Telephone 319-356-2922 or 800-272-6477 (statewide)
Kentucky	Kentucky Regional Poison Center of Kosair-Children's Hospital NKC, Inc. P.O. Box 35070 Louisville, KY 40232 Telephone:502-589-8222 or 800-722-5725 (statewide)
Maryland	Maryland Poison Center 20 North Pine Street Baltimore, MD 21201 Telephone: 301-528-7701 or 800-492-2414 (statewide)
Michigan	Southeast Regional Poison Center Children's Hospital of Michigan 3901 Beaubien St. Detroit, MI 48201 Telephone: 313-494-5711 or 800-572-1655 (statewide); 800-462-6642 (greater Detroit area)
Minnesota	Minnesota Poison Information Center St. Paul-Ramsey Medical Center 640 Jackson Street

	St. Paul, MN 55101 Telephone: 612-221-2113 or 800-222-1222 (statewide)
Nebraska	Mid-Plains Regional Poison Center Children's Memorial Hospital 8301 Dodge Omaha, NE 68114 Telephone: 402-390-5400, or 800-642-9999 (statewide); 800-228-9515 (surrounding states)
New Jersey	New Jersey Poison Information and Education System Beth Israel Medical Center 201 Lyons Avenue Newark, NJ 07112 Telephone: 201-926-8005 or 800-962-1253 (statewide)
New Mexico	New Mexico Poison, Drug Information and Medical Crisis Center University of New Mexico Albuquerque, NM 87131 Telephone: 505-843-2551 or 800-432-6866 (statewide)
New York	Long Island Regional Poison Center Nassau County Medical Center 2201 Hempstead Turnpike East Meadow, NY 11554 Telephone: 516-542-2324
	New York City Regional Poison Center Department of Health Bureau of Laboratories 455 First Avenue New York, NY 10016 Telephone: 212-340-4494 or 212-764-7667
	Finger Lakes Poison Center LIFELINE University of Rochester Medical Center Rochester, NY 14642 Telephone: 716-275-5151
Utah	Intermountain Regional Poison Control Center 50 North Medical Drive Salt Lake City, UT 84132 Telephone: 801-581-2151

Index

Page numbers followed by *f* indicate figures; *t* following a page number indicates tabular material.